Clinical Neuropsychiatry

Clinical Neuropsychiatry

Jeffrey L. Cummings, M.D.

Director, Neurobehavior Unit
West Los Angeles
Veterans Administration Medical Center (Brentwood Division)

Assistant Professor of Neurology in Residence
UCLA School of Medicine
Los Angeles, California

Grune & Stratton, Inc.

(Harcourt Brace Jovanovich, Publishers)

Orlando   San Diego   New York
London   Toronto   Montreal   Sydney   Tokyo

Library of Congress Cataloging in Publication Data

Cummings, Jeffrey L., 1948-
  Clinical Neuropsychiatry.

  Includes bibliographies and index.
  1. Neuropsychiatry. I. Title. [DNLM: 1. Mental
Disorders. 2. Nervous System Diseases.
3. Neuropsychology. WL 100 C971c]
RC341.C846   1985   616.89   85-842
ISBN 0-8089-1722-6

Grune & Stratton, Inc.
Orlando, FL 32887

Distributed in the United Kingdom by
Grune & Stratton, Ltd.
24/28 Oval Road, London NW 1

Library of Congress Catalog Number 85-842
International Standard Book Number 0-8089-1722-6

Printed in the United States of America
85 86 87 88   10 9 8 7 6 5 4 3 2 1

Contents

Acknowledgments

Clinical Neuropsychiatry reflects the influence of many individuals throughout my career. During my college years, instructors in zoology, physiology, and philosophy contributed to my emerging interest in behavior. In medical school at the University of Washington, John Green, John Sundsten, and Patrick Friel further inspired my interest in neurology and the neurosciences. At the Boston University School of Medicine, where I completed my residency in neurology and fellowship in behavioral neurology, my interests were molded and encouraged by D. Frank Benson, Martin Albert, Norman Geschwind, Simeon Locke, and Paul Yakovlov. At the National Hospital for Nervous Diseases in London, Michael Trimble and Leo Duchen supported and reinforced my enthusiasm for understanding human behavior and its neurologic correlates. In my current post as Director of the Neurobehavior Unit at the West Los Angeles VAMC (Brentwood Division), I have enjoyed the unflagging support of Ransom Arthur, Chief of Staff, and Mark Mills, Chief of Psychiatry. In addition, the psychiatrists at Brentwood have generously allowed me to work with many of their patients. Finally the staff of the Neurobehavior Unit—Stephen Read, Michael Mahler, Jill Shapira, among many others—have responded to my interests and have risen admirably to the challenge of caring for these taxing patients. The unique combination of devoted staff and instructive patients has provided the clinical experience on which this volume is based.

Two people deserve special acknowledgment. My mentor, colleague, and friend, D. Frank Benson has been an inspirational model of enthusiasm and clinical excellence. Our current collaboration is a continuing source of pleasure and learning, and many of the ideas developed in this book are products of our mutual efforts. My wife, Inese Verzemnieks, has been supportive and self-sacrificing, allowing me to devote uninterrupted hours to my work.

I am indebted to Norene Hiekel for typing much of the manuscript and coordinating its completion. I am also grateful to Murt Thompson, Joan Lopez, and Joanne Sandilands for typing portions of the book.

Susan Gay, the Grune & Stratton editor responsible for *Clinical Neuropsychiatry*, has proven to be a good friend and responsible professional who guided many aspects of the development of the book.

Preface

Clinical Neuropsychiatry is intended for psychiatrists, neurologists, psychologists, and other clinicians who are faced with the difficult challenge of diagnosing, treating, and trying to understand disorders of human behavior. The book presents a comprehensive approach emphasizing the structural, toxic, and metabolic conditions that produce behavioral alterations and also attempts to forge a link between the neurobiology of brain disorders that cause disturbances of behavior and the emerging psychobiology of major psychiatric illnesses. It is a guide to the unification of the neurologic and psychiatric approaches to behavior, integrating information derived from both contemporary neuroscience and biological psychiatry. *Clinical Neuropsychiatry* provides a compendium of differential diagnostic information not readily available in other sources and also stimulates consideration of the wider and more basic issues involving brain-behavior relationships.

The first chapter briefly summarizes the historical background, terminology, and philosophical premises of neuropsychiatry. In Chapter 2, the neuropsychiatric mental status examination is presented in detail; the approach to deficit detection and the history taking presen-

ted will be utilized throughout the remaining portions of the book. Chapters 3 through 6 discuss abnormalities of verbal output, memory alterations, visuospatial disorders, and frontal lobe disturbances. Chapters 7 and 8 present acute confusional states and the dementias, respectively. Whenever possible, both the neurologic and psychiatric disorders that enter into the differential diagnosis of the specific behavioral alterations are discussed. Chapters 9, 10, and 11 present the paroxysmal and episodic behavioral disturbances. Chapter 12 is concerned with movement disorders and discusses both the movement abnormalities that accompany idiopathic psychiatric disorders and the psychiatric abnormalities that commonly occur in conjunction with primary movement disorders. Chapters 13 through 17 involve the disorders classically considered in the realm of psychiatry—psychosis; affective disturbances; personality alterations; hallucinations; and disorders of sleep, appetite, and sexual behavior.

Clinical Neuropsychiatry provides a comprehensive overview of disorders that have often been divided between neurology and psychiatry but share many neurobiologic features and profit from conceptual unification.

Chapter 1

Introduction
to Clinical Neuropsychiatry

HISTORICAL ANTECEDENTS

Neurology and psychiatry arose from common origins, and many early neuropsychiatrists harbored the belief proffered in this volume, specifically, that it will eventually be possible to explain behavioral alterations in terms of altered neural structure or function. In a few cases, notably general paresis, this promise was fulfilled, and a major psychiatric illness was determined to be a product of neurological dysfunction and later was found to be treatable with specific agents. For many diseases (e.g., schizophrenia, mania, depression), however, no neurological correlates could be found and extraneural explanatory factors were sought. Progressively, neurology concentrated more exclusively on diseases of muscles, nerves, spinal cord, and brain where pathological changes were obvious, whereas psychiatry pursued those disorders manifest predominantly or exclusively by behavioral alterations. To a large extent, neurology abandoned behavior and psychiatry abandoned the brain.

Two developments began to close the schism between neurology and psychiatry and provide the scientific framework for a reunification of the disciplines: one was the emergence of biological psychiatry as a movement within psychiatry, and the other was the development of behavioral neurology as a discipline within neurology. Together these two fields form the basis for contemporary neuropsychiatry. Biological psychiatry received its primary impetus from the success of biological treatment of psychiatric disorders. The usefulness of drugs that increase monoamines at the synaptic junction in relieving depression or block dopamine receptors in ameliorating many of the symptoms of schizophrenia implied that these neurotransmitters were in some way involved in the mediation of the behavioral disturbances. Although complete confirmation of the amine hypotheses of affective disorders and schizophrenia is still lacking, accumulating information supports

a major role for transmitter system disturbances in these disorders, and this line of inquiry has been very fruitful in generating new psychobiological information concerning mood and thought disturbances and new therapeutic strategies useful in treating these devastating disorders. Biological psychiatry, however, has depended heavily on assumptions derived from psychopharmacology and has focused primarily on the role of synapses and neurotransmitters in psychiatric disorders. Information from this branch of psychiatry has rarely been integrated with observations concerning the anatomic distribution of transmitter systems in the brain, the effects of focal lesions that may interrupt transmitter function, or the nature of neurological diseases in which psychiatric disturbances are manifest as part of the clinical expression. Although biological psychiatry contributes essential information, it is not synonymous with neuropsychiatry and has not provided a comprehensive approach to brain–behavior relationships.

Behavioral neurology is the other cornerstone of neuropsychiatry. Modern behavioral neurology began in the 1960s with the intensive investigation of the aphasias and amnesias resulting from focal brain injuries and the revelations concerning hemispheric specialization based on observations of brain-injured and commissurotomized patients. Drawing heavily on techniques developed simultaneously by the nascent discipline of neuropsychology, behavioral neurology provided detailed clinical descriptions of language disorders, memory abnormalities, visuospatial disturbances, agnosias, and dementias associated with focal brain damage or degenerative central nervous system (CNS) disorders. In addition, behavioral neurology was largely responsible for the reintroduction of thorough mental status examinations that afforded more specific characterizations of deficits exhibited by brain-injured patients. Behavioral neurology maintained the traditional link between clinical findings and neuroanatomy and emphasized the specific relationships between localized lesions and the resulting clinical deficits. Behavioral neurology, however, has been concerned primarily with the study of deficit syndromes (aphasia, amnesia, agnosia, dementia, etc.) and has not pursued the study of other behavioral disorders such as hallucinations and delusions that can also result from brain injuries. Psychoses, depression, mania, and personality alterations have remained outside of the domain of interest of most behavioral neurologists. Behavioral neurology has thus developed important techniques and concepts applicable to many types of behavioral disturbance but has ignored others. Like biological psychiatry, it is not sufficiently comprehensive by itself to provide a broad-based understanding of brain-related behavioral alterations.

Neuropsychiatry, as reflected in this volume, attempts to integrate and build on the advances of biological psychiatry and behavioral neurology. For example, specific focal lesions (i.e., left frontal infarctions) and certain neurological disorders (i.e., Parkinson's disease) have been discovered to be associated with unusually high frequencies of depression (Chapter 14). The depression appears to reflect an interruption of the source or distribution of monoamine neurotransmitters essential to maintenance of a normal mood state. Likewise, schizophrenialike psychoses have been discovered to be associated with neurological disorders affecting subcortical and limbic structures (Chapter 13). These anatomic areas are innervated by dopaminergic neurotransmitter systems, and dopamine is the transmitter primarily implicated in idiopathic schizophrenia. Involvement of dopaminergic function in both schizophrenia and schizophrenialike psychoses thus provides a possible explanation for the similarity of symptoms in the two disorders. In both these examples, the importance of lesion localization emphasized in behavioral neurology is retained but is modified by information from neuroanatomy and biological psychiatry, indicating that focal lesions may disrupt neurotransmitter tracts, produce transmitter deficiencies in brain areas remote from the lesion site, and result in depression or psychosis. Similar approaches are being applied to the neurobiology of obsessive–compulsive disorders, mania, and the interictal behavioral disturbances of epilepsy.

Neuropsychiatry is an emerging discipline, and its techniques, hypotheses, and conclusions are relatively untried. No doubt some lesion–symptom complexes that now appear to have a causative relationship will be shown to be merely associations reflecting some more basic common pathogenetic mechanism. Nevertheless, as a new approach to disorders of human behavior and brain–behavior relationships, neuropsychiatry is already generating important information useful to neurologists, psychiatrists, and psychologists in more established branches of their respective disciplines.

TERMINOLOGY

A new discipline often generates a new vocabulary, but neuropsychiatry is a product of long-standing neurological and psychiatric traditions and must retain some of the vocabulary of its progenitors. Unfortunately, much of this established terminology is based on assumptions specifically rejected by neuropsychiatry. For example, it is traditional to divide behavioral disorders into those that are "organic" and those that are "functional." Many "functional" illnesses such as psychosis and depression, however, appear now to be products of "organic" processes, and "organic" disorders such as epilepsy and tic syndromes produce significant functional alterations with few or no structural changes. An alternative nomenclature is adopted in this volume in order to rectify this terminological confusion. Although still imperfect, the term "idiopathic" is used in this volume to describe the psychiatric disorders such as schizophrenia, mania, and depression traditionally referred to as "functional." This usage avoids the nonbiologic connotation of the previous terminology but admittedly underemphasizes the fact that some of the idiopathic disturbances, particularly the affective disorders, appear to be genetically determined. The term "organic" is abandoned here. Instead, brain disturbances are referred to as *neurological* or *toxic– metabolic* disorders. When regarded as a class, they are called "symptomatic" or "secondary" disorders. "Secondary" here refers to the fact that a diagnosable neurological, toxicologic, or metabolic disorder is present. These terms escape some of the burden of objectionable assumptions associated with the more traditional terminology but are not entirely satisfactory, and improved terminology should be sought.

CLINICAL APPROACH

The emphasis in *Clinical Neuropsychiatry* is on information with clinical utility. Although this volume has important theoretical and philosophical implications, its principal purpose is to aid clinicians in the diagnosis and management of patients with neuropsychiatric disorders. A method for thorough clinical examination is presented early in the book, and each chapter emphasizes neuropsychiatric differential diagnosis. The mental status examination is borrowed largely from behavioral neurology, with emphasis on characterization of the patient's verbal output, memory, calculations, constructional skills, and abstracting abilities. This is augmented by interview techniques taken from psychiatry emphasizing anamnesis and disclosure of subjective phenomena such as delusions and hallucinations. The interview and mental state examination are combined with elementary neurological and general physical examinations. Some may regard this approach as overdetailed, but the large number of neurological and metabolic diseases that may present with "psychiatric" symptoms, and the potential consequences for the patient of overlooking these disturbances more than justify the additional investment of time and resources.

Dynamically oriented psychiatrists and psychologists may object to the absence of dynamic considerations in this volume. Some have charged that neuropsychiatry attempts to turn a brainless psychiatry into a mindless neurology. The past excesses of classical analytic psychiatry are now apparent, however, and balance is being restored with respect to the sphere of activity of dynamic, genetic, and neurological factors in behavioral disturbances. CNS changes have been found to be etiologically significant in an increasing number of behavioral disorders, and the relative importance of dynamic and neurological factors is gradually being clarified. This volume emphasizes the neurological correlates of human behavior.

A principal that is emerging from neuropsychiatric investigations is that features of a behavioral disturbance that are unique to the individual are more likely to be dynamically influenced and representative of social and cultural influences, whereas aspects of behavior that are relatively invariant from individual to individual are more likely to be neurologically determined. Neuropsychiatric investigations attempt to identify these invariant characteristics and relate them to an underlying neurobiologic disturbance. For example, the *content* of schizophrenic delusions varies from individual to individual, culture to culture, and historical age to age and reflects the individual's unique dynamic-experential background. On the other hand, the *occurrence* of schizophrenia is relatively stable from culture to culture and from historical age to age. The occurrence of the psychotic disorder may thus be related to genetic or acquired CNS abnormalities, whereas the content of schizophrenic delusions has dynamic determinants. Likewise, the obsessions and compulsions in Gilles de la Tourette syndrome appear to be an expression of the basic neurobiology of the disorder, but the content of the obsessional concerns and compulsive actions is highly individualized and dynamically relevant. This volume emphasizes the neurological, toxicologic, and metabolic aspects of behavioral disturbances because they influence the occurrence of the behavioral disorders. Dynamic factors contribute mostly to the content of behavioral disturbances and receive less emphasis in neuropsychiatry.

Treatment, particularly the development and application of somatic therapies, is also a major area of interest in neuropsychiatry, and the attention to etiologic factors in neuropsychiatric disorders corresponds to this therapeutic concern. Somatic therapies have produced the greatest treatment advances in psychiatry, providing relief to thousands of patients and comprehension of the neural mechanisms producing and mediating behavioral disturbances is likely to lead to the discovery of new avenues for intervention.

THE PRACTICE OF NEUROPSYCHIATRY

The care of patients with neuropsychiatric illnesses differs markedly from that provided to patients with medical illnesses and varies in some respects from that of patients with other neurological and psychiatric disorders. Brain disorders, unlike medical illnesses, are manifest by alterations in the behavior and experience of the victim; in many ways they are disorders *of* the person, rather than disorders that simply happen *to* the individual. Patients may *have* pneumonia or congestive heart failure, but they *are* demented, psychotic, or depressed.

The difference in the way neuropsychiatric disturbances affect patients necessitates a change in the way the clinician responds. Although patients with affective disorders and some reversible dementing illnesses can be completely restored to their premorbid levels of function, most other neuropsychiatric disorders produce changes that are at least partially irreversible. After head trauma or stroke or following the onset of a schizophrenic illness, the patient is unlikely to be completely restored to the same "person" as in the premorbid state; thus the patient has become a "new" person. The clinician is obligated to respect this change and is responsible for helping to formulate goals appropriate for the patient's new situation. The goals and expectations of the brain-disordered patient must be reconciled with the limits imposed by altered brain function. The patient has entered a new state of being, and the clinician must accept and respond to this change by attempting to optimize function within the new existential context. For many neuropsychiatric patients, the role of the clinician is to aid in accommodating the expectations of the patient, the patient's family, and society to the patient's new capacities. This does not imply that all goals for the brain-disordered patient must be abandoned, but it does indicate that expectations must be adjusted to the realistic capacities of the patient. Knowledge of the course and impact of neuropsychiatric illness will provide the clinician with the ability to broker appropriate expectations.

Despair arises in novice clinicians when they cannot cure their patients, but the notion of "cure" must be modified in neuropsychiatry. Most neuropsychiatric illnesses cannot be cured and are likely to modify the patient's behavior and experience throughout life. In the case of degenerative disorders, the disease will progress and eventually bring death to the patient, whereas other disorders will leave unaltered the duration of life but will profoundly change its substance. For such patients and their families, the clinician must be prepared to enter a long-term relationship. The guidance and support provided by the clinician will often be as important as the nostrums dispensed.

In addition to the role of the neuropsychiatrist in advising family and patients, there is an exciting opportunity and a pressing obligation to learn from the patient. The victim of a neuropsychiatric illness is traversing an uncharted landscape, and each pilgrim-patient is the source of information that can be utilized to help guide others whose nervous system has been violated. The patient's observations, verbal descriptions, and motoric expression of personal experiences are invaluable bits of information that contribute to the science of neuropsychiatry but, perhaps more importantly, also help us to understand our patients and, ultimately, ourselves.

PHILOSOPHICAL PREMISES

Contemporary neuroscience has established a fundamental correlation between brain function and mental activity. Few would deny the basic monistic premise that human intellectual and emotional life is dependent on neuronal operations, but this postulate has not yet been integrated into clinical practice. Most current psychiatric nosologies, as discussed earlier, divide behavioral disorders into "functional" and "organic" types utilizing terminology based on a dualistic philosophy. Dualism distinguishes "mental" and "physical" as separate entities and correspondingly divides behavioral disturbances into mental ("functional") or physical ("organic"). This dualistic approach is inconsistent with current information derived from the neurosciences and biological psychiatry demonstrating that mental activities are inseparable from brain function. The dependence of human psychologic life on CNS integrity is most consistent with a materialistic monism, and this basic postulate has been adopted and applied consistently

throughout this volume. The terminology chosen and presented in this introductory chapter is part of the attempt at philosophical consonance, and throughout this book it is emphasized that all behavior reflects CNS activity—including normal behavior, behavioral alterations associated with neurological illnesses, or idiopathic psychiatric disorders.

The two principal objections raised against the monist position are that it (1) commits one to a determinism that disallows any role for free will and (2) undermines respect for human beings by approaching them as machines or automatons. Although a complete philosophical position cannot be developed here, it may be noted that neither objection challenges the fundamental monist position, but rather that both objections are directed at possible consequences of monism. Neither objection is necessarily true. Free will in human behavior is not the ability to have random activity: it is the ability to direct one's behavior according to one's preferences, and brain function provides the neurophysiological basis of preference-motivated behavior. In addition, although many aspects of CNS structure and, consequently, CNS function and behavior are genetically influenced, it is also obvious that behavior is modified by experience and that there is a constant commerce between the CNS and the environment. Behavior is a summary product of genetic, historical–experiential, and environmental influences, and CNS structure provides the physical basis for integrating and mediating these coexisting behavioral determinants. Once this potential for environmental influence and preference-motivated behavior is accommodated within the monist proposition, the free-will objection to monism loses force. Likewise, the ability to integrate ongoing experience and environmental interaction with monism deflates the objection that monism inevitably leads to treating human beings like machines. Indeed, monism can provide the basis for increasing respect for human individuality by emphasizing that each individual is the product of a unique blend of genetic, experiential, and environmental influences, all mediated through a unique CNS structure.

Chapter 2

The Neuropsychiatric Interview
and Mental Status Examination

The purpose of the neuropsychiatric interview and mental status examination is to elicit information concerning the patient's complaint or reason for referral; to assess the patient's psychological and intellectual function, seeking disturbances relevant to the presenting difficulties; and to establish a basis for a subsequent working relationship with the patient (Hill et al., 1973). The characteristics of the errors made during mental status testing yield important localizing information and indicate which areas of the central nervous system (CNS) are dysfunctional.

The examination begins as soon as the clinician encounters the patient and continues as long as the two are together. Often, the patient's spontaneous behavior gives as much insight into the neuropsychiatric disorder as the more formal aspects of mental state testing. Appearance and behavior yield information that may not be accessible to exploration through conversational means. Observations concerning the patient's behavior as well as the content and form of the spontaneous conversation will generate hypotheses about the patient's mental functioning that can be probed and extended by specific questioning during the more formal mental status testing. Any separation between the interview and mental status examination is artificial, therefore, as the latter is simply a more explicit and stylized method of exploring specific aspects of intellectual function. For convenience, this chapter begins by presenting those observations usually made during the initial portion of the interview such as the appearance and behavior of the patient, the patient's affect, and the form and content of the patient's spontaneous conversation. The mental status examination is then presented with a discussion of each specific area to be explored, including language, memory, visuospatial skills, calculation, abstraction, praxis, and frontal systems tasks. Finally, a brief overview of additional tests that may yield information in specific clinical circumstances is presented.

NEUROPSYCHIATRIC INTERVIEW

Table 2-1 lists the major components of the neuropsychiatric interview and mental status examination. Each of these elements is described and potential abnormalities briefly discussed.

Appearance and Behavior

An assessment of the patient's general appearance is the first observation made in the neuropsychiatric examination. The patient's manner of dressing may reveal much about any existing neuropsychiatric disorder. Dishevelment reflecting a lack of self-care is most striking in the dementia syndromes and in schizophrenic illnesses. Unilateral dressing disturbances occur in conjunction with hemispatial neglect. Specific dressing disturbances wherein patients are unable to correctly orient themselves with regard to their garments and thus fail to dress appropriately occurs with right parietal lesions. Dressing with multiple layers of clothing may be seen in the dementias, acute confusional states, and occasionally in schizophrenia. Unusual combinations of styles and colors of dress occur in schizophrenic and manic syndromes (Leff and Isaacs, 1981).

Disturbances of motor function are among the most revealing of all aspects of the neuropsychiatric examination. No interview is without its behavioral components, and the observed motor characteristics should be part of all diagnostic formulations. Characteristic abnormalities of gait, posture, and spontaneous movement occur in most neuropsychiatric disorders. Table 2-2 presents the major motor disturbances observed during the neuropsychiatric examination. Depression is characterized by psychomotor retardation, long latency to replies, paucity of verbal output, hypophonia, and bowed posture (Marsden et al., 1975). Agitated depressions produce abnormal pacing, hand wringing, and an akathis-

TABLE 2–1. Components of the Neuropsychiatric Interview and Mental Status Examination

Interview	Mental Status examination
Appearance and motoric behavior	Attention and concentration
Mood and affect	Language
Verbal Output	Memory
Thought	Constructions
Perception	Abstraction
	Insight and judgment
	Praxis
	Frontal system tasks
	Miscellaneous tests
	Right–left orientation
	Finger identification

icalike inability to sit calmly. The motor manifestations of mania include psychomotor hyperactivity, agitation, pressure of speech, and rapid talking (tachyphemia). Catatonic behavior (stereotypy, mannerisms, waxy flexibility, passivity, negativism, sustained posturing) may occur in affective disorders, in schizophrenic syndromes, or as part of neurological and toxic–metabolic disturbances (Chapter 12). Anxiety is reflected by a rigid posture, widened palpebral fissures, dilated pupils, and action tremor (Leff and Isaacs, 1981). Obsessions and compulsions are manifested by compulsory stereotyped acts, checking, cleaning, and rituals. Drugs used in the treatment of psychiatric disorders commonly produce motor system abnormalities such as tremor, dystonia, parkinsonism, dyskinesias, and akathisia (Chapter 12.) The extrapyramidal diseases frequently have concomitant psychiatric abnormalities, and in such cases the motor examination will reveal rigidity, tremors, ballismus, athetosis, chorea, dystonia, tics, myoclonus, or bradykinesia.

TABLE 2-2. Motor Disturbances Characteristic of Neuropsychiatric Syndromes

Hypokinesias	
Bradykinesia (psychomotor retardation)	
Paresis	
Catatonia: waxy flexibility, passivity, negativism, and sustained posturing	
Hyperkinesias	
Akathisia	Tics
Tremor	Myoclonus
Tardive dyskinesia	Mannerisms and stereotype
Ballismus	Agitation
Chorea	Psychomotor hyperactivity
Athetosis	Compulsive acts and rituals

Mood and Affect

Mood and affect, like behavior, permeate the entire neuropsychiatric interview and are assessed in an ongoing manner throughout the examination. *Mood* refers to emotion as experienced by the patient, whereas *affect* refers to the emotion manifested by the patient in speech, facial expression, and behavioral demeanor. The two aspects of emotion are usually congruent but may become dissociated in pathologic states such as pseudobulbar palsy, when the patient may laugh in spite of feeling depressed or cry even when in a good mood (Chapter 14). It is, therefore, necessary to verify observations about affect by inquiring specifically about the patient's mood. Euphoria, of course, characterizes mania, and sadness is characteristic of depression, but either may be accompanied by irritability, and euphoria with silly facetiousness occurs with certain frontal lobe disturbances (Chapter 6). Eutonia, a feeling of physical well-being, is particularly common among patients with multiple sclerosis (Trimble and Grant, 1982). Uncontrollable anger and rage are one manifestation of some dyscontrol syndromes (Chapter 11). Apathy and emotional blunting characterize the mood state of many patients with frontal lobe disturbances, schizophrenic syndromes, and extrapyramidal disorders. Patients with epileptogenic lesions of the limbic system may experience a heightening and intensification of their emotional states (Chapter 9).

When depressed mood is evident, other evidence of a depressive disorder such as decreased appetite and weight loss, diminished libido, constipation, and sleep disturbances should be sought.

Verbal Output

Table 2-3 lists the principal abnormalities of verbal output encountered during the neuropsychiatric interview, and these are presented in more detail in Chapter 3. Mutism occurs in a wide variety of clinical circumstances, including catatonic states, conversion reactions,

TABLE 2-3. Disorders of Verbal Output

Mutism	Reiterative disturbances
Speech disorders	Stuttering
	Echolalia
Dysarthria	Palilalia
Hypophonia	Verbigeration
Slow speech (bradyphemia)	
Rapid speech (tachyphemia;	Miscellaneous
press of speech)	
Aprosodia	Word salad
	Coprolalia
Aphasic syndromes	
Nonfluent	
Fluent	

pseudobulbar syndromes, early in the course of some aphasic syndromes, and in advanced stages of many neurological syndromes (Cummings et al., 1983a). Speech disturbances include abnormally rapid speech occurring in mania and in many fluent aphasias; slow speech characteristic of depression and nonfluent aphasias; dysarthria secondary to mechanical disruption of articulation; and abnormalities of loudness, particularly in the hypophonia of many depressive and extrapyramidal syndromes. *Aprosodia* (also termed *dysprosody*) refers to the loss of melody, rhythm, and emotional inflection that accompanies nonfluent aphasia, extrapyramidal disturbances, and anterior right hemispheric lesions (Ross, 1981).

Abnormalities of verbal fluency occur in the aphasias. Nonfluent aphasias are characterized by a halting sparse output with dysarthria, whereas fluent aphasias have a normal or increased verbal output with prominent paraphasia. Nonfluent aphasias correlate with lesions located anteriorly in the left hemisphere and fluent aphasias, with lesions located posteriorly in the left hemisphere (Chapter 3) (Benson, 1979a).

Reiterative speech disturbances occur in a variety of clinical settings. *Stuttering*, the repetition of single syllables, is seen as a congenital abnormality, in extrapyramidal syndromes, in the recovery phases of aphasia, and with bilateral cerebral insults. *Palilalia*, the repetition of the patient's own output, is seen primarily in extrapyramidal syndromes; and *echolalia*, the repetition of the examiner's output, occurs in some aphasic syndromes, dementia, and Gilles de la Tourette syndrome. *Verbigeration* refers to the constant repetition of a word or phrase sometimes noted in schizophrenic disorders (Boller et al., 1975).

''Word salad'' is a rare disorder occurring in schizophrenia when the derailment of thought and loosening of associations become so profound that the individual words in a sentence bear little relationship to each other (Leff and Isaacs, 1981).

Coprolalia, the involuntary utterance of curse words, occurs primarily in Gilles de la Tourette syndrome, where it is usually accompanied by other involuntary vocalizations such as grunting, snorting, and barking (Chapter 12). Coprolalia is occasionally reported in other clinical disorders such as choreic syndromes, Lesch-Nyhan syndrome, and schizophrenia.

Thought Characteristics

No absolute distinctions can be drawn between disorders of verbal output and thought disorders since the latter must necessarily be inferred from abnormalities of what the patient says. Nevertheless, there are a number of disorders that appear to reflect disturbances in the form or content of thought and seem independent of speech of language disorders. Abnormalities in the form of thought are presented first, followed by a discussion of disturbances of thought content.

Disorders of the Form of Thought

Table 2-4 lists disorders in the form and content of thought. Disturbances of the form of thought refers to abnormal relationships between ideas in the flow of

TABLE 2-4. Disturbances of Thought

Alterations in the form of thought

Autistic thinking
Loosening of associations
Poverty of thought (small quantity or vague quality)
Thought blocking
Tangentiality
Circumstantiality
Derailment
Condensation
Illogicality
Neologisms
Word salad
Flight of ideas

    clang association (association by rhyming)
    assonance (association by similar sounds)
    punning (association by double meaning)
    word association (association by semantic meaning)

Racing thoughts
Incoherence
Thought retardation
Perseveration

Alterations in thought content

Delusions
Obsessions
Phobias
Hypochondria
Confabulation
Approximate answers

tangentialty = digress = returning
circumstanctiality = digression = returning

conversation (loose associations, flight of ideas, perseveration, abnormally slow or fast thinking). Autistic thinking (personally idiosyncratic thought unrelated to reality) and loosening of associations are classical findings in schizophrenic disorders. However, schizophrenic conversation may also include tangentiality (digression without returning to the point of departure), thought blocking, vagueness and poverty of thinking, self-reference, derailment, illogicality, condensation of thoughts and sentences, and abnormal word and sentence construction with resulting neologisms or word salad (Andreasen, 1979; Kaplan and Saddock, 1980; Leff and Isaacs, 1981). Circumstantiality (digression from the topic with eventual return to the intended point) is a frequent finding in some patients with epileptogenic lesions in the limbic system and associated personality alterations. Circumstantiality must be distinguished from circumlocution (talking around a word or defining without naming it because of word-finding difficulties).

Flight of ideas is characteristic of mania and is characterized by a rapid flow of ideas in which the direction is determined by specific word characteristics such as rhyming, assonance, punning, or sematic meaning (Leff and Isaacs, 1981).

Perseveration is seen in many disorders that disrupt normal thought patterns, including dementia, aphasia, and acute confusional states. Likewise, incoherence of thought occurs in schizophrenia and dementia and may be particularly striking in toxic–metabolic confusional states. Retardation of thought occurs in depression and in the extrapyramidal syndromes.

Disorders of Thought Content

Delusions are the most flagrant abnormalities of thought content. They reflect the patient's loss of ability to correctly assess external consensually validated reality. Ideas of reference, delusions of passivity, mind reading, thought broadcasting, grandiose beliefs, and so on occur in schizophrenic syndromes, in neurological and toxic delusional disorders, and during some manic and depressive episodes. Delusions should be specifically sought in the course of the interview, but the patient may be guarded about revealing them. Delusions are usually either persecutory or grandiose in nature, although apparently benign delusions are occasionally reported. Patients should be questioned about fears of surveillance, threats against their lives, or special powers that they or others may possess. Concerns spontaneously voiced by the patient are explored to determine whether they are based on verifiable observations and realistic possibilities or are the product of delusional fears and misinterpretations. Delusions are discussed in more detail in Chapter 13.

Less severe disturbances of thought content include abnormal preoccupations or ruminations, obsessions, phobias, and hypochondriasis.

Confabulation refers to fabrication of responses concerning situations that are unrecalled because of an impaired memory. The facts may be benign and trivial or fantastic productions generated without restraint by the patient (Chapter 4) (Berlyne, 1974). Confabulations, unlike delusions, lack stability and vary from day to day. They also lack the affective investment characteristic of many delusional beliefs.

The syndrome of approximate answers, or the Ganser syndrome, is an hysterical pseudodementia that usually occurs in patients with head trauma or toxic–metabolic encephalopathies but may also occur in schizophrenia. The pathognomonic sign of the syndrome is the approximate answer given in response to even trivially simple questions (e.g., "How many legs does a dog have?") (Whitlock, 1967).

Perception

Abnormalities of perception may be classified according to modality (visual, auditory, touch, olfactory, gustatory) or according to whether positive or negative abnormalities occur. Table 2-5 presents positive and negative visual perceptual disturbances. Positive visual phenomena include hallucinations and illusions (Chapter 16). The former may be either formed or unformed and occur without a corresponding external stimulus; the latter are distortions or misinterpretations of existing stimuli (Linn, 1980). Negative visual phenomena include unilateral neglect in which one half of the visual universe is ignored; blindness, which in some cases may be denied by the blind patient; central color blindness or achromatopsia associated with occipital lobe lesions; and agnosia, or the inability to recognize objects, faces, or places, despite intact perceptual and naming functions (Chapter 5) (Benton, 1979; Cummings et al., 1983b; Heilman, 1979; Rubens, 1979). Agnosias

TABLE 2-5. Abnormalities of Visual Perception

Positive phenomena

    Hallucinations
    Illusions (metamorphopsia, macropsia, micropsia)

Negative phenomena

    Unilateral neglect
    Blindness
    Achromatopsia
    Agnosia
        Visual object agnosia
        Prosopagnosia (agnosia for familiar faces)
        Environmental agnosia (agnosia for familiar places)

may occur in auditory as well as visual modalities. The subject with auditory agnosia is able to perceive auditory stimuli but is unable to decode or recognize them. The condition is usually associated with bilateral temporal lobe lesions (Rubens, 1979).

Hallucinations may occur in all sensory modalities, including hearing, touch (formication hallucinations), smell, and taste. They may be recognizable (formed) or unformed. Some specific types of auditory hallucination, such as hearing two voices discussing one or hearing one's own thoughts, occur primarily in schizophrenic conditions (Chapters 13 and 16).

MENTAL STATUS EXAMINATION

The mental status examination augments and refines the observations made during the neuropsychiatric interview. The emphasis changes from an anamnesis concerning the patient's past and observations about spontaneous conversation and behavior to a systematic testing of individual neuropsychological functions. Information allowing localization of lesions in the nervous system is based primarily on observing the types of failure made by the patient in response to questions on the mental status examination. Not all the tests presented in the following paragraphs need be done with each patient; clinical experience guides the decision as to which aspects of the mental status require most thorough exploration in any particular patient. Nevertheless, the major areas of neuropsychological function should be screened in most patients.

Attention and Concentration

Attention and concentration must be assessed in all patients since any disturbance in this sphere will result in failures throughout the mental status examination. For example, the drowsy or inattentive patient is likely to have particular difficulty with memory tests, calculations, and tests of language comprehension that might be misinterpreted as amnesia, acalculia, or aphasia if the attentional deficit is unrecognized. When the patient is unable to attend to or concentrate on the given task, any failure to perform may be attributable to the attentional disturbance, and interpretation of the performance deficit must take the attentional difficulties into account. Most often, the patient must be retested later when attention and concentration have improved.

Three major types of attentional disturbance may be identified: (1) deficits of alertness or drowsiness, (2) deficits in concentration with distractibility and wandering attention, and (3) unilateral neglect or hemispatial inattention (Table 2-6). The neurophysiological

and neuroanatomic aspects of attention are normally integrated into a functional unit mediating arousal, concentration, and sensory awareness (Mesulam, 1981). Deficits of alertness are usually evident during the interview and are manifested by drowsiness and the need for repeated stimulation to keep the patient engaged with the examiner. Drowsiness reflects dysfunction of the reticular activating system on a toxic–metabolic or structural basis. The digit span test—asking the patient to repeat a list of numbers dictated by the examiner (normal 7 ± 2 digits forward and 5 ± 1 digits in reverse)—is a useful test of alertness and arousal (Lezak, 1976; Strub and Black, 1977).

Distractibility and ability to consistently sustain vigilance is best assessed by a continuous performance task such as the "A" test where patients are asked to respond by lifting their hands whenever they hear the letter "A" in a list of letters read aloud by the examiner (Strub and Black, 1977). Errors of omission usually reflect distractibility or loss of set for the task; errors of commission are usually perseverative, with patients raising their hands for letters other than the letter "A." Disturbances of sustained concentration and vigilance most often reflect frontal lobe dysfunction or toxic–metabolic encephalopathy.

Unilateral disturbances of attention or hemispatial neglect may involve unilateral sensory attention (hemi-inattention) or unilateral motor activity (hemi-inintention). Behaviorally, patients may ignore all stimuli on the side contralateral to the lesion and will perceive or respond only to those stimuli in the hemispatial universe receiving their attention. They will perceive only one of two simultaneous auditory clicks (finger snaps) and will feel only one of two simultaneous somatosensory stimuli (touching each side of the body at the same time). Visually, they may read only half of written words ("northwest" as "north" or "west" depending on which side is neglected), will draw only half of constructions they are asked to copy, and will ignore half of vertically written mathematical problems. A useful test of visual neglect is the line-crossing test in which patients are given a piece of paper with a number of short straight lines scattered across the page in a variety of orientations and are asked to cross each line in the middle (Albert, 1973). All or a portion of the lines in the neglected field will be missed, and the middle of each line may be misjudged with the line crossings systematically displaced away from the neglected field (See Fig. 5-1 in Chapter 5). The occurrence of a hemianopa is independent of hemispatial neglect: patients with hemianopsias may or may not have unilateral neglect, and neglect may occur with or without a hemianopsia. Unilateral sensory neglect occurs primarily with parietal lobe lesions and is more profound and more persistent in pa-

TABLE 2-6. Major Types of Attentional Deficit and Their Anatomic Correlates

Type of Attentional Deficit	Anatomic Basis
Drowsiness	Reticular activating system
Distractibility	Frontal lobe
Unilateral neglect	
Sensory (hemi-inattention)	Thalamus or parietal lobe
Motor (hemi-inintention)	Thalamus, basal ganglia, frontal lobe

tients with right parietal lesions than with left-sided insults (Battersby et al., 1956; Gainotti et al., 1972). When motor neglect is present (hemi-inintention), the patient may appear to be hemiparetic because of lack of use of an extremity, but normal motor and sensory function can be demonstrated when the patient's attention is specifically directed to the neglected limb (Heilman and Valenstein, 1972; Watson and Heilman, 1979). Motor neglect occurs with frontal lobe, thalamic, and striatal lesions.

In addition to structural and toxic disorders, other neuropsychiatric syndromes, including depression, mania, anxiety, and schizophrenia, may produce prominent concentration and attentional disturbances, particularly during periods of acute psychosis.

Language

Language disturbances, like attentional deficits, may profoundly influence the patient's ability to perform in many areas of the mental status examination. Memory testing, calculation, abstraction, and indeed comprehension of instructions for all other aspects of testing depend on intact language capabilities, and the integrity of linguistic capabilities must be determined early in the course of assessing the patient's mental state. A systematic approach to language evaluation and in-

TABLE 2-7. Principal Aspects of Language Function Tested in Mental Status, Examination

Spontaneous speech

Comprehension

Repetition

Naming

Reading

Writing

Word-list generation

Speech prosody

Miscellaneous

  Automatic speech
  Completion phenomenon
  Singing

terpretation is presented in more detail in Chapter 3, but the principal areas to be tested are presented here (Table 2-7). Language disturbances (aphasia) must be distinguished from alterations in the mechanical aspects of sound production (dysarthria) and from thought disturbances (outlined previously in this chapter).

Spontaneous Speech

A major change in the spontaneous speech of language-disordered patients is a disturbance in language fluency. Nonfluent aphasias are characterized by decreased verbal output, effortful speech, dysarthria, decreased phrase length, dysprosody (loss of melody and rhythm), and agrammatism (omission of the small relational or "functor" words). Fluent aphasias have a normal or increased verbal output, normal articulation, normal phrase length, preserved prosody, empty speech, circumlocution, and paraphasia (Benson, 1979a). In nearly all right-handed individuals and a majority of left-handed subjects, nonfluent aphasia reflects structural changes in the left frontal lobe, whereas fluent aphasia is indicative of damage to the left posterior temporal, inferior parietal, or temporoparietooccipital junction region (Benson, 1967, 1979a). Speech prosody may also be disrupted by right-sided frontal lobe lesions and subcortical dysfunction in extrapyramidal disturbances (Darley et al., 1975; Ross, 1981; Ross and Mesulam, 1979).

Comprehension

Language comprehension is a difficult function to assess with precision. It is heavily dependent on attention, concentration, and cooperation as well as linguistic abilities. Comprehension should be tested in a graded fashion beginning with one-, two-, and then three-step pointing to room objects. ("Point to the door, the window, and the chair.") Then a series of easy to difficult yes/no questions should be administered. (Easy:"Is your name 'Green'?" Difficult: "Do you put your shoes on before your socks?") Finally, comprehension of more sophisticated linguistic structures can be assessed such as sentences with passive constructions ("If a lion and a tiger are in a fight and the lion is killed by the tiger, which animal is dead?") and possessives ("Is my wife's brother a man or a woman?'') (Goodglass and Kaplan, 1972). Disruption of language comprehension occurs with involvement of the left posterior temporal and temporoparietooccipital junction regions (Chapter 3). Left-sided anterior lesions generally spare most aspects of language comprehension, although some patients with left frontal lesions have difficulty following commands that depend on correct interpretation of sequential information. (''Touch the pen with the pencil,'' in contrast to ''With the pen touch the pencil.'')

Repetition

Repetition, like comprehension, should be tested with a graded series of sentences of increasing complexity. The patient is requested to repeat each sentence exactly as spoken by the examiner. From simple phrases such as ''He is here'' they proceed to longer and more difficult sentences such as ''The quick brown fox jumped over the lazy dog'' and finally include more complex and linguistically irregular sentences such as ''No ifs, ands, or buts'' (Goodglass and Kaplan, 1972). Again, concentration and attention span may interfere with all but the most simple tests of repetition, and interpretation of repetition failures must take this into account. Patients with disturbances of repetition as a result of aphasia characteristically omit words, alter the word sequence, and have paraphasic intrusions when trying to reproduce the test sentence. Anatomically, failure of repetition occurs in aphasias with lesions situated adjacent to the left Sylvian fissure. Aphasics with preserved repetition have intact peri-Sylvian structures (Benson, 1979a).

Naming

Naming disturbances are a sensitive indication of language impairment but lack specificity for the type of linguistic compromise. Anomia may be manifested in spontaneous speech by word-finding pauses, emptiness, and circumlocution or may be identified by tests of confrontation naming. High- and low-frequency names should be tested (in general object names; e.g., ''wristwatch'' indicates high frequency and object parts, e.g., ''stem,'' ''crystal,'' ''band,'' represent lower frequency), as well as names in several linguistic categories (e.g., colors, body parts, room objects, actions). Naming errors may take the form of literal paraphasias (phonemic substitutions such as ''greel'' for ''green''), verbal paraphasias (semantic substitutions such as ''blue'' for ''green''), neologisms (completely new constructions), or failure to make any response. Anomia is most often one aspect of an aphasia syndrome but may occasionally be evident in toxic–confusional states, with

increased intracranial pressure, and with other nonfocal disturbances (Benson, 1979b; Cummings et al., 1980; Weinstein and Kahn, 1952).

Reading

Reading is a complex neurological function that must be learned and is subject to many cultural and educational influences. Literacy is still uncommon in most of the world, and the significance of an individual's reading difficulties must be based at least partially on an assessment of that person's level of educational achievement. The ability to read aloud and reading comprehension must be tested individually since some lesions may disrupt oral reading, leaving reading comprehension intact, whereas other lesions may impair reading comprehension but spare the ability to read aloud. Letter, word, and sentence reading should be systematically tested. Failures may include an inability to read letters, an inability to read words, ignoring one-half of the word, or substitution of one word for another (Benson, 1979a). Alexias may occur with anterior or posterior left-sided lesions as discussed in Chapter 3.

Writing

Writing is also an acquired task heavily dependent on one's educational experience and occupational demands. Agraphia, an acquired disturbance of writing, may be on an aphasic basis secondary to an interruption of linguistic function or on a nonaphasic basis produced by an impairment of the motor system and mechanical aspects of writing. All aphasics will make errors in their written as well as their oral productions, and the characteristics of the written language will resemble those of the spoken output (Benson and Cummings, in press). Peripheral, corticospinal, extrapyramidal, and cerebellar disturbances all disrupt the motoric aspects of writing and produce distinctive agraphic syndromes. The differential diagnosis of agraphia is presented in Chapter 3.

Word List Generation

Word list generation, sometimes referred to as verbal fluency, is a sensitive but nonspecific test of language function. In the two common versions of the test, the patient is asked to name as many animals as possible in 1 minute (normal 18 ± 6) (Goodglass and Kaplan, 1972) or as many words beginning with the letter ''F,'' then ''A,'' and then ''S'' with 1 minute allowed per letter (mean of 15 ± 5 per letter or mean total of 45 for the test). All aphasics do poorly on the test, and, in addition, patients with left frontal lobe lesions, subcortical hemispheric disturbances, or psychomotor retardation fail to produce the expected number of words per minute.

Prosody

Prosody refers to the melodic, rhythmic, and inflectional elements of speech, and aprosodic output is typically monotonic, amelodic, and affectless. Two aspects of prosody should be assessed: spontaneous prosody and prosodic comprehension. Spontaneous prosody is judged simply by listening to verbal utterances occurring during the course of conversation. Prosodic comprehension is tested by having the patient, with eyes closed, listen to a neutral sentence executed in four prosodic styles (surprised, happy, angry, sad). The patient is then asked to identify the emotional state of the examiner based on the way the sentence was inflected. Impaired spontaneous prosody is produced by right frontal lesions, left frontal lesions, and extrapyramidal disturbances, whereas prosodic comprehension is most disturbed by right temporoparietal injuries (Heilman et al., 1975, 1984; Ross, 1981; Ross and Mesulam, 1979; Tucker et al., 1977).

Miscellaneous Language Tests

In addition to the standard language tests described in the preceding paragraphs, other types of linguistic probes may be used in specific circumstances. In profoundly aphasic patients, remnants of intact language function may be elicited by having the patient produce automatic speech (counting, reciting the alphabet, naming the days of the week, reciting the months of the year), attempting to complete overlearned sequences (filling in the last line of nursery rhymes or prayers), or singing. The latter is dependent on right hemispheric structures and may be preserved even in the face of marked aphasia.

Memory

Memory is often divided into three functions—immediate, recent, and remote—with immediate memory representing the ultra-short-term memory tested with digit span, recent memory representing the ability to learn new information, and remote memory representing the recall of material learned in the distant past. As noted earlier, immediate memory is better considered as an attentional capacity since the information is not memorized or committed to memory for later recall. Attention, however, is a necessary prerequisite for all aspects of memory, and the presence of intact attention

must be demonstrated before conclusions about memory can be drawn.

Recent memory refers to the ability to learn and recall new information. Amnesia is the result of disruptions of this process (Benson, 1978) (Chapter 4). Two types of test are commonly used to assess recent memory: orientation and the recall of recently presented verbal or nonverbal information. Orientation in time and space must be learned on a daily basis and inquiring whether one knows the correct year, month, day, date, and time of day as well as one's current location will reveal important information about learning and recent memory abilities.

A more structured assessment of verbal learning can be performed by asking patients to learn three or four unrelated words and then asking them to recall them after 3 minutes (Strub and Black, 1977). Amnesia, the inability to learn new information, can be distinguished from forgetfulness, the inability to spontaneously recall what has been learned, by providing the patient with clues about the unrecalled words. Both category clues ("one of the words I asked you to remember was a color") and multiple choices ("the color I asked you to remember was either red, green, or blue") can be provided. Amnestic patients seldom are aided by prompting of this sort, whereas the additional hints often substantially help the forgetful patient. Testing nonverbal memory is more difficult than assessment of verbal memory, but an assessment can be made by warning patients when they are copying constructions (discussed in the next section) that they will have to reproduce them later. After a 3 minute delay, the patient is asked to redraw the figures from memory. If failures occur, recognition of forgotten figures can be tested by presenting a number of constructions and asking which ones had been shown previously. Unfortunately, many patients spontaneously develop verbal descriptions of the drawings, converting the test into an assessment of verbal memory. A more precise evaluation of nonverbal learning demands use of more specialized and sophisticated neuropsychological techniques. Verbal memory is mediated by the left temporal lobe, whereas nonverbal memory is dependent on the functional integrity of right-sided temporal lobe structures (Hécaen and Albert, 1978).

Remote memory abilities are revealed during the neuropsychiatric interview by the patient's ability to recapitulate personal history. Such historical information, however, may be unverifiable by the clinician, and a review of public knowledge (past political leaders, dates of historical events, etc.) may add another dimension to the testing. Information of this type is dependent on the educational background of the patient and intact language abilities.

Constructions

Assessment of visuoconstructive abilities is performed by asking the patient to copy drawings provided by the examiner (e.g., circle, cross, cube). The drawings should be a graded series of figures of increasing complexity and should include at least one three-dimensional representation. Relatively normal motor skills are an obvious prerequisite for performance of the task. Tests of constructional abilities are an excellent method of screening for acquired CNS dysfunction. Most idiopathic psychiatric disorders spare constructional skills, whereas lesions of the frontal or parietooccipital regions of either hemisphere may disrupt visuoconstructive abilities (Arena and Gainotti, 1978; Benson and Barton, 1970; Nahor and Benson, 1970). Neglect of one side of the figures is most consistent with a posterior hemispheric lesion contralateral to the neglected hemispace (Fig. 5-2), whereas a fragmented and disorganized approach to complex constructions occurs most often with frontal lobe lesions or in acute confusional states (Fig. 6-3) (Albert and Kaplan, 1980; Luria, 1980; Walsh, 1978).

Calculation

Calculating abilities are tested by asking the patient to solve arithmetic problems (usually addition and multiplication) presented either orally or in written form. Attention must be intact, and previous competency in calculation must be assured before failures in calculating abilities can be interpreted. At least three types of acalculia are described: (1) patients with fluent aphasias may make paraphasic errors when reading, writing, or saying numbers, making correct calculation impossible; (2) patients with right-sided parietal lesions may have a visuospatial acalculia, resulting from an inability to correctly align columns of written numbers; and (3) a primary anarithmetria may occur with left-sided posterior lesions. This last type of acalculia is evident in Gerstmann's syndrome and reflects an inability to perform the actual numerical manipulations (Levin, 1979).

Abstraction

The ability to abstract provides a good index of general intellectual function and, like calculation, is dependent on the patient's level of educational achievement and cultural experience. Most English-speaking individuals will be able to abstract idioms such as "cold shoulder," "heavy heart," and "level headed" regardless of their educational history, and impairment of this skill usually indicates a disturbance of abstracting abilities. Proverbs can be understood by most individuals

with a high school education, and an inability to interpret proverbs by patients with more advanced educational achievement is evidence of compromised intellectual function. Both simple proverbs ("don't cry over spilled milk") and complex proverbs ("people who live in glass houses shouldn't throw stones") should be tested (Cummings and Benson, 1983). In addition to testing the ability to abstract, proverb interpretation often elicits bizarre, paranoid, or idiosyncratic responses from patients with psychoses and macabre, pessimistic, or hopeless interpretations from depressed patients.

Insight and Judgment

The traditional "insight" questions such as "What would you do if you found an addressed stamped envelope?" or "What would you do if you were the first to see a fire in a crowded theater?" are so simplistic that they provide little information in most circumstances. Instead, more information can be obtained by inquiring about what one understands of one's illness, intends to do after leaving the hospital, or perceives about current personal medical and psychosocial needs. Answers reveal the patient's judgment, foresight, motivation, and depth of insight.

Praxis

Ideomotor apraxia refers to the inability to perform on command volitional acts that can be performed spontaneously (Geschwind, 1975). To test praxis, the patient is asked to perform limb, whole-body, and oral–lingual movements. Limb commands include "show me how you comb your hair" or "show me how you brush your teeth"; whole-body commands include "take a bow" and "show me how you swing a golf club"; and oral–lingual commands include "show me how you blow out a match," "show me how you suck through a straw," and "cough." The presence of ideomotor apraxia reflects focal dysfunction in the left hemisphere of right-handed individuals (Chapter 3).

Frontal Systems Tasks

These tests are called "frontal systems" tasks rather than "frontal lobe" tests because patients with lesions in either the frontal lobes or the connections between the frontal lobes and subcortical structures may exhibit difficulties in their performance. Patients with Parkinson's disease, Huntington's disease, or other subcortical disorders may thus exhibit abnormalities similar to those found in patients with frontal lobe dysfunction (Cummings and Benson, 1983).

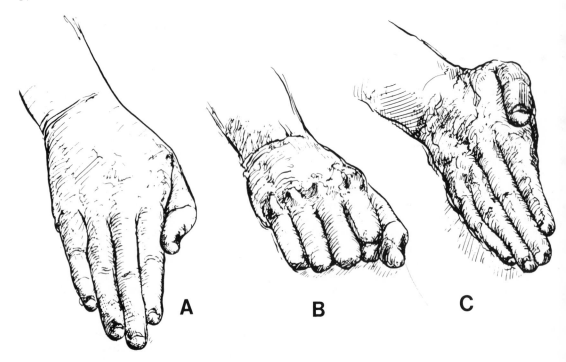

Figure 2–1.   Serial hand sequence: **(A)** ''slap,'' **(B)** ''fist,'' and **(C)** ''cut.'' Reprinted from Benson DF and Stuss DT. *Neurology,* 1982, *32,* 1353–1357, Figure 2. With permission of the publisher.

Many of the tests just presented will already have given some indication of frontal systems function. Attention and concentration depend on the integrity of frontal systems; patients with frontal disturbances are often distractible. Word list generation assesses left-sided frontal function if the patient is not aphasic and does not exhibit psychomotor retardation. Complex constructional tasks are often approached in a segmented and fragmented manner by patients with frontal system lesions, and abstraction, insight, judgment, and categorization also depend on frontal system function.

Additional frontal systems tasks include alternating programs, reciprocal programs, multiple loops, serial hand sequences, and rhythm tapping (Albert and Kaplan, 1980; Luria, 1980). All these tests have in common a dependence on the patient's ability to program motor responses in specific repeating or alternating sequences. Failures include an inability to achieve the specific behavioral set required to perform the task, rapid extinction of the appropriate set with consequent deterioration of the expected sequence, or inability to change set with perseveration or intrusion of unwanted activities. Figures 6-1 and 6-2 present examples of alternating programs and multiple loops. The patient is

asked to copy the alternating sequence or looped figure provided by the examiner and then to continue the same repeating pattern across the page. Reciprocal programs are performed by having the patient and examiner execute reciprocal maneuvers. For example, the patient is requested to tap once each time the examiner taps twice and twice whenever the examiner taps once. The examiner then proceeds to tap once or twice in random order and observes whether the patient is able to respond reciprocally. Similarly, rhythm tapping abilities are assessed by asking the patient to imitate a rhythmic sequence of taps performed by the clinician. Serial hand sequences are tested by requiring that the patient execute a series of repeating hand postures while announcing aloud the name of each posture (fist–slap–cut) (Fig. 2-1). A dissociation between the verbal sequence and the manual sequence indicates a frontal system disturbance. Performance of these tests of motor programming is often impaired in patients with prefrontal convexity or subcortical lesions. Injury to the orbitofrontal cortex, medial frontal lobe or frontal pole may not disturb these functions, and a normal performance on frontal systems tasks does not exclude the presence of a frontal lobe lesion (Chapter 6).

Additional Tests and Miscellaneous Observations

Right–Left Orientation

The inability to distinguish right from left usually occurs as part of a symptom complex with dysgraphia, acalculia, and finger agnosia (Gerstmann's syndrome), a reliable indication of a lesion in the dominant angular gyrus (Gerstmann, 1940). When it occurs in other circumstances, its localizing value is less certain. Right–left orientation is tested by asking the patient to raise the right hand, touch the right ear with the left hand, and then indicate the examiner's right hand as the examiner and the patient face each other. Deficits in attention or in language comprehension must be excluded before a failure can be attributed to a specific impairment of right–left orientation.

Finger Agnosia

Finger agnosia, like right–left disorientation, has localizing significance when it occurs as part of the Gerstmann syndrome. In its simplest form, finger agnosia can be detected by asking the patient to point to the little finger, middle finger, ring finger, or index finger. More subtle forms can be detected by touching an individual finger on the patient's hand while it is held out of sight above head level and asking the patient to indicate the corresponding finger on the other hand. In another version, the examiner touches any combination of two fingers on one hand and asks the patient how many digits there are between those touched (Kinsbourne and Warrington, 1962).

Miscellaneous Observations

During the course of the interview and testing many additional observations will be made that may require more detailed exploration or may, in themselves, have localizing significance. For example, inability to perceive two objects simultaneously occurs with bilateral parietal lesions, and anosognosia or denial or illness may occur with lesions of either parietal lobe, although it is more profound and more persistent with right-sided lesions (Chapter 5) (Hécaen and Albert, 1978).

SUPPLEMENTARY EVALUATIONS

After completion of the neuropsychiatric interview and mental status examination, additional diagnostic and therapeutic information may be gained from supplementary evaluations. A neurological examination will contribute information about focal lesions, degenerative conditions, and movement disorders, and the general physical examination may reveal clues to a systemic illness or toxic disturbance. The importance of detecting neuromedical illnesses in patients with behavioral disturbances is emphasized by studies revealing a 30–60 percent prevalance of physical illness among patients referred for psychiatric hospitalization (Hall et al., 1982).

Neuropsychological testing will aid in the identification and characterization of intellectual deficits and provide quantitative data that can be followed during the course of the patient's illness. Projective testing may reveal information concerning the patient's mood and thought processes, and personality testing yields information regarding the patient's personality functioning.

Laboratory tests, including EEG, computerized tomography of the head, neuroendrocrinologic testing, and tests for systemic illness and intoxications will be useful in specific circumstances. These are discussed in the appropriate sections of the following chapters.

REFERENCES

Albert ML. A simple test of visual neglect. *Neurology,* 1973, *23,* 658–664.

Albert MS and Kaplan E. Organic implications of neuropsychological deficits in the elderly. In Poon LW, Fozard JL, Cermak LS, Arenberg D, and Thompson LW (Eds.): *New Directions in Memory and Aging.* Hillsdale, New Jersey, Lawrence Erlbaum Associates, 1980, pp. 403–432.

Andreasen NC. Thought, language, and communication disorders. I. Clinical assessment, definition of terms, and evaluation of their reliability. *Arch Gen Psychiat,* 1979, *36,* 1315–1321.

Arena R and Gainotti G. Constructional apraxia and visuoperceptive disabilities in relation to laterality of cerebral lesions. *Cortex,* 1978, *14,* 463–473.

Battersby WS, Bender MB, Pollack M, and Kahn RL. Unilateral "spatial agnosia" ("inattention") in patients with cerebral lesions. *Brain,* 1956, *79,* 68–83.

Benson DF. Fluency in aphasia: correlation with radioactive scan localization. *Cortex,* 1967, *3,* 373–394.

Benson DF. Amnesia. *South Med J,* 1978, *71,* 1221–1228.

Benson DF. *Aphasia, alexia, and agraphia.* New York, Churchill Livingston, 1979a.

Benson DF. Neurologic correlates of anomia. In Whitaker H and Whitaker HA (Eds.): *Studies in neurolinguistics*, Vol. 4. New York, Academic Press, 1979b, pp. 293–328.

Benson DF and Barton MI. Disturbances in constructional ability. *Cortex*, 1970, *6*, 19–46.

Benson DF and Cummings JL. Agraphia. In Vinken PJ and Bruyn GW (Eds.): *Handbook of clinical neurology*, Vol. 1, 2nd ed., *Disorders of speech, perception and symbolic behavior*. New York, American Elsevier Publishing Company, in press.

Benton A. Visuoperceptive, visuospatial, and visuoconstructive disorders. In Heilman KM and Valenstein E (Eds.): *Clinical neuropsychology*. New York, Oxford University Press, 1979, pp. 186–232.

Berlyne N. Confabulation. *Br J Psychiat*, 1972, *120*, 31–39.

Boller F, Albert M, and Denes F. Palilalia. *Br J Dis Commun*, 1975, *10*, 92–97.

Cummings JL and Benson DF. *Dementia: a clinical approach*. Boston, Butterworths Publishers, 1983.

Cummings JL, Benson DF, Houlihan JP, and Gosenfeld LF. Mutism: loss of neocortical and limbic vocalization. *J Nerv Ment Dis*, 1983a, *171*, 255–259.

Cummings JL, Hebben NA, Obler L, and Leonard P. Nonaphasic misnaming and other neurobehavioral features of an unusual toxic encephalopathy: case study. *Cortex*, 1980, *16*, 315–323.

Cummings JL, Landis T, and Benson DF. Environmental disorientation: clinical and radiologic findings. *Neurology*, 1983b, *33*(2), 103–104.

Darley FL, Aronson AE, and Brown JR. *Motor speech disorders*. Philadelphia, WB Saunders Company, 1975.

Gainotti G, Messerli P, and Tissot R. Qualitative analysis of unilateral spatial neglect in relation to laterality of cerebral lesions. *J Neurol Neurosurg Psychiat*, 1972, *35*, 545–550.

Gerstmann J. Syndrome of finger agnosia, disorientation for right and left, agraphia, and acalculia. *Arch Neurol Psychiat*, 1940, *44*, 398–408.

Geschwind N. The apraxias: neural mechanisms of disorders of learned movement. *Am Sci*, 1975, *63*, 188–195.

Goodglass H and Kaplan E. *The assessment of aphasia and related disorders*. Philadelphia, Lea & Febiger, 1972.

Hall RCW, Beresford TP, Gardner ER, and Popkin MK. The medical care of psychiatric patients. *Hosp Commun Psychiat*, 1982, *33*, 25–34.

Hécaen H and Albert ML. *Human neuropsychology*. New York, John Wiley & Sons, 1978.

Heilman KM. Neglect and related disorders. In Heilman KM and Valentein E (Eds.): *Clinical neuropsychology*. New York, Oxford University Press, 1979, pp. 268–307.

Heilman KM, Scholes R, and Watson RT. Auditory affective agnosia. *J Neurol Neurosurg Psychiat*, 1975, *38*, 69–72.

Heilman KM and Valenstein E. Frontal lobe neglect in man. *Neurology*, 1972, *22*, 660–664.

Heilman KM, Bowers D, Speedie L, and Coslett HB. Comprehension of affective and nonaffective prosody. *Neurology*, 1984, *34*, 917–921.

Hill D, Birley JLT, Cawley RH, Kendell RE, Lishman WA, Post F, Rutter ML, Wing JK, and Wolff HH. *Notes on eliciting and recording clinical information*. London, Oxford University Press, 1973.

Kaplan HI and Saddock BJ. Typical signs and symptoms of psychiatric illness. In Kaplan HI, Freedman AM, and Saddock BJ (Eds.): *Comprehensive textbook of psychiatry III*, 3rd ed. Baltimore, Williams & Wilkins, 1980, pp. 923–926.

Kinsbourne M and Warrington EK. A study of finger agnosia. *Brain*, 1962, *85*, 47–66.

Leff JP and Isaacs AD. *Psychiatric examination in clinical practice*, 2nd ed. London, Blackwell Scientific Publications, 1981.

Levin HS. The acalculias. In Heilman KM and Valenstein (Eds.): *Clinical neuropsychology*. New York, Oxford University Press, 1979, pp. 128–140.

Lezak MD. *Neuropsychological assessment*. New York, Oxford University Press, 1976.

Linn L. Clinical manifestations of psychiatric disorders. In Kaplan HI, Freedman AM, and Saddock BJ (Eds.): *Comprehensive textbook of psychiatry III*, 3rd ed. Baltimore, Williams & Wilkins, 1980, pp. 990–1034.

Luria AR. *Higher cortical functions in man*. New York, Basic Books, 1980.

Marsden CD, Tarsy D, and Baldessarini RJ. Spontaneous and drug-induced movement disorders in psychotic patients. In Benson DF and Blumer D (Eds.): *Psychiatric aspects of neurologic disease*. New York, Grune & Stratton, 1975, pp. 219–265.

Mesulam M-M. A cortical network for directed attention and unilateral neglect. *Ann Neurol*, 1981, *10*, 309–325.

Nahor A and Benson DF. A screening test for organic brain disease in emergency psychiatric evaluation. *Behav Psychiat*, 1970, *2*, 23–26.

Ross ED. The aprosodias. *Arch Neurol*, 1981, *38*, 561–569.

Ross ED and Mesulam M-M. Dominant language functions of the right hemisphere? *Arch Neurol*, 1979, *36*, 144–148.

Rubens AB. Agnosia. In Heilman KM and Valenstein E (Eds.): *Clinical neuropsychology*. New York, Oxford University Press, 1979, pp. 233–267.

Strub RL and Black FW. *The mental status examination in neurology*. Philadelphia, F. A. Davis Company, 1977.

Trimble MR and Grant I. Psychiatric aspects of multiple sclerosis. In Benson DF and Blumer D (Eds.): *Psychiatric aspects of neurologic diseases*, Vol. 2. New York, Grune & Stratton, 1982, pp. 279–298.

Tucker DM, Watson RT, and Heilman KM. Discrimination and evocation of affectively intoned speech in patients with right parietal disease. *Neurology*, 1977, *27*, 947–950.

Walsh KW. *Neuropsychology: a clinical approach*. New York, Churchill Livingstone, 1978.

Watson RT and Heilman RM. Thalamic neglect. *Neurology*, 1979, *29*, 690–694.

Weinstein EA and Kahn RL. Nonaphasic misnaming (paraphasia) in organic brain disease. *Arch Neurol Psychiat*, 1952, *67*, 72–79.

Whitlock FA. The Ganser syndrome. *Br J Psychiat*, 1967, *113*, 19–29.

Chapter 3

Disorders of Verbal Output: Mutism, Aphasia, and Psychotic Speech

Verbal interchange accounts for a major part of all neuropsychiatric interviews, and characteristics of the patient's verbal output are among the most diagnostically revealing clues available to the clinician. In this chapter, three principal disorders of verbal output are presented: mutism, aphasia and related disturbances, and psychotic speech.

MUTISM

Mutism has been used to refer both to the loss of all verbal output (but with the retained ability to grunt, cough, sing, etc.) and to the complete obliteration of all sound-producing abilities. Table 3-1 presents the differential diagnosis of mutism and lists the wide variety of disorders that may abolish sound production.

Structural Disturbances Producing Mutism

The most common cause of mutism is laryngitis with local inflammation of the larynx. Local throat pain is often present in addition to the mutism. Laryngeal neoplasms and disruption of vocal cord function by myopathies, neuromuscular junction disorders, peripheral neuropathies, or lower motor neuron involvement in the brainstem (amyotrophic lateral sclerosis, poliomyelitis, cerebrovascular disease, neoplasm) are also capable of producing complete mutism by interfering with largyngeal function. In many cases the mutism will be preceded by hoarseness, and laryngoscopy will reveal local inflammation, neoplastic involvement of the vocal cords, or paralysis of cord movement. When bulbar musculature or brainstem neurons are involved, dysphagia and tongue and facial weakness are often prominent.

Central nervous system (CNS) lesions rostral to the brainstem (pseudobulbar) can produce mutism when the corticobulbar tracts are involved bilaterally. In most cases, verbal output is preferentially affected, whereas nonverbal vocalization such as laughing and crying is spared or may even be pathologically exaggerated (Chapter 14) (Davison and Kelman, 1939; Ironside, 1956; Langworthy and Hesser, 1940; Lieberman and Benson, 1977; Wilson, 1924). Deficits commonly accompanying the mutism of the pseudobulbar syndrome include dysphagia, facial weakness, brisk jaw jerk and facial muscle stretch reflexes, impaired tongue movements, and an exaggerated gag reflex. The bilateral supranuclear lesions responsible for pseudobulbar palsy may be produced by cerebrovascular disease, neoplasms, multiple sclerosis, inflammatory or infectious disorders, or amyotrophic lateral sclerosis. When the lesions involve limbic as well as corticobulbar connections, the mutism may include both verbal and nonverbal emotional vocalizations (Cummings et al., 1983).

Advanced neurological disease of practically any type can produce mutism, but it is particularly common with the bradykinetic and dystonic extrapyramidal syndromes, where progressive dysarthria and hypophonia eventually lead to mutism. Extrapyramidal syndromes capable of producing mutism include Parkinson's disease, progressive supranuclear palsy, Wilson's disease, and the dystonias. Occasionally, the facial and laryngeal involvement is out of proportion to limb and truncal involvement, resulting in mutism early in the course of the disease. In some cases the mutism may be overcome when the patient is extremely excited or angry (Yakovlev, 1966), and singing may be possible even when expository vocalization is not.

Mutism precludes the recognition of aphasia since mutism indicates the absence of language production, whereas *aphasia* refers to the presence of an abnormal language output. Nevertheless, mutism may be present in the initial phases of some patients with nonfluent aphasias (Broca's aphasia, global aphasia) and is a standard feature early in the course of thalamic aphasia and of transcortical motor aphasia (Alexander and LoVerme, 1980). In these cases the mutism is transient, and aphasic agraphia is evident in the patient's writing. Childhood aphasia, unlike aphasic disturbances in adults, is

TABLE 3-1.   Differential Diagnosis of Mutism

Structural disturbances

  Pheripheral

    Local laryngeal disorders
    Myopathies
    Neuromuscular junction disturbances
    Neuropathies

  Central nervous system disorders

    Bulbar (brainstem) abnormalities
    Pseudobulbar disorders

      Cerebrovascular disease
      Amyotrophic lateral sclerosis
      Neoplasms
      Multiple sclerosis

    Advanced extrapyramidal disorders

      Parkinson's disease
      Progressive supranuclear palsy
      Wilson's disease
      Dystonia

    Trangent mutism with aphasia

      Broca's aphasia
      Transcortical motor aphasia
      Global aphasia
      Thalamic aphasia

    Aphemia
    Supplementary motor area lesions
    Akinetic mutism

Idiopathic neuropsychiatric disorders

  Depression

  Mania

  Schizophrenia

  Hysterical conversion reactions

  Elective mutism

Reprinted from Cummings JL, Benson DF, Houlihan JP, and Gosenfeld LF. Mutism: loss of neocortical and limbic vocalization. *J Nerv Ment Dis*, 1983, *171*, p. 257. Copyright © 1984, The Williams & Wilkins Company, Baltimore. With permission.

commonly associated with an initial mute period regardless of the type of aphasia (Alajouanine and Lhermitte, 1965; Geschwind, 1964; Guttmann, 1942).

Aphemia is an uncommon disorder that presents with an acute right hemiparesis and mutism, but with preserved ability to write. When speech is restored, it has a hoarse, breathy, dysarthric, and often hypophonic quality, but there is no aphasia (Bastian, 1887; Benson, 1979a). The lesion producing aphemia is usually an infarction limited to the Broca area in the left frontal cortex or the white matter immediately subtending it, and the lesion is usually an embolic infarction (Schiff et al., 1983).

Lesions of the supplementary motor area on the medial aspect of the left hemisphere commonly produce mutism in the acute stages. During recovery, the patient may manifest a transcortical motor type aphasia (discussed later) or may exhibit a paucity of speech output without aphasia (Alexander and Schmitt, 1980; Arseni and Botez, 1961; Chusid et al., 1954; Laplane et al., 1977; Masdeu et al., 1978; Rubens, 1975). The lesions are most commonly infarctions in the territory of the left anterior cerebral artery, but parasagittal tumors and medial cortical surgical excisions have also produced the syndrome.

Akinetic mutism is a state of nearly complete motionlessness combined with total mutism. Two varieties of akinetic mutism have been distinguished: a "vigilant coma" variety in which the patient is immobile yet seemingly alert, has full extraocular movements, and can occasionally be aroused to move or may even have brief agitated periods; the other is a somnolent variant in which the patient appears asleep most of the time and has oculomotor abnormalities. In the former, the lesion is usually situated at the base of the brain anteriorly in the region of the optic chiasm, medial forebrain bundle, or anterior hypothalamus; in the latter, the lesion is located more posteriorly in the anterior midbrain or mesodiencephalic junction (Segarra, 1970). The syndrome may be produced by vascular lesions (Barris and Schuman, 1953; Segarra, 1970), but most cases have been produced by tumors in the region of the third ventricle (Cairns et al., 1941; Daly and Love, 1958; Klee, 1961; Lavy, 1959; Ross and Stewart, 1981).

Idiopathic Neuropsychiatric Disorders with Mutism

In addition to the structural disorders, a variety of idiopathic neuropsychiatric conditions may also produce mutism. Depression with psychomotor retardation can produce mutism as one manifestation of the motor disorder, and catatonia with mutism (Chapter 12) is most common among patients with affective disorders of either the depressed or manic type (Abrams and Taylor, 1976; Akhtar and Buckman, 1972; Morrison, 1973).

Mutism can occur in the course of catatonic schizophrenia and is usually accompanied by other catatonic signs such as negativism, passivity, echopraxia, automatic obedience, or waxy flexibility and sustained postures (Hamilton, 1976; Smith, 1959).

Mutism may occur as a conversion symptom and can take the form of either aphonia with whispered speech or complete mutism, sometimes with apparent inability to comprehend as well as to produce spoken language. In most cases the patient is able to read and write normally, and normal vocal cord function can be demonstrated by having the patient cough (Weintraub,

1983). Normal coughing is impossible if the vocal cords are paretic, and patients with paretic cords produce a distorted, bovine sound. Hysterical mutism is more common in children than in adults and, like all conversion reactions, may be the harbinger of a major neurological or psychiatric illness (Chapter 15) (Slater, 1965; Stefansson et al., 1976).

Elective mutism is a syndrome occurring in children in their preadolescent years who do not speak in specific circumstances—usually while in school—but are capable of talking in other situations. In some cases, the mutism appears to be an anxiety-reducing maneuver, whereas in others articulation defects contribute to the development of the behavior (Herbert, 1969; Reed, 1963; Salfield, 1950; Wright, 1968).

APHASIA AND RELATED DISORDERS

Aphasia refers to an impairment of language produced by brain dysfunction (Benson, 1979a). It is an acquired syndrome that can be caused by a wide variety of cerebral insults, including cerebrovascular accidents, intracranial neoplasms, cerebral trauma, and degenerative conditions. Aphasia must be distinguished from mutism, disorders of speech volume and articulation (dysarthria), disturbances of speech melody and inflection (dysprosody), and thought disorders with abnormal verbal output. Several different patterns of aphasic output have been identified and correlated with lesions in specific anatomic areas. Each aphasia syndrome is presented along with its correlative anatomy. The individual aphasias have different neuropsychiatric complications, prognosis, treatment, and etiology, and these are also described. The discussion that follows focuses on aphasia syndromes associated with relatively discreet CNS lesions associated with infarctions, neoplasms, or trauma; aphasia associated with dementia syndromes is presented in Chapter 8.

Types of Aphasia and Their Anatomic Correlates

Examination techniques for detecting and assessing language abnormalities were presented in Chapter 2. The observations concerning language function made during the neuropsychiatric interview and mental state assessment are utilized in this chapter to identify individual types of aphasia and to infer the underlying lesion.

The first localization principle to be invoked with regard to aphasia concerns lateralization of language function. In right-handed individuals, aphasia will be correlated with a left hemispheric lesion 99 percent of the time. In left-handed patients, the situation is more complex and variable. Approximately 60 percent of left-handed individuals will have a dominance pattern similar to right-handers with language represented in the left hemisphere. A considerable number of left-handers, however, particularly those with a family history of left-handedness, appear to have cerebral ambilaterality with some degree of language competence present in both hemispheres (Benson, 1979a; Hécaen and Sauguet, 1971). This relative lack of lateralization among non-right-handers is manifest by their tendency to develop an aphasia regardless of which hemisphere is injured, their better prognosis for language recovery, and the poor correlation between pattern of aphasic deficits and lesion site (Benson, 1979a; Gloning et al., 1969; Goodglass and Quadfasel, 1954). The aphasia patterns presented in Fig. 3-1 and Table 3-2 are those observed in right-handed individuals.

Figure 3-1 presents a systematic approach to aphasia diagnosis based on the cardinal observations of fluency of spontaneous speech, integrity of linguistic comprehension, and ability to repeat phrases and sentences provided by the examiner. Table 3-2 summarizes the principal clinical features of each type of aphasia, and Figure 3-2 is a composite drawing showing the common location of lesions producing the different aphasic syndromes. The first step in aphasia assessment involves determination of the fluency of verbal output. Table 3-3 presents the principal features of nonfluent and fluent verbal output (Benson, 1967, 1979a). Nonfluent output is characterized by a paucity of verbal output (usually 10-50 words per minute), whereas fluent aphasics have a normal or even exaggerated verbal output (up to 200 words or more per minute) with tachyphemia, logorrhea, press of speech, and an intrusive lack of regard for the usual rules of conversational interchange. Nonfluent aphasics have difficulty initiating and producing speech and tend to produce one-word replies or to utilize short phrases. There is an omission of the short grammatical connecting words, and the resultant output has an amelodic, dysrhythmic loss of prosody. The words produced are usually meaningful, and there is little paraphasia. Fluent aphasics have nearly the opposite pattern of verbal output, producing large amounts of well-articulated, prosodic phrases of normal length but with little information content. Grammatical words are not omitted, but errors in the use of grammar (paragrammatism) may occur. Paraphasias are prominent, and in the acute phases there is a tendency for the patient to be unaware of or to deny any language deficit. Not all these distinguishing features are present in every case, and phrase length, agrammatism, and paraphasia are then the most useful parameters for differentiation of fluent from nonfluent verbal output. In adults, fluent aphasias correspond to lesions in the posterior left hemisphere, whereas nonfluent aphasias are produced by lesions of

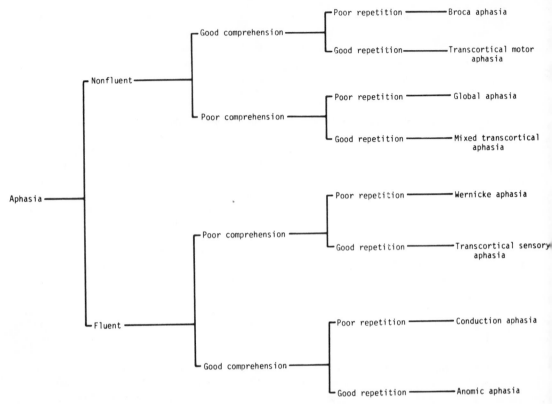

Figure 3-1. Systematic approach to differential diagnosis of the aphasia syndromes. (The clinical characteristics of thalamic aphasia are somewhat variable and are not included in the schema; see text for description).

the left frontal lobe. In children, however, nonfluent aphasia may occur regardless of the location of the lesion (Alajouanine and Lhermitte, 1965; Guttmann, 1942).

Assessment of language comprehension is the second step in evaluation of the aphasic patient. Comprehension deficits may be mild or severe, and a hierarchy of increasingly difficult tests of linguistic understanding must be utilized in aphasia testing (Chapter 2). In general, patients with focal lesions limited to the left frontal lobe have preserved comprehension (Broca's and transcortical motor aphasia), whereas patients with left posterior temporal or parietal involvement suffer some degree of comprehension impairment (Wernicke's, global, transcortical sensory, and isolation aphasias).

The third step in a systematic examination of the aphasic patient is to determine the ability to correctly repeat words and sentences. For accurate assessment of this ability, the length of the presented material must not exceed the attention span of the subject. Failures in repetition take the form of paraphasic intrusions, alterations in the presented sequence of words, omission of words, or a tendency to alter the content of the presented sentence. Aphasic syndromes with impaired repetition

(Wernicke's, Broca's, and conduction aphasias) have lesions involving structures immediately adjacent to the Sylvian fissure of the left hemisphere, whereas aphasia syndromes with intact repetition abilities (transcortical aphasias) are associated with lesions that spare the peri-Sylvian areas (Albert et al., 1981).

After the initial observations regarding fluency, comprehension, and repetition have been made, further refinements regarding characterization of the aphasic syndromes and lesion localization depend on tests of naming, reading, and writing (Table 3-2).

Broca's Aphasia

Broca's aphasia is a nonfluent aphasic syndrome characterized by effortful, dysarthric, dysprosodic, and agrammatical verbal output. Although comprehension is largely intact in patients with Broca's aphasia, patients often have difficulty in mastering material that involves sequential manipulation based on specific grammatical relationships. This deficit in grammatical comprehension is present for both oral and written material and corresponds to the agrammatism of the individual's spoken language (Goodglass, 1973). Repetition, reading aloud, naming, and writing are also impaired. The lesion responsible for Broca's aphasia usually involves the inferior frontal gyrus and adjacent areas of the operculum and insula in the territory of the upper division of the middle cerebral artery (Benson, 1979a; Mohr et al., 1978; Tonkonogy and Goodglass, 1981). A right-sided hemiparesis involving the face and the arm more than the leg usually accompanies the aphasia, and a sympathetic apraxia may affect buccolingual and left-sided limb function.

Transcortical Motor Aphasia

Transcortical motor aphasia is characterized by nonfluent verbal output, good auditory comprehension, preserved repetition despite nonfluent spontaneous speech, intact ability to read aloud, variable reading comprehension, and poor naming and writing ability (Albert et al., 1981; Benson, 1979a). Mutism is common in the early phases of the disorder. The syndrome resembles Broca's aphasia except that repetition is preserved and reading aloud is less impaired. The usual pathology involves infarction of the supplementary motor area and adjacent cingulate gyrus in the distribution of the anterior cerebral artery of the left frontal lobe (Alexander and Schmitt, 1980; Rubens, 1975), but occasional cases with lesions of the frontal convexity sparing the Broca area or of the dominant thalamus have been reported (Albert et al., 1981; Benson, 1979a; Kertesz, 1979; McFarling et al., 1982). In most cases, a right hemiparesis involving the leg more than arm and face will be present.

Global Aphasia

Patients with global aphasia have impairments in virtually all aspects of language function, including spontaneous verbal output, comprehension, repetition, naming, reading aloud, reading comprehension, and writing (Albert et al., 1981; Benson, 1979a). Often the only spontaneous verbalizations will be stereotyped nonsense productions such as "za, za, za," although some patients may have a small repertoire of overlearned stock phrases ("hello," "I can't," etc.) that can be uttered fluently, and many global aphasics can curse with ease when angered. Automatic speech (counting, reciting the days of the week or months of the year), and humming of learned tunes ("Happy Birthday," "Jingle Bells") may be possible despite the severe defect in expressive propositional language. Poor comprehension of language distinguishes global aphasia from Broca's aphasia, and poor repetition distinguishes it from mixed transcortical aphasia (isolation aphasia). Even when comprehension is severely impaired, many global aphasics will be able to follow whole-body commands ("stand up," "sit down"), can distinguish foreign language and nonsense speech from their native tongues, can judge inflection sufficiently to differentiate questions and commands, and will reject written language that is presented upside down (Boller and Green, 1972).

Pathologically, the usual lesion producing global aphasia is a large left-sided infarction involving the entire territory of the middle cerebral artery, and there is usually an accompanying hemiparesis, hemisensory defect, and homonymous hemianopsia. Rarely, multiple emboli to anterior and posterior language-mediating areas will produce global aphasia without major motor deficits (Van Horn and Hawes, 1982).

Mixed Transcortical (Isolation) Aphasia

Mixed transcortical or isolation aphasia is a rare aphasic syndrome in which the findings of transcortical motor aphasia and transcortical sensory aphasia are combined, leaving only a paradoxical preservation of the ability to repeat. In some cases, repeating whatever the examiner says (echolalia) is virtually the sole verbal output, whereas in others nonfluent verbalization and even some naming may be intact (Geschwind et al., 1968; Heilman et al., 1976; Ross, 1980). The usual lesion responsible for producing isolation aphasia is a large sickle-shaped infarction in the carotid borderzone territory of the left hemisphere or a large medial lesion involving anterior and posterior parasagittal structures.

Wernicke's Aphasia

Wernicke's aphasia entails fluent, paraphasic output with poor comprehension, repetition, and naming. The patient's colorful, often nonsensical, logorrhea frequently combined with an unawareness or denial of any deficit creates one of the most striking syndromes in clinical neurology (Albert et al., 1981; Benson, 1979a). The patient exhibits press of speech with accelerated output and often has a demanding, intrusive, even quarrelsome conversational style. Spontaneous speech contains primarily semantic paraphasias and neologisms, whereas literal paraphasias may dominate attempts to respond to naming tests. The production of logorrheic, paraphasic speech with multiple substitutions and incomprehensible gibberish is called *jargon aphasia,* a verbal output disorder that may also occur in conduction aphasia and transcortical sensory aphasia (Albert et al., 1981; Kertesz and Benson, 1970). The relative preservation of comprehension in conduction aphasia and repetition in transcortical sensory aphasia distinguishes the three disorders.

Although the cardinal features of Wernicke's aphasia (fluent output, poor comprehension, poor repetition) describe a basic syndrome, there are many variations

TABLE 3-2. Characteristics of the Aphasia Syndromes

Aphasia Type	Fluency	Comprehension	Repetition	Naming
Broca	Nonfluent	+[a]	−[b]	−
Transcortical motor	Nonfluent	+	+	−
Global	Nonfluent	−	−	−
Mixed transcortical (isolation aphasia)	Nonfluent	−	+	−
Wernicke	Fluent	−	−	−
Transcortical sensory	Fluent	−	+	−
Conduction	Fluent	+	−	−
Anomic	Fluent	+	+	−
Thalamic	Fluent	±	+	−

[a] Intact.
[b] Impaired.

in the clinical presentation. Comprehension may be mildly impaired with preserved ability to interpret moderately complex sentences, or it may be severely involved, sparing only simple midline and whole-body commands ("close your eyes," "open your mouth," "stand up," "sit down"). Comprehension of orally presented material may be relatively spared whereas written information is severely affected, or the reverse may occur. Greater involvement of auditory comprehension corresponds to more extensive involvement of temporal lobe structures, including primary auditory cortex, and greater compromise of reading comprehension may reflect extension of the lesion superiorly into inferior parietal lobe and angular gyrus (Benson, 1979a; Sevush et al., 1983).

Pathologically, the lesion corresponding to Wernicke's aphasia involves the posterior third of the left superior temporal gyrus but rarely is limited to this region and frequently involves adjacent posterior temporal and inferior parietal areas (Benson, 1979a; Kertesz et al., 1977). A superior quadrantanopsia and cortical sensory loss in the face and the arm are common associated findings, and if the lesion extends into the posterior limb of the internal capsule, a hemiparesis will result. Occlusion of a branch of the middle cerebral artery on an embolic or thrombotic basis is the usual cause of the disorder, although it may also occur with neoplasms or trauma.

Transcortical Sensory Aphasia

Transcortical sensory aphasia shares many features with Wernicke's aphasia but is distinguished by the retained ability to repeat. The ease with which the patient repeats long sentences and phrases, but cannot comprehend them, is a notable finding. Spontaneous speech is empty, circumlocutory, and paraphasic, and there is a mild to marked tendency to spontaneously repeat (echo) whatever the examiner says. The patient may be able to read aloud, but both reading and auditory comprehension are impaired (Albert et al., 1981; Benson, 1979a).

Transcortical sensory aphasia is produced by focal lesions involving the dominant angular gyrus and adjacent areas or the medial parietal lobule (Benson, 1979a; Kertesz et al., 1982; Ross, 1980). When it results from involvement of the angular gyrus, it is frequently accompanied by the Gerstmann syndrome, constructional disturbances, and other evidence of the angular gyrus syndrome (Benson et al., 1982). Transcortical sensory aphasia may also be seen during one stage of the evolution of dementia of the Alzheimer type (Cummings and Benson, 1983).

Conduction Aphasia

Conduction aphasia is a unique fluent aphasic syndrome in which comprehension is relatively intact and repetition is disproportionately impaired. Spontaneous speech is characterized by word-finding pauses and a predominance of phonemic or literal paraphasias. Often the patient is aware of making errors and makes sequentially closer approximations to the intended word (conduit d'approche). Reading aloud is impaired, but reading comprehension is intact. Naming and writing are both abnormal and contain phonemic paraphasic substitutions (Albert et al., 1981; Benson, 1979a). Although comprehension is relatively preserved in conduction aphasia, some patients have syntactic comprehension

Reading Aloud	Reading Comprehension	Writing	Special Features
−	±	−	Comprehension of grammatically dependent constructions impaired
+	±	−	Onset with mutism
−	−	−	Automatic speech (e.g., counting) and singing may be preserved
−	−	−	Echolalia
−	−	−	Semantic and neologistic paraphasia
±	−	−	Repeat without comprehending
−	+	−	Literal paraphasia most common
±	+	±	
−	±	−	Onset with mutism; rapid fatigue of fluent output

defects similar to those described in Broca's aphasia (Rothi et al., 1982).

The anatomic location of the lesions responsible for conduction aphasia involves primarily the arcuate fasciculus in the region of the left parietal operculum. Adjacent cortical areas mediating language comprehension are sometimes involved, and it is suggested that in such cases the right hemisphere has been able to assume auditory comprehension functions (Benson et al., 1973; Damasio and Damasio, 1980).

Anomic Aphasia

Anomia is a ubiquitous finding in disorders affecting the cerebral hemispheres and is present in all types of aphasia as well as in toxic–metabolic encephalopathies and with increased intracranial pressure. In the latter circumstances, anomia is a nonspecific indicator of cerebral dysfunction and has no localizing significance (Benson, 1979a,b). Anomic aphasia, on the other hand, refers to a specific aphasic syndrome in which anomia is the principal finding and in which the other possible causes of anomia have been excluded. Spontaneous speech has an empty, circumlocutory quality with frequent word-finding pauses, many words of indefinite reference ("it," "thing," etc.), and little paraphasia. Comprehension is relatively preserved, and repetition, reading aloud, and reading comprehension are spared. Anomia will be present on tests of confrontation naming and in spontaneous writing. The patient can usually, but not invariably recognize the correct word when it is presented by the examiner (Albert et al., 1981; Benson, 1979a,b). When it occurs in this pure form, anomic aphasia indicates a lesion in the left angular gyrus or adjacent areas of the posterior second temporal gyrus. Anomic aphasia is frequently the residual deficit following recovery from more extensive aphasic syndromes (Wernicke's aphasia, conduction aphasia).

Thalamic Aphasia

The advent of computerized tomography revealed that some aphasic deficits previously considered pathognomonic of cerebral cortical involvement could be produced by focal subcortical lesions. The aphasic syndrome associated with hemorrhage in the dominant thalamus is the best known subcortical aphasia and consists of a fluent paraphasic output, variable compromise of comprehension (mild in some, severe in others), good repetition, poor naming ability, impairment of reading aloud and writing, and relatively preserved reading comprehension. The syndrome may closely resemble transcortical sensory aphasia, but there is often an initial mute period at the time of onset, and articulatory deficits may persist throughout the clinical course. The aphasia is often transient and is usually associated with attentional deficits, right-sided neglect, lack of appropriate concern, perseveration, and right hemiparesis (Alexander and LoVerme, 1980; Ciemens, 1970; Fazio et al., 1973; Mohr et al., 1975). The transient nature of the aphasia associated with thalamic hemorrhage along with the relatively modest language deficits that follow nonhemorrhagic types of thalamic insult (infarct, stereotactic thalamotomy) suggest that the aphasia may be primarily a product of pressure exerted by the hemorrhagic mass on distant cortical structures.

Hemorrhage into left-sided basal ganglia structures adjacent to the thalamus produce aphasic syndromes sim-

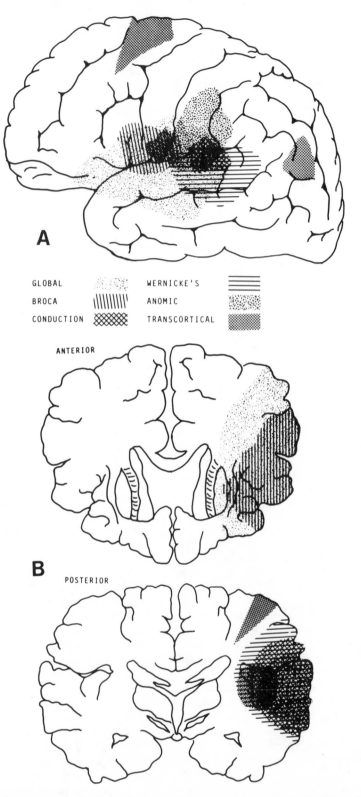

Figure 3-2. Composite drawings showing locations of lesions producing six major types of aphasia: **(A)** lateral and **(B)** anterior and posterior coronal views. Reproduced from Kertesz A, Lesk D, and McCabe P. Isotope localization of infarcts in aphasia. *Arch Neurol*, 1977, *34*, 590–601, Figures 20 and 21. Copyright 1977, American Medical Association. With permission.

TABLE 3-3. Characteristics of Nonfluent and Fluent Aphasic Output

Nonfluent aphasia	Fluent aphasia
Decreased output	Normal or increased verbal output
Effortful; difficulty with speech initiation	Little or no effort in initiating or producing speech
Dysarthria	Normal articulation
Decreased phrase length	Normal phrase length
Dysprosody	Melody and inflection preserved
Agrammatism	Low information content (empty speech)
High information content	Paraphasias present
Paraphasias rare	
	Literal pharaphasias (phonemic substitution)
	Verbal paraphasia (semantic or word substitution)
	Neologism (substitution of a nonsense word)

ilar to that associated with thalamic hemorrhage, but dysarthria and hypophonia are more prominent (Albert et al., 1981). Nonhemorrhagic lesions may produce atypical aphasic syndromes by disrupting subcortical white matter tracts and radiations or by extending to involve adjacent cortical regions (Damasio et al., 1982; Naeser et al., 1982).

Neuropsychiatric Complications, Prognosis, and Treatment of Aphasia

Prognosis and treatment of the aphasic patient depend not only on the nature of the aphasia syndrome itself, but also on the associated neuropsychiatric complications. Table 3-4 lists the neurological and neuropsychiatric disturbances commonly associated with anterior or posterior left hemisphere lesions. Catastrophic reactions may occur with either anterior or posterior lesions but are more prominent in patients with anterior disturbances and Broca's aphasia (Gainotti, 1972). Patients with posterior lesions, particularly Wernicke aphasics, may be unaware of their language deficits, and these patients exhibit the greatest tendency to become suspicious and paranoid during the course of their illness (Ben-

son, 1973). Anxiety is most often found in patients with anomic aphasia and retrorolandic lesions (Gainotti, 1972). Depression is more common and more profound among patients with anterior than posterior lesions. Depression is not correlated with severity of physical or cognitive impairment but is related to the proximity of the lesion to the anterior pole of the frontal lobe, and Robinson and colleagues have suggested that anterior polar lesions disrupt ascending catecholaminergic tracts, depleting brain norepinephrine levels and producing the depressed mood (Chapter 14) (Robinson and Benson, 1981; Robinson and Bloom, 1977; Robinson and Szetela, 1981). Moderate to severe depression in aphasics is associated with neurovegetative disturbances (sleep and appetite alterations) and an abnormal dexamethasone suppression test (Finklesteine et al., 1982).

Prognosis for language recovery varies with etiology of the aphasia and the type of linguistic deficit. The outcome of aphasias associated with neoplasms depends directly on the success of treating the tumor. Traumatic aphasias recover more completely than do aphasias produced by cerebrovascular disease, and among vascular aphasias, the greatest amount of recovery occurs within the first 3–6 months, although minor degrees of recov-

TABLE 3-4. Neurological and Neuropsychiatric Disturbances Associated with Anterior and Posterior Left Hemisphere Lesions

Clinical Features	Anterior Lesion	Posterior Lesion
Aphasia	Nonfluent	Fluent
Neurological deficits		
Hemiparesis	+	+/−
Hemisensory loss	−	+/−
Hemianopsia	−	+/−
Behavioral alterations		
Depression	+	−
Denial and/or unawareness	−	+
Anxiety	−	+
Paranoia, suspiciousness	−	+
Catastrophic reactions	+	+/−

ery may continue for 5 or more years (Kertesz and McCabe, 1977; Thomsen, 1975). Global aphasics have the worst prognosis for recovery of useful language skills; Broca and Wernicke aphasics have an overall fair prognosis for recovery with sizable variations from patient to patient; anomic, conduction, and transcortical aphasics have a relatively good prognosis, with some patients recovering completely (Kertesz and McCabe, 1977; Lomas and Kertesz, 1978). In many cases, patients with more extensive linguistic deficits evolve into a stage of residual anomic aphasia. Younger patients with aphasia tend to recover more language skills than do older patients, and left-handed patients have a better prognosis than do dextrals (Kertesz and McCabe, 1977; Subirana, 1958). In general, comprehension of language improves more than fluency of expressive output (Cummings et al., 1979; Prins et al., 1978).

Aphasia therapy facilitates language recovery and should be pursued in all patients. Results are best if therapy is initiated soon after onset of the aphasic disturbance, but improvement can occur even in patients who have had language deficits for prolonged periods and regardless of the type of aphasic syndrome (Basso et al., 1979; Benson, 1979c; Butfield and Zangwill, 1946; Vignolo, 1964). In addition to traditional reeducation techniques, recent efforts have been made to develop individualized techniques for specific types of aphasia such as utilization of melodic intonation therapy in patients with Broca's aphasia and the use of visual communication symbols by patients with global aphasic syndromes (Gardner et al., 1976; Sparks et al., 1974).

Aphasia-Related Syndromes

Alexia

Alexia refers to an acquired inability to read caused by brain damage and must be distinguished from dyslexia, a developmental abnormality in which the individual is unable to learn to read, and from illiteracy reflecting a poor educational background (Benson, 1979a). Most aphasics are also alexic, but alexia may occur in the absence of aphasia and may occasionally be virtually the sole disability resulting from specific

TABLE 3-5.   Classification of the Alexias

Alexia without agraphia
Alexia with agraphia
Without aphasia
With fluent aphasia
With nonfluent aphasia (frontal alexia)
Deep dyslexia (deep alexia, paralexia)
Hemialexia

CNS lesions. The ability to read aloud and reading comprehension may be dissociated by some lesions and must be assessed independently. Table 3-5 presents a classification of alexia, and each alexic syndrome is discussed in the following paragraphs.

Alexia without agraphia.   Alexia without agraphia is a classic disconnection syndrome in which the usual lesion includes an infarction in the left occipital cortex and the posterior aspect of the corpus callosum. The occipital lesion produces a right homonymous hemianopsia, making reading in the right visual field impossible. At the same time the callosal lesion makes it impossible to transfer visual information from the left visual field (perceived by the intact right occipital region) across the corpus callosum to the left posterior hemispheric region, where graphic decoding can occur (Benson, 1979a; Geschwind, 1965). In the alexia without agraphia syndrome, letter reading is superior to word reading, the patient retains the ability to spell and to recognize words spelled aloud, there is greater difficulty in copying words than writing spontaneously, and a color anomia is frequently present (Benson, 1979a; Geschwind and Fusillo, 1966). In some cases a right hemiparesis, right hemisensory loss, and mild naming ability disturbance accompany the syndrome (Benson and Tomlinson, 1971). Occasionally, alexia without agraphia has been produced by a small lesion beneath the angular gyrus and is then unaccompanied by a visual field defect or other neurological impairment (Greenblatt, 1973, 1976).

Alexia with agraphia.   Alexia with agraphia may occur with no significant associated aphasia, with fluent aphasia, or with nonfluent aphasia. Alexia with agraphia in the absence of aphasia occurs with lesions in the region of the angular gyrus and often coexists with elements of the Gerstmann syndrome (discussed later). Both letter and word reading are impaired, and the patient cannot spell aloud or recognize spelled words—the syndrome is equivalent to an acquired illiteracy. Word copying is superior to spontaneous writing (Albert, 1979; Benson, 1979a). The syndrome is usually produced by occlusion of the angular branch of the middle cerebral artery but may occur as part of a borderzone syndrome following carotid occlusion or with trauma or neoplasms.

Alexia with agraphia and fluent aphasia occurs with Wernicke's aphasia or transcortical sensory aphasia; in the latter, reading aloud may be preserved despite impaired reading comprehension.

Alexia with agraphia and nonfluent aphasia is found in some patients with Broca's aphasia. Not all Broca aphasics are alexic, but when alexia is present, the reading disturbance has several distinctive characteristics. Word reading is superior to letter reading, and the words recognized are almost exclusively substantive nouns and

TABLE 3-6. Classification of the Agraphias

Aphasic agraphias	Nonaphasic agraphias
Agraphia with fluent aphasia	Motor agraphia
Agraphia with nonfluent aphasia	Paretic agraphia
Alexia with agraphia	Hypokinetic agraphia
Gerstmann syndrome agraphia	Micrographia with parkinsonism
Pure agraphia	Hyperkinetic agraphia
Agraphia in confusional states	Tremor
Deep agraphia	Chorea, athetosis, tics
Disconnection agraphia	Dystonia (writer's cramp)
	Reiterative agraphia
	Perseveration
	Paligraphia
	Echographia
	Coprographia
	Visuospatial agraphia
	Hysterical agraphia

Adopted from Benson DF and Cummings JL. Agraphia. In Vinken PJ and Bruyn GW (Eds.): *Disorders of speech, perception, and symbolic behavior*, Vol. 4, 2nd ed., *Handbook of clinical neurology*, New York, American Elsevier Publishing Company, in press, Table 34-1. With permission from Excerpta Medica, Elsevier Science Publishers.

verbs. The reading disability is comparable to other aspects of Broca's aphasia where syntactic comprehension and spontaneous production of the small grammatical functor words are impaired and comprehension and production of substantives is preserved. Spontaneous writing and copying of verbal material are also abnormal (Benson, 1977; Benson et al., 1971; Nielsen, 1939).

Deep dyslexia. Deep dyslexia (deep alexia, paralexia) refers to a syndrome that evolves in some aphasics with severe reading impairments in which semantically related paralexias are produced in response to written stimuli. The patient may read "automobile" as "car" or "infant" as "baby." Such reading is thought to be mediated by the right hemisphere on the basis of iconic recognition (Coltheart, 1980; Marshall and Newcombe, 1980).

Hemialexia. Alexia may occur with hemispheric lesions that produce profound unilateral neglect. The syndrome usually occurs in patients with right hemispheric lesions and severe hemispatial inattention. The left half of words is ignored so that "northwest" is read as "west" or "baseball" as "ball"; or the left half may be misjudged so that "navigator" is read as "indicator," "match" as "hatch," or "alligator" as "narrator" (Henderson et al., 1982; Kinsbourne and Warrington, 1962a).

Agraphia

Agraphia indicates an acquired impairment of the ability to write (Benson, 1979a; Benson and Cummings, in press). It may reflect an aphasic disturbance with a writing deficit similar to that of oral language, or it may be a consequence of a motor system abnormality. Like alexia, agraphia must be distinguished from illiteracy where writing was never within the patient's intellectual domain. Table 3-6 presents the classification to be followed here. Aphasic agraphias are discussed first, and then nonaphasic agraphias are presented.

Aphasic agraphia. As shown in Table 3-2, all aphasias are accompanied by writing disturbances. The type of writing disturbance usually closely parallels the disturbances of oral language, and in some cases the language abnormalities may be more marked in written than spoken language. In the nonfluent aphasias there is sparse graphic output, with clumsy calligraphy, agrammatism, and poor spelling. Fluent agraphias, on the other hand, have a normal quantity of well-formed letters, but with a lack of substantive words and insertion of literal, verbal, or neologistic paragraphias similar to oral paraphasias (Benson and Cummings, in press).

Alexia with agraphia was discussed earlier with the alexias. The writing disturbance of alexia with agraphia is severe and has the characteristics of agraphias accompanying fluent aphasias. Similarly, the agraphia of Gerstmann's syndrome (discussed later) is a fluent form of agraphia but in its pure form lacks an accompanying disturbance of reading.

Pure agraphia is a controversial entity originally posited to occur with left frontal lobe lesions. No convincing cases with isolated pathologic involvement in this region have been described, but there are cases of relatively pure agraphia with left parietal lobe lesions (Auerbach and Alexander, 1981).

Chedru and Geschwind (1972a,b) observed that

writing disturbances are among the most sensitive measures of confusional states associated with toxic and metabolic encephalopathies, and in some cases a relatively pure agraphia was the most prominent neuropsychological manifestation of the encephalopathy. The characteristics of the writing disturbance occurring in acute confusional states include poor coordination and mild tremor, spatial misalignment, agrammatism, omission and substitution of letters (especially consonants), and reduplication of letters and words. Errors were concentrated at the endings of words.

Deep agraphia refers to a syndrome similar to deep dyslexia involving writing rather than reading. Concrete imageable words are written much better than abstract or nonsense words, and semantic paragraphias, similar to the semantic paralexias of deep dyslexia, are present (Benson and Cummings, in press; Bub and Kertesz, 1982). The syndrome usually occurs in patients with severe alexia and left parietal lobe lesions.

Disconnection agraphia occurs with other aspects of callosal ideomotor apraxia (discussed later) in patients with lesions resulting in disconnection of the writing hand from the necessary input of the left hemisphere. The agraphia occurs in the left hand of right-handed patients with callosal lesions. The lesion prevents the transfer of linguistic information from the left to the right hemisphere controlling the left hand. Copying is usually superior to spontaneous writing or writing to dictation (Bogen, 1969; Geschwind and Kaplan, 1962).

Nonaphasic agraphia. Writing depends on a complex array of motor and visuospatial skills in addition to language abilities. Disruption of any aspect of the motor system—peripheral, corticospinal, extrapyramidal, cerebellar—will produce agraphia, and in each case the writing disturbance will have distinctive abnormalities. Lesions of the muscles, peripheral nerves, or corticospinal tracts produce a clumsy, uncoordinated agraphia secondary to limb paralysis. Micrographia is a common manifestation of parkinsonism and occurs in idiopathic, postencephalitic, and drug-induced parkinsonian disorders (Benson and Cummings, in press). Extrapyramidal micrographia is characterized by a progressive diminution in the size of the letters, often accompanied by increased crowding (Fig. 12-1). The micrographia may be most apparent in writing but eventually includes all written productions including constructions. Tests of micrographia that make the deficit apparent include obtaining the patient's current signature and comparing it with past signatures on licenses or legal documents, asking the patient to write serial productions such as the alphabet or consecutive digits, or having the patient draw repeated connected oval loops.

Action tremors (Chapter 12) of either the cerebellar or postural type produce disturbances in writing and may make written productions unintelligible. Postural tremor is a high-frequency (8–12 Hz), low-amplitude tremor that is precipitated by movement and disappears at rest (Critchley, 1972). Postural tremors are very evident in written material (Fig. 12-2), and in some cases writing is the only maneuver that elicits the tremor (Klawans et al., 1982). Cerebellar tremors are usually large-amplitude, intention tremors that are worsened by attempts to produce fine writing movements. Often the patient can make only a few sweeping marks on the page.

Chorea, athetosis, and tics are hyperkinetic movement disorders that influence writing in the same way that they affect all other volitional motor activity. In severe cases writing is impossible, and even in mild cases the output will be visibly distorted. The differential diagnosis and treatment of these disorders is discussed in Chapter 12.

"Writer's cramp" is among the most well known and most misunderstood of all agraphias. The syndrome of progressive cramping of the hand and forearm among individuals in professions demanding fine finger movements—writers, telegraphers, pianists, and violinists—was treated as a neurotic disorder by early psychoanalysts and as a learned disturbance by behavioral therapists. The progression of writer's cramp to a segmental dystonia involving the entire limb or even to generalized dystonia musculorum deformans, however, along with the absence of a consistent psychopathology among its victims, indicate that the disorder is a focal dystonia (Sheehy and Marsden, 1982). The cramping begins between age 20 and 50, and there may be inconspicuous associated neurological deficits, including abnormal posturing or tremor of the affected limb, diminished arm swing, or increased limb tone.

Reiterative agraphias refer to the abnormal repetition of letters, words, or phrases in writing. Perseveration is a continuation of activity after the appropriate stimulus has stopped; paligraphia is the rewriting of phrases generated by the patient; and echographia is the rewriting of phrases produced by the examiner. These disorders occur in severely deteriorated patients, including those with advanced degenerative, vascular, or traumatic conditions and in catatonic disturbances (Benson and Cummings, in press). Coprographia occurs primarily in Gilles de la Tourette syndrome, where the patient occasionally has a compulsion to express coprolalic tendencies in writing (Eriksson and Persson, 1969).

Visuospatial agraphia is manifested by a tendency to neglect one portion of the writing page; slanting of the lines upward or downward; and abnormal spacing between letters, syllables, or words. It is seen most often with right-sided lesions in the region of the temporoparietooccipital junction and is accompanied by other evidence of left-sided neglect (Hécaen and Albert, 1978; Marcie and Hécaen, 1979).

Agraphia may occasionally occur as an hysterical conversion symptom. The agraphia is usually part of a monoparesis in which the limb is weak throughout with slightly diminished tone and normal muscle stretch reflexes. Sensation may or may not be affected (Ziegler, 1967). The disorder typically is short-lived, and the psychogenic cause seldom is subtle. Like all conversion symptoms, it often indicates the presence of a major psychiatric or neurological disturbance (Slater, 1965; Stefansson et al., 1976).

Acalculia

There are three principal types of acalculia: (1) acalculia associated with language disturbances, including number paraphasia, number agraphia, or number alexia; (2) acalculia secondary to visuospatial dysfunction with malalignment of numbers and columns; and (3) a primary anarithmetria entailing disruption of the computation process (Levin, 1979) (Table 3-7). A fourth type of acalculia—symbol agnosia—in which the patient loses the ability to understand the operational symbols that determine the mathematical process to be performed ($+$, $\div$, $\times$, $-$), has occasionally been observed but has not been well studied and is rare (Grewel, 1952).

Aphasia-related disturbances of calculation include paraphasic errors wherein the patient makes a verbal paraphasic error, substituting one number for another (Benson and Denckla, 1969). Number alexia and number agraphia may also occur and, in some cases, may be disproportionately greater than letter reading and writing disturbances (Levin, 1979). All these disorders occur with lesions located in the posterior left hemisphere usually involving the parietal lobe and angular gyrus areas.

Visuospatial acalculia may occur with lesions of either hemisphere but is most common with right parietal dysfunction. Spacing of multidigit numbers, placeholding values, and column alignment are disrupted (Grewel, 1969).

Primary anarithmetria occurs mainly in the context of Gerstmann's syndrome with lesions in the region of the dominant angular gyrus, but it may occasionally be seen as an isolated abnormality with disturbances of the

TABLE 3-7.   Classification of the Acalculias

Language-related acalculias

    Number paraphasia
    Number alexia
    Number agraphia

Visuospatial acalculia

Anarithmetria

Symbol agnosia

same region (Benson and Wier, 1972). In this case there is no significant aphasic or visuospatial disturbance, but errors are made in the computation process (Grewel, 1952, 1969).

Gerstmann's Syndrome and Angular Gyrus Syndrome

In 1924, Josef Gerstmann described a syndrome occurring with discrete left angular gyrus lesions and consisting of a tetrad of clinical findings including dysgraphia, finger agnosia, inability to distinguish left from right, and acalculia. In 1940 Gerstmann reviewed the considerable literature that had evolved concerning the syndrome and concluded that the findings did have clinical validity and localizing value (Gerstmann, 1940). The prominence of the different components varies in each individual case, and specific testing may be necessary in order to elicit subtle deficits (Hécaen and Albert, 1978; Kinsbourne and Warrington, 1962b; Roeltgen et al., 1983). When one or more of the elements of the syndrome is missing, the localizing implications of the remaining members is doubtful (Benton, 1961).

In many cases a lesion of the dominant angular gyrus produces deficits in addition to the Gerstmann syndrome. Some degree of aphasia frequently is present, alexia with agraphia may occur, and constructional disturbances often accompany the Gerstmann syndrome (Benson, 1979a). This combination of deficits may closely imitate the clinical findings of Alzheimer's disease (Benson et al., 1982).

Apraxia

Apraxia refers to disorders of learned movement that cannot be accounted for on the basis of weakness, sensory loss, inattention, or failure to understand the requested action (Geschwind, 1975; Heilman, 1979). Two principal types of apraxia have been recognized: (1) ideational apraxia, in which the patient fails to correctly pantomime a multicomponent sequence such as folding a letter, inserting it in an envelope, and stamping the envelope (Denny-Brown, 1958) and (2) ideomotor apraxia, in which the patient fails to perform on command actions that can be done spontaneously, such as waving good-bye, hammering, thumbing a ride, sawing, sucking through a straw, or whistling. Ideational apraxias occur in dementias and in acute confusional states. Ideomotor apraxias occur with specific left hemisphere lesions (De Renzi et al., 1968; Geschwind, 1975; Haaland et al., 1977; Kimura and Archibald, 1974).

Table 3-8 presents the three principal types of ideomotor apraxia and their associated clinical findings. Parietal apraxia refers to the occurrence of apraxic movements in patients with lesions involving the inferior parietal lobule and the adjacent arcuate fasciculus. The patients have a fluent aphasia (usually conduction apha-

TABLE 3-8. Ideomotor Apraxias and Accompanying Clinical Findings

Characteristic	Type of Apraxia		
	Parietal	Sympathetic	Callosal
Apraxia distribution	Bilateral limb, buccolingual	Left limbs, buccolingual	Left limbs
Aphasia	Conduction	Broca's	None or transcortical motor
Hemiparesis	± right-sided weakness	Right hemiparesis	None
Lesion location	Inferior parietal lobule (arcuate fasciculus)	Left premotor cortex	Callosal fibers
Associated findings	± right hemisensory loss		Commissurotomy syndrome[a]

[a]Involving left tactile anomia, left agraphia, poor crossed tactile matching, poor intermanual position matching, and right-hand constructional disturbance.

sia), may have a mild right hemiparesis and a hemisensory defect, and frequently fail to recognize that the apraxic movements are incorrectly performed (Heilman et al., 1982; Kertesz and Hooper, 1982).

Sympathetic apraxia is the apraxia of the left limbs and buccolingual structures noted in patients with left frontal lesions. The apraxic limbs are "in sympathy" with the right hemiparesis produced by the frontal lesion (Geschwind, 1963, 1975). The patients also manifest a nonfluent Broca-type aphasia, have more prominent involvement of buccolingual than limb movements, and are likely to perceive that the apraxic movements are faulty (De Renzi et al., 1966; Geschwind, 1975; Heilman et al., 1982; Nathan, 1948).

Callosal apraxia occurs when verbal directions mediated by the left hemisphere cannot cross the corpus callosum for execution of left-sided limb commands. The apraxia involves only the left arm and leg, and in most cases there is no associated aphasia or hemiparesis (Ettlinger, 1969; Gazzaniga et al., 1967; Gersh and Damasio, 1981; Volpe et al., 1982; Watson and Heilman, 1983). Disruption of interhemispheric communication is manifested in a variety of disturbances in addition to the left limb apraxia, including left-hand tactile anomia, left-hand aphasic agraphia, right-hand constructional disturbances, and a variety of somesthetic disorders such as failure of intermanual tactile matching and intermanual matching of hand positions (Bogen, 1979; Geschwind and Kaplan, 1962). Corpus callosum injury may be produced by surgical sectioning for the control of intractable epilepsy, anterior cerebral artery occlusion, trauma, or neoplasm (Bogen, 1979; Geschwind and Kaplan, 1962; Rubens et al., 1977).

DISORDERED VERBAL OUTPUT IN PSYCHOSIS

Severe thought disturbances in psychosis may result in disordered verbal output that can occasionally be difficult to distinguish from fluent aphasia. Tangentiality,

derailment, circumstantiality, and perseveration may occur in the speech of manics, but the patient usually provides sufficient associative links to allow the content to be followed, and there is an accompanying press of speech (Andreasen, 1979a,b, 1982; Wykes and Leff, 1982). These features usually allow manic speech to be differentiated from aphasia.

The verbal output of a small percentage of schizophrenics, however, can sometimes closely resemble jargon aphasia and can be distinguished only with difficulty (Faber and Reichstein, 1981; Faber et al., 1983; Gerson et al., 1977; Rausch et al., 1980). Furthermore, the tendency for some fluent aphasics to develop paranoid syndromes resembling schizophrenia (Benson, 1973) makes the differential task even more challenging. The two disorders share many features, including fluent output, poverty of information content, relative preservation of syntax and phonology, paraphasia, perseveration, incoherence, and impairment of the pragmatic aspects of discourse (Andreasen, 1982; Chaika, 1974; Critchley, 1964; Lecours and Vanier-Clement, 1976; Maher, 1972; Rochester et al., 1977). Despite these similarities, there are differences between jargon aphasia and the disordered verbal output of schizophrenics (Table 3-9). In spontaneous speech, schizophrenics tend to have more extended replies to inquiries than do fluent aphasics. They are less aware of their communication deficit and become less engaged in conversational exchange, and the ideational content of their output is more bizarre with a tendency to return to a few main themes and to use a restricted vocabulary (Andreasen, 1982; Gerson et al., 1977). Neologisms and paraphasia are common in fluent aphasia and rare in schizophrenia. When they occur in schizophrenia, however, they may be highly distinctive in that the new word may acquire a stable meaning within the schizophrenic's idiosyncratic vocabulary. For instance, one of the present author's patients believed he had a "seisometer" behind his right eye that could receive and transmit instructions; Forrest reported a patient with a thesaurus of neologisms such as "semitiertology" or the study of half hundreds; one of Bleuler's

TABLE 3-9.   Clinical Features that Distinguish Fluent Aphasia from the Verbal Output of Schizophrenia

Clinical Characteristic	Fluent Aphasia	Schizophrenia
Spontaneous speech		
Length of response	Shorter	Extended
Awareness of deficit	Present	Absent
Participation in conversation	Present	Absent
Content	Empty	Impoverished; bizarre; restricted themes
Neologisms and paraphasias	Common	Rare (stable meaning)
Language testing		
Comprehension	±	Intact
Repetition	±	Intact
Naming	Impaired	Intact
Word-list generation	Diminished	May be normal or bizarre
Reading	Impaired	Intact
Writing	Aphasic	Resembles spoken output
Associated characteristics		
Medical history	+	−
Psychiatric history	−	+
Age at onset	>50	<30
Family history	−	±
Neurological examination	± focal findings	± "soft" signs

patients used the word "snortse" to mean "to talk through the walls"; and a patient studied by Hamilton used a process of condensation to construct words such as "esamaxrider" meaning "he's a married man" (Bleuler, 1950; Forrest, 1969; Hamilton, 1976; Kraepelin, 1971). The stability of the paraphasic usage in schizophrenia differs markedly from fluent aphasia, wherein patients rarely make the same paraphasic substitution consistently.

Language testing in the course of the mental status examination can also be helpful in distinguishing aphasia from schizophrenic verbal output if the patient can be engaged in the testing process (Faber et al., 1983; Gerson et al., 1977; Rausch et al., 1980). Naming ability will invariably be impaired to some extent in aphasia and normal in schizophrenia. Likewise, comprehension and repetition may be impaired in aphasia depending on the type of language deficit present, whereas they are preserved in schizophrenia. Generation of word lists such as the maximum number of animals one can name in a minute is diminished in aphasia and may be normal or contain bizarre entries in schizophrenia. For example, one patient examined by the present author

included "vaginal monster" and "Phoenician circus woman" among his animals. Reading and writing are impaired in aphasia; in schizophrenia reading is preserved and writing may be normal or may resemble the disordered spoken output. For example, when one patient was asked to describe the weather, he wrote: "Rumors of a fiercer nature were let out about the phloral trumps of our Lord." Preliminary studies suggest that erroneous use of language increases with increased duration of the schizophrenia (Silverberg-Shalev et al., 1981).

Finally, the clinical circumstances in which the verbal output disorder occurs may also facilitate differentiation of aphasia and schizophrenia. Onset before age 30, history of psychosis, and absence of known medical illness all favor the diagnosis of schizophrenia; whereas onset after age 50 years, presence of a predisposing medical illness, absence of previous psychiatric disturbances, and focal findings on neurological examination all indicate a hemispheric insult and support a diagnosis of aphasia. These features are not infallible, however, and it must be remembered that schizophrenics are at the same risk as the general population for the development of cerebrovascular or neoplastic disease.

REFERENCES

Abrams R and Taylor MA. Catatonia: a prospective clinical study. *Arch Gen Psychiat*, 1976, *33*, 579–581.

Akhtar S and Buckman J. The differential diagnosis of mutism: a review and report of three unusual cases. *Dis Nerv Syst*, 1972, *38*, 558–563.

Alajouaine TH and Lhermitte F. Acquired aphasia in children. *Brain*, 1965, *88*, 653–662.

Albert ML. Alexia. In Heilman KM and Valenstein E (Eds.): *Clinical neuropsychology*. New York, Oxford University Press, 1979, pp. 59–91.

Albert ML, Goodglass H, Helm NA, Rubens AB, and Alexander MP. *Clinical aspects of dysphasia*. New York, Springer-Verlag, 1981.

Alexander MP and LoVerme SR, Jr. Aphasia after left hemispheric intracerebral hemorrhage. *Neurology*, 1980, *30*, 1193–1202.

Alexander MP and Schmitt MA. The aphasia syndrome of stroke in the left anterior cerebral artery territory. *Arch Neurol*, 1980, *37*, 97–100.

Andreasen NC. Thought, language, and communication disorders. I. Clinical assessment, definition of terms, and evaluation of their reliability. *Arch Gen Psychiat*, 1979a, *36*, 1315–1321.

Andreasen NC. Thought, language, and communication disorders. II. Diagnostic significance. *Arch Gen Psychiat*, 1979b, *36*, 1325–1330.

Andreasen NC. The relationship between schizophrenic language and the aphasias. In Henn FA and Nasrallah HA (Eds.): *Schizophrenia as a brain disease*. New York, Oxford University Press, 1982, pp. 99–111.

Arseni C and Botez MI. Speech disturbances caused by tumours of the supplementary motor area. *Acta Psychiat Scand*, 1961, *36*, 279–299.

Auerbach SH and Alexander MP. Pure agraphia and unilateral optic ataxia associated with left superior parietal lobe lesion. *J Neurol Neurosurg Psychiat*, 1981, *44*, 430–432.

Barris RW and Schuman HR. Bilateral anterior cingulate gyrus lesions. *Neurology*, 1953, *3*, 44–52.

Basso A, Capitani E, and Vignolo LA. Influence of rehabilitation on language skills in aphasic patients. *Arch Neurol*, 1979, *36*, 190–196.

Bastian HC. On different kinds of aphasia, with special reference to their classification and ultimate pathology. *Br Med J*, 1887, *2*, 931–936, 985–990.

Benson DF. Fluency in aphasia: correlation with radioactive scan localization. *Cortex*, 1967, *3*, 373–394.

Benson DF. Psychiatric aspects of aphasia. *Br J Psychiat*, 1973, *123*, 555–566.

Benson DF. The third alexia. *Arch Neurol*, 1977, *34*, 327–331.

Benson DF. *Aphasia, alexia, and agraphia*. New York, Churchill Livingston, 1979a.

Benson DF. Neurologic correlates of anomia. In Whitaker H and Whitaker HA (Eds.): *Studies in neurolinguistics*, Vol. 4. New York, Academic Press, 1979b, pp. 293–328.

Benson DF. Aphasia rehabilitation. *Arch Neurol*, 1979c, *36*, 187–189.

Benson DF, Brown J, and Tomlinson EB. Varieties of alexia. *Neurology*, 1971, *21*, 951–957.

Benson DF, Cummings JL, and Tsai SY. Angular gyrus syndrome simulating Alzheimer's disease. *Arch Neurol*, 1982, *39*, 616–620.

Benson DF and Cummings JL. Agraphia. In Vinken PJ and Bruyn GW (Eds.): *Disorders of speech, perception, and symbolic behavior*, Vol. 4, 2nd ed., *Handbook of clinical neurology*. New York, American Elsevier Publishing Company, in press.

Benson DF and Denckla MB. Verbal paraphasia as a source of calculation disturbance. *Arch Neurol*, 1969, *21*, 96–102.

Benson DF, Sheremata WA, Bouchard R, Segarra JM, Price D, and Geschwind N. Conduction aphasia. A clinicopathological study. *Arch Neurol*, 1973, *28*, 339–346.

Benson DF and Tomlinson EB. Hemiplegic syndrome of the posterior cerebral artery. *Stroke*, 1971, *2*, 559–564.

Benson DF and Wier WF. Acalculia: acquired anarithmetia. *Cortex*, 1972, *8*, 465–472.

Benton AL. The fiction of the "Gerstmann syndrome." *J Neurol Neurosurg Psychiat*, 1961, *24*, 176–181.

Bleuler E. In Zinken J (Translator): *Dementia praecox or the group of schizophrenias*. New York, International Universities Press, 1950.

Bogen JE. The other side of the brain. I: Dysgraphia and dyscopia following cerebral commissurotomy. *Bull LA Neurol Soc*, 1969, *34*, 73–105.

Bogen JE. The callosal syndrome. In Heilman KM and Valenstein E (Eds.): *Clinical neuropsychology*. New York, Oxford University Press, 1979, pp. 308–359.

Boller F and Green E. Comprehension in severe aphasics. *Cortex*, 1972, *8*, 382–394.

Bub D and Kertesz A. Deep agraphia. *Brain Lang*, 1982, *17*, 146–165.

Butfield E and Zangwill OL. Re-education in aphasia: a review of 70 cases. *J Neurol Neurosurg Psychiat*, 1946, *9*, 75–79.

Cairns H, Oldfield RC, Pennybacker JB, and Whitteridge D. Akinetic mutism with an epidermoid cyst of the 3rd ventricle. *Brain*, 1941, *64*, 273–290.

Chaika E. A linguist looks at "schizophrenic" language. *Brain Lang*, 1974, *1*, 257–276.

Chedru F and Geschwind N. Disorders of higher cortical functions in acute confusional states. *Cortex*, 1972a, *8*, 395–411.

Chedru F and Geschwind N. Writing disturbances in acute confusional states. *Neuropsychologia*, 1972b, *10*, 343–353.

Chusid JG, de Gutierrez-Mahoney CG, and Margules-Lavergne MP. Speech disturbances in association with parasagittal frontal lesions. *J Neurosurg*, 1954, *11*, 193–204.

Ciemens VA. Localized thalamic hemorrhage. A cause of aphasia. *Neurology*, 1970, *20*, 776–782.

Coltheart M. Deep dyslexia: a review of the syndrome. In Coltheart M, Patterson K, and Marshall JC (Eds.): *Deep dyslexia*. Boston, Routledge and Kegan Paul, 1980, pp. 22–47.

Critchley E. Clinical manifestations of essential tremor. *J Neurol Neurosurg Psychiat*, 1972, *35*, 365–372.

Critchley M. The neurology of psychotic speech. *Br J Psychiat*, 1964, *110*, 353–364.

Cummings JL and Benson DF. *Dementia: a clinical approach*. Boston, Butterworths, 1983.

Cummings JL, Benson DF, Houlihan JP, and Gosenfeld LF. Mutism: loss of neocortical and limbic vocalization. *J Nerv Ment Dis*, 1983, *171*, 255–259.

Cummings JL, Benson DF, Walsh MJ, and Levine HL. Left-to-right transfer of language dominance: a case study. *Neurology*, 1979, *29*, 1547–1550.

Daly DD and Love JG. Akinetic mutism. *Neurology*, 1958, *8*, 238–242.

Damasio H and Damasio AR. The anatomical basis of conduction aphasia. *Brain*, 1980, *103*, 337–350.

Damasio AR, Damasio H, Rizzo M, Varney N, and Gersh F. Aphasia with nonhemorrhagic lesions in the basal ganglia and internal capsule. *Arch Neurol*, 1982, *39*, 15–20.

Davison C and Kelman H. Pathologic laughing and crying. *Arch Neurol Psychiat*, 1939, *42*, 595–643.

Denny-Brown D. The nature of apraxia. *J Nerv Ment Dis*, 1958, *126*, 9–32.

De Renzi E, Pieczuro A, and Vignolo LA. Oral apraxia and aphasia. *Cortex*, 1966, *2*, 50–73.

De Renzi E, Pieczuro A, and Vignolo LA. Ideational apraxia: a quantitative study. *Neuropsychologia*, 1968, *6*, 41–52.

Eriksson B and Persson T. Gilles de la Tourette's syndrome. *Br J Psychiat*, 1969, *115*, 351–353.

Ettlinger G. Apraxia considered as a disorder of movements that are language dependent: evidence from cases of brain bisection. *Cortex*, 1969, *5*, 285–289.

Faber R, Abrams R, Taylor MA, Kasprison A, Morris C, and Weis R. Comparison of schizophrenic patients with formal thought disorder and neurologically impaired patients with aphasia. *Am J Psychiat*, 1983, *140*, 1348–1351.

Faber R and Reichstein MB. Language dysfunction in schizophrenia. *Br J Psychiat*, 1981, *139*, 519–522.

Fazio C, Sacco G, and Bugiani O. The thalamic hemorrhage. An anatomoclinical study. *Europ Neurol*, 1973, *9*, 30–43.

Finklestein S, Benowitz LI, Baldessarini RJ, Arana GW, Leine D, Woo E, Bear D, Moya K, and Stoll AL. Mood, vegetative disturbance, and dexamethasone suppression test after stroke. *Ann Neurol*, 1982, *12*, 463–468.

Forrest DV. New words and neologisms. With a thesaurus of coinages by a schizophrenic savant. *Psychiatry*, 1969, *32*, 44–73.

Gainotti G. Emotional behavior and hemispheric side of lesion. *Cortex*, 1972, *8*, 41–55.

Gardner H, Zurif EB, Berry T, and Baker E. Visual communication in aphasia. *Neuropsychologia*, 1976, *14*, 275–292.

Gazzaniga MS, Bogen JE, and Sperry RW. Dyspraxia following division of the cerebral commissures. *Arch Neurol*, 1967, *16*, 606–612.

Gersh F and Damasio AR. Praxis and writing of the left hand may be served by different callosal pathways. *Arch Neurol*, 1981, *38*, 634–636.

Gerson SN, Benson DF, and Frazier SH. Diagnosis: schizophrenia versus posterior aphasia. *Am J Psychiat*, 1977, *134*, 966–969.

Gerstmann J. Syndrome of finger agnosia, disorientation for right and left, agraphia, and acalculia. *Arch Neurol Psychiat*, 1940, *44*, 398–408.

Geschwind N. Sympathetic dyspraxia. *Trans Am Neurol Assoc*, 1963, *88*, 219–220.

Geschwind N. Non-aphasic disorders of speech. *Internat J Neurol*, 1964, *4*, 207–214.

Geschwind N. Disconnexion syndrome in animals and man. *Brain*, 1965, *88*, 237–294, 585–644.

Geschwind N. The apraxias: neural mechanisms of disorders of learned movement. *Am Sci*, 1975, *63*, 188–195.

Geschwind N and Fusillo M. Color-naming defects in association with alexia. *Arch Neurol*, 1966, *15*, 137–146.

Geschwind N and Kaplan E. A human cerebral deconnection syndrome. *Neurology*, 1962, *12*, 675–685.

Geschwind N, Quadfasel FA, and Segarra JM. Isolation of the speech area. *Neuropsychologia*, 1968, *6*, 327–340.

Gloning I, Gloning K, Haub G, and Quatember R. Comparison of verbal behavior in right-handed and non-right-handed patients with anatomically verified lesion of one hemisphere. *Cortex*, 1969, *5*, 43–52.

Goodglass H. Studies on the grammar of aphasics. In Goodglass H and Blumstein S (Eds.): *Psycholinguistics and aphasia*. Baltimore, Johns Hopkins University Press, 1973, pp. 183–215.

Goodglass H and Quadfasel FA. Language literality in left-handed aphasics. *Brain*, 1954, *77*, 521–548.

Greenblatt SH. Alexia without agraphia or hemianopsia. *Brain*, 1973, *96*, 307–316.

Greenblatt SH. Subangular alexia without agraphia or hemianopsia. *Brain Lang*, 1976, *3*, 229–345.

Grewel F. Acalculia. *Brain*, 1952, *75*, 397–407.

Grewel F. The acalculias. In Vinken PJ and Bruyn GW (Eds.): *Disorders of speech, perception, and symbolic behavior*, Vol. 4. *Handbook of clinical neurology* New York, American Elsevier Publishing Company, 1969, pp. 181–194.

Guttmann E. Aphasia in children. *Brain*, 1942, *65*, 205–219.

Haaland KY, Cleeland CS, and Carr D. Motor performance after unilateral hemisphere damage in patients with tumor. *Arch Neurol*, 1977, *34*, 556–559.

Hamilton M. *Fish's schizophrenia*. Bristol, England, John Wright and Sons, Ltd., 1976.

Hécaen H and Albert ML. *Human neuropsychology*. New York, John Wiley & Sons, 1978.

Hécaen H and Sauguet J. Cerebral dominance in left-handed subjects. *Cortex*, 1971, *7*, 19–48.

Heilman KM. Apraxia. In Heilman KM and Valenstein E (Eds.): *Clinical neuropsychology*. New York, Oxford University Press, 1979, pp. 159–185.

Heilman KM, Rothi LJ, and Valenstein E. Two forms of ideomotor apraxia. *Neurology*, 1982, *32*, 342–346.

Heilman KM, Tucker DM, and Valenstein E. A case of mixed transcortical aphasia with intact naming. *Brain*, 1976, *99*, 415–426.

Henderson VW, Alexander MP, and Naesser MA. Right thalamic injury, impaired visuospatial perception, and alexia. *Neurology*, 1982, *32*, 235–240.

Herbert EL. Analysis of six cases of voluntary mutism. *J Speech Hear Dis*, 1959, *24*, 55–58.

Ironside R. Disorders of laughter due to brain lesions. *Brain*, 1956, *79*, 589–609.

Kertesz A. *Aphasia and associated disorders: taxonomy, localization, and recovery*. New York, Grune & Stratton, 1979.

Kertesz A and Benson DF. Neologistic jargon: a clinicopathologic study. *Cortex*, 1970, *6*, 362–387.

Kertesz A and Hooper P. Praxis and language: the extent and variety of apraxia in aphasia. *Neuropsychologia*, 1982, *20*, 275–286.

Kertesz A, Lesk D, and McCabe P. Isotope localization of infarcts in aphasia. *Arch Neurol*, 1977, *34*, 590–601.

Kertesz A and McCabe P. Recovery patterns and prognosis in aphasia. *Brain*, 1977, *100*, 1–18.

Kertesz A, Sheppard A, and Mackenzie R. Localization in transcortical sensory aphasia. *Arch Neurol*, 1982, *39*, 475–478.

Kimura D and Archibald Y. Motor functions of the left hemisphere. *Brain*, 1974, *97*, 337–350.

Kinsbourne M and Warrington EK. A variety of reading disability associated with right hemispheric lesions. *J Neurol Neurosurg Psychiat*, 1962a, *25*, 339–344.

Kinsbourne M and Warrington EK. A study of finger agnosia. *Brain*, 1962b, *85*, 47–66.

Klawans HL, Glantz R, Tanner CM, and Goetz CG. Primary writing tremor: a selective action tremor. *Neurology*, 1982, *32*, 203–206.

Klee A. Akinetic mutism: review of the literature and report of a case. *J Nerv Ment Dis*, 1961, *133*, 536–553.

Kraepelin E. In Barclay RM (Translator) and Robertson GM (Ed.): *Dementia praecox and paraphrenia*. Huntington, New York, Robert E. Krieger Publishing Company, 1971.

Langworthy OR and Hesser FH. Syndrome of pseudobulbar palsy. *Arch Int Med*, 1940, *65*, 106–121.

Laplane D. Talairoch J. Meininger V, Bancaud J, and Orgogozo JM. Clinical consequences of corticetomies involving the supplementary motor area in man. *J Neurol Sci*, 1977, *34*, 301–314.

Lavy S. Akinetic mutism in a case of craniopharyngioma. *Psychiat Neurol* (Basel), 1959, *138*, 369–374.

Lecours AR and Vanier-Clement M. Schizophrenia and jargonaphasia. *Brain Lang*, 1976, *3*, 516–565.

Levin HS. The acalculias. In Heilman KM and Valenstein E (Eds.): *Clinical neuropsychology*. New York, Oxford University Press, 1979, pp. 128–140.

Lieberman A and Benson DF. Control of emotional expression in pseudobulbar palsy. *Arch Neurol*, 1977, *34*, 717–719.

Lomas J and Kertesz A. Patterns of spontaneous recovery in aphasic groups: a study of adult stroke patients. *Brain Lang*, 1978, *5*, 388–401.

Maher B. The language of schizophrenia: a review and interpretation. *Br J Psychiat*, 1972, *120*, 3–17.

Marcie P and Hécaen H. Agraphia: writing disorders associated with unilateral cortical lesions. In Heilman KM and Valenstein E (Eds.): *Clinical neuropsychology*. New York, Oxford University Press, 1979, pp. 92–127.

Marshall JC and Newcombe F. The conceptual status of deep dyslexia: an historical perspective. In Coltheart M, Patterson K, and Marshall JC (Eds.): *Deep dyslexia*. Boston, Routledge and Kegan Paul, 1980, pp. 1–21.

Masdeu JC, Schoene WC, and Funkenstein H. Aphasia following infarction of the left supplementary motor area. *Neurology*, 1978, *28*, 1220–1223.

McFarling D, Rothi LJ, and Heilman KM. Transcortical aphasia from ischemic infarcts of the thalamus: a report of two cases. *J Neurol Neurosurg Psychiat*, 1982, *45*, 107–112.

Mohr JP, Pessin MS, Finkelstein S, Funkenstein HH, Duncan GW, and Davis KR. Broca aphasia: pathologic and clinical. *Neurology*, 1978, *28*, 311–324.

Mohr JP, Watters WC, and Duncan GW. Thalamic hemorrhage and aphasia. *Brain Lang*, 1975, *2*, 3–17.

Morrison JR. Catatonia: retarded and excited types. *Arch Gen Psychiat*, 1973, *28*, 39–41.

Naeser MA, Alexander MP, Helm-Estabrooks N, Levine HL, Laughlin SA, and Geschwind N. Aphasia with predominantly subcortical lesion sites. *Arch Neurol*, 1982, *39*, 2–14.

Nathan PW. Facial apraxia and apraxic dysarthria. *Brain*, 1948, *70*, 449–478.

Nielsen JM. The unsolved problems in aphasia. I. Alexia in "motor" aphasia. *Bull LA Neurol Soc*, 1939, *4*, 114–122.

Prins RS, Snow CE, and Wagenaar E. Recovery from aphasia: spontaneous speech comprehension. *Brain Lang*, 1978, *6*, 192–211.

Quitkin F, Rifkin A, and Klein DF. Neurologic soft signs in schizophrenia and character disorders. *Arch Gen Psychiat*, 1976, *33*, 845–853.

Rausch MA, Prescott TE, and De Wolfe AS. Schizophrenic and aphasic language: discriminable or not? *J Consult Clin Psychol*, 1980, *48*, 63–70.

Reed GF. Elective mutism in children: a re-appraisal. *J Child Psychol Psychiat*, 1963, *4*, 99–107.

Robinson RG and Benson DF. Depression in aphasic patients: frequency, severity, and clinical-pathological correlations. *Brain Lang*, 1981, *14*, 282–291.

Robinson RG and Bloom FE. Pharmacological treatment following experimental cerebral infarction: implications for understanding psychological symptoms of human stroke. *Biol Psychiat*, 1977, *12*, 669–680.

Robinson RG and Szetela B. Mood change following left hemispheric brain injury. *Ann Neurol*, 1981, *9*, 447–453.

Rochester SR, Martin JR, and Thurston S. Thought-process disorder in schizophrenia: the listener's task. *Brain Lang*, 1977, *4*, 95–114.

Roeltgen DP, Sevush S, and Heilman K. Pure Gerstmann's syndrome from a focal lesion. *Arch Neurol*, 1983, *40*, 46–47.

Ross ED. Left medial parietal lobe and receptive language functions: mixed transcortical sensory aphasia after left anterior cerebral artery infarction. *Neurology*, 1980, *30*, 144–151.

Ross ED and Stewart RM. Akinetic mutism from hypothalamic damage: successful treatment with dopamine agnosists. *Neurology*, 1981, *31*, 1435–1439.

Rothi LJ, Farling D, and Heilman KM. Conduction aphasia,

syntactic alexia and the anatomy of syntactic comprehension. *Arch Neurol,* 1982, *39,* 272–275.

Rubens AB. Aphasia with infarction in the territory of the anterior cerebral artery. *Cortex,* 1975, *11,* 239–250.

Rubens AB, Geschwind N, Mahowald MW, and Mastri A. Post-traumatic cerebral hemispheric disconnection syndrome. *Arch Neurol,* 1977, *34,* 750–755.

Salfield DJ. Observations on elective mutism in children. *J Ment Sci,* 1950, *96,* 1024–1032.

Schiff HB, Alexander MP, Naeser MA, and Galaburda AM. Aphemia. *Arch Neurol,* 1983, *40,* 720–727.

Segarra JM. Cerebral vascular disease and behavior. I. The syndrome of the mesencephalic artery (basilar artery bifurcation). *Arch Neurol,* 1970, *22,* 408–418.

Sevush S, Roeltgen DP, Campanella DT, and Heilman KM. Preserved oral reading in Wernicke's aphasia. *Neurology,* 1983, *33,* 916–920.

Sheehy MP and Marsden CD. Writers cramp—a focal dystonia. *Brain,* 1982, *105,* 461–480.

Silverberg-Shalev R, Gordon HW, Bentin S, and Aranson A. Selective language deterioration in chronic schizophrenia. *J Neurol Neurosurg Psychiat,* 1981, *44,* 547–551.

Slater E. Diagnosis of "hysteria." *Br Med J,* 1965, *1,* 1395–1399.

Smith S. An investigation and survey of 27 cases of akinesis with mutism (stupor). *J Ment Sci,* 1959, *105,* 1088–1094.

Sparks R. Helms N, and Albert M. Aphasia rehabilitation resulting from melodic intonation therapy. *Cortex,* 1974, *10,* 303–316.

Stefansson JG, Messina JA, and Meyerowitz S. Hysterical neurosis, conversion type: clinical and epidemiologic considerations. *Acta Psychiat Scand,* 1976, *53,* 119–138.

Subirana A. The prognosis in aphasia in relation to cerebral dominance and handedness. *Brain,* 1958, *81,* 415–425.

Thomsen IV. Evaluation and outcome of aphasia in patients with severe closed head trauma. *J Neurol Neurosurg Psychiat,* 1975, *38,* 713–718.

Tonkonogy J and Goodglass H. Language function, foot of the third frontal gyrus, and rolandic operculum. *Arch Neurol,* 1981, *38,* 486–490.

Van Horn G and Hawes A. Global aphasia without hemiparesis: a sign of embolic encephalopathy. *Neurology,* 1982, *32,* 403–406.

Vignolo LA. Evolution of aphasia and language rehabilitation: a retrospective exploratory study. *Cortex,* 1964, *1,* 344–367.

Volpe BT, Sidtis JJ, Holtzman JD, Wilson DH, and Gazzaniga MS. Cortical mechanisms involved in praxis: observations following partial and complete section of the corpus callosum in man. *Neurology,* 1982, *32,* 645–650.

Watson RT and Heilman KM. Callosal apraxia. *Brain,* 1983, *106,* 391–403.

Weintraub MI. *Hysterical conversion reactions.* New York, SP Medical and Scientific Books, 1983.

Wilson SAK. Pathological laughing and crying. *J Neurol Psychopathol,* 1924, *4,* 299–333.

Wykes T and Leff J. Disordered speech: differences between manics and schizophrenics. *Brain Lang,* 1982, *15,* 117–124.

Wright HL. A clinical study of children who refuse to talk in school. *J Am Acad Child Psychiat,* 1968, *7,* 603–617.

Yakovlev PI. The central "paradox" of Parkinson's disease. *J Neurosurg,* 1966 (Suppl.), 292–296.

Ziegler DK. Neurological disease and hysteria—the differential diagnosis. *Internat J Neuropsychiat,* 1967, *3,* 388–395.

Chapter 4

Amnesia, Paramnesia, and Confabulation

Disturbed memory function is a ubiquitous finding in central nervous system (CNS) diseases, and identification of the presence and characteristics of a memory disorder provides important information regarding the nature and location of brain dysfunction. Several different processes mediate aspects of memory function, and all must be intact for normal memory to occur. Attention is necessary to ensure proper registration of data; recent memory mediates the learning of new materials; and remote memory allows the recollection of information from the more distant past. Disturbances of arousal and attention are produced by acute confusional states and frontal lobe disorders. *Amnesia* refers to a specific defect in new learning and occurs with lesions in the medial hemispheric hippocampal–fornix–mamillary body–thalamus circuit. Abnormalities in the recollection of remote information occur in dementia syndromes with relatively widespread cerebral cortical involvement. *Forgetfulness* is a cardinal feature of subcortical dementing disorders (Chapter 8) and indicates a disturbance in the spontaneous recall of stored information. *Confabulation* is closely related to amnesia and indicates the production of incorrect answers in response to questions regarding unremembered information. *Paramnesias* are systematic distortions of memory that typically occur during the recovery phase of amnesic syndromes. Each of these memory-related disturbances is presented in more detail in this chapter. Recurrent episodic disturbances of memory are considered in Chapter 9 with the epilepsies and in Chapter 10 with the dissociative states and fugues.

AMNESIA

Amnesia refers to a specific clinical condition in which there is an impairment in the ability to learn new information despite normal attention, preserved ability to recall remote information, and intact cognitive functions (Benson, 1978). The amnestic patient has a nor-

mal or even supernormal digit span, indicating intact attention and immediate memory, and has normal linguistic and cognitive functions, including language comprehension, naming, reading, writing, calculating, drawing, and abstracting but is unable to learn such new information as the current day, month, or year or the current geographic location. The patient cannot recall 3 words after 3 minutes or reproduce constructions after a brief delay and may not be aided by memory clues and prompting. In addition to the difficulty with new learning (anterograde amnesia), the patient often has a period of from a few minutes to a few years of retrograde amnesia for which remote recall is also impaired. If recent memory recovers, the retrograde amnesia may progressively shrink to some finite period prior to the amnesia-inciting event, and the patient will be left with a period of permanent memory loss that extends from the beginning of the retrograde amnesia to the end of the anterograde amnesia (Benson and Geschwind, 1967). Table 4-1 lists the principal causes of amnesia and presents distinguishing findings commonly associated with each amnestic syndrome (Benson, 1978; Symonds, 1966).

Clinical Syndromes with Amnesia

The Wernicke–Korsakoff Syndrome

The Wernicke–Korsakoff syndrome was one of the earliest recognized amnestic syndromes and continues to be among the most common causes of isolated recent memory impairment. Wernicke described the acute phase of the illness characterized classically by ophthalmoplegia, ataxia, and confusion and included it in his three-volume handbook published in 1881–1883 (Brody and Wilkins, 1968). Korsakoff, a Russian neuropsychiatrist, called attention to the chronic amnestic phase of the illness and to the frequent coexistence of peripheral neuropathy (Victor and Yakovlev, 1955). Consequently, in contemporary usage, *Wernicke's en-*

TABLE 4-1. Distinguishing Clinical Features Associated with Each of the Principal Causes of Amnesia

Wernicke–Korsakoff syndrome	Nystagmus, ataxia, peripheral neuropathy
Temporal lobectomy	Superior quadrantansopia (contralateral to lobectomy)
Head trauma	Frontal lobe dysfunction
Hippocampal infarction (posterior cerebral artery occlusion)	Homonymous hemianopsia or cortical blindness
Anoxia	History of acute cardiopulmonary arrest
Herpes simplex encephalitis	Klüver-Bucy syndrome, aphasia, seizures
Neoplasms	Homonymous hemianopsia, hemiparesis, headache
Basal frontal lesions (rupture of anterior communicating artery aneurysm)	Personality alterations, diabetes insipidus, hypothermia
Electroconvulsive therapy	Depression with recent ECT
Transient global amnesia	Vascular etiology most common; there may be associated evidence of cerebrovascular disease
Hypoglycemia	Insulin overdose
Psychogenic amnesia	Personal identity lost; may be amnesic for specific personal information

cephalopathy denotes the acute changes such as ataxia, neuroophthalmic abnormalities, autonomic disturbances, and confusional state, whereas *Korsakoff's syndrome* refers to the more enduring memory deficit. A personality change, usually placidity or apathy, frequently accompanies the amnesia. The Wernicke–Korsakoff syndrome results from chronic thiamine deficiency and is characterized pathologically by hyperplasia of the small vessels with occasional hemorrhages, hypertrophy of the astrocytes, and mild axonal and neuronal changes (Cravioto et al., 1961; Liss, 1958; Malamud and Skillicorn, 1956; Rosenblum and Feigin, 1965; Victor et al., 1971). These pathological alterations are distributed preferentially in the periventricular regions surrounding the third and fourth ventricles and the Sylvian aqueduct. Involvement of the thalamus and mammillary bodies accounts for the amnesia, whereas changes near the aqueduct and floor of the fourth ventricle account for the ophthalmoplegia, vestibular ataxia, and autonomic symptoms, respectively (Birchfeld, 1964; Victor et al., 1971; Vogel and Lee, 1967).

Korsakoff syndrome patients have difficulty learning new information and usually have a retrograde amnesia that extends backward 3–20 years prior to the onset of the amnesia (Albert et al., 1979; Butters and Cermak, 1980; Seltzer and Benson, 1974). Typically, patients remain amnestic for 1–3 months after onset and then begin to recover over a 1–10-month period. Of these patients, 25 percent recover completely, 50 percent show slight to moderate improvement, and 25 percent have no demonstratable recovery (Victor et al., 1971). Confabulation is common during the early phases of the Korsakoff syndrome but is unusual in the chronic phase of the condition. In some cases, administration

of thiamine during the acute Wernicke phase prevents emergence of the chronic amnestic syndrome. Once established, however, thiamine has little effect on the memory defect except to prevent further deterioration.

Chronic nutritional deprivation associated with alcoholism is the most common cause of the thiamine deficiency producing Korsakoff syndrome, but other causes of thiamine deficiency may also cause the disorder. One of Korsakoff's original patients developed the syndrome from pyloric stenosis associated with intentional sulfuric acid ingestion, and other cases have been attributed to gastric carcinoma, hemodialysis, hyperemesis gravidarum, prolonged intravenous (IV) hyperalimentation, gastric plication, and dietary deprivation in prisoner of war (POW) camps (Brody and Wilkins, 1968; Cummings and Benson, 1983; de Wardener and Lennox, 1947, Haid et al., 1982). Preliminary observations suggest that an inherited abnormality of transketolase activity may render some patients vulnerable to the development of the Wernicke–Korsakoff syndrome under conditions where dietary thiamine is inadequate (Blass and Gibson, 1977).

Alcoholic Korsakoff syndrome must be distinguished from alcoholic dementia where deficits involve attention, word-list generation, abstraction, and constructions as well as recent memory (Cummings and Benson, 1983; Cutting, 1978).

Temporal Lobectomy, Fornicotomy, and Related Surgeries

The search for an anatomy of memory was greatly stimulated when, in 1954, Scoville removed both temporal lobes of a patient with intractible seizures and produced a profound and lasting amnesia (Scoville and Milner, 1957). The epileptic patient, H.M., has become one of the most thoroughly studied cases in neuropsychology, and the results of extensive testing carried out on the patient have contributed significantly to understanding the role of temporal lobe structures in memory (Milner et al., 1968). Amnesia complicates temporal lobectomy when the hippocampal formations are removed bilaterally or when one hippocampus is removed and the other is dysfunctional (Penfield and Mathieson, 1974; Penfield and Milner, 1958; Scoville and Milner, 1957). When one hippocampus is removed and the other is normal, the functioning member can compensate to a large extent for the missing structures, and the resulting deficits are relatively mild. In such cases the identifiable memory impairments are specific for the side of the lesion: left temporal lobectomy impairs learning and retention of verbal material, whereas right temporal lobe removal produces deficits in the recognition and recall of visual and auditory patterns that are not verbally coded (places, faces, melodies, nonsense patterns) (Milner, 1968, 1971).

In addition to temporal lobectomy, several other surgical procedures have resulted in amnestic syndromes. Bilateral sectioning of the fornix has produced deficits in recent memory in several reported cases (Heilman and Sypert, 1977; Sweet et al., 1959). [In some patients with sectioned fornices, no memory deficit was noted, but systematic testing was not performed and pathological verification of the extent of fornix interruption was not available (Bengochea et al., 1954; Umbach, 1966).] Surgical injury to the mamillary bodies at the time of removal of pituitary tumors has also produced amnesia (Kahn and Crosby, 1972), and a transient Korsakoff-like syndrome affecting primarily orientation in time and learning of temporal sequences has been observed in the postcingulumotomy state (Whitty and Lewin, 1960).

Posttraumatic Amnesia

Traumatic brain injuries are undoubtedly the most common cause of amnesia syndromes seen in clinical practice. The position of the temporal lobe in the middle cranial fossa, suspended between the petrous pyramid inferiorly and the greater wing of the sphenoid anteriorly and medially, renders them vulnerable to contusions with both coup and contrecoup injuries (Courville, 1950; Lindenberg and Freytag, 1960). The amnesia induced by head injury includes a period of retrograde memory loss extending for a few minutes to a few years prior to the injury, a variable period of unconsciousness caused by the injury, and a period of anterograde amnesia that lasts for a few hours to a few months or longer following recovery from coma (Levin et al.,

1982). In cases with resolution of the anterograde amnesia, there is often a concomitant shrinking of the period of retrograde amnesia to within a few minutes or hours of the trauma (Benson and Geschwind, 1967). The duration of the posttraumatic amnesia is a good index of the severity of head trauma with the incidence of motor disturbances, language changes, and cognitive deficits increasing with the length of amnesia (Russell, 1971; Russell and Smith, 1961; von Wowern, 1966).

Hippocampal Infarction

The hippocampus receives its blood supply from penetrating branches of the posterior cerebral artery, and occlusion of the basilar artery or proximal portions of both posterior cerebral arteries with bilateral hippocampal infarction will produce an amnestic syndrome (Benson et al., 1974; Muller and Shaw, 1965). The infarction is rarely limited to the hippocampal formation, and extension of the injury to include other occipital structures results in the frequent occurrence of visual field defects, prosopagnosia, central achromatopsia, alexia without agraphia, hemiparesis, or hemisensory loss with the amnesia (Benson et al., 1974; DeJong et al., 1969; Victor et al., 1961; Woods et al., 1982). Although most cases of amnesia secondary to hippocampal infarction have had bilateral lesions, a few cases appear to have undergone damage limited to the hippocampal formation of the left hemisphere, suggesting that a unilateral infarction of the language-dominant hemisphere can produce at least transient amnesia (Benson et al., 1974; Mohr et al., 1971). Occlusion of the posterior cerebral artery may be produced by embolism, thrombosis, or compression against the tentorium by an expanding hemispheric lesion (Lindenberg, 1955).

Anoxia and Hypoglycemia

The widespread application of emergency cardiopulmonary resuscitation procedures has resulted in the emergence of a population of patients who have had profound but short-lived episodes of cerebral anoxia. Under such circumstances only those areas of the brain that are most vulnerable to acute lack of oxygen become symptomatic, and in many cases it is the hippocampus that sustains the greatest injury (Cummings et al., 1984; McNeil et al., 1965; Turner, 1950; Volpe and Hirst, 1983a). The resulting clinical syndrome is a profound amnesia with preserved performance in other realms of intellectual activity. The amnesia is often permanent, but a few cases have shown gradual resolution over a period of months to nearly normal levels of function. In addition to its occurrence following cardiopulmonary arrest, postanoxic amnesia has occurred following anesthetic accidents, carbon monoxide intoxication, and strangulation due to hanging (Allison, 1961; Berlyne and Strachan, 1968; Brierly and Cooper, 1962; Muramoto et al., 1979). When the period of oxygen deprivation is more prolonged, widespread damage is incurred, and a post anoxic dementia ensues if the patient survives (Cummings and Benson, 1983).

Acute hypoglycemia, like acute anoxia, has its greatest impact on hippocampal function, and subacute or chronic recurrent hypoglycemia often produces a memory disturbance. In many cases, however, other intellectual functions are also impaired and a dementia syndrome results (Lishman, 1978; Pallis and Lewis, 1974).

Herpes Simplex Encephalitis

Herpes encephalitis is the most common severe nonepidemic encephalitis and is unique in its tendency to preferentially involve orbitofrontal and medial temporal areas of the brain (Johnson, 1982; Lishman, 1978). The virus apparently gains access to the brain by way of the olfactory nerves or through trigeminal nerves innervating the meninges of the anterior and middle cranial fossa. After entering the inferior frontal and medial temporal lobes, further spread of the virus is limited by immunologic control (Davis and Johnson, 1979; Johnson, 1982). Once in the brain, the virus initiates a destructive hemorrhagic process that may prove fatal. Among survivors, the most common neuropsychological deficit is a profound amnesia. The deficit in learning new information may be accompanied by other evidence of temporal lobe dysfunction, including aphasia, partial complex seizures, or the Klüver-Bucy syndrome (Drachman and Adams, 1962; Gascon and Gilles, 1973; Lilly et al., 1983; Marlowe et al., 1975; Rose and Symonds, 1960). Compared with patients with thiamine deficiency–induced Korsakoff syndrome, individuals rendered amnestic from herpes encephalitis appear to exhibit less confabulation, are more aware of their memory deficits, profit less from cues, and are more adept at learning logically ordered spatial arrangements and sequentially presented material (Walsh, 1978).

Neoplasms

Neoplasms producing amnestic syndromes fall into two general categories: extracerebral tumors such as craniopharyngiomas that produce pressure on the base of the brain, and intracerebral tumors, particularly gliomas, that involve structures in the wall and floor of the third ventricle (Kahn and Crosby, 1972; McEntee et al., 1976; Williams and Pennybacker, 1954; Ziegler et al., 1977). The extracerebral compressive lesions exert upward pressure on the mamillary bodies and adjacent tracts, and the gliomas invade the nuclei of the thalamus and hypothalamic structures to produce the disruption of memory function.

Basal Frontal Lesions

Amnesia is not commonly associated with frontal lobe lesions. In most cases where memory disturbances are prominent, the patient is markedly distractible, and learning impairment is a product of impaired attention (Stuss and Benson, 1984). Occasionally, however, a true amnesia is observed following frontal lobe injuries. In nearly all cases, the amnesia has been associated with rupture and/or surgical repair of an anterior communicating artery aneurysm located medially in the basal forebrain region (Gade, 1982; Lindqvist and Norlen, 1966; Talland et al., 1967; Volpe and Hirst, 1983b). In the acute phase, the patients are confused and tend to deny all deficits; as the confusion resolves they are left with amnesia and mild personality changes including disinhibition and excessive jocularity (Alexander and Freedman, 1984). Unilateral grasp reflexes, hemipareses, diabetes insipidus, and hypothermia may coexist with the amnesia.

The pathological anatomy of the lesion responsible for the amnesia has not been fully determined. Penetrating branches from the anterior communicating artery supply the anterior hypothalamus, septal nucleus, lamina terminalis, portions of the head of the caudate nucleus, columns of the fornix, ventromedial corpus callosum, and anterior cingulate gyrus (Alexander and Freedman, 1984; Taren, 1965). Some of these structures (e.g., the columns of the fornix) are known to play a major role in anatomical circuits mediating memory functions, and the other structures may make as yet undetermined contributions to the process of learning new information.

Electroconvulsive Therapy

Electroconvulsive therapy (ECT) produces both a retrograde amnesia for items learned a few minutes prior to the treatment and an anterograde amnesia for information introduced immediately after the treatment. The anterograde amnesia usually subsides within 4–6 hours of the most recent treatment, but mild memory deficits may persist for several weeks following termination of a full course of therapy (6–12 treatments) (Task Force Report 14, 1978; Williams, 1977). Long-term follow-up studies show no objective evidence of memory impairment 6–9 months following a standard course of ECT (Squire and Chace, 1975). Use of bilateral electrodes induces impairment of both verbal and nonverbal learning; right unilateral ECT produces less memory disruption and preferentially affects nonverbal material (Task

TABLE 4-2.   Etiologies of Transient Global Amnesia

Seizures

Migraine

Drug intoxication (diazepam)

Hypoglycemia

Cerebrovascular disease

   Vertebrobasilar insufficiency
   Embolism (vertebrobasilar circulation)
   Vertebral angiography
   Circulatory disturbances in specific circumstances

      Highly emotional situations
      Sexual intercourse
      Abrupt temperature variations
      Pain

Neoplasms (left hemisphere)

Force Report 14, 1978). The pathopysiology of the amnesia induced by ECT is unknown. The discharge is most likely mediated by nonspecific reticulothalamocortical circuits and may have a preferential affect on limbic mechanism rendered vulnerable by their low seizure threshold (Volavka, 1972).

Transient Global Amnesia

Transient global amnesia (TGA) refers to a distinct clinical syndrome consisting of an acute transient period of amnesia. The amnesia consists of an ongoing anterograde amnesia that usually persists for several hours and a retrograde amnesia of a few weeks' duration. As the anterograde learning deficit subsides, the retrograde amnesia shrinks to within a few minutes of the onset of the episode. During the amnestic period the patients usually recall their own identities and recognize familiar people but cannot remember recent occurrences or current circumstances and do not remember what they are told. Frequent repetition of the same question is one of the hallmarks of the syndrome and is the behavior that usually leads to recognition by family members or friends that something is wrong. The patients appear bewildered and recognize that a problem exists. No other neurological deficit or behavioral disturbances are present during the attack (Evans, 1968; Heathfield et al., 1973; Shuping et al., 1980a; Shuttleworth and Morris, 1966; Steinmetz and Vroom, 1972; Whitty, 1977). Most patients have a single attack of TGA and suffer no further amnestic episodes, but a few, particularly those with underlying cerebrovascular disease, have repeated attacks and eventually have infarctions in the vertebrobasilar or posterior cerebral arterial territories (Matthew and Meyer, 1974). In some cases specific circumstances such as intense emotional excitement, pain, sexual intercourse, or abrupt variations in temperature

may acutely alter circulation and precipitate TGA in vulnerable individuals (Fisher, 1982a; Mayeux, 1979). In addition to cerebrovascular disease, a variety of other causes of TGA have been reported, including migraine, valium overdose, seizures, and tumors (Table 4-2) (Caplan et al., 1981; Cochran et al., 1982; Crowell et al., 1984; Damasio et al., 1983; Fisher, 1982a; Gilbert and Benson, 1972; Lisak and Zimmerman, 1977; Longridge et al., 1974; Mayeux, 1979; Shuping et al., 1980b; Shuttleworth and Wise, 1973).

Cerebral blood flow studies of patients with transient global amnesia reveal diminished blood flow in the posterior hemispheric or inferior temporal regions (Crowell et al., 1984).

Psychogenic Amnesia

There are several types of psychogenic memory disturbances, including psychogenic amnesia, fugue states, and multiple personality. The latter two entities entail the partial or total assumption of different identities for a finite period (usually days to weeks) that the patient has difficulty recalling later (*Diagnostic and statistical manual of mental disorders*, 1980). The patients do not appear amnestic in the sense of having an inability to learn new information. Fugues and multiple personality are considered in Chapter 10.

Psychogenic amnesia or psychogenic loss of personal identity can, however, be confused with amnesias associated with dysfunction of medial limbic structures. Psychogenic amnesia is an hysterical conversion symptom in which patients suddenly forget their personal identities and life situations. They may not recall their names, addresses, families, or any other personal information. In some cases there is a selective loss of specific emotionally charged information such as whether one is married or the identity and whereabouts of one's parents. In other cases there is a failure to recall all past information. The amnesia is usually of short duration (24–48 hours) and either stops spontaneously or is terminated by hypnosis, suggestion, or an amobarbital (®Amytal) interview. Unlike other types of conversion reaction, there is an equal preponderance of men and women among patients exhibiting psychogenic amnesia. The causes of psychogenic amnesia are variable. The most common underlying condition is depression, usually punctuated by a recent severe psychological stress. There also appears to be a high incidence of malingering, particularly among "absconding treasurers, reluctant bridegrooms, and other criminals and wrongdoers seeking to evade the consequences of their actions" (Kennedy and Neville, 1957). Schizophrenics and manics occasionally exhibit psychogenic amnesia, and, like other conversion symptoms, there is a high incidence of CNS disorders among patients with psy-

TABLE 4-3.   Characteristics that Distinguish Psychogenic Amnesia from Transient Global Amnesia

Psychogenic Amnesia	Transient Global Amnesia
Personal identity lost	Personal identity retained
Ability to learn new information preserved	Inability to learn new information
Memory loss may be selective for specific personal information	Amnesia not selective
Temporal gradient absent	Temporal gradient present
Depression common	Depression infrequent
Indifference to amnesia	Distress caused by amnesia
Most common in younger patients (2nd–4th decades)	More common in older patients (6th–7th decades)

chogenic amnesia. Several authors have noted a high prevalence of headache and other somatic complaints among the patients (Abeles and Schilder, 1935; Croft et al., 1973; Kanzer, 1939; Kennedy and Neville, 1957; Kiersch, 1962; Merskey, 1979; Wilson et al., 1950).

Psychogenic amnesia is most likely to be confused with TGA, but there are several characteristics that aid in the differentiation of psychogenic amnesia from TGA and from other types of amnesia associated with hippocampal, hypothalamic, or thalamic dysfunction (Table 4-3). Transient global amnesia almost never entails a loss of personal identity, whereas it is one of the hallmarks of psychogenic amnesia. By definition, patients with TGA have difficulty learning and retaining new information, whereas patients with psychogenic amnesia may be able to learn many details about their current situation at a time that they cannot recall information concerning their remote histories. The pattern of memory loss in TGA patients includes a temporal gradient with relative preservation of remote memory beyond the period of retrograde amnesia; patients with psychogenic amnesia do not exhibit a temporal gradient, and memory loss may be highly specific for selected personal information. Depression is common among patients with psychogenic amnesia, and they are usually indifferent to their memory losses, whereas TGA patients show no preponderance of any associated psychopathology and are frequently distressed by their memory deficits. Psychogenic amnesia patients are usually in their teens, twenties, or thirties, whereas TGA is most common in patients in their sixth or seventh decade with underlying vascular disease.

Differential Diagnosis of Amnesia

Amnesias must be distinguished from a variety of other types of memory disturbance (Table 4-4). For clinical purposes, memory disturbances can conveniently be divided into those that are short-lived (usually less than 24–48 hours), those that are either more prolonged or are stable (lasting for more than 48 hours), and those that are progressive.

Transient, short-duration episodes of memory loss include psychogenic amnesia, some cases of posttraumatic amnesia, and transient global amnesia. These must be distinguished from other brief interruptions of consciousness with memory lapses, including complex partial seizures, alcoholic blackout spells, migraine, and toxic–metabolic confusional states. Seizures as a cause of memory lapses should be considered in individuals with a history of head trauma or other predisposing circumstances, a known history of epilepsy, or other symptoms suggestive of an epileptic ictus such as an aura, incontinence, or postictal confusion. Most seizure-related

TABLE 4-4.   Differential Diagnosis of Memory Disturbances

Transient episodes of memory loss (< 48 hours)

  Amnesias (nonmemory functions intact)

    Transient global amnesia
    Psychogenic amnesia
    Posttraumatic amnesia

  Memory Lapses with altered attention, cognition

    Seizures
    Alcoholic blackouts
    Migraine
    Toxic–metabolic confusional states

Prolonged periods of memory loss syndromes (> 48 hours)

  Amnestic syndromes (Table 4-1)

  Dissociative States

    Fugues
    Multiple personality

Progressive memory dysfunction

  Forgetfulness (subcortical dementias)

  Recent and remote memory loss (cortical dementias)

episodes are short-lived, lasting for only minutes, but automatic behavior may occasionally persist for hours or even several days. Integrated, purposeful behavior is rare during seizures (Andermann and Robb, 1972; Escueta et al., 1974; Geier, 1978; Goldensohn and Gold, 1960; Lennox, 1943; Saper and Lossing, 1974). Automatic behavior during alcoholic blackouts occurs in patients with chronic alcoholism who have neglected eating, are fatigued, or rapidly ingest a large quantity of alcohol (Goodwin et al., 1969). Migraine as a cause of confusional states with memory lapses is usually accompanied by other migrainous symptoms such as photophobia, visual hallucinations, nausea, and headache, although the latter need not be prominent (Moersch, 1924; Selby and Lance, 1960). Toxic and metabolic encephalopathies, particularly those associated with drug ingestion and transient hypoglycemia, must also be considered in the differential diagnosis of transient memory alterations.

Memory disturbances lasting for more prolonged periods include the amnesia syndromes discussed earlier (Table 4-1) and the more long lasting dissociative states, including fugues and multiple personality. The latter are not amnesias as defined here in that there is no disturbance of recent memory. Rather, on recovering from the dissociative state, the patient is unable to recall all or most of the events transpiring during the dissociated period.

Progressive memory dysfunction occurs in the dementias where two principal types of memory impairment are described: forgetfulness occurring in the subcortical dementias and combined impairment of recent and remote memory in the cortical dementias. Forgetfulness or forgetting to remember describes the type of memory impairment associated with extrapyramidal syndromes, multiple subcortical infarctions, depression, and chronic confusional states. The patient is able to learn and store new information as demonstrated by the ability to recall the material when given cues. Spontaneous access to the information, however, is diminished and the patient is unable to retrieve and utilize learned material without substantial prompting. Forgetfulness is a normal occurrence and becomes more prominent during the aging process, but it is exaggerated to a pathological extent in dementing disorders affecting subcortical structures (Chapter 8) (Benson, 1978; Cummings and Benson, 1983; Hécaen and Albert, 1978).

Dementing processes affecting the hippocampus and cerebral cortex produce a profound memory disturbance consisting of an inability to learn new information and impairments in the retrieval of remote material. In the early stages of Alzheimer's disease, recent memory may be preferentially affected and the syndrome resembles an amnesia. As the disease progresses, aphasia, visuospatial disturbances, and impairment of remote memory evolve to complete the picture of a chronic progressive dementing disorder. Pick's disease, the other principal cortical dementia, tends to spare memory function early in its clinical course, but both new learning and remote recall are impaired in the later stages (Cummings, 1982; Cummings and Benson, 1983).

Neuroanatomy and Neurochemistry of Amnesia

The location of the lesions capable of producing amnestic syndromes are all concentrated within a single cohesive medial limbic circuit that has come to be regarded as the anatomic basis of new learning and recent memory (Fig. 4-1) (Barbizet, 1963; Benson, 1978). This system originates in the hippocampal formations that are located on the medial surface of each temporal lobe. The hippocampi receive their major input from parahippocampal temporal lobe neurons (entorhinal cortex), which, in turn, receive projections from widespread cortical regions, particularly association areas of the parietal and frontal cortex. Axons of efferent neurons of each hippocampus converge to form the fimbria, an enlarging tract of fibers located on medial surface of the hippocampus. The fimbria becomes the fornix when the tract leaves the hippocampus and curves superiorly beneath the corpus callosum. The fornices converge soon after exiting from the hippocampi and exchange fibers in a commissure known as the *psalterium*. The fornix then continues anteriorly to the anterior commissure, where it splits into a precommissural portion destined for the septal area and a postcommissural portion bound for the mamillary bodies. Neurons from the mamillary bodies then project through the mamillothalamic tracts (Vicq d'Azyr's tracts) to the anterior nucleus of the thalamus (Isaacson, 1974; Truex and Carpenter, 1969). Interruption of this circuit anywhere between the hippocampus and the thalamus will produce an amnestic syndrome. Head trauma, anoxia, herpes encephalitis, and posterior cerebral artery occlusion disrupt the circuit at the level of the hippocampi; the Wernicke–Korsakoff syndrome produces lesions of the mamillary bodies and medial thalamic nuclei; neoplasms produce amnesia by invading the hypothalamus (mamillary bodies) or thalamus; and surgical amnesias have resulted from bilateral temporal lobectomy and sectioning of the fornices. Horel (1978), in a challenge to the role of the hippocampus in new memory, suggested that lesions involving the hippocampus also involve the temporal stem (a large band of fibers connecting the temporal lobe with the thalamus) and that the stem lesions were responsible for the amnesia. Experimental evidence in nonhuman primates with limited hippocampal excisions and

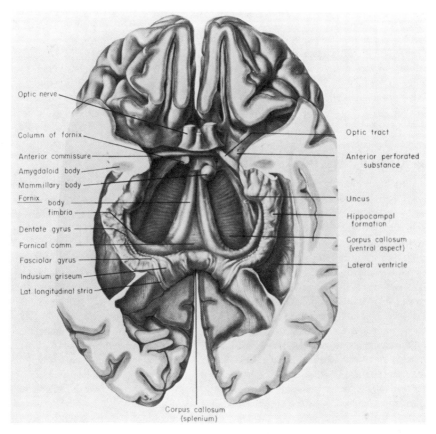

Optic nerve

Column of fornix

Anterior commissure

Amygdaloid body

Mammillary body

Fornix body
      fimbria

Dentate gyrus

Fornical comm

Fasciolar gyrus

Indusium griseum

Lat. longitudinal stria

Optic tract

Anterior perforated
substance

Uncus

Hippocampal
formation

Corpus callosum
(ventral aspect)

Lateral ventricle

Corpus callosum
(splenium)

Figure 4-1. Drawing of the inferior aspect of the brain showing structures of the medial limbic-memory circuit, including the hippocampus, fornix, and mamillary bodies. Reproduced from Truex RC and Carpenter MB., *Human neuroanatomy,* 6th ed. Baltimore, Williams & Wilkins Company, 1969, Figure 21-7. Copyright 1969, The Williams & Wilkins Company, Baltimore. With permission of the publisher and author.

clinical evidence from anoxic lesions confined to the hippocampus and sparing the temporal stem indicate, however, that amnesia does occur with isolated hippocampal lesions (Cummings et al., 1984; Zola-Morgan et al., 1982).

Lateralization and hemispheric specialization effects are evident with both hippocampal and thalamic lesions: left-sided lesions preferentially disrupt verbal learning and recall, and right-sided lesions have a greater effect on nonverbal memory functions (Milner, 1971; Ojemann et al., 1971; Speedie and Heilman, 1983).

The occurrence of a retrograde amnesia with most amnestic syndromes suggests that the medial limbic circuit is involved in some aspects of retrieval of remote information, but the existence of a temporal gradient and preservation of some remote material indicates that remote memory is at least partially independent of these structures. The neuroanatomic basis of remote memory has not been determined.

Neurochemical investigations of memory and learning processes have concentrated on the role of acetylcholine and have demonstrated a significant association between integrity of the cholinergic system and the ability to perform on tests of recent memory. Scopolamine, a cholinergic blocking agent, produces deficits in recent memory without impairing attention. Physostigmine, an anticholinesterase agent, reverses the scopolamine effects (Drachman, 1978; Drachman and Leavitt, 1974). Modest improvement in posttraumatic and postencephalitic amnesias has been achieved by increasing the availability of synaptic acetylcholine (Goldberg et al., 1982; Peters and Levin, 1977). A role for adrenergic mechanisms in recent memory has been suggested by the small but measurable beneficial effects of clonidine, an alpha-adrenergic agonist, on memory function of patients with the Wernicke–Korsakoff syndrome (McEntee and Mair, 1980), and by the discovery of the low levels of CSF monoamine metabolites of Korsakoff patients (McEntee et al., 1984). Despite those advances in understanding the neurochemical basis of recent memory and small gains in the treatment of amnesia, most improvement in the amnestic syndromes results from spontaneous recovery following the initial insult, and no compelling pharmacotherapy is yet available.

REDUPLICATIVE PARAMNESIA

Reduplicative paramnesia or *double orientation* refers to a peculiar disorientation syndrome in which the patient claims to be present simultaneously in two locations. One of the locations is usually correct, whereas the other is typically in the vicinity of the patient's home or even a room inside the home. For example, a patient reported by Benson et al. (1976) and hospitalized in the Boston Veterans Hospital maintained that the hospital was located in Great Falls, Montana (his home). The reduplicative paramnesia may take the form of believing that the location has two names, that the two locations are contiguous, or that the patient has recently made a journey from one to the other (Paterson and Zangwill, 1944). Reduplicative paramnesia most commonly occurs during the recovery phase of posttraumatic encephalopathy, but it has been observed in patients with tumors, infarctions, and arteriovenous malformations as well as in metabolic and toxic encephalopathies (Benson et al., 1976; Fisher, 1982b; Levin, 1956; Paterson and Zangwill, 1944; Ruff and Volpe, 1981). In most cases with focal lesions, there has been damage to the right hemisphere and to both frontal lobes. A possible explanation for the unique phenomenon is that the right hemispheric lesion makes it difficult for patients to integrate spatially significant information whereas concomitant frontal lobe dysfunction or the confusional state impairs patients' abilities to appreciate and correct the discrepancy in their beliefs (Benson et al., 1976; Ruff and Volpe, 1981).

Alexander et al. (1979) have suggested that the Capgras syndrome, the delusional belief that people have been replaced by identical-appearing imposters, shares many features with reduplicative paramnesia, including the combination of right hemispheric and frontal dysfunction, and might be regarded as a similar paramnestic syndrome. The Capgras syndrome is presented more thoroughly in Chapter 13.

REFERENCES

Ables M and Schilder P. Psychogenic loss of personal identity. *Arch Neurol Psychiat*, 1935, *34*, 587–604.
Albert MS, Butters N, and Levin T. Temporal gradients in

CONFABULATION

Confabulation refers to the production of erroneous answers by patients with memory defects and represents a failure of self-monitoring rather than a desire to deliberately mislead (Stuss et al., 1978; Talland, 1961). Two basic forms of confabulation have been distinguished: (1) confabulation of embarrassment, in which the amnestic patient provides incorrect answers based on personal past experience, and (2) fantastic confabulation, in which patients with impaired judgment and current or recent amnesia spontaneously describe impossible, adventurous, and often gruesome experiences (Berlyne, 1972; Stuss et al., 1978; Talland, 1961). Confabulation of embarrassment typically occurs in the active stages of the Wernicke–Korsakoff syndrome. Patients respond to questions regarding the date, location, and their employment with answers derived from their pasts. The answers are usually coherent or possible, but incorrect. If the syndrome enters its more chronic phases, confabulation diminishes and may ultimately disappear altogether. Studies of confabulation demonstrate that it represents a failure of self-monitoring and self-criticism and most likely reflects frontal lobe dysfunction (Mercer et al., 1977; Shapiro et al., 1981). Confabulation frequently coexists with other evidence of a frontal lobe disturbance such as perseveration and apathy. Confabulation of embarrassment may occur in other amnestic states and in degenerative dementias as well as in the Korsakoff syndrome, but appears to be most common in patients with lesions in the mamillary bodies or thalamus (Parkin, 1984).

Fantastic confabulation is a more rare and more colorful syndrome. One of the present author's patients described how he had been taken into a spaceship by extraterrestrial visitors and taught how to drive their ship, and on another occasion he told how he had single-handedly decapitated 39 enemy soldiers as they were lined up shooting from behind a log. Most patients with fantastic confabulation have obvious frontal lobe syndromes, but their amnesias may be mild (Berlyne, 1972; Stuss et al., 1978). The syndrome has been observed in posttraumatic encephalopathy, the Wernicke–Korsakoff syndrome, and degenerative dementias.

Confabulation must be distinguished from prevarication, where the patient attempts to deliberately mislead the examiner and from delusions where the false responses are stable and represent unusual beliefs held by the patient.

the retrograde amnesia of patients with alcoholic Korsakoff's disease. *Arch Neurol*, 1979, *36*, 211–216.
Alexander MP and Freedman M. Amnesia after anterior com-

municating artery aneurysm rupture. *Neurology,* 1984, *34,* 752–757.

Alexander MP, Stuss DT, and Benson DF. Capgras syndrome: a reduplicative phenomenon. *Neurology,* 1979, *29,* 334–339.

Allison RS. Chronic amnesic syndromes in the elderly. *Proc Roy Soc Med,* 1961, *54,* 961–965.

Andermann F and Robb JP. Absence status. A reappraisal following review of thirty-eight patients. *Epilepsia,* 1972, *13,* 177–187.

Barbizet J. Defect of memorizing of hippocampal-mammillary origin: a review. *J Neurol Neurosurg Psychiat,* 1963, *26,* 127–135.

Bengochea FG, de la Torre O, Esquivel O, Vieta R, and Fernandez C. The section of the fornix in the surgical treatment of certain epilepsies. *Trans Am Neurol Assoc,* 1954, *79,* 176–178.

Benson DF. Amnesia. *South Med J,* 1978, *71,* 1221–1228.

Benson DF, Gardner H, and Meadows JC. Reduplicative paramnesia. *Neurology,* 1976, *26,* 147–151.

Benson DF and Geschwind N. Shrinking retrograde amnesia. *J Neurol Neurosurg Psychiat,* 1967, *30,* 539–544.

Benson DF, Marsden CD, and Meadows JC. The amnesic syndrome of posterior cerebral artery occlusion. *Acta Neurol Scand,* 1974, *50,* 133–145.

Berlyne N. Confabulation. *Br J Psychiat,* 1972, *120,* 31–39.

Berlyne N and Strachan M. Neuropsychiatric sequelae of attempted hanging. *Br J Psychiat,* 1968, *114,* 411–422.

Birchfield RI. Postural hypotension in Wernicke's disease. *Am J Med,* 1964, *36,* 404–414.

Blass JP and Gibson GE. Abnormality of a thiamine-requiring enzyme in patients with Wernicke–Korsakoff syndrome. *New Engl J Med,* 1977, *297,* 1367–1370.

Brierly JB and Cooper JE. Cerebral complications of hypotensive anesthesia in a healthy adult. *J Neurol Neurosurg Psychiat,* 1962, *25,* 24–30.

Brody IA and Wilkins RH. Wernicke's encephalopathy. *Arch Neurol,* 1968, *19,* 228–232.

Butters N and Cermak LS. *Alcoholic Korsakoff's syndrome.* New York, Academic Press, 1980.

Caplan L, Chedru F, Lhermitte T, and Mayman C. Transient global amnesia and migraine. *Neurology,* 1981, *31,* 1167–1170.

Cochran JW, Morrell F, Hackman MS and Chochran EJ. Transient global amnesia after cerebral angiography. *Arch Neurol,* 1982, *39,* 593–594.

Courville CB. The mechanism of coup-contrecoup injuries of the brain. *Bull Los Angeles Neurol Soc,* 1950, *15,* 72–86.

Cravioto H, Korein J, and Silberman J. Wernicke's encephalopathy. *Arch Neurol,* 1961, *4,* 510–519.

Croft PB, Heathfield KWG, and Swash M. Differential diagnosis of transient amnesia. *Br Med J,* 1973, *4,* 593–596.

Crowell GF, Stump DA, Biller J, McHenry LC Jr, and Toole JF. The transient global amnesia–migraine connection. *Arch Neurol,* 1984, *41,* 75–79.

Cummings JL. Cortical dementias. In Benson DF and Blummer D (Eds.): *Psychiatric aspects of neurologic disease,* Vol. 2. New York, Grune & Stratton, 1982, pp. 93–120.

Cummings JL and Benson DF. *Demantia: a clinical approach.* Boston, Butterworths, 1983.

Cummings JL, Tomiyasu U, Reed S, and Benson DF. Amnesia with hippocampal lesions after cardiopulmonary arrest. *Neurology,* 1984, *34,* 679–681.

Cutting J. The relationship between Korsakov's syndrome and "alcoholic dementia." *Br J Psychiat,* 1978, *132,* 240–251.

Damasio AR, Graff-Radford NR, and Damasio H. Transient partial amnesia. *Arch Neurol,* 1983, *40,* 656–657.

Davis LE and Johnson RT. An explanation for the localization of herpes simplex encephalitis? *Ann Neurol,* 1979, *5,* 2–5.

DeJong RN, Itabashi HH, and Olson JR. Memory loss due to hippocampal lesions. *Arch Neurol,* 1969, *20,* 339–348.

de Wardener HE and Lennox B. Cerebral beriberi (Wernicke's encephalopathy). *Lancet,* 1947, *1,* 11–17.

Diagnostic and statistical manual of mental disorders, 3rd ed. American Psychiatric Association, Washington, D.C., 1980.

Drachman DA. Memory, dementia, and the cholinergic system. In Katzman R, Terry RD, and Bick KL (Eds.): *Alzheimer's disease: senile dementia and related disorders.* New York, Raven Press, 1978, pp. 141–148.

Drachman DA and Adams RD. Herpes simplex and acute inclusion-body encephalitis. *Arch Neurol,* 1962, *7,* 45–63.

Drachman DA and Leavitt J. Human memory and the cholinergic system. *Arch Neurol,* 1974, *30,* 113–121.

Escueta AV, Boxley J, Stubbs N, Waddell G, and Wilson WA. Prolonged twilight state and automatisms: a case report. *Neurology,* 1974, *24,* 331–339.

Evans JH. Transient loss of memory, an organic mental syndrome. *Brain,* 1968, *89,* 539–548.

Fisher CM. Transient global amnesia. Precipitating activities and other observations. *Arch Neurol,* 1982a, *39,* 605–608.

Fisher CM. Disorientation for place. *Arch Neurol,* 1982b, *30,* 33–36.

Gade A. Amnesia after operation on aneurysms of the anterior communicating artery. *Surg Neurol,* 1982, *18,* 46–49.

Gascon GG and Gilles F. Limbic dementia. *J Neurol Neurosurg Psychiat,* 1973, *36,* 421–430.

Geier S. Prolonged psychic epileptic seizures: a study of the absence status. *Epilepsia,* 1978, *19,* 431–445.

Gilbert JJ and Benson DF. Transient global amnesia: report of two cases with definite etiologies. *J Nerv Ment Dis,* 1972, *154,* 461–464.

Goldberg E, Gerstman LJ, Mattis S, Hughes JEO, Bilder RM Jr, and Sirio CA. Effects of cholinergic treatment of posttraumatic anterograde amnesia. *Arch Neurol,* 1982, *39,* 581.

Goldensohn ES and Gold AP. Prolonged behavioral disturbances as ictal phenomena. *Neurology,* 1960, *10,* 1–9.

Goodwin DW, Crane JB, and Guze SB. Alcoholic "blackouts": a review and clinical study of 100 alcoholics. *Am J Psychiat,* 1969, *126,* 191–198.

Haid RW, Gutmann L, and Crosby TW. Wernicke-Korsakoff encephalopathy after gastric plication. *JAMA,* 1982, *247,* 2566–2567.

Heathfield KWG, Croft PB and Swash M. The syndrome of transient global amnesia. *Brain,* 1973, *96,* 729–736.

Hécaen H and Albert ML. *Human neuropsychology*. New York, John Wiley & Sons, 1978.

Heilman KM and Sypert GW. Korsakoff's syndrome resulting from bilateral fornix lesions. *Neurology*, 1977, *27*, 490–493.

Horel JA. The neuroanatomy of amnesia. A critique of the hippocampal memory hypothesis. *Brain*, 1978, *101*, 403–445.

Isaacson RL. *The limbic system*. New York, Plenum Press, 1974.

Johnson RT. *Viral infections of the nervous system*. New York, Raven Press, 1982.

Kahn EA and Crosby EC. Korsakoff's syndrome associated with surgical lesions involving the mammillary bodies. *Neurology*, 1972, *22*, 117–125.

Kanzer M. Amnesia: a statistical study. *Am J Psychiat*, 1939, *96*, 711–716.

Kennedy A and Neville J. Sudden loss of memory. *Br Med J*, 1957, *2*, 428–433.

Kiersch TA. Amnesia: a clinical study of ninety-eight cases. *Am J Psychiat*, 1962, *116*, 57–60.

Lennox WC. Amnesia, real and feigned. *Am J Psychiat*, 1943, *99*, 732–743.

Levin HS, Benton AL, and Gassman RG. *Neurobehavioral consequences of closed head injury*. New York, Oxford University Press, 1982.

Levin M. Varieties of disorientation. *J Ment Sci*, 1956, *102*, 619–623.

Lilly R, Cummings JL, Benson DF, and Frankel M. The human Klüver-Bucy syndrome. *Neurology*, 1983, *33*, 1141–1145.

Lindenberg R. Compression of brain arteries as pathogenetic factor for tissue necroses and their areas of prediliction. *J Neuropath Exp Neurol*, 1955, *14*, 223–243.

Lindenberg R and Freytag E. The mechanisms of cerebral contusions. *Arch Pathol*, 1960, *69*, 440–469.

Lindqvist G and Norlen G. Korsakoff's syndrome after operation on ruptured aneurysm of the anterior communicating artery. *Acta Psychiat Scand*, 1966, *42*, 24–34.

Lisak RP and Zimmerman RA. Transient global amnesia due to a dominant hemisphere tumor. *Arch Neurol*, 1977, *34*, 317–318.

Lishman WR. *Organic psychiatry*. London, Blackwell Scientific Publications, 1978.

Liss L. Histopathology of the mammillary bodies in alcoholic psychosis. *Neurology*, 1958, *8*, 832–838.

Longridge NS, Hachinski V, and Barber HO. Brain stem dysfunction in transient global amnesia. *Stroke*, 1979, *10*, 473–474.

Malamud N and Skillicorn SA. Relationship between Wernicke and Korsakoff syndrome. *Arch Neurol Psychiat*, 1956, *76*, 585–596.

Marlowe WB, Mancall EL, and Thomas JJ. Complete Klüver-Bucy syndrome in man. *Cortex*, 1975, *11*, 53–59.

Mathew NT and Meyer JS. Pathogenesis and natural history of transient global amnesia. *Stroke*, 1974, *5*, 303–311.

Mayeux R. Sexual intercourse and transient global amnesia. *New Engl J Med*, 1979, *300*, 864.

McEntee WJ, Biber MP, Perl DP, and Benson DF. Diencephalic amnesia: a reappraisal. *J Neurol Neurosurg Psychiat*, 1976, *39*, 436–441.

McEntee WJ and Mair RG. Memory enhancement in Korsakoff's psychosis by clonidine: further evidence for a noradrenergic deficit. *Ann Neurol*, 1980, *7*, 466–470.

McEntee WJ, Mair RG, and Langlais PJ. Neurochemical pathology in Korsakoff's psychosis: implications for other cognitive disorders. *Neurology*, 1984, *34*, 648–652.

McNeill DL, Tidmarsh D, and Rastall ML. A case of dysmnesic syndrome following cardiac arrest. *Br J Psychiat*, 1965, *111*, 697–699.

Mercer B, Wapner W, Gardner H, and Benson DF. A study of confabulation. *Arch Neurol*, 1977, *34*, 429–433.

Merskey H. *The analysis of hysteria*. London, Bailliere Tindall, 1979.

Milner B. Visual recognition and recall after right temporal lobe excision in man. *Neuropsychologia*, 1968, *6*, 191–209.

Milner B. Interhemispheric differences in the localization of psychological processes in man. *Br Med Bull*, 1971, *27*, 272–277.

Milner B, Corkin S, and Teuber H-L. Further analysis of the hippocampal amnesic syndrome; 14 year follow-up study of H.M. *Neuropsychologia*, 1968, *6*, 215–234.

Moersch FP. Psychic manifestations in migraine. *Am J Psychiat*, 1924, *80*, 697–716.

Mohr JP, Leicester J, Stoddard LT, and Sidman M. Right hemianopia with memory and color deficits in circumscribed left posterior cerebral artery territory infarction. *Neurology*, 1971, *21*, 1104–1112.

Muller J and Shaw L. Arterial vascularization of the human hippocampus. *Arch Neurol*, 1965, *13*, 45–47.

Muramoto O, Kuru Y, Sugishita M, and Toyokura Y. Pure memory loss with hippocampal lesions. *Arch Neurol*, 1979, *36*, 54–56.

Ojemann GA, Blick KI, and Ward AA Jr. Improvement and disturbance of short-term verbal memory with human ventrolateral thalamic stimulation. *Brain*, 1971 *94*, 225–240.

Pallis CA and Lewis PD. *The neurology of gastrointestinal disease*. Philadelphia, WB Saunders Company, 1974.

Parkin AJ. Amnesic syndrome: a lesion-specific disorder? *Cortex*, 1984, *20*, 479–508.

Paterson A and Zangwill OL. Recovery of spatial orientation in the posttraumatic confusional state. *Brain*, 1944, *67*, 54–68.

Penfield W and Mathieson G. Memory. Autopsy findings and comments on the role of hippocampus in experiential recall. *Arch Neurol*, 1974, *31*, 145–154.

Penfield W and Milner B. Memory deficit produced by bilateral lesions in the hippocampal zone. *Arch Neurol Psychiat*, 1958, *79*, 475–497.

Peters BH and Levin HS. Memory enhancement after physostigmine treatment in the amnesic syndrome. *Arch Neurol*, 1977, *34*, 215–219.

Rose FC and Symonds CP. Persistent memory deficit following encephalitis. *Brain*, 1960, *83*, 195–212.

Rosenblum WI and Feigin I. The hemorrhagic component of

Wernicke's encephalopathy. *Arch Neurol*, 1965, *13*, 627–632.

Ruff RL and Volpe BT. Environmental reduplication associated with right frontal and parietal lobe injury. *J Neurol Neurosurg Psychiat*, 1981, *44*, 382–386.

Russell WR. *The traumatic amnesias*. London, Oxford University Press, 1971.

Russell WR and Smith A. Post-traumatic amnesia in closed head injury. *Arch Neurol*, 1961, *5*, 4–17.

Saper JR and Lossing JH. Prolonged trance-like stupor in epilepsy. *Arch Int Med*, 1974, *134*, 1079–1082.

Scoville WB and Milner B. Loss of recent memory after bilateral hippocampal lesions. *J Neurol Neurosurg Psychiat*, 1957, *20*, 11–21.

Selby G and Lance JW. Observations on 500 cases of migraine and allied vascular headache. *J Neurol Neurosurg Psychiat*, 1960, *23*, 23–32.

Seltzer B and Benson DF. The temporal pattern of retrograde amnesia in Korsakoff's disease. *Neurology*, 1974, *24*, 527–530.

Shapiro BE, Alexander MP, Gardner H, and Mercer B. Mechanisms of confabulation. *Neurology*, 1981, *31*, 1070–1076.

Shuping JR, Rollinson RD, and Toole JF. Transient global amnesia. *Ann Neurol*, 1980a, *7*, 281–285.

Shuping JR, Toole JF, and Alexander E Jr. Transient global amnesia due to glioma in the dominant hemisphere. *Neurology*, 1980b, *30*, 88–90.

Shuttleworth EC and Morris CE. The transient global amnesia syndrome. *Arch Neurol*, 1966, *15*, 515–520.

Shuttleworth EC and Wise GR. Transient global amnesia due to arterial embolism. *Arch Neurol*, 1973, *29*, 340–342.

Speedie LJ and Heilman KM. Antero-grade memory deficits for visuospatial material after infarction of the right thalamus. *Arch Neurol*, 1983, *40*, 183–186.

Squire LR and Chace PM. Memory functions six to nine months after electroconvulsive therapy. *Arch Gen Psychiat*, 1975, *32*, 1557–1564.

Steinmetz EF and Vroom FQ. Transient global amnesia. *Neurology*, 1972, *22*, 1193–1200.

Stuss DT, Alexander MP, Lieberman A, and Levine H. An extraordinary form of confabulation. *Neurology*, 1978, *28*, 1166–1172.

Stuss DT and Benson DF. Neuropsychological studies of the frontal lobes. *Psychol Bull*, 1984, *95*, 3–28.

Sweet WH, Talland GA, and Ervin FR. Loss of recent memory following section of fornix. *Trans Am Neurol Assoc*, 1959, *84*, 76–78.

Symonds C. Disorders of memory. *Brain*, 1966, *89*, 625–644.

Talland GA. Confabulation in the Wernicke-Korsakoff syndrome. *J Nerv Ment Dis*, 1961, *132*, 361–381.

Talland GA, Sweet WH, and Ballantine HT Jr. Amnesic syndrome with anterior communicating artery aneurysm. *J Nerv Ment Dis*, 1967, *145*, 179–192.

Taren TA. Anatomical pathways related to clinical findings in aneurysms of the anterior communicating artery. *J Neurol Neurosurg Psychiat*, 1965, *28*, 228–234.

Task Force Report 14. *Electroconvulsive therapy*. Washington, D.C., American Psychiatric Association, 1978.

Truex RC and Carpenter MB. *Human neuroanatomy*, 6th ed. Baltimore, Williams & Wilkins Company, 1969.

Turner H. Case report: the mental state during recovery after heart arrest during anaesthesia. *J Neurol Neurosurg Psychiat*, 1950, *13*, 153–155.

Umbach W. Long-term results of fornicotomy for temporal epilepsy. *Confin Neurol*, 1966, *27*, 121–123.

Victor M and Yakovlev PI. SS Korsakoff's psychic disorder in conjunction with peripheral neuritis. *Neurology*, 1955, *5*, 394–406.

Victor M, Adams RD, and Collins GH. *The Wernicke–Korsakoff syndrome*. Philadelphia, FA Davis Company, 1971.

Victor M, Angevine JB Jr, Mancall EL, and Fisher CM. Memory loss with lesions of hippocampal formation. *Arch Neurol*, 1961, *5*, 244–263.

Vogel RM and Lee RV. Bilateral ptosis in Wernicke's disease. *Neurology*, 1967, *17*, 85–86.

Volavka J. Neurophysiology of ECT. *Semin Psychiat*, 1972, *4*, 55–65.

Volpe BT and Hirst W. The characterization of an amnesic syndrome following hypoxic ischemic injury. *Arch Neurol*, 1983a, *40*, 436–440.

Volpe BT and Hirst W. Amnesia following the rupture and repair of an anterior communicating artery aneurysm. *J Neurol Neurosurg Psychiat*, 1983b, *46*, 704–709.

von Wowern F. Posttraumatic amnesia and confusion as an index of severity of head injury. *Acta Neurol Scand*, 1966, *42*, 373–378.

Walsh KW. *Neuropsychology. A clinical approach*. New York, Churchill Livingstone, 1978.

Whitty CWM. Transient global amnesia. In Whitty CWM and Zangwill OL (Eds.): *Amnesia*. Boston, Butterworths, 1977, pp. 93–103.

Whitty CWM and Lewin W. A Korsakoff syndrome in the post-cingulectomy confusional state. *Brain*, 1960, *83*, 648–653.

Williams M. Memory disorders associated with electroconvulsive therapy. In Whitty CWM and Zangwill OL (Eds.): *Amnesia*. Boston, Butterworths, 1977, pp. 183–198.

Williams M and Pennybacker J. Memory disturbances in third ventricular tumours. *J Neurol Neurosurg Psychiat*, 1954, *17*, 115–123.

Wilson G, Rupp C, and Wilson WW. Amnesia. *Am J Psychiat*, 1950, *106*, 481–485.

Woods BT, Schoene W, and Knisley L. Are hippocampal lesions sufficient to cause lasting amnesia? *J Neurol Neurosurg Psychiat*, 1982, *45*, 243–247.

Ziegler DK, Kaufman A, and Marshall HE. Abrupt memory loss associated with thalamic tumor. *Arch Neurol*, 1977, *34*, 545–548.

Zola-Morgan S, Squire LR, and Mishkin M. The neuroanatomy of amnesia: amygdala–hippocampus versus temporal stem. *Science*, 1982, *218*, 1337–1339.

Chapter 5

Visuospatial and Visual-Perceptual Disturbances

Despite their unique highly developed linguistic abilities, humans remain heavily reliant on vision for spatial orientation and environmental interaction. When portions of the brain mediating visuospatial and visuoperceptual function are injured, significant disability results. This chapter presents three types of visuospatial disability: (1) disorders of visual recognition— the agnosias; (2) disorders of spatial attention—neglect, denial, and anosognosia; and (3) visuoconstructive deficits. In a final section, a miscellaneous group of visuospatial deficits including dressing disturbances, central achromatopsia, and Balint syndrome is discussed.

VISUAL AGNOSIAS

Agnosia refers to a clinical syndrome in which the patient has intact sensory functions and is able to perceive sensory stimuli but recognition of perceived material is impaired. The patient has a percept stripped of its meaning (Rubens, 1979). The process of visual recognition is a multistep chain of events that begins with elementary perceptual activities and gradually results in a central nervous system (CNS) construct that is a neural "representation" of the stimulus. Interruption of the transmission of information at the level of the retina produces blurred vision; interruption of connections between the optic chiasm and occipital cortex produces homonymous visual field defects; and lesions in visual association cortex or in tracts connecting the association regions with other cortical areas produce high-level recognition deficits, including the agnosias. The specific characteristics of the agnosia will reflect the stage of recognition disrupted and the class of stimulus object most involved (Table 5-1).

Visual Object Agnosia

The existence of visual object agnosia has been denied (Bay, 1953; Critchley, 1964a), but a sufficient number of credible cases have been reported to estab-

lish the syndrome as a clinical entity. When carefully sought in patients with diffuse or multifocal brain damage (dementia of the Alzheimer type, posttraumatic encephalopathy, postanoxic states, multi-infarct conditions) it may not be rare (Adler, 1944; Benson and Greenberg, 1969; Kertesz, 1979; Levine, 1978; Rubens and Benson, 1971; Wapner et al., 1978). Following Lissauer's 1889 suggestion, the visual object agnosias are divided into two principal types: apperceptive visual agnosias and associative visual agnosias (Benson and Greenberg, 1969). The former involve deficits at a lower level of visual analysis at the boundary between perception and recognition; the latter involve higher levels of visual processing and are almost purely recognition deficits. In apperceptive visual agnosia, the patient is able to see to the extent of identifying color, movement and direction of movement, line direction and dimension, and light intensity. The patient cannot, however, distinguish one form from another (e.g., a cross from a circle) and cannot draw presented objects. Identification through other sensory modalities—auditory, tactile, and olfactory—is intact. Most patients have had extensive bilateral posterior cerebral insults (Brown, 1972; Benson and Greenberg, 1969; Rubens, 1979).

Associative visual agnosia is a disturbance of visual recognition with intact visual perception. The integrity of perceptual processes is attested to by the ability of the patient to make drawings or copies of objects that cannot be visually identified. The preservation of the ability to copy and match similar visual stimuli are the primary clinical characteristics that distinguish associative from apperceptive visual agnosia. Impairment of facial recognition (prosopagnosia), color recognition (color agnosia), and reading (alexia) usually accompany the associative visual agnosias, although there have been rare cases of agnosia for nonverbal material with preserved reading abilities (Albert et al., 1975a; Gomori and Hawryluk, 1984). Associative visual agnosia can be distinguished from anomia by the intact ability of anomic patients to select the correct name from a list of

TABLE 5-1.   The Visual Agnosias

Visual object agnosia

  Apperceptive type
  Associative type

Prosopagnosia

Environmental agnosia

Color agnosia

Simultanagnosia

---

choices or to describe the correct use of the object. Apraxia can similarly be distinguished by the ability of the apraxic patients to describe the use of the object and to state whether the examiner is using it correctly. Pathologically, nearly all autopsied cases of associative visual agnosia have had bilateral medial occiptotemporal lesions involving the medial longitudinal fasciculi connecting occipital and temporal lobes (Albert et al., 1979; Benson et al., 1974; Brown, 1972).

Prosopagnosia

Prosopagnosia is a unique syndrome in which the patient's major difficulty is the identification of familiar faces. Although able to see normally and demonstrating no visual agnosia for most other classes of objects, patients with prosopagnosia are unable to recognize spouses, friends, or relatives. They may be able to correctly describe the face, but no sense of recognition ensues, and they must develop alternate strategies to compensate for the visual recognition deficit (e.g., the sound of the unrecognized person's voice or specific identifying features such as mustache, hair color, etc. are used to aid identification) (Damasio et al., 1982; Hécaen and Angelergues, 1962; Meadows, 1974a; Shuttleworth et al., 1982). Although the defect in prosopagnosia involves primarily recognition of familiar faces, some patients have deficits in recognizing individual members of other classes of objects such as specific animals or specific automobiles with which the patient was previously familiar (Bornstein et al., 1969; Damasio et al., 1982). Prosopagnosia patients may be able to discriminate and to match unfamiliar faces normally, but they cannot learn new faces and recognize them at a later time (Malone et al., 1982). Likewise, difficulty with discriminating and matching unfamiliar faces is a ubiquitous abnormality among patients with posterior right hemisphere lesions, and such patients seldom have concomitant prosopagnosia (De Renzi and Spinnler, 1966; De Renzi et al., 1969; Hamsher et al., 1979).

The anatomic basis of prosopagnosia is controversial. All autopsied cases to date have had bilateral medial occipital lesions, and many take this as evidence that bilateral lesions are necessary to produce the syndrome (Cohn et al., 1977; Damasio et al., 1982; Gloning et al., 1970; Meadows, 1974a; Nardelli et al., 1982; Pevzner et al., 1962). Several cases studied by computerized axial tomography, however, appear to have unilateral right-sided posteromedial lesions, suggesting that a unilateral right-sided lesion may be sufficient to interrupt recognition of familiar faces (Whiteley and Warrington, 1977).

Environmental Agnosia

Environmental agnosia (also called *topographagnosia, topagnosia,* and *topographic memory loss*), like prosopagnosia, involves loss of recognition of a specific class of visual stimuli, in this case the environment. The patient can see adequately, can usually describe the environment correctly, can often correctly utilize maps to find directions, and may even be able to draw an accurate map; when faced with the actual environment, however, the patient has no sense of familiarity or recognition (Ettlinger et al., 1957; Hécaen et al., 1980; McFie et al., 1950; Pallis, 1955; Peterson and Zangwill, 1945; Whiteley and Warrington, 1978). Most patients capitalize on their intact linguistic capacities and adopt verbal strategies to help compensate for their deficits. For example, they use street names and house numbers to find their way around, and they may not even recognize their own houses except in this way! Environmental agnosia frequently occurs as part of a clinical triad with prosopagnosia and central achromatopsia, although a variety of concomitant deficits have been described, including palinopsia, absent mental revisualization, dressing disturbances, visual allesthesia, and disturbances of brightness modulation (Cummings et al., 1983; Pallis, 1955). Although many patients with environmental agnosia have had bilateral medial occipital lesions, there are well-documented autopsy-verified cases of unilateral right-sided occipitotemporal lesions producing the syndrome (Cogan, 1979; Cummings et al., 1983; Ettlinger et al., 1957; Hécaen and de Ajuriaguerra, 1954; Hemphill and Klein, 1948; McFie et al., 1950). The underlying defect in environmental agnosia appears to be an inability to relate current perceptions to stored memories that would allow environmental recognition to occur.

Color Agnosia

Color agnosia accompanies alexia without agraphia and results from disconnection of the "color-seeing" right hemisphere from the "color-naming" left hemisphere by a lesion destroying the medial left occipital cortex and the splenium of the corpus callosum (Geschwind and Fusillo, 1966). In such cases the patients have intact color perception as demonstrated by pseudoisochromatic plates and color matching tests and intact color memory as shown by correct responses to questions concerning colors of named objects. They cannot, however, name colors correctly in confrontation testing or point to named colors. Color agnosia must be distinguished from central achromatopsia and color anomia (Brown, 1972; Hécaen and Albert, 1978; Kinsbourne and Warrington, 1964; Rubens, 1979).

Simultanagnosia

Simultanagnosia refers to a curious neuropsychological deficit in which the patient is unable to simultaneously perceive more than one stimulus item or more than one part of a complex visual pattern. For example, if shown a piece of paper with a circle and a cross on it, the patient will see only one of the items; or, if shown a complex picture, only one portion of it is visible to the patient (Hécaen and Albert, 1978; Kinsbourne and Warrington, 1962; Luria, 1959). The disorder cannot be attributed to elementary visual abnormalities or to hemispatial neglect. Luria and coworkers (1963) demonstrated that the patients have abnormal ocular movements when exploring visual stimuli but considered these to be a product of the underlying deficit rather than the cause. The disorder is thought to be due to an impaired ability to integrate more than one stimulus item at a time or to an inability to use visual cues that allow rapid analysis of complex figures (Kinsbourne and Warrington, 1962; Luria, 1959; Weigel, 1964). Most patients with simultanagnosia have had bilateral parietooccipital lesions, although Kinsbourne and Warrington (1962) suggested that a left-sided occipital lesion might be sufficient to produce the syndrome.

NEGLECT, DENIAL, AND ANOSOGNOSIA

Hemispatial Neglect

Unilateral neglect refers to a hemi-inattention syndrome in which the patient fails to notice, report, or respond to stimuli in one-half of space. All sensory modalities can be included in a neglect syndrome, and the severity of the attentional deficit varies considerably among patients. In severe cases the patient will see nothing in the neglected half field; will draw only one-half of constructions; may dress, shave, or apply make-up to only one-half of the body; and will frankly deny the presence of any motor or sensory deficit of the involved side. In milder cases there will be a less pronounced ten-

TABLE 5-2. Location of Lesions that May Produce Unilateral Hemi-inattention

Inferior parietal lobule
Dorsolateral frontal lobe
Cingulate gyrus
Neostriatum (caudate, putamen)
Thalamus

dency to ignore stimuli on the involved side, the patient's attention can be directed to the affected hemispace and the patient will not overtly deny the deficits. In its least severe form, the neglect will be revealed only by extinguishing one of a pair of stimuli during double simultaneous sensory stimulations (Battersby et al., 1956; Gilliatt and Pratt, 1952; Heilman, 1979; Lawson, 1962; Willanger et al., 1981).

Classically, neglect was attributed to lesions of the right parietal lobe, and the most frequent, profound, and enduring examples of hemispatial neglect do occur with lesions in this region (Critchley, 1953; Gilliatt and Pratt, 1952; Oxbury et al., 1974). Neglect syndromes have also been observed with lesions of either hemisphere involving the dorsolateral frontal lobe, cingulate gyrus, neostriatum, and thalamus, however, and these observations have been synthesized to suggest that hemispatial attention is the product of an organized network of reticulosubcortical–limbic–neocortical structures (Table 5-2) (Healton et al., 1982; Heilman and Valenstein, 1972; Mesulam, 1978, 1981; Perani et al., 1982; Stein and Volpe, 1983; Watson and Heilman, 1979; Watson et al., 1981). Within this network, right-sided lesions produce more pronounced hemispatial neglect than do the corresponding left-sided lesions, but neglect is not uncommon in the acute phases of a left hemisphere injury (Denny-Brown and Banker, 1954).

Tests for unilateral neglect should include all sensory modalities. The line-crossing test (Fig. 5-1) is one simple and effective way of demonstrating visual neglect (Albert 1973). The patient is presented with a sheet of paper with random lines on it and asked to mark the center of each line. If neglect is present, all or a portion of the lines in the neglected field will not be marked. Drawings and copying tasks may also reveal hemispatial neglect. The patient will reproduce only the portion of the drawing that appears in the nonneglected half of space (Fig. 5-2). Neglect is not a product of any coexisting visual field defect: many patients with homonymous hemianopia do not have neglect syndromes, and many with neglect syndromes do not have hemianopias.

Extinction of one stimulus during double simultaneous sensory stimulation can be demonstrated in the visual sphere by stimulating homonymous portions of

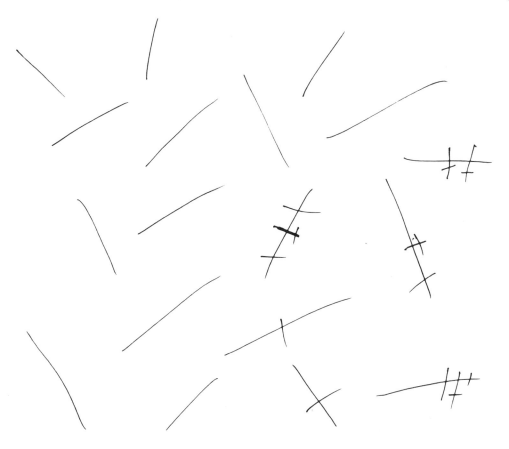

Figure 5-1. Line-crossing test. The patient neglected the lines on the left side of the sheet, crossed only lines on the right side, and perseverated on the crossing task.

the visual fields during confrontation testing (a visual field defect will, if present, also obliterate perception of one stimulus and invalidate this test), in the auditory sphere by snapping one's fingers behind the ears on each side, and in the somatosensory sphere by simultaneously stimulating both sides of the body (Bender and Furlow, 1944; Bender and Teuber, 1946; Denny-Brown et al., 1952; Heilman, 1979).

Neglect is most pronounced during the acute phases of an acquired cerebral insult and, in the case of static lesions, gradually improves. Subtle evidence of neglect may persist for months or even longer, however, and may be one of the factors most limiting to the rehabilitation of the brain-injured patient (Colombo et al., 1982; Heilman, 1979; Leicester et al., 1969).

Anosognosia

The term "anosognosia" was originally used by Babinski to describe patients with denial of illness, of which the two best studied examples are denial of hemi-

paresis and denial of blindness. Denial of hemiparesis is nearly always part of a profound unilateral neglect syndrome. The patient may deny that any deficit exists and when shown the paralyzed limbs, may even deny owning them (Critchley, 1964b; Nathanson et al., 1952; Roth, 1949; Sandifer, 1946; Ullman et al., 1960; Weinstein and Kahn, 1950.) In less pronounced cases, the patients may experience a variety of anosognosic phenomena, including a feeling of nonownership of the limb, indifference to the disability (anosodiaphoria), hatred of the paralyzed side (misoplegia), personification (naming the limb, addressing it as a person), or even a feeling that a third upper or lower extremity has appeared (Cutting, 1978; Weinstein et al., 1954). Anosognosia and associated phenomena, like neglect, are most profound and enduring when produced by right-sided parietal lesions, but it is not unusual for fluent aphasics with posterior left-sided lesions to deny their language deficits and any accompanying motor or sensory impairment in the acute period of the illness (Cutting, 1978; Weinstein et al., 1964; Welman, 1969).

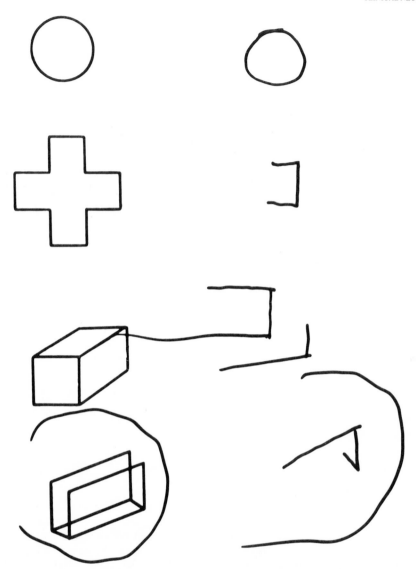

Figure 5-2.   Constructions show severe neglect of the leftside of the models.

The other classic example of denial of illness is the syndrome of denial of blindness (Anton's syndrome). The patient is blind but denies sightlessness and readily confabulates answers to questions concerning visual information. If pressed, the patient may admit to having vision that is "slightly blurred" or that "the light is dim" but gives no other hint concerning the presence or severity of the deficit. The syndrome most commonly occurs with cerebral blindness produced by bilateral lesions of the occipital cortex or retrogeniculate visual radiations, but it has also been described in patients with anterior blindness who have an associated dementia or confusional state (Bergman, 1957; Redlich and Dorsey,

1945; Symonds and MacKenzie, 1957). Cerebral blindness is usually a product of vertebrobasilar or bilateral posterior cerebral artery disease and may be accompanied by a profound amnesia secondary to simultaneous infarction of the hippocampi. The Anton syndrome must be distinguished from bilateral hemianopias with macular sparing where the patient has a tiny area of preserved central vision and from blindness as a conversion symptom (Kearns et al., 1955; Merskey, 1979; Minor et al., 1959; Weintraub, 1983). In the former, the examiner may be able to demonstrate intact vision by situating very small targets within the diminutive visual field; in the latter, both pupillary responses and optokinetic nystagmus (produced by moving a striped target in front of the patient's eyes) are intact (Table 5-3).

Constructional Disturbances

Constructional disturbances have traditionally been called *apraxias* in the neurological and neuropsychological literature, but they do not fit the definition of apraxia adopted in Chapter 3 and are referred to simply as constructional disturbances in this discussion. The evaluation of constructional abilities is a rapid and discriminating technique for assessment of the integrity of visuospatial skills and should be included in all neuropsychiatric assessments. Constructional abilities are impaired by a wide variety of hemispheric lesions, and the presence of a constructional deficit usually indicates an acquired CNS disturbance. Most idiopathic neuropsychiatric disorders, including schizophrenia, mania, and depression, have minimal impact on constructional skills (Nahor and Benson, 1970). Constructional deficits may be demonstrated by asking the patient to make spontaneous drawings, copy model figures, or reproduce matchstick designs.

The presence of constructional disturbances per se has limited localizing value. Isolated temporal lobe lesions appear not to impair the ability to copy figures, but frontal and parietooccipital lesions of either hemisphere can impair copying and drawing abilities (Arena and Gainotti, 1978; Benson and Barton, 1970; Benton, 1979; Gainotti et al., 1977; Piercy and Smyth, 1962). Analysis of the approach to reproducing the constructions and of the type of errors made, however, may yield circumstantial localizing information. When neglect of one-half of the model is present, the lesion is nearly always in the contralateral hemisphere and usually in the posterior hemispheric regions (Gainotti et al., 1972; Heilman, 1979). Similarly, normal right-handed individuals typically begin a construction in the upper left-hand corner and proceed rightward; patients with right-sided lesions are likely to begin on the right side of the construction and work toward the left, perhaps neglecting some aspects of the left side of the model (Albert and Kaplan, 1980). Left-sided lesions are more likely to result in omissions and simplifications of the construction, whereas right-sided lesions produce a loss of perspective and inappropriate relationships among the constituent parts. Right hemispheric lesions tend to produce more profound deficits than do those associated with left-sided lesions (Bogen, 1979; Gainotti et al., 1977; Piercy and Smyth, 1962). Frontal lobe disorders, particularly those affecting the right frontal lobe, disrupt drawings by imposing an unplanned segmented approach that results in a poorly integrated product (Figure 6-3) (Albert and Kaplan, 1980). Perseveration may also be evident. In addition to discrete lesions, multifocal and widespread processes such as multi-infarct dementia, dementia of the Alzheimer type, and chronic and acute confusional states produce profound constructional disturbances (Chapters 7 and 8).

MISCELLANEOUS VISUOPERCEPTUAL AND VISUOSPATIAL DISORDERS

In addition to the agnosias, neglect syndromes, and constructional disturbances presented previously in this chapter, hemispheric lesions may produce a wide variety of other visuoperceptual and visuospatial disorders. A few of these syndromes and their pathological correlates are discussed in the following sections.

Balint's Syndrome

Balint's syndrome is a complex disturbance including (1) "psychic paralysis of visual fixation," in which the patient cannot volitionally shift gaze from one object to another; (2) "optic ataxia," manifest by an inability to execute visually guided manual movements;

TABLE 5-3. Distinguishing Characteristics of Cerebral Blindness, Anterior Blindness, and Blindness as a Conversion Symptom

Type of Blindness	Pupillary Responses	Optokinetic Nystagmus	Comment
Cerebral blindness	Present	Absent	Bilateral retrogeniculate lesions
Anterior blindness	Absent	Absent	Bilateral lesions in optic tracts of eyes
Conversion reaction with blindness	Present	Present	Underlying neurological or psychiatric illness common (see Chapter 15)

and (3) a disturbance of visual attention characterized by an inability to see all but the most prominent visual stimuli (Allison et al., 1969; Hécaen and Albert, 1978; Hécaen and de Ajuriaguerra, 1954). The latter disability may be equivalent to simultanagnosia (discussed earlier). The psychic paralysis of visual fixation is reflected in abnormalities of eye movements on exploration of novel stimuli (Tyler, 1968). Pathologically, Balint's syndrome is produced by bilateral parietooccipital lesions involving the lateral aspects of the hemispheres. Fractions of the syndrome have been reported in patients with circumscribed bilateral or unilateral lesions (Auerbach and Alexander, 1981; Damasio and Benton, 1979).

Central Achromatopsia

Central achromatopsia refers to loss of color vision produced by occipital lobe lesions. It must be distinguished from inherited abnormalities of color vision, acquired disorders of the optic nerves that impair color vision, and color agnosia and color anomia. Central processing of color perception in the occipital lobes occurs inferior to the calcarine sulcus anterior to the region mediating visual field information. Bilateral injury to this area produces complete color blindness, whereas unilateral damage produces contralateral hemiachromatopsia (Albert et al., 1975b; Damasio et al., 1980; Green and Lessell, 1977; Meadows, 1974b; Pearlman et al., 1979).

Dressing Disturbances

Dressing disturbances may be produced by a variety of CNS lesions and occur in the context of several different clinical syndromes: (1) in syndromes with profound unilateral neglect, only the nonneglected side of the body may be bathed, toileted, and dressed; (2) in acute confusional states, dementing disorders, and schizophrenia, patients may don multiple layers of clothing when such bundling is inappropriate for the weather; and (3) a syndrome of true body-garment disorientation may occur. In the third case one may be unable to correctly orient one's arm to the sleeve, may try to wear one's shirt on one's legs, or may put pants on backward. The syndrome appears to be uniquely associated with right parietal lesions and is more prevalent with damage to the parietal convexity (Hemphill and Klein, 1948).

REFERENCES

Adler A. Disintegration and restoration of optic recognition in visual agnosia. *Arch Neurol Psychiat*, 1944, *51*, 243–259.

Albert ML. A simple test of visual neglect. *Neurology*, 1973, *23*, 658–664.

Albert ML, Reches A, and Silverberg R. Associative visual agnosia without alexia. *Neurology*, 1975a, *25*, 322–326.

Albert ML, Reches A, and Silverberg R. Hemianopic color blindness. *J Neurol Neurosurg Psychiat*, 1975b, *38*, 546–549.

Albert ML, Soffer D, Silverberg R, and Reches A. The anatomic basis of visual agnosia. *Neurology*, 1979, *29*, 876–879.

Albert MS and Kaplan E. Organic implications of neuropsychological deficits in the elderly. In Poon LW, Fozard JL, Cermak LS, Arenberg D, and Thompson LW (Eds.): *New directions in memory and aging*. Hillsdale, New Jersey, Lawrence Erlbaum Associates, 1980, pp. 403–432.

Allison RS, Hurwitz LJ, White JG, and Wilmot TJ. A follow-up study of a patient with Balint's syndrome. *Neuropsychologia*, 1969, *7*, 319–333.

Arena R and Gainotti G. Constructional apraxia and visuoperceptive disabilities in relation to laterality of cerebral lesions. *Cortex*, 1978, *14*, 463–473.

Auerbach SH and Alexander MP. Pure agraphia and unilateral optic ataxia associated with a left superior parietal lobule lesion. *J Neurol Neurosurg Psychiat*, 1981, *44*, 430–432.

Battersby WS, Bender MB, Pollack M, and Kahn RL. Unilateral "spatial agnosia" ("inattention") in patients with cerebral lesions. *Brain*, 1956, *79*, 68–83.

Bay E. Disturbances of visual perception and their examination. *Brain*, 1953, *76*, 515–550.

Bender MB and Furlow LT. Phenomenon of visual extinction and binocular rivalry mechanism. *Trans Am Neurol Assoc*, 1944, *70*, 87–89.

Bender MB and Teuber HL. Phenomena of fluctuation, extinction, and completion in visual perception. *Arch Neurol Psychiat*, 1946, *55*, 627–658.

Benson DF and Barton MI. Disturbances in constructional ability. *Cortex*, 1970, *6*, 19–46.

Benson DF and Greenberg JP. Visual form agnosia. *Arch Neurol*, 1969, *20*, 82–89.

Benson DF, Segarra J, and Albert ML. Visual agnosia–prosopagnosia. A clinicopathologic correlation. *Arch Neurol*, 1974, *30*, 307–310.

Benton A. Visuoperceptive, visuospatial and visuoconstructive disorders. In Heilman KM and Valenstein E (Eds.): *Clinical neuropsychology*. New York, Oxford University Press, 1979, pp. 186–232.

Bergman PS. Cerebral blindness. *Arch Neurol Psychiat*, 1957, *78*, 568–584.

Bogen JE. The callosal syndrome. In Heilman KM and Valenstein E (Eds.): *Clinical neuropsychology*. New York, Oxford University Press, 1979, pp. 308–359.

Bornstein B, Sroka H, and Munitz H. Prosopagnosia with animal face agnosia. *Cortex*, 1969, *5*, 164–169.

Brown JW. *Aphasia, apraxia, and agnosia*. Springfield, Illinois, Charles C Thomas, Publisher, 1972.

Cogan DG. Visuospatial dysgnosia. *Am J Opthalmol*, 1979, *88*, 361–368.

Cohn R, Neumann MA, and Wood DH. Prosopagnosia: a clinicopathological study. *Ann Neurol*, 1977, *1*, 177–182.

Columbo A, De Renzi E, and Gentilini M. The time course of visual hemi-inattention. *Acta Psychiat Nervenkr*, 1982, *231*, 539–546.

Critchley M. *The parietal lobes*. New York, Hafner Press, 1953.

Critchley M. The problem of visual agnosia. *J Neurol Sci*, 1964a, *1*, 274–290.

Critchley M. Psychiatric symptoms and parietal disease: differential diagnosis. *Proc Roy Soc Med*, 1964b, *57*, 422–428.

Cummings JL, Landis T, and Benson DF. Environmental disorientation: clinical and radiologic findings. *Neurology*, 1983, *33* (Suppl. 2), 103–104.

Cutting J. Study of anosognosia. *J Neurol Neurosurg Psychiat*, 1978, *41*, 548–555.

Damasio AR and Benton AL. Impairment of hand movements under visual guidance. *Neurology*, 1979, *29*, 170–178.

Damasio AR, Damasio H, and Van Hoesen GW. Prosopagnosia: anatomic basis and behavioral mechanisms. *Neurology*, 1982, *32*, 331–341.

Damasio A, Yamada T, Damasio H, Corbett J, and McKee J. Central achromatopsia: behavioral, anatomic, and physiologic aspects. *Neurology*, 1980, *30*, 1064–1071.

Denny-Brown D and Banker BQ. Amorphosynthesis from left parietal lesion. *Arch Neurol Psychiat*, 1954, *71*, 302–313.

Denny-Brown D, Meyer JS, and Horenstein S. The significance of perceptual rivalry resulting from parietal lesion. *Brain*, 1952, *75*, 433–471.

De Renzi E, Scotti G, and Spinnler H. Perceptual and associative disorders of visual recognition. *Neurology*, 1969, *19*, 634–642.

De Renzi E and Spinnler H. Facial recognition in brain-damaged patients. *Neurology*, 1966, *16*, 145–152.

Ettlinger G, Warrington E, and Zangwill OL. A further study of visualspatial agnosia. *Brain*, 1957, *80*, 335–361.

Gainotti G, Messerli P, and Tissot R. Qualitative analysis of unilateral spatial neglect in relation to laterality of cerebral lesions. *J Neurol Neurosurg Psychiat*, 1972, *35*, 545–550.

Gainotti G, Miceli G, and Caltagirone C. Constructional apraxia in left brain-damaged patients: a planning disorder? *Cortex*, 1977, *13*, 119–130.

Geschwind N and Fusillo M. Color-naming deficits in association with alexia. *Arch Neurol*, 1966, *15*, 137–146.

Green GJ and Lessell S. Acquired cerebral dyschromatopsia. *Arch Ophthalmol*, 1977, *95*, 121–128.

Gilliatt RW and Pratt RTC. Disorders of perception and performance in a case of right-sided cerebral thrombosis. *J Neurol Neurosurg Psychiat*, 1952, *15*, 264–271.

Gloning I, Gloning K, Jellinger K, and Quatember R. A case of "prosopagnosia" with necropsy findings. *Neuropsychologia*, 1970, *8*, 199–204.

Gomori AJ and Hawryluk GA. Visual agnosia without alexia. *Neurology*, 1984, *34*, 947–980.

Hamsher K de S, Levin HS, and Benton AL. Facial recognition in patients with focal brain lesions. *Arch Neurol*, 1979, *36*, 837–839.

Healton EB, Navarro C, Bressman S, and Brust JCM. Subcortical neglect. *Neurology*, 1982, *32*, 776–778.

Hécaen H and Albert ML. *Human neuropsychology*. New York, John Wiley & Sons, 1978.

Hécaen H and Angelergues R. Agnosia for faces (prosopagnosia). *Arch Neurol*, 1962, *7*, 92–100.

Hécaen H and de Ajuriaguerra J. Balint's syndrome (psychic paralysis of visual fixation) and its minor forms. *Brain*, 1954, *77*, 373–400.

Hécaen H, Tzortzis C, and Rondot P. Loss of topographic memory with learning deficits. *Cortex*, 1980, *16*, 525–542.

Heilman KM. Neglect and related disorders. In Heilman KM and Valenstein E (Eds.): *Clinical neuropsychology*. New York, Oxford University Press, 1979, pp. 268–307.

Heilman KM and Valenstein E. Frontal lobe neglect in man. *Neurology*, 1972, *22*, 660–664.

Hemphill RE and Klein R. Contribution to the dressing disability as a focal sign and to the imperception phenomenon. *J Ment Sci*, 1948, *94*, 611–622.

Kearns TP, Wagner HP, and Millikan CH. Bilateral homonymous hemianopia. *Arch Ophthalmol*, 1955, *53*, 560–565.

Kertesz A. Visual agnosia: the dual defect of perception and recognition. *Cortex*, 1979, *15*, 403–419.

Kinsbourne M and Warrington EK. A disorder of simultaneous form perception. *Brain*, 1962, *85*, 461–486.

Kinsbourne M and Warrington EK. Observations on color agnosia. *J Neurol Neurosurg Psychiat*, 1964, *27*, 296–299.

Lawson IR. Visual-spatial neglect in lesions of the right cerebral hemisphere. *Neurology*, 1962, *12*, 23–33.

Leicester J, Sidman M, Stoddard LT, and Mohr JP. Some determinants of visual neglect. *J Neurol Neurosurg Psychiat*, 1969, *32*, 580–587.

Levine DN. Prosopagnosia and visual object agnosia. *Brain Lang*, 1978, *5*, 341–365.

Luria AR. Disorders of "simultaneous perception" in a case of bilateral occipito-parietal brain injury. *Brain*, 1959, *82*, 437–449.

Luria AR, Pravdina-Vinarskaya EN, and Yarbuss AL. Disorders of ocular movement in a case of simultanagnosia. *Brain*, 1963, *86*, 219–228.

Malone DR, Morris HH, Kay MC, and Levin HS. Prosopagnosia: a double dissociation between the recognition of familiar and unfamiliar faces. *J Neurol Neurosurg Psychiat*, 1982, *45*, 820–822.

McFie J, Piercy MF, and Zangwill OL. Visual-spatial agnosia associated with lesions of the right cerebral hemisphere. *Brain*, 1950, *73*, 167–190.

Meadows JC. The anatomical basis of prosopagnosia. *J Neurol Neurosurg Psychiat*, 1974a, *37*, 489–501.

Meadows JC. Disturbed perception of colors associated with localized cerebral lesions. *Brain*, 1974b, *97*, 615–632.

Merskey H. *The analysis of hysteria*. London, Bailliere Tindall, 1979.

Mesulam M-M. Attention and its disorders. *Weekly update: Neurol Neurosurg*, 1978, *1*(7), 1–7.

Mesulam M-M. A cortical network for directed attention and unilateral neglect. *Ann Neurol*, 1981, *10*, 309–325.

Minor RH, Kearns TP, Millikan CH, Siekert RG, and Sayre GP. Ocular manifestations of occlusive disease of the vertebral-basilar arterial system. *Arch Ophthalmol*, 1959, *62*, 84–96.

Nahor A and Benson DF. A screening test for organic brain disease in emergency psychiatric evaluation. *Behav Psychiat*, 1970, *2*, 23–26.

Nardelli E, Buonanno F, Coccia G, Fiaschi A, Terzian H, and Rizzuto N. Prosopagnosia. Report of four cases. *Europ Neurol*, 1982, *21*, 289–297.

Nathanson M, Bergman PS, and Gordon GG. Denial of illness. *Arch Neurol Psychiat*, 1952, *68*, 380–387.

Oxbury JM, Campbell DC, and Oxbury SM. Unilateral spatial neglect and impairments of spatial analysis and visual perception. *Brain*, 1974, *97*, 551–564.

Pallis CA. Impaired identification of faces and places with agnosia for colors. *J Neurol Neurosurg Psychiat*, 1955, *18*, 218–224.

Paterson A and Zangwill OL. A case of topographic disorientation associated with a unilateral cerebral lesion. *Brain*, 1945, *68*, 188–212.

Pearlman AL, Birch J, and Meadows JC. Cerebral color blindness: an acquired defect in hue discrimination. *Ann Neurol*, 1979, *5*, 253–261.

Perani D, Nardocci N, and Braggi G. Neglect after right unilateral thalamotomy. A case report. *Ital J Neurol Sci*, 1982, *1*, 61–64.

Pevzner S, Bornstein B, and Loewenthal M. Prosopagnosia. *J Neurol Neurosurg Psychiat*, 1962, *25*, 336–338.

Piercy M and Smyth VOG. Right hemisphere dominance for certain nonverbal intellectual skills. *Brain*, 1962, *85*, 775–790.

Redlich FC and Dorsey JF. Denial of blindness by patients with cerebral disease. *Arch Neurol Psychiat*, 1945, *53*, 407–417.

Roth M. Disorders of the body image caused by lesions of the right parietal lobe. *Brain*, 1949, *79*, 89–111.

Rubens AB. Agnosia. In Heilman KM and Valenstein E (Eds.): *Clinical neuropsychology*. New York, Oxford University Press, 1979, pp. 233–267.

Rubens AB and Benson DF. Associative visual agnosia. *Arch Neurol*, 1971, *24*, 305–316.

Sandifer PH. Anosognosia and disorders of body scheme. *Brain*, 1946, *69*, 122–137.

Shuttleworth EC Jr, Syring V, and Allen N. Further observations on the nature of prosopagnosia. *Brain Cognit*, 1982, *1*, 307–322.

Stein S and Volpe BT. Classical ''parietal'' neglect syndrome after right frontal lobe infarction. *Neurology*, 1983, *33*, 797–799.

Symonds C and MacKenzie I. Bilateral loss of vision from cerebral infarction. *Brain*, 1957, *80*, 415–455.

Tyler HR. Abnormalities of perception with defective eye movements (Balint's syndrome). *Cortex*, 1968, *4*, 154–171.

Ullman M, Ashenhurst EM, Hurwitz LJ, and Gruen A. Motivational and structural factors in the denial of hemiplegia. *Arch Neurol*, 1960, *3*, 306–318.

Wapner W, Judd T, and Gardner H. Visual agnosia in an artist. *Cortex*, 1978, *14*, 343–364.

Watson RT and Heilman KM. Thalamic neglect. *Neurology*, 1979, *29*, 690–694.

Watson RT, Valenstein E, and Heilman KM. Thalamic neglect. Possible role of the medial thalamus and nucleus reticularis in behavior. *Arch Neurol*, 1981, *38*, 501–506.

Weigel E. Some critical remarks concerning the problem of so-called simultanagnosia. *Neuropsychologia*, 1964, *2*, 189–207.

Weinstein EA, Cole M, Mitchell MS, and Lyerly OG. Anosognosia and aphasia. *Arch Neurol*, 1964, *10*, 376–386.

Weinstein EA and Kahn RL. The syndrome of anosognosia. *Arch Neurol Psychiat*, 1950, *64*, 772–791.

Weinstein EA, Kahn RL, Malitz S, and Rozanski J. Delusional reduplication of parts of the body. *Brain*, 1954, *77*, 45–60.

Weintraub MI. *Hysterical conversion reactions*. New York, SP Medical and Scientific Books, 1983.

Welman AJ. Right-sided visual spatial agnosia, asomatagnosia, and anosognosia with left hemisphere lesions. *Brain*, 1969, *92*, 571–580.

Whiteley AM and Warrington EK. Prosopagnosia: a clinical, psychological, and anatomical study of three patients. *J Neurol Neurosurg Psychiat*, 1977, *40*, 395–403.

Whiteley AM and Warrington EK. Selective impairment of topographical memory: a single case study. *J Neurol Neurosurg Psychiat*, 1978, *41*, 575–578.

Willanger R, Danielson UT, and Ankerhus J. Visual neglect in right-sided apopleptic lesions. *Acta Neurol Scand*, 1981, *64*, 327–336.

Chapter 6

Behavioral Disorders Associated with Frontal Lobe Injury

The frontal lobe is the largest lobe of the human brain, comprising approximately one-third of the total cortex. It is among the most recent phylogenetic acquisitions and is one of the last regions to mature and myelinate in ontogenetic development (Fuster, 1980). It is not a homogenous entity but is divided into functionally specialized subregions, and injury to different areas will produce clinically distinct psychosyndromes and behavioral alterations. This chapter presents the recognized syndromes resulting from restricted frontal damage and describes additional behavioral symptoms that are related to frontal dysfunction. The anatomic correlates of the principal syndromes and the common etiologies of frontal damage are also discussed.

FRONTAL LOBE SYNDROMES AND SYMPTOMS

Three principal frontal lobe syndromes have been identified (Table 6-1): an orbitofrontal syndrome dominated by disinhibited and impulsive behavior, a frontal convexity syndrome that has apathy as its major behavioral correlate, and a medial frontal syndrome associated with variable degrees of akinesia. Each syndrome has distinct behavioral alterations and can be correlated with different anatomic systems within the frontal lobe. Clinically, however, a mixture of frontal lobe symptoms and behavioral characteristics is more common than the pure expression of a single frontal psychosyndrome. The occurrence of mixed syndromes and bilateral frontal lobe involvement reflects the immediate anatomic juxtaposition of the two frontal lobes and the tendency for most pathological processes to involve both frontal lobes. Traumatic, neoplastic, and other central nervous system (CNS) disorders are unlikely to be confined to a restricted region within a frontal lobe or even to a single lobe. The principal characteristics of each specific frontal syndrome are presented separately, but the likelihood of encountering mixed syndromes in the clinical setting cannot be underemphasized.

Orbitofrontal Syndrome

Behaviorally, the outstanding feature of the orbitofrontal syndrome is disinhibition. The patients lack social tact, make tasteless and socially inappropriate comments, may commit antisocial acts, and exhibit a general coarsening of interpersonal style. Emotionally the patients are irritable and labile with a tendency to an inane euphoria and inappropriate jocularity (witzelsucht). The patients may be hyperactive, and hypomanic behavior is not uncommon. Sexual preoccupations, inappropriate sexual jesting, and improper sexual comments are frequent, but overt sexual aggression is rare (Arseni et al., 1966; Blumer and Benson, 1975; Faust, 1966; Hunter et al., 1968; Jarvie, 1954; Reitman, 1946).

Neuropsychological deficits are surprisingly difficult to identify in patients with orbitofrontal lesions. Impulsiveness, distractibility, and lack of concern for correct performance may interfere with intellectual assessment; however, when these can be contained, basic language, memory, and cognitive skills are usually found to be intact (Faust, 1966; Luria, 1980). Insight, especially into the social or emotional consequences of actions, is limited, and interpersonal judgment is poor.

Elementary neurological deficits are not prominent in patients with lesions limited to the orbitofrontal cortex. The olfactory nerves lie immediately beneath the frontal lobes and can be damaged by any process injuring or compressing the inferior frontal surface. A grasp reflex and involuntary grasping of presented objects ("utilization behavior") may be present in some patients (Lhermitte, 1983). Primary motor, somatosensory, and visual functions are normal if the lesion is limited to the orbitofrontal region.

Frontal Convexity Syndrome

The dominant behavioral characteristic of a patient with the frontal convexity syndrome is apathy. The patient is indifferent, is unmotivated, and lacks initia-

TABLE 6-1. Clinical Characteristics of the Three Principal
Frontal Lobe Syndromes

Orbitofrontal Syndrome (disinhibited)

Disinhibited, impulsive behavior (''pseudopsychopathic'')
Inappropriate jocular affect, euphoria
Emotional lability
Poor judgment and insight
Distractibility

Frontal Convexity Syndrome (apathetic)

Apathetic
   (occasional brief angry or aggressive outbursts common)
Indifference
Psychomotor retardation
Motor preservation and impersistence
Loss of set
Stimulus boundedness
Discrepant motor and verbal behavior
Motor programming deficits

   Three-step hand sequence
   Alternating programs
   Reciprocal programs
   Rhythm tapping
   Multiple loops

Poor word-list generation
Poor abstraction and categorization
Segmented approach to visuospatial analysis

Medial Frontal Syndrome (akinetic)

   Paucity of spontaneous movement and gesture
   Sparse verbal output (repetition may be preserved)
   Lower extremity weakness and loss of sensation
   Incontinence

tive. Psychomotor retardation of at least moderate severity is usually present, and the patient may give a
superficial impression of depression (Blumer and Benson, 1975; Faust, 1966). When irritated, the patient
may have brief outbursts of verbal or physical aggression that interrupt the overall apathetic demeanor, but
the anger is short-lived and the apathy quickly supervenes.

Many of the most striking abnormalities observed
in patients with frontal convexity lesions reflect an inability to program novel motor activity and to use verbal functions to guide motor actions. There may be a
complete dissociation between the patient's verbal and
motor performance. When given verbal instructions, the
patient may be able to comprehend and even reiterate
the directions but be unable to use the information for
guiding or correcting behavior (Drewe, 1975; Luria,
1980; Stuss and Benson, 1984; Zangwill, 1960). This
deficit is evident in the daily behavior of the patient who
performs incorrectly despite clear instructions and in the
testing situation where the patient is unable to use ver-

bal cues to guide the three-step hand sequence (reciting
aloud ''fist,'' ''slap,'' and ''side,'' while simultaneously
putting the hand through the same sequence of positions)
(Fig. 2-1), alternating programs (Fig. 6-1), or reciprocal programs (tapping once each time the examiner taps
twice and vice versa).

There is a tendency toward distractibility and inability to maintain a behavioral set. This may be demonstrated on continuous performance tests such as
requesting that the patient's hand be raised each time the
letter ''A'' occurs in a list of letters recited by the examiner. The patient may be able to repeat the instructions but looses set during test performance and may
make either errors of omission (does not detect an ''A'')
or commission (responds to letters other than ''A''). Distractibility is also evident in the stimulus boundedness
of the patient. The patient's attention is easily redirected
by novel or concrete stimuli. For example, when the
patient is asked to draw, number, and set a clock for
11:10, the clock is often drawn and numbered correctly,
but one hand will be placed on the 10 (stimulus bounded)
and the other on the 11.

Other behavioral characteristics include perservera-
tion or impersistence in the execution of motor acts (e.g.,
the patient may not persist in maintaining tongue protrusion or may perseverate on eye closure). Perservera-
tion may also be evident in copying multiple loop figures
(Fig. 6-2) and when one portion of the examination in-
trudes into the next (e.g., the patient will continue to
attempt serial hand sequences when asked to do rhythm-
tapping tasks). Patients show a marked inflexibility in
behavior and an inability to profit from their mistakes
and are unable to inhibit inappropriate responses (Kolb
and Whishaw, 1980).

Primary linguistic functions are not disturbed by
frontal convexity lesions sparing the Broca area, but
word-list generation (also called word fluency) is impaired by left-sided frontal insults. The easiest version
of this task involves asking the patient to name as many
animals as possible in one minute. The mean score for
normal controls is 18 (Goodglass and Kaplan, 1972).
A more difficult variant of the task is to ask the patient
to name as many words as possible beginning with a
specified letter (usually ''F,'' ''A,'' and ''S'' with a
normal mean consisting of 15 words per minute for each
letter) (Borkowski et al., 1967; Perret, 1974). Subcortical lesions and lesions producing aphasia also disrupt
word-list generation, and these must be excluded before an impaired performance is attributed to a left frontal lesion. Word-list generation is one of the few available
tests that distinguish left and right frontal lobe dysfunction (Benton, 1968; Perret, 1974; Walsh, 1978).

Visuospatial functions are altered by frontal convexity lesions. The aberrant strategies used by patients

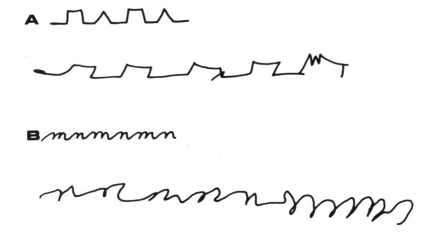

Figure 6–1. Examples of alternating programs used to elicit motor programming deficits and typical types of error committed: [Please note: in both A&B the model is above and the copy is below.]

with frontal lesions in attempting to copy figures are best revealed by complex stimuli such as the Rey-Osterrieth Complex Figure (Figure 6-3). Rather than analyzing the figure as an overall configuration with individual subunits, the patient simply begins copying individual elements without regard to their relationship to other parts. Stimulus boundedness and attraction to novel stimuli are often apparent in the drawings. The final product may be a reasonable facsimile of the model, but the approach is abnormal and more frequently results in a poor reproduction of the original (Albert and Kaplan, 1980; Walsh, 1978).

Abstraction and categorization skills also depend on the integrity of the frontal lobes. Interpretation of idioms and metaphors and recognition of features that determine likenesses and differences among classes of objects are impaired. Performance on tests of abstract reasoning (i.e., the Wisconsin Card Sorting Test) and interpretation of proverbs (i.e., the Gorham Proverbs Test) is abnormal (Lezak, 1976; Walsh, 1978).

Unlike the orbitofrontal syndrome where behav-

ioral alterations predominate and there is little evidence of neuropsychologic dysfunction, therefore, the frontal convexity syndrome has both personality disturbances (particularly apathy) and prominent neuropsychological abnormalities. In both syndromes, elementary motor and sensory functions as well as primary language and memory skills are intact.

Medial Frontal Syndrome

The orbitofrontal and frontal convexity syndromes have been identified as separable behavioral syndromes with corresponding anatomic lesions for many years, but recently sufficient evidence has accumulated to suggest a third frontal lobe syndrome associated with medial frontal dysfunction. The principal behavioral symptom of the medial frontal syndrome is akinesia. With acute bilateral medial lesions, the patient is in an akinetic mute state manifested by lack of spontaneous movement, absent verbalization, and failure to respond to commands. The lesions are located on the medial surfaces

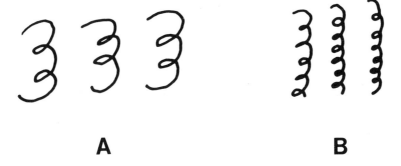

A   **B**

Figure 6-2. Multiple loops and examples of errors elicited from patients with frontal lobe lesions: **(A)** sample; **(B)** copy.

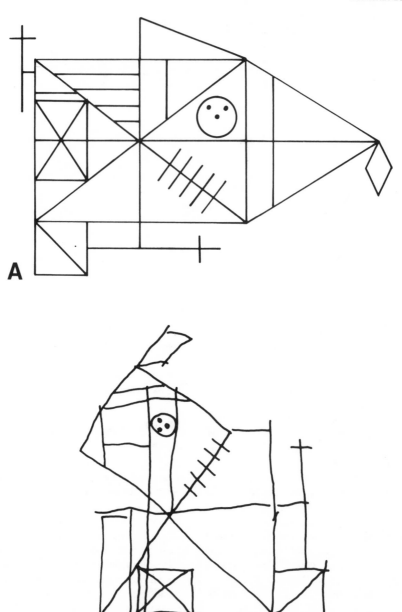

Figure 6-3. Copy of Rey-Osterrieth figure showing stimulus boundedness and attraction to novel stimuli by patient with frontal lobe damage: **(A)** model; **(B)** copy.

of the frontal lobes in the cingulate gyri (Barris and Schuman, 1953; Nielsen and Jacobs, 1951) or more inferiorly in the medial basal region inferior and anterior to the third ventricle (Ross and Stewart, 1981; Segarra, 1970).

Transcortical motor aphasia and its accompanying

behavioral alterations appear to be a limited expression of the medial frontal akinetic mute state. The patient is agestural and largely mute but is able to repeat what is said. The associated lesion is usually an infarction in the territory of the anterior cerebral artery involving the cingulate gyrus and the adjacent supplementary motor area of the left hemisphere (Alexander and Schmitt, 1980; Masdeu et al., 1978; Rubens, 1975).

Other neuropsychological correlates of the medial frontal syndrome have not been determined. Gait disturbances and sensory impairment of the lower extremity are common if the lesion extends posteriorly to involve the medial pre- and postcentral gyri. Incontinence frequently accompanies bilateral medial frontal lesions (Andrew and Nathan, 1964).

Behavioral Symptoms Associated with Frontal Lobe Dysfunction

In addition to the three primary frontal lobe syndromes, there are a variety of individual behavioral symptoms that occur with frontal lobe dysfunction (Table 6-2). They may accompany one of the three fundamental syndromes or occur independently of them. Broca's aphasia and aphemia (presented in Chapter 3) and elementary motor disorders associated with precentral gyrus lesions are not discussed here.

Although memory impairment has been attributed to frontal lobe dysfunction, true amnesia is uncommon with frontal lobe lesions. Inattention, distractibility, poor motivation, segmented approach to problem solving, and impaired strategy generation disturb the patient's approach to learning, but memory processes per se are intact in most patients with frontal lobe dysfunction. In rare cases, medial basal forebrain lesions associated with anterior communicating artery aneurysms have been associated with amnesia syndromes (Chapter 4) (Alexander and Freedman, 1984). Frontal lobe lesions may contribute to symptoms associated with memory impairment, particularly confabulation and reduplicative paramnesia. Confabulation may be of either the "embarrassment" or "momentary" type, in which the patient fabricates answers based on past experience, or it may be the "fantastic" type in which the patient elaborates bizarre, macabre, and impossible stories (Berlyne, 1972). Experimental studies have demonstrated that confabulation correlates better with lack of self-monitoring than with memory impairment, and clinicopathological correlations suggest that confabulation is likely when memory disturbances occur in patients with concomitant frontal lobe dysfunction (Chapter 4) (Kapur and Coughlan, 1980; Mercer et al., 1977; Shapiro et al., 1981; Stuss et al., 1978).

Reduplicative paramnesia is a disorder of spatial orientation wherein the patients insist that their current environments are relocated elsewhere, usually nearer to their homes (Chapter 4). In most cases the patients are recovering from posttraumatic encephalopathy or other acute cerebral insults and usually have combined fron-

TABLE 6-2.   Behavioral Symptoms Associated with Frontal Lobe Lesions

Confabulation
Reduplicative paramnesia
Depression
Secondary mania
Catatonia
Dysprosody
Callosal disconnection syndrome
Eye movement abnormalities
Hemispatial neglect

tal and right parietal lesions (Benson et al., 1976; Ruff and Volpe, 1981).

A variety of neuropsychiatric disorders have been associated with frontal lobe dysfunction, including depression, mania, and catatonia. These are discussed in detail in Chapters 12 and 14 but are mentioned briefly here to emphasize their relationship to frontal lobe injuries. Depression among patients with left frontal strokes and nonfluent aphasia has been compared with mood disturbances in those with left parietal strokes and fluent aphasia. Depression was found to be significantly more common among patients with frontal infarctions (Robinson and Benson, 1981; Robinson and Szetela, 1981). Depression has also been associated with mass lesions of both left and right frontal lobes (Chapter 14) (Avery, 1971; Lin et al., 1952; Strauss and Keschner, 1935) and with traumatic injuries to the frontal lobes (Lishman, 1978).

Euphoria and inappropriate jocularity is common among patients with frontal disorders, particularly when the orbital cortex is involved (Botez, 1974), and a few patients develop mania or hypomania in association with frontal lobe dysfunction. Lesions producing manic behavior have been located in the posteroinferior and medial regions of the frontal lobe near the third ventricle and have included tumors, infarctions, trauma, and degenerative changes (Chapter 14) (Cohn et al., 1977; Cummings and Mendez, 1984; Oppler, 1950).

Catatonia occurs in schizophrenia, affective illnesses, metabolic and toxic encephalopathies and with focal CNS lesions (Chapter 12) (Gelenberg, 1976). Frontal lobe lesions are among the localized disorders producing catatonia, and the lesions are typically located in the inferior and medial regions, suggesting a close relationship to the akinetic syndrome discussed earlier (Belfer and d'Autremont, 1971; Roberts, 1965; Thompson, 1970).

Dysprosody, the loss of the inflectional, rhythmic, and melodic aspects of speech, occurs with lesions of the right frontal region analogous to the Broca area of the left hemisphere (Ross, 1981; Ross and Mesulam, 1979).

Frontal lobe lesions frequently involve the corpus callosum and may produce callosal disconnection syndromes. The anterior cerebral artery supplies the medial frontal lobe and the anterior four-fifths of the corpus callosum, rendering the callosum vulnerable to infarction with anterior cerebral artery occlusion. Intrinsic frontal lobe tumors frequently spread through the corpus callosum to involve both frontal lobes as well as the connecting fibers. Traumatic frontal lesions frequently include contusions of the corpus callosum produced by contact with the hard fibrous falx cerebri extending vertically between the hemispheres. Behavioral manifestations of callosal interruption in the frontal region include apraxia of the left hand (Chapter 3), left-hand agraphia, tactile anomia of the left hand, constructional disturbances, and impaired cross-replication of hand postures (Bogen, 1979; Geschwind and Kaplan, 1962; Rubens et al., 1977).

Several eye movement disorders have been associated with frontal lobe lesions. With acute destructive prefontal lesions, the eyes are deviated toward the side of the lesion (away from an accompanying hemiparesis). In addition, the patient will have difficulty generating saccadic (volitional) eye movements in the direction opposite to the tonic deviation. Saccadic movements in response to moving targets and vestibular stimulation may be absent and volitional movements away from the side of the lesion will be executed in a series of hypometric saccades (Hoyt and Daroff, 1971). These abnormalities usually remit within a few weeks, although minimum deficits may persist. Visual exploration of complex stimuli is also defective (Luria et al., 1966; Tyler, 1969).

Unilateral spatial neglect may occur with frontal lobe lesions (Chapter 5) (Heilman and Valenstein, 1972; Mesulam, 1981; Stein and Volpe, 1983). The patients neglect all stimuli from the contralateral space and fail to direct actions into the neglected hemispace. The limbs of the neglected side may or may not be paretic but are not utilized.

ANATOMIC CORRELATES OF FRONTAL LOBE SYNDROMES

The frontal lobe is conveniently divided into four general areas: (1) the precentral area or primary motor area anterior to the central sulcus (area 4 of Brodmann), (2) the premotor area immediately anterior to the precentral cortex (area 6 of Brodmann), (3) the prefrontal area occupying the rest of the frontal lobe anterior to

the premotor cortex, and (4) the limbic cortex of the cingulate gyrus on the medial aspects of the frontal lobe anterior and superior to the corpus callosum (Damasio, 1979; Truex and Carpenter, 1969). The supplementary motor area is a subregion of the precentral cortex on the medial aspect of the hemisphere anterior to premotor and posterior to prefrontal cortex (DeVito and Smith, 1959; Penfield and Welch, 1951; Truex and Carpenter, 1969). The behavioral syndromes described in the preceding section occur primarily with lesions of the prefrontal cortex (dorsal convexity or orbitofrontal regions) or the medial limbic areas. These regions have different afferent and efferent connections, and these anatomic distinctions provide a basis for the distinctive behavioral alterations that accompany lesions in each area.

The dorsolateral convexity region of the prefrontal cortex has diverse connections to other cortical areas and to subcortical structures. Cortical afferents to the polar-convexity region arise from sensory association cortices in the inferior parietal and temporal lobes (Fuster, 1980; Jones and Powell, 1970; Nauta, 1971). The principal subcortical afferents to prefrontal convexity originate in the dorsomedial nucleus of the thalamus (Kievit and Kuypers, 1977; McLardy, 1950; Nauta, 1971). Prefrontal cortical efferents project to the areas from which they receive afferents and, in addition, connect with the hypothalamus, hippocampus, and basal ganglia (Beck et al., 1951; Fuster, 1980; Goldman and Nauta, 1977; Johnson et al, 1968).

The orbitofrontal cortex is much more closely linked with the limbic system than is the dorsolateral frontal convexity. The orbital regions are reciprocally connected with the dorsomedial nucleus and the amygdala (Damasio, 1979; Fuster, 1980; Nauta, 1961). The orbital cortex also projects through the medial forebrain bundle to rostral brainstem regions (French et al., 1955). The orbitofrontal cortex is reciprocally connected to the frontal polar regions and the dorsolateral frontal convexity.

The frontal limbic cortex located in the cingulate gyrus on the medial aspect of the frontal lobe is connected to amygdala, anterior thalamus, and septum. It projects to the midbrain, supplementary motor cortex, premotor cortex, and basal ganglia and receives projections from sensory association cortices (Baleydier and Mauguiere, 1980; Damasio and Van Hoesen, 1983; Ward, 1948).

The anatomic relationships provide the basis for tentative structure–function correlations underlying the frontal lobe syndromes. The dorsolateral convexity receives highly integrated sensory information from sensory systems mediating external perception. It also receives internal and "emotional" information from the adjacent orbitofrontal cortex and its limbic system connections. This portion of the frontal lobe is thus optimally situated to monitor ongoing sensory input, to simultaneously assess the emotional significance of "external" events and the internal emotional state, and to initiate appropriate motor responses (Damasio, 1979; Jouandet and Gazzaniga, 1979; Nauta, 1971). Disruption results in an apathetic lack of response, impaired motor programming, and poor self-monitoring—the principal components of the dorsolateral frontal syndrome. Acute unilateral lesions produce contralateral sensory–motor neglect.

The orbitofrontal cortex has its primary connections with the limbic system, thalamus, and frontal convexity. It is the neocortical representation of the limbic system (Nauta, 1971). Lesions in this region appear to divorce frontal monitoring systems from limbic input, resulting in a disinhibited behavioral syndrome where impulses are acted on without consideration of consequences, antisocial actions occur, and emotional lability is marked. Sensory, motor, and cognitive processes are not mediated in this region and lesions do not produce neuropsychologic deficits such as those occurring with convexity lesions.

Medial frontal lesions affect both the supplementary motor area and the limbic–cingulate cortex. These two areas are heavily interconnected, and the latter is also integrated with limbic system through projections to amygdala and anterior thalamus. Connections with dopaminergic limbic midbrain regions provide an anatomochemical basis for the similarity between the akinesia of parkinsonism and the akinesia associated with medial frontal lesions (Damasio and Van Hoesen, 1983; Ross and Stewart, 1981).

Inspection of anatomic connections of the frontal lobes also provides an explanation for the similarities in behavior of patients with frontal lobe lesions and those with subcortical disorders affecting thalamus and basal ganglia. Frontal convexity regions project to anterodorsal caudate, lateral globus pallidus, subthalamic nucleus, and hippocampus, whereas the orbital cortex projects to ventrolateral caudate, medial globus pallidus, centromedian nucleus of thalamus, hypothalamus, and septum. Lesions on either end of these cortical–subcortical projections produce similar behavioral alterations. This may acount for the behavioral similarities of patients with frontal disorders and those with subcortical diseases such as Huntington's disease, Parkinson's disease, and other extrapyramidal syndromes (Rosvold, 1972).

ETIOLOGIES OF FRONTAL LOBE SYNDROMES

As noted earlier, most conditions affecting the frontal lobes—trauma, neoplasms, infections, and demyelinating disorders—affect both lobes, and most fron-

tal syndromes reflect bilateral frontal dysfunction. Vascular occlusions involving the anterior cerebral artery are capable of producing unilateral frontal lesions.

The orbitofrontal syndrome arises from damage to the inferior frontal lobe overlying the bony roofs of the orbits. The orbital roofs comprise the floor of the anterior cranial fossa. The most common injury to the orbitofrontal cortex results from blunt head trauma with contusion of the inferior frontal cortex and adjacent white matter connections by the irregular bony surface (Arseni et al., 1966; Blumer and Benson, 1975; Courville, 1950; Lindenberg and Freytag, 1960). A second common etiology is compression by a subfrontal neoplasm arising from the pituitary fossa, olfactory groove, or sphenoid ridge. Meningiomas and chromophobe adenomas are particularly frequent in these locations (Hunter et al., 1968; Russell and Rubinstein, 1977). Aneurysms arising from the anterior communicating artery can also act as mass lesions or rupture into the orbitofrontal and medial frontal areas (Logue et al., 1968). Intrinsic brain tumors, vascular infarctions, degenerative disorders, encephalitis, psychosurgery, and demyelinating diseases are less frequent causes of the orbitofrontal syndrome (Blumer and Benson, 1975; Reitman, 1946).

Frontal convexity lesions result from disorders similar to those producing the orbitofrontal syndrome, accounting for the frequent simultaneous occurrence of orbitofrontal and convexity symptoms. The differential diagnosis of etiologies of the frontal convexity syndrome includes trauma, hydrocephalus, external compressive neoplasms (meningiomas) and intrinsic tumors (gliomas), demyelinating disorders, and degenerative diseases (Blumer and Benson, 1975; Direkze et al., 1971; Fisher, 1969; Frazier, 1936; Kolodny,1929; Sachs, 1950; Strauss and Keschner, 1935). Among the degenerative dementias, Alzheimer's disease has greater involvement of the frontal convexity region, whereas Pick's disease preferentially affects the orbitofrontal cortex (Brun and Gustafson, 1978; Cummings and Benson, 1983).

The akinetic frontal lobe syndrome and its variants are associated with medial lesions, usually of a vascular nature (Barris and Schuman, 1953; Critchley, 1930; Nielsen and Jacobs, 1951). The syndrome has also been produced by deep medial tumors and by hydrocephalus (Lavy, 1959; Messert et al., 1966; Ross and Stewart, 1981).

Psychosurgery may produce either an orbitofrontal syndrome or a frontal convexity syndrome depending on the site and extent of the neurosurgical lesions. Medial frontal and orbitofrontal lesions may produce marked personality changes manifested by euphoria, increased motor activity, and impulsiveness (Reitman, 1946). Neuropsychological testing reveals deficits on the Wisconsin Card Sorting Test reflecting abnormali-

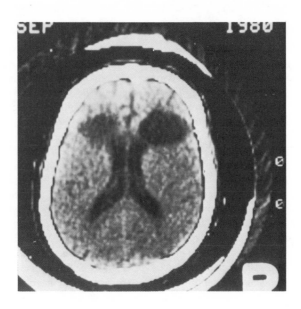

Figure 6-4. Computerized axial tomogram demonstrating bilateral frontal lobotomy lesions lateral to the frontal horns of the lateral ventribles.

ties in abstracting and maintaining and shifting mental sets appropriately (Benson and Stuss, 1982; Benson et al., 1981; Kelly and Mitchell-Heggs, 1973; Knight, 1969; Scherer, 1961; Scherer et al., 1957; Stuss et al., 1981a,b, 1983; Wehler and Hoffman, 1978). More laterally placed lesions (Fig. 6-4) produce different personality alterations and more extensive neuropsychological deficits. The personality changes include loss of drive, stimulus boundedness, and impaired ability to elaborate experiences (Greenblatt and Solomon, 1958). Neuropsychological assessment reveals difficulty with abstraction as well as deteriorated performance on tests of intelligence (Hamlin, 1970; Poppen et al., 1965; Smith and Kinder, 1959).

Frontal lobe syndromes are usually the result of overt structural changes, but some chronic toxic encephalopathies appear to involve primarily frontal lobe functions. Chronic alcholic dementia (Chapter 8) has a predilection for affecting neuropsychological abilities mediated by the frontal lobes or related subcortical structures. Typical personality changes include an irritable apathy, and cognitive deficits include impaired word-list generation, poor attention, visuospatial abnormalities, impaired memory, and poor abstraction (Brandt et al., 1983; Brewer and Perrett, 1971; Cutting, 1978; Jones and Parsons, 1971; Lishman, 1981; Ron, 1977; Tarter, 1975). The deficits may partially or completely remit if the patient remains abstinent.

TREATMENT OF FRONTAL LOBE SYNDROMES

No specific treatments have been devised for the successful management of either the orbitofrontal syndrome or the frontal convexity syndrome. In all cases the preliminary management is directed at discovering the underlying etiology and treating the causative process. Behavioral improvement may follow resection of a neoplasm or shunting of hydrocephalus, and considerable spontaneous resolution may follow vascular or traumatic insults to the frontal lobes. A variety of pharmacological agents have been tried in an attempt to modify the disinhibited behavior of the patient with an orbitofrontal injury. Major tranquilizers, minor tranquilizers, lithium, propranolol, and carbamazepine have all been used with some success in individual patients, but none has proved to be uniformly reliable. Psychostimulants (amphetamines, methylphenidate) have been used in patients with the frontal convexity syndrome because they are apathetic and also because their impairments are similar to those of children with attention deficit disorders. Response to such treatment has been variable. Patients with the akinetic syndrome associated with medial frontal lesions have occasionally responded to dopamine agonists (levodopa, bromocriptine) (Ross and Stewart, 1981).

REFERENCES

Albert MS and Kaplan E. Organic implications of neuropsychological deficits in the elderly. In Poon LW, Focard JL, Cermak LS, Arenberg D, and Thompson LW (Eds.): *New directions in memory and aging*. Hillsdale, New Jersey, Lawrence Erlbaum Associates, 1980. pp. 403–432.

Alexander MP and Freedman M. Amnesia after anterior communicating artery aneurysm rupture. *Neurology* 1984, *34*, 752–757.

Alexander MP and Schmitt MAS. The aphasia syndrome of stroke in the left anterior cerebral artery territory. *Arch Neurol*, 1980, *37*, 97–100.

Andrew J and Nathan PW. Lesions of the anterior frontal lobes and disturbances of micturition and defaecation. *Brain*, 1964, *87;* 233–262.

Arseni C, Botez MI, Alexandru S, and Simionescu MD. Bilateral defect of frontal and orbital lobes. *Internat J Neurol*, 1966, *5*, 430–441.

Avery TL. Seven cases of frontal tumour with psychiatric presentation. *Br J Psychiat*, 1971, *119*, 19–23.

Baleydier C and Mauguiere F. The duality of the cingulate gyrus in monkey. *Brain*, 1980, *103*, 525–554.

Barris RW and Schuman HR. Bilateral anterior cingulate gyrus lesions. *Neurology*, 1953, *3*, 44–52.

Beck E, Meyer A, and LeBeau J. Efferent connexions of the human prefrontal region with reference to fronto-hypothalamic pathways. *J Neurol Neurosurg Psychiat*, 1951, *14*, 295–302.

Belfer ML and d'Autremont CC. Catatonia-like symptomatology. *Arch Gen Psychiat*, 1971, *24*, 119–120.

Benson DF, Gardner H, and Meadows JC. Reduplicative paramnesia. *Neurology*, 1976, *26*, 147–151.

Benson DF and Stuss DT. Motor abilities after frontal leukotomy. *Neurology*, 1982, *32*, 1353–1357.

Benson DF, Stuss DT, Naeser MA, Weir WS, Kaplan EF, and Levine HL. The long-term effects of prefrontal leukotomy. *Arch Neurol*, 1981, *38*, 165–169.

Benton AL. Differential effects in frontal lobe disease. *Neuropsychologia*, 1968, *6*, 53–60.

Berlyne N. Confabulation. *Br J Psychiat*, 1972, *120*, 130–139.

Blumer D and Benson DF. Personality changes with frontal and temporal lobe lesions. In Benson DF and Blumer D (Eds.): *Psychiatric aspects of neurologic disease*. New York, Grune & Stratton, 1975, pp. 151–169.

Bogen JE. The callosal syndrome. In Heilman KM and Valenstein E (Eds.): *Clinical neuropsychology*. New York, Oxford University Press, 1979, pp. 308–359.

Borkowski JG, Benton AL, and Spreen O. Word fluency and brain damage. *Neuropsychologia*, 1967, *5*, 135–140.

Botez MI, Frontal lobe tumours. In Vinken PJ and Bruyn GW (Eds.): *Tumors of the brain and skull*, Vol. 17. *Handbook of clinical neurology*. 1974, pp. 234–280.

Brandt J, Butters N, Ryan C, and Bayog R. Cognitive loss and recovery in long-term alcohol abusers. *Arch Gen Psychiat*, 1983, *40*, 435–442.

Brewer C and Perrett L. Brain damage due to alcohol consumption: an air-encephalographic, psychometric and electroencephalographic study. *Br J Addict*, 1971, *66*, 170–182.

Brun A and Gustafson L. Limbic lobe involvement in presenile dementia. *Arch Psychiat Nervenkr*, 1978, *226*, 79–93.

Cohn CK, Wright JR III, and Devaul RA. Post head trauma syndrome in an adolescent treated with lithium carbonate—case report. *Dis Nerv Syst*, 1977, *38*, 630–631.

Courville CB. The mechanism of coup-contrecoup injuries of the brain. *Bull Neurol Soc.*, 1950, *15*, 72–86.

Critchley M. The anterior cerebral artery, and its syndromes. *Brain*, 1930, 53, 120–165.

Cummings JL and Benson DF. *Dementia: a clinical approach*. Boston, Butterworths, 1983.

Cummings JL and Mendez MF. Secondary mania with focal cerebrovascular lesions. *Am J Psychiat*, 1984, *14*, 1084–1087.

Cutting J. Specific psychological deficits in alcoholism. *Br J Psychiat*, 1978, *133*, 119–122.

Damasio A. The frontal lobes. In Heilman KM and Valenstein E (Eds.):*Clinical neuropsychology*. New York, Oxford University Press, 1979, pp. 360–412.

Damasio AR and Van Hoesen GW. Emotional disturbances associated with focal lesions of the limbic frontal lobe. In Heilman KM and Satz P (Eds.): *Neuropsychology of human emotion*. New York, Guilford Press, 1983, pp. 85–110.

DeVito JL and Smith OA, Jr. Projections from the mesial frontal cortex (supplementary motor area) to the cerebral hemispheres and brain stem of the macaca mulatta. *J Comp Neurol*, 1959, *111*, 261–278.

Direkze M, Bayliss SG, and Cutting JC. Primary tumours of the frontal lobe. *Br J Clin Pract*, 1971, *25*, 207–213.

Drewe EA. Go–no go learning after frontal lobe lesions in humans. *Cortex*, 1975, *11*, 8–16.

Faust CR. Different psychological consequences due to superior frontal and orbito-basal lesions. *Internat J Neurol*, 1966, *5*, 410–421.

Fisher A. On meningioma presenting with dementia. *Proc Aust Assoc Neurol*, 1969, *6*, 29–38.

Frazier CH. Tumor involving the frontal lobe alone. *Arch Neurol Psychiat*, 1936, *35*, 525–571.

French JD, Hernandez-Peon R, and Livingston RB. Projections from cortex to cephalic brain stem (reticular formation) in monkey. *J Neurophysiol*, 1955, *18*, 74–95.

Fuster JM. *The prefrontal cortex*. New York, Raven Press, 1980.

Gelenberg AJ. The catatonic syndrome. *Lancet*, 1976, *1*, 1339–1341.

Geschwind N and Kaplan E. A human cerebral deconnection syndrome. *Neurology*, 1962, *12*, 675–685.

Goldman PS and Nauta WJH. An intricately patterned prefronto-caudate projection in the rhesus monkey. *J Comp Neurol*, 1977, *171*, 369–386.

Greenblatt M and Solomon HC. Studies of lobotomy. *Assn Res New Ment Dis*, 1958, *36*, 19–34.

Goodglass H and Kaplan E. *The assessment of aphasia and related disorders*. Philadelphia, Lea & Febiger, 1972.

Hamlin RM. Intellectual function 14 years after frontal lobe surgery. *Cortex*, 1970, *6*, 299–307.

Heilman KM and Valenstein E. Frontal lobe neglect in man. *Neurology*, 1972, *22*, 660–664.

Hoyt WF and Daroff RB. Supranuclear disorders of ocular control systems in man. In Bach-y-Rita P and Collins CC (Eds.): *The control of eye movements*. New York, Academic Press, 1971, pp. 175–235.

Hunter R, Blackwood W, and Bull J. Three cases of frontal meningiomas presenting psychiatrically. *Br Med J*, 1968, *3*, 9–16.

Jarvie HF. Frontal lobe wounds causing disinhibition. *J Neurol Neurosurg Psychiat*, 1954, *17*, 14–32.

Johnson TN, Rosvold HE, and Mishkin M. Projections from behaviorally-defined sectors of the prefrontal cortex to the basal ganglia, septum, and diencephalon of the monkey. *Exp Neurol*, 1968, *21*, 20–34.

Jones B and Parsons A. Impaired abstracting ability in chronic alcoholics. *Arch Gen Psychiat*, 1971, *24*, 71–75.

Jones EG and Powell TPS. An anatomic study of converging sensory pathways within the cerebral cortex of the monkey. *Brain*, 1970, *93*, 793–820.

Jouandet M and Gazzaniga MS. The frontal lobes. In Gazzaniga MS (Ed.): *Handbook of behavioral neurobiology*, Vol. 2, *Neuropsychology*. New York, Plenum Press, 1979, pp. 25–59.

Kapur N and Coughlan AK. Confabulation and frontal lobe dysfunction. *J Neurol Neurosurg Psychiat*, 1980, *43*, 461–463.

Kelly D and Mitchell-Heggs N. Stereotactic limbic leucotomy—a follow-up study of thirty patients. *Postgrad Med J*, 1973, *49*, 805–882.

Kievit J and Kuypers HGJM. Organization of the thalamo-cortical connections to the frontal lobe in the rhesus monkey. *Brain Res*, 1977, *29*, 229–322.

Knight GC. Bifrontal stereotactic tractotomy: an atraumatic operation of value in the treatment of intractable psychoneurosis. *Br J Psychiat*, 1969, *115*, 257–266.

Kolb B and Whishaw IQ. *Fundamentals of human neuropsychology*. San Francisco, WH Freeman & Company, 1980.

Kolodny A. Symptomatology of tumor of the frontal lobe. *Arch Neurol Psychiat*, 1929, *21*, 1107–1127.

Lavy S. Akinetic mutism in a case of craniopharyngioma. *Psychiat Neurol* (Basel), 1959, *138*, 369–374.

Lezak MD. *Neuropsychological assessment*. New York, Oxford University Press, 1976.

Lhermitte F. "Utilization behavior" and its relation to lesions of the frontal lobes. *Brain*, 1983, *106*, 237–255.

Lin T-Y, Greenblatt M, and Solomon HC. Agitated depression associated with arteriovenous aneurysm of left frontal lobe. *New Engl J Med*, 1952, *247*, 631–633.

Lindenberg R and Freytag E. The mechanism of cerebral contusions. *Arch Pathol*, 1960, *69*, 440–469.

Lishman WA. *Organic psychiatry*. London, Blackwell Scientific Publications, 1978.

Lishman WA. Cerebral disorder in alcoholism. *Brain*, 1981, *104*, 1–20.

Logue V, Durward M, Pratt RTC, Piercy M, and Nixon WLB. The quality of survival after rupture of an anterior cerebral aneurysm. *Br J Psychiat*, 1968, *114*, 137–160.

Luria AR. *Higher cortical functions in man*, 2nd ed., New York, Basic Books, 1980.

Luria AR, Karpov BA, and Yarbuss AL. Disturbances of active visual perception with lesions of the frontal lobes. *Cortex*, 1966, *2*, 202–212.

Masdeu JC, Schoene WC, and Fuukenstein H. Aphasia following infarction of the left supplementary motor area. *Neurology*, 1978, *28*, 1220–1223.

McLardy T. Thalamic projection to frontal cortex in man. *J Neurol Neurosurg Psychiat*, 1950, *13*, 198–202.

Mercer B, Wapner W, Gardner H, and Benson DF. A study of confabulation. *Arch Neurol*, 1977, *34*, 429–433.

Messert B, Henke TK, and Langheim W. Syndrome of akinetic mutism associated with obstructive hydrocephalus. *Neurology*, 1966, *16*, 635–649.

Mesulam M-M. A cortical network for directed attention and unilateral neglect. *Ann Neurol*, 1981, *10*, 309–325.

Nauta WJH. Fibre degeneration following lesions of the amygdaloid complex in the monkey. *J Anat*, 1961, *95*, 515–531.

Nauta WJH. The problem of the frontal lobe: a reinterpretation. *J Psychiat Res*, 1971, *8*, 167–187.

Neilsen JM and Jacobs LL. Bilateral lesions of the anterior cingulate gyri. *Bull Neurol Soc.*, 1951, *16*, 231–234.

Oppler W. Manic psychosis in a case of parasagittal meningioma. *Arch Neurol Psychiat*, 1950, *64*, 417–430.

Penfield W and Welch K. The supplementary motor area of the cerebral cortex. *Arch Neurol Psychiat*, 1951, *66*, 289–317.

Perret E. The left frontal lobe of man and the suppression of habitual responses in verbal categorical behavior. *Neuropsychologia*, 1974, *12*, 323–330.

Poppen RL, Pribram KH, and Robinson RS. Effects of frontal lobotomy in man on the performance of the multiple choice task. *Exp Neurol*, 1965, *11*, 217–229.

Reitman F. Orbital cortex syndrome following leucotomy. *Am J Psychiat*, 1946, *103*, 238–241.

Roberts DR. Catatonia in the brain: a localization study. *Internat J Neuropsychiat*, 1965, *1*, 395–403.

Robinson RG and Benson DF. Depression in aphasic patients: frequency, severity, and clinical-pathological correlations. *Brain Lang*, 1981, *14*, 282–291.

Robinson RG and Szetela B. Mood change following left hemispheric brain injury. *Ann Neurol*, 1981, *9*, 447–453.

Ron MA. Brain damage in chronic alcoholism: a neuropathological, neuroradiological and psychological review. *Psychol Med*, 1977, *7*, 103–112.

Ross ED. The aprosodias. *Arch Neurol*, 1981, *38*, 561–569.

Ross ED and Mesulam M-M. Dominant language functions of the right hemisphere? *Arch Neurol*, 1979, *36*, 144–148.

Ross ED and Stewart RM. Akinetic mutism from hypothalamic damage: successful treatment with dopamine agonists. *Neurology*, 1981, *31*, 1435–1439.

Rosvold HE. The frontal lobe system: cortical-subcortical interrelationships. *Acta Neurobiol Exp*, 1972, *32*, 435–460.

Rubens AB. Aphasia with infarction in the territory of the anterior cerebral artery. *Cortex*, 1975, *11*, 239–250.

Rubens AB, Geschwind N, Mahowald MW, and Mastri A. Post traumatic cerebral hemispheric disconnection syndrome. *Arch Neurol*, 1977, *34*, 750–755.

Ruff RL and Volpe BT. Environmental reduplication associated with right frontal and parietal lobe injury. *J Neurol Neurosurg Psychiat*, 1981, *44*, 382–386.

Russell DS and Rubinstein LJ. *Pathology of tumours of the nervous system*. Baltimore, Williams & Wilkins Company, 1977.

Sachs E Jr. Meningiomas with dementia as the first presenting feature. *J Ment Sci*, 1950, *96*, 998–1007.

Scherer IW. Prognoses and psychological scores in electro-convulsive therapy, psychosurgery, and spontaneous remission. *Am J Psychiat*, 1961, *107*, 926–931.

Scherer IW, Klett CJ, and Winne JF. Psychological changes over a five year period following bilateral prefrontal lobotomy. *J Consult Psychol*, 1957, *21*, 291–295.

Segarra JM. Cerebral vascular disease and behavior. I. The syndrome of the mesencephalic artery (basilar artery bifurcation). *Arch Neurol*, 1970, *22*, 408–418.

Shapiro BE, Alexander MP, Gardner H. and Mercer B. Mechanisms of confabulation. *Neurology*, 1981, *31*, 1070–1076.

Smith A and Kinder EF. Changes in psychological test performances of brain operated schizophrenics after 8 years. *Science*, 1959, *129*, 145–150.

Stein S and Volpe BT. Classical "parietal" neglect syndrome after subcortical right frontal lobe infarction. *Neurology*, 1983, *33*, 797–799.

Strauss I and Keschner M. Mental symptoms in cases of tumor of the frontal lobe. *Arch Neurol Psychiat*, 1935, *33*, 986–1105.

Stuss DT, Alexander MP, Lieberman A, and Levine H. An extraordinary form of confabulation. *Neurology*, 1978, *28*, 1166–1072.

Stuss DT, Benson DF, Kaplan EF, Weir WS, and Della Malva

C. Leucotomized and nonleucotomized schizophrenics: comparison on tests of attention. *Biol Psychiat*, 1981a, *16*, 1085–1100.

Stuss DT, Kaplan EF, Benson DF, Weir WS, Naeser MA, and Levine HL. Long-term effects of prefrontal leuctomy—an overview of neuropsychologic residuals. *J Clin Neuropsychol*, 1981b, *3*, 13–32.

Stuss DT, Benson DF, Kaplan EF, Weir WS, Naeser MA, Lieberman I, and Ferrill D. The involvement of orbitofrontal cerebrum in cognitive tasks. *Neuropsychologia*, 1983, *21*, 235–248.

Stuss DT and Benson DF. Neuropsychological studies of the frontal lobes. *Psychol Bull*, 1984, *95*, 3–28.

Tarter RE. Psychological deficits in chronic alcoholics: a review. *Internat J Addict*, 1975, *10*, 327–368.

Thompson GN. Cerebral lesions simulating schizophrenia: three case reports. *Biol Psychiat*, 1970, *2*, 59–64.

Truex RC and Carpenter MB. *Human neuroanatomy*, 6th ed. Baltimore, Williams & Wilkins Company, 1969.

Tyler HR. Defective stimulus exploration in aphasic patients. *Neurology*, 1969, *19*, 105–112.

Walsh KW. *Neuropsychology. A clinical approach*. New York, Churchill Livingston, 1978.

Ward AA JR. The cingular gyrus: area 24. *J Neurophysiol*, 1948, *11*, 12–23.

Wehler R and Hoffman H. Intellectual functioning in lobotomized and non-lobotomized long term chronic schizophrenia patients. *J Clin Psychol*, 1978, *34*, 449–451.

Zangwill OL. Psychological deficits associated with frontal lobe lesions. *Internat J Neurol*, 1960, *5*, 395–402.

Chapter 7

Acute Confusional States

The acute confusional state (ACS) is synonymous with "delirium" and in this volume is used specifically to denote a state of relatively abrupt onset and short duration whose major behavioral characteristic is altered attention (Berrios, 1981; Chedru and Geschwind, 1972a; Lipowski, 1967, 1980). Other behavioral abnormalities frequently coexist with the clouded, reduced, or shifting attention, including cognitive disturbances, hallucinations and delusions, sleep cycle abnormalities, and autonomic dysfunction. In most cases the EEG reveals diffuse slowing (Cadilhac and Ribstein, 1961; Engel et al., 1946; Pro and Wells, 1977; Romano and Engel, 1944).

"Confusion" is among the most misused of all behavioral terms. It is often applied vaguely and indiscriminately to patients whose behavior is erratic, incoherent, os psychotic. Confusion is often linked to disorientation, dementia, delirium, or psychosis without specifying the behavior to which it refers. When used in this vague and undefined way, "confusion" loses all meaning as a behavioral descriptor and fails to communicate any relevant information about the state of the patient. In this chapter, "confusion" is used to refer only to states characterized predominantly by attentional alterations. The terms "ACS" and "delirium" are used synonymously, whereas "chronic confusional state" is one of the etiologies of the dementia syndrome and is considered in Chapter 8.

CLINICAL CHARACTERISTICS

Table 7-1 lists the principal behavioral manifestations of the ACS. The behavioral change that defines the syndrome and determines many of the other clinical alterations is an alteration of attention (Chedru and Gerschwind, 1972a). The level of consciousness may be reduced or may fluctuate between drowsiness and hypervigilance, but the patient is unable to maintain attention for any substantial period of time. Even when arousal and level of consciousness per se are not abnormal, subtle attentional deficits can usually be elicited on examination. Digit span (number of digits the patient can repeat forward or backward after presentation by the examiner) and continuous performance tests (asking patients to raise their hands each time they hear an "A" within a sequence of spoken letters) are among the best mental status tests for detecting attentional deficits and should be performed on all patients in whom an ACS is a consideration.

The attentional impairment is associated with and contributes to alterations in language, memory, constructions, perceptions, and mood (Simon and Cahan, 1963). Language abnormalities noted during the ACS include abnormal spontaneous speech, anomia, the syndrome of nonaphasic misnaming, and agraphia. Spontaneous speech is often incoherent, rambling, and shifts from topic to topic. Intelligibility is further limited by the hypophonia and slurring of speech that frequently coexist with the language changes. Anomia may be noted in the course of spontaneous speech or on tests of confrontation naming. Paraphasia is rare, and the anomia is usually manifested as a simple failure to recall the correct name (Benson, 1979; Chedru and Geschwind, 1972a). In the syndrome of nonaphasic misnaming, naming errors are most pronounced for illness-related items, the anomia propagates (i.e., all misnamed items are named according to a specific theme), the speech style is pedantic or bombastic, and there is a tendency to make facetious and bizarre responses (Cummings et al., 1980; Curran and Schilder, 1935; Geschwind, 1964; Weinstein and Kahn, 1952; Weinstein and Keller, 1963). In almost all reported cases, patients manifesting nonaphasic misnaming have experienced ACSs and have had anomia in association with their "nonaphasic" abnormalities.

Agraphia is sometimes particularly marked in the ACS, and writing errors may be out of proportion to other behavioral and linguistic alterations. Writing abnormalities include illegibility and abnormal spatial alignment, abbreviated agrammatical sentences, and spelling errors. The latter tend to involve small grammatical words and ends of words, and omissions, substitutions,

TABLE 7-1.   Principal Clinical Characteristics of Acute Confusional States

Alertness
  Clouded or fluctuating consciousness
	Other behavioral alterations
	  Perseveration and/or impersistence
	  Occupational pantomime

Attention
  Impaired attention, distractible
	Neurosychiatric disorders
	  Hallucinations

Language
  Incoherent spontaneous speech
  Anomia
  Agraphia
  Variable comprehension defect
  Nonaphasic misnaming
	Delusions
	  Mood alterations
	
	Motor system abnormalities
	  Psychomotor retardation and/or hyperactivity
	  Action tremor
	  Asterixis

Memory
  Disoriented, poor recent memory
	Myoclonus
	  Dysarthria

Constructions Visuoconstructive deficits	Tone and reflex abnormalities Miscellaneous

Cognition
  Incoherent thought
  Concrete thinking
  Dyscalculia
	Sleep disturbances
	  Autonomic dysfunction
	
	Electroencephalogram
	  Diffuse slowing

and duplication errors are particularly common (Chedru and Geschwind, 1972b).

Memory and learning abnormalities are virtually always present in the ACS, although their severity may vary. The learning deficits are attributed to abnormalities of registration produced by the attentional limitations. Memory abnormalities are evident in the patient's inability to recall three words after 3 minutes, and the patient may even be unable to repeat the three words immediately after hearing them. The patients are usually disoriented with regard to time and place and may exhibit reduplicative paramnesia (the belief that the hospital has been relocated closer to one's home) (Chapter 4) (Levin, 1955). Disorientation, however, is a nonspecific finding occurring in amnesia, dementia, and a variety of other disorders, and its occurrence does not necessarily imply the presence of an ACS.

Constructional tasks, like writing, are also abnormal in the ACS. The drawings may be distorted or unrecognizable. Three-dimensional aspects are lost, and lines and angles are omitted (Chedru and Geschwind, 1972a).

Cognitive abnormalities are also pervasive in the ACS. Errors in calculation occur, particularly when the problem requires the patient to "carry" one sum to the next column. There is a lack of coherent thought with loss of normal associations and intrusion of abnormal associative connections. Discrepancies do not trouble the patient, who is unlikely to recognize incongruities when they are pointed out (Chedru and Geschwind, 1972a; Levin, 1956). Thinking is concrete, and abstraction and categorization skills are limited.

Perseveration is common in all aspects of behavior of patients in ACSs. It contributes to the duplication errors in writing and speaking, is apparent in recurrent but irrelevant themes of conversation, and contaminates the motor system examination (Levin, 1968). Paradoxically, impersistence may occur in the same patient with some tasks completed and perseverated while others go unfinished.

Occupational delirium refers to elaborate pantomimes performed by the patient in an ACS (Wolff and Curran, 1935). Patients act as if they are continuing their usual occupations of sweeping, driving, or working despite being, in fact, in a hospital bed. Patients in ACSs may remove nonexistent glasses, take nonexistent pills, and pantomime other activities of everyday life.

Neuropsychiatric abnormalities, including hallucinations, delusions, and mood alterations, are common in ACSs. In some cases, these disturbances dominate the clinical picture to such an extent that the patient is thought to be suffering from an idiopathic psychiatric disorder and is referred for psychiatric care. The hallucinations of the ACS tend to be silent visual images that may be fully formed, such as dogs walking through the room or people standing at the bedside or peering in through the window (Lipowski, 1980; Strub, 1982; Wolff and Curran, 1935). Tactile (formication) hallucinations are not unusual in some ACSs, particularly alcohol and cocaine withdrawal syndromes. Auditory hallucinations (voices, sounds) may occur but are less common than visual hallucinations.

The delusions occurring in ACSs may be simple, transient, and loosely held or may be complex, intricately structured, and rigidly endorsed (Chapter 13) (Cummings, 1985; Nash, 1983). Occasionally, specific delusional beliefs such as the Capgras syndrome (the belief that significant others have been replaced by identical-appearing impostors) may be the principal manifestation of an ACS (Cummings, 1985; Hay et al., 1974; Madakasira and Hall, 1981; Pies, 1982). Delusions can motivate combative, self-destructive, or paranoid behavior and can be among the most difficult aspects of an ACS to manage. Improvement in the underlying condition usually leads to resolution of the false beliefs, but in some cases small doses of a major tranquilizer may have to be used to treat the delusions, limit abnormal behavior related to the delusions, and facilitate management of the etiologic disorder.

A diverse array of mood alterations has also been observed in patients in ACSs. The most common is a labile, perplexed, excitable state. Affective alterations ranging from euphoria to depression and fearful paranoia to indifference and apathy also occur (Doty, 1946; Lipowski, 1980; Wolff and Curran, 1935). Mood changes are often congruent with the belief content of delusions in delusional patients.

Patients in ACSs may be entirely devoid of motor system abnormalities, but more commonly they manifest alterations in general activity level, tremor, asterixis, myoclonus, or tone and reflex alterations. Changes in activity level may be in the direction of hypo- or hyperactivity. Myxedema is most likely to lead to diminished psychomotor activity, whereas hyperthyroidism and delirium tremens are characterized by increased activity and motor restlessness. Not all ACSs, however, have such predictable alterations, and many factors such as rate of change in metabolic status, age of the patient, and severity of the encephalopathy influence the behavioral manifestations. In some cases, the patient may have alternating periods of hypoactivity and hyperactivity.

Tremor is one of the most frequent concomitants of toxic–metabolic disturbances. The typical tremor is a slightly irregular, oscillating, distal movement that is absent at rest and precipitated by action (Chapter 12) (Fahn, 1972; Jankovic and Fahn, 1980). It is visible in the outstretched hands and may also be apparent in the neck, lids, tongue, or jaw.

Asterixis is the sudden jerk produced by brief interruptions of the muscular activity involved in sustaining a fixed posture. Although it is common in hepatic encephalopathy and has been called "liver flap," it occurs in many toxic and metabolic conditions and is an etiologically nonspecific sign of encephalopathy (Bodensteiner et al., 1981; Conn, 1958; Davis et al., 1982; Leavitt and Tyler, 1964; Murphy and Goldstein, 1974; Rubin et al., 1980). Focal lesions involving the mid-brain, thalamus, and parietal cortex may produce unilateral asterixis affecting the contralateral limb and must be excluded before asterixis can be attributed to a metabolic disorder (Bril et al., 1979; Degos et al., 1979; Donat, 1980; Massey et al., 1979; Tarsy et al., 1977; Vallat et al., 1981; Young et al., 1976).

Myoclonus is common in uremic and postanoxic encephalopathy but, like asterixis, is a nonspecific finding and occurs in a large number of toxic and metabolic disturbances (Lance, 1968; Swanson et al., 1962). Alterations in muscle tone and reflexes are also frequent in metabolic encephalopathies. The tone is symmetrically increased, imparting a plastic resistance to passive movement, and reflex changes include generalized hyperreflexia and extensor plantar responses.

Sleep disturbances comprise an important part of the ACS. There may be a disruption of the normal circadian cycle with excessive drowsiness during the day and restless wakefulness at night (Henry and Mann, 1965; Lipowski, 1980). When the ACS results from withdrawal from alcohol or other agents that suppress rapid eye movement (REM) sleep, REM rebound may occur and the nocturnal sleep pattern will be dominated by REM sleep (Greenberg and Pearlman, 1967).

Autonomic disturbances, including tachycardia, diaphoresis, and pupillary dilatation, are common in some ACSs, particularly those associated with alcohol and drug withdrawal (Henry and Mann, 1965).

The EEG is the most useful laboratory tool for the identification of metabolic encephalopathies. The tracing reveals a generalized symmetrical slowing in the theta or delta range (Cadilhac and Ribstein, 1961; Engel et al., 1946; Moure, 1967; Obrecht et al., 1979; Otomo and Mikami, 1965; Pro and Wells, 1977; Romano and Engel, 1944).

ETIOLOGIES

The ACS state reflects acute interruption of cerebral function and as such can be produced by a large number of metabolic, toxic, and intracranial conditions (Table 7-2). It is particularly likely to occur in patients with preexisting intellectual impairment and in the elderly (Lipowski, 1967, 1980; Liston, 1982; Purdie et al., 1981; Wahl et al., 1967).

Intracranial disorders presenting as ACSs include head trauma, cerebral edema, hypertensive encephalopathy, intracranial inflammatory diseases, acute cerebrovascular accidents, meningitis, encephalitis, epilepsy, and migraine. Confusional behavior in epilepsy occurs in the ictal and postictal stages and may last for hours or (rarely) days in complex partial status epileptitus or petit

TABLE 7-2. Etiologies of Acute Confusional States

Systemic conditions	Withdrawal syndromes
Cardiac failure	Drugs
Pulmonary disease	Alcohol
Uremia	Infections
Hepatic encephalopathy	Systemic infections with fever
Electrolyte disturbances	Meningitis
Hypoglycemia	Encephalitis
Inflammatory disorders	
Anemia	Intracranial disorders
Porphyria	Head trauma
Carcinoid syndrome	Cerebral edema
	Epilepsy (ictal and postictal confusion)
Endocrinopathies	Hypertensive encephalopathy
Thyroid dysfunction	Intracranial inflammatory disease
Parathyroid dysfunction	Cerebrovasular accident (acute phase)
Adrenal dysfunction	Migraine
Pituitary dysfunction	Subdural hematoma
Nutritional deficiencies	Focal cerebral lesions
Thiamine (Wernicke's encephalopathy)	Right parietal lesions
Niacin	Bilateral occipitotemporal lesions
B_{12}	
Folic acid	Miscellaneous conditions
Protein	Heatstroke
	Radiation
Intoxications	Electrocution
Drugs	Hypersensitivity reaction
Iatrogenic	Sleep deprivation
Self-administered	Postoperative confusion
Alcohol	Idiopathic psychiatric disorders
Metals	Mania (particularly in elderly individuals)
Industrial agents	Schizophrenia
Biocides	Depression

mal status epilepticus (Ellis and Lee, 1978; Escueta et al., 1974; Goldensohn and Gold, 1960; Niedermeyer and Khalifeh, 1965; Saper and Lossing, 1974; Somerville and Bruni, 1983). Acute confusional migraine occurs almost exclusively in children and adolescents and is characterized by confused behavior occurring as a prodrome to the migraine headache (Bickerstaff, 1961; Ehyai and Fenichel, 1978).

The metabolic and toxic disorders producing ACSs include systemic disturbances, endocrinopathies, nutritional deficiencies, drug intoxications, withdrawal syndromes, and infections. Among the most common metabolic conditions producing the ACS are infections, dehydration and electrolyte abnormalities, cardiopulmonary failure, uremia, and hepatic encephalopathy (Liston, 1982; Purdie et al., 1981; Seymour et al., 1980).

Drug-induced ACSs are also common. Encephalopathies are particularly likely to be produced by anticholinergic agents but may occur with virtually any drug reaching high serum concentrations (Blazer et al., 1983; Itil and Fink, 1966). Altered drug metabolism and dis-

position in the elderly renders them vulnerable to developing an iatrogenic ACS even when conventional dosages of medications are prescribed (Vestal, 1978).

Postoperative confusion deserves special consideration because of its frequency and because its etiology is often perplexing. Acute confusional states presenting immediately after surgery are usually due to anoxia or persistent medication effects, particularly the effects of anticholinergic medication (Strub, 1982). When the ACS appears later in the postoperative course, it is likely to be a product of multiple factors, including metabolic abnormalities, sleep deprivation, pain, and sensory isolation (Kornfeld et al., 1965; Morse, 1980; Morse and Litin, 1969; Wilson, 1972; Witoszka and Tamura, 1980).

In addition to the acute disruption of cellular function produced by metabolic and toxic encephalopathies and the disturbances of arousal resulting from epilepsy, migraine, and sleep deprivation, ACSs can also be produced by specific focal central nervous system (CNS) lesions and, rarely, by idiopathic psychiatric disorders.

The common manifestation of all these conditions is a disturbance of attention, the hallmark of the ACS. Two focal lesions that have been associated with acute confusional behavior are (1) right parietal lesions and (2) bilateral medial occipitotemporal lesions (Horenstein et al., 1967; Medina et al., 1974; Mesulam et al., 1976).

Idiopathic psychiatric disorders usually present with distinctive behavioral alterations indicative of schizophrenia, mania, or depression. Rarely, however, such patients appear to have an ACS as a major feature of their psychiatric disorder. The most frequent circumstance in which this is noted is in the course of a manic or depressive episode in an elderly individual (Lipowski, 1983; Roberts, 1963). The patients manifest a significant attentional impairment in addition to the typical symptoms of mania or depression, and the attentional deficits resolve with successful treatment of the psychiatric disorder. Other medical and drug-induced causes of ACSs must be carefully excluded in these patients, but the evaluation will frequently be unrevealing, and the ACS will be determined to be a product of the psychiatric illness.

DIFFERENTIAL DIAGNOSIS

The differential diagnosis of the ACS includes dementia, amnesia, catatonic stupor, and hysterical unresponsiveness (Henry and Mann, 1965; Lipowski, 1980; Strub, 1982; Wahl et al., 1967). The only definitive criterion distinguishing ACS from dementia is duration: the ACS persists for hours, days, or rarely weeks, whereas dementia usually implies persistence of intellectual deficits for months or years (Cummings and Benson, 1983). Other features that may facilitate differentiation between the two syndromes include greater attentional impairment in the ACS, along with more frequent delusions and hallucinations. The EEG is also more abnormal in the ACS than in most dementias (Chapter 8) (Harner, 1975).

Amnesia enters the differential diagnosis of ACS because disorientation is a prominent feature of both. *Amnesia,* however, refers to an impairment of new learning with intact attention and intellect (Chapter 4) (Benson, 1978). *Acute confusional state,* on the other hand, has prominent attentional deficits along with impairment of language, memory, cognition, visuospatial skills, and personality. Disorientation in ACSs is a product of inattention and is one among a host of deficits. The amnesic patient is not ''confused'' when ''confusion'' implies an attentional disturbance, and the disorienta-

tion accompanying amnesia is a product of the failure to retain spatial and temporal information.

Catatonia, including catatonic stupor, can occur in affective disorders and schizophrenia as well as in a variety of neurological and metabolic disturbances (Chapter 12) (Gelenberg, 1976; Stoudemire, 1982). When stupor is a manifestation of an idiopathic psychiatric disturbance, it usually persists for less than 1 week and is distinguished from other causes of stupor by normal reflex function and a normal EEG (Henry and Woodruff, 1978; Hopkins, 1973; Joyston-Bechal, 1966; Smith, 1959). Similarly, hysterical unresponsiveness is characterized by normal reflex responses and a normal EEG (Garmany, 1955; Guze et al., 1971; Weintraub, 1983).

MANAGEMENT

The principal effort in the management of the patient in an ACS is directed at identifying and treating the underlying disease process. Once the presence of an ACS is recognized by careful mental status testing and identification of the attentional deficits, the clinician must immediately search for the etiology of the encephalopathy. In most cases a reversible metabolic or toxic condition will be discovered. A careful history may suggest the presence of drug intoxication, a medical illness resulting from exposure to industrial toxins, or alcoholism. Hypoxia, uremia, hepatic encephalopathy, electrolyte disorders, and endocrine disturbances can be identified by the appropriate laboratory studies. In addition to these measures, there are general management strategies that apply to most patients in ACSs, including maintaining proper nutrition, hydration, and electrolyte balance; ensuring adequate sleep; providing an appropriate amount of sensory and social stimulation; and sedating patients whose agitation prevents evaluation and management of the underlying condition (Lipowski, 1980; Strub, 1982). Drugs should be used sparingly since they may exaggerate the ACS. When drug management is necessary in order to control agitation, small doses of a major tranquilizer should be utilized (Bayne, 1978). Restoration of the metabolic milieu of the CNS lags behind normalization of the peripheral blood and serum values, and the ACS may persist for several days or more after appropriate treatment of the etiologic condition. In the elderly, the ACS may endure for several weeks after improvement of the underlying disorder. Death is not an uncommon outcome of ACS because of the seriousness of many of the etiologic conditions (Flint and Richards, 1956; Liston, 1982).

REFERENCES

Bayne JRD. Management of confusion states in elderly persons. *Canad Med Assoc J*, 1978, *118*, 139–141.

Benson DF. Amnesia. *South Med J*, 1978, *71*, 1221–1228.

Benson DF. *Aphasia, alexia, and agraphia*. New York, Churchill Livingston, 1979.

Berrios GE. Delirium and confusion in the 19th century: a conceptual history. *Br J Psychiat*, 1981, *139*, 439–449.

Bickerstaff ER. Impairment of consciousness in migraine. *Lancet*, 1961, *2*, 1057–1059.

Blazer DG II, Federspiel CF, Ray WA, and Schaffner W. The risk of anticholinergic toxicity in the elderly: a study of prescribing practices in two populations. *J Gerontol*, 1983, *38*, 31–35.

Bodensteiner JB, Morris HH, and Golden GS. Asterixis associated with sodium valproate. *Neurology*, 1981, *31*, 186–190.

Bril V, Sharpe JA, and Ashby P. Midbrain asterixis. *Ann Neurol*, 1979, *6*, 362–364.

Cadilhac J and Ribstein M. The EEG in metabolic disorders. *World Neurol*, 1961, *2*, 296–308.

Chedru F and Geschwind N. Disorders of higher cortical functions in acute confusional states. *Cortex*, 1972a, *10*, 395–411.

Chedru F and Geschwind N. Writing disturbances in acute confusional states. *Neuropsychologia*, 1972b, *10*, 343–353.

Conn HO. Asterixis. Its occurrence in chronic pulmonary disease, with a commentary on its general mechanism. *New Engl J Med*, 1958, *259*, 564–569.

Cummings JL. Organic delusions: phenomenology, anatomic correlations, and review. *Br J Psychiat*, 1985, *46*, 184–197.

Cummings JL and Benson DF. *Dementia: a clinical approach*. Boston, Butterworths, 1983.

Cummings J, Hebben NA, Obler L, and Leonard P. Nonaphasic misnaming and other neurobehavioral features of an unusual toxic encephalopathy: case study. *Cortex*, 1980, *16*, 315–323.

Curran FJ and Schilder P. Paraphasic signs in diffuse lesions of the brain. *J Nerv Ment Dis*, 1935, *82*, 613–636.

Davis CE, Smith C, and Harris R. Persistent movement disorders following metrizamide myelography. *Arch Neurol*, 1982, *39*, 128.

Degos JD, Verroust J, Bouchareine A, Serdaru M, and Barbizet J. Asterixis in focal brain lesions. *Arch Neurol*, 1979, *36*, 705–707.

Donat JR. Unilateral asterixis due to thalamic hemorrhage. *Neurology*, 1980, *30*, 80–84.

Doty EJ. The incidence and treatment of delirious reactions in later life. *Geriatrics*, 1946, *1*, 21–26.

Ehyai A and Fenichel GM. The natural history of acute confusional migraine. *Arch Neurol*, 1978, *35*, 368–369.

Ellis JM and Lee SI. Acute prolonged confusion in later life as an ictal state. *Epilepsia*, 1978, *19*, 119–128.

Engel GL, Romano J, and Goldman L. Delirium. *Arch Neurol Psychiat*, 1946, *56*, 659–664.

Escueta AV, Boxley J, Stubbs N, Waddell G, and Wilson WA. Prolonged twilight state and automatisms: a case report. *Neurology*, 1974, *24*, 331–339.

Fahn S. Differential diagnosis of tremors. *Med Clin Am*, 1972, *56*, 1363–1375.

Flint FJ and Richards SM. Organic basis of confusional states in the elderly. *Br Med J*, 1956, *2*, 1537–1539.

Garmany G. Acute anxiety and hysteria. *Br Med J*, 1955, *2*, 115–117.

Gelenberg AJ. The catatonic syndrome. *Lancet*, 1976, *1*, 1339–1341.

Geschwind N. Non-aphasic disorders of speech. *Internat J Neurol*, 1964, *4*, 207–214.

Goldensohn ES and Gold AP. Prolonged behavioral disturbances as ictal phenomena. *Neurology*, 1960, *10*, 1–9.

Greenberg R and Pearlman C. Delirium tremens and dreaming. *Am J Psychiat*, 1967, *124*, 133–142.

Guze SB, Woodruff RA, and Clayton PJ. A study of conversion symptoms in psychiatric outpatients. *Am J Psychiat*, 1971, *128*, 643–646.

Harner RN. EEG in evaluation of the patient with dementia. In Benson DF and Blumer D (Eds.): *Psychiatric aspects of neurologic disease*. New York, Grune & Stratton, 1975, pp. 63–82.

Hay GG, Jolley DJ, and Jones RG. A case of the Capgras Syndrome in association with pseudo-hypoparathyroidism. *Acta Psychiat Scand*, 1974, *50*, 73–77.

Henry JA and Woodruff GHA. A diagnostic sign in states of apparent unconsciousness. *Lancet*, 1978, *2*, 920–921.

Henry WD and Mann AM. Diagnosis and treatment of delirium. *Canad Med Assoc J*, 1965, *93*, 1156–1166.

Hopkins A. Pretending to be unconscious. *Lancet*, 1973, *2*, 312–314.

Horenstein S, Chapmberlain W, and Conomy J. Infarction of the fusiform and calcarine regions: agitated delirium and hemianopia. *Trans Am Neurol Assoc*, 1967, *92*, 85–87.

Itil L and Fink M. Anticholinergic drug-induced delirium; experimental modification, quantitative EEG, and behavioral correlations. *J Nerv Ment Dis*, 1966, *143*, 492–507.

Jankovic J and Fahn S. Physiologic and pathologic tremors. *Ann Int Med*, 1980, *93*, 460–465.

Joyston-Bechal MP. The clinical features and outcome of stupor. *Br J Psychiat*, 1966, *112*, 967–981.

Kornfeld DS, Zimberg S, and Malm JR. Psychiatric complications of open heart surgery. *New Engl J Med*, 1965, *273*, 287–292.

Lance JW. Myoclonic jerks and falls: aetiology, classification, and treatment. *Med J Aust*, 1968, *1*, 113–120.

Leavitt S and Tyler R. Studies in asterixis. *Arch Neurol*, 1964, *10*, 360–365.

Levin M. Perseveration at various levels of complexity, with comments on delirium. *Arch Neurol Psychiat*, 1955, *73*, 439–444.

Levin M. Delirium: an experience and some reflections. *Am J Psychiat*, 1968, *124*, 1120–1123.

Lipowski ZJ. Delirium, clouding of consciousness and confusion. *J Nerv Ment Dis*, 1967, *145*, 227–255.

Lipowski ZJ, *Delirium. Acute brain failure in man*. Springfield, Illinois, Charles C Thomas, Publisher, 1980.

Lipowski ZJ. Transient cognitive disorders (delirium, acute confusional states) in the elderly. *Am J Psychiat*, 1983, *140*, 1426–1436.

Liston EH. Delirium in the aged. *Psychiat Clin N Am*, 1982, *5*, 49–66.

Madakasira S and Hall TB III. Capgras syndrome in a patient with myxedema. *Am J Psychiat*, 1981, *138*, 1506–1508.

Massey EW, Goodman JC, Stewart C, and Brannon WL. Unilateral asterixis: motor integrative dysfunction in focal vascular disease. *Neurology*, 1979, *29*, 1188–1190.

Medina JL, Chokroverty S, and Rubino FA. Syndrome of agitated delirium and visual impairment: a manifestation of medial temporo-occipital infarction. *J Neurol Neurosurg Psychiat*, 1977, *40*, 861–864.

Medina JL, Rubino FA, and Ross E. Agitated delirium caused by infarctions of the hippocampal formation and fusiform and lingual gyri: a case report. *Neurology*, 1974, *24*, 1181–1183.

Mesulam M-M, Waxman SG, Geschwind N, and Sabin TD. Acute confusional states with right middle cerebral artery infarctions. *J Neurol Neurosurg Psychiat*, 1976, *39*, 84–89.

Morse RM. The relationship between psychopathology (delirium) and somatic-organic-pharmacologic factors following open-heart surgery. In Speidel H and Rodewald G (Eds):*Psychic and neurological dysfunctions after open-heart surgery*. New York, Thieme Stratton, Inc., 1980. pp. 111–117.

Morse RM and Litin EM. Post-operative delirium: a study of etiologic factors. *Am J Psychiat*, 1969, *126*, 388–395.

Moure JM. The electroencephalogram in hypercalcemia. *Arch Neurol*, 1967, *17*, 34–51.

Murphy MJ and Goldstein MN. Diphenylhydantoin-induced asterixis. *JAMA*, 1974, *229*, 538–540.

Nash JL. Delusions. In Cavenar JO Jr and Brodie HKH (Eds.): *Signs and symptoms in psychiatry*. Philadelphia, JB Lippincott, 1983, pp. 455–481.

Niedermeyer E and Khalifeh R. Petit mal status ("spike-wave stupor"). *Epilepsia*, 1965, *6*, 250–262.

Obrecht R, Okhomina FOA, and Scott DF. Value of EEG in acute confusional states. *J Neurol Neurosurg Psychiat*, 1979, *42*, 75–77.

Otomo E and Mikami R. Clinical studies on the relationship of the electroencephalogram to pH and pCO2 in arterial blood. *Neurology*, 1965, *15*, 1063–1070.

Pies R. Capgras phenomenon, delirium, and transient hepatic dysfunction. *Hosp Commun Psychiat*, 1982, *33*, 382–383.

Pro JD and Wells CE. The use of the electroencephalogram in the diagnosis of delirium. *Dis Nerv Syst*, 1977, *38*, 804–808.

Purdie FR, Honigman B, and Rosen P. Acute organic brain syndrome: a review of 100 cases. *Ann Emerg Med*, 1981, *10*, 455–461.

Roberts AH. The value of ECT in delirium. *Br J Psychiat*, 1963, *109*, 653–655.

Romano J and Engel GL. Delirium. *Arch Neurol Psychiat*, 1944, *51*, 356–377.

Rubin B, Horowitz G, and Katz RI. Asterixis following metrizamide myelography. *Arch Neurol*, 1980, *37*, 522.

Saper JR and Lossing JH. Prolonged trance-like stupor in epilepsy. *Arch Intern Med*, 1974, *134*, 1079–1082.

Seymour DG, Henschke PJ, Cape RDT, and Campbell AJ. Acute confusional states and dementia in the elderly: the role of dehydration/volume depletion, physical illness and age. *Age Ageing*, 1980, *9*, 137–146.

Simon A and Cahan RB. The acute brain syndrome in geriatric patients. *Psychiat Res Rep*, 1963, *16*, 8–21.

Smith S. An investigation and survey of 27 cases of akinesis and mutism (stupor). *J Ment Sci*, 1959, *105*, 1088–1094.

Somerville ER and Bruni J. Tonic status epilepticus presenting as confusional state. *Ann Neurol*, 1983, *13*, 549–551.

Stoudemire A. The differential diagnosis of catatonic states. *Psychosomatics*, 1982, *23*, 245–252.

Strub RL. Acute confusional state. In Benson DF and Blumer D (Eds.): *Psychiatric aspects of neurologic disease*. Vol. 2. New York, Grune & Stratton, 1982, pp. 1–21.

Swanson PD, Luttrell CN, and Magladery JW. Myoclonus—a report of 67 cases and review of the literature. *Medicine*, 1962, *42*, 339–356.

Tarsy D, Lieberman B, Chirico-Post J, and Benson DF. Unilateral asterixis associated with a mesencephalic syndrome. *Arch Neurol*, 1977, *34*, 446–447.

Vallat JM, Rkina M, and Bokor J. Unilateral asterixis due to subdural hematoma. *Arch Neurol*, 1981, *38*, 535.

Vestal RE. Drug use in the elderly: a review of problems and special considerations. *Drugs*, 1978, *16*, 358–382.

Wahl, CW, Golden JS, Liston EH Jr, Rimer DG, Rose AS, Soghor D, and Solomon DH. Toxic and functional psychosis. *Ann Int Med*, 1967, *66*, 989–1007.

Weinstein EA and Kahn RL. Nonaphasic misnaming (paraphasia) in organic brain disease. *Arch Neurol Psychiat*, 1952, *67*, 72–79.

Weinstein EA and Keller NJA. Linguistic patterns of misnaming in brain injury. *J Neuropsychol*, 1963, *1*, 79–90.

Weintraub MI. *Hysterical conversion reactions*. New York, SP Medical and Scientific Books, 1983.

Wilson LM. Intensive care delirium. *Arch Int Med*, 1972, *130*, 225–226.

Witoszka MM and Tamura H. Neurological dysfunction and behavior disorder following open-heart surgery. In Speidel H and Rodewald G (Eds.): *Psychic and neurological dysfunction after open-heart surgery*. New York, Thieme Stratton, Inc., 1980, pp. 37–41.

Wolff HG and Curran D. Nature of delirium and allied states. *Arch Neurol Psychiat*, 1935, *33*, 1175–1215.

Young RR, Shahani BJ, and Kjellberg RT. Unilateral asterixis produced by a discrete CNS lesion. *Trans Am Neurol Assoc*, 1976, *101*, 306–307.

Chapter 8

Dementia

Dementia is a syndrome of acquired intellectual impairment characterized by persistent deficits in at least three of the following areas of mental activity: memory, language, visuospatial skills, personality or emotional state, and cognition (abstraction, mathematics, judgment) (Cummings et al., 1980a). Its acquired nature distinguishes dementia from mental retardation, whereas its persistence differentiates it from acute confusional states (ACSs). The requirement that the intellectual alterations include multiple areas of mental function distinguishes dementia from aphasic, amnesic, and other monosymptomatic cognitive deficits. Dementia is a clinical syndrome with many etiologies and may be reversible or irreversible.

Dementia is a rapidly growing public health concern. It is largely a problem of elderly individuals, and the size of the aged population is expanding more rapidly than any other segment of the population. Approximately 5 percent of individuals over age 65 are severely demented, and an additional 10–15 percent are mildly to moderately intellectually impaired (Cummings and Benson, 1983; Gunner-Svensson and Jensen, 1976; Mortimer et al., 1981; Nielsen, 1962). In 1950, 8 percent of the population was over age 65 (12.3 million individuals), and by 1978 the proportion had increased to 11 percent (22 million), and it is estimated that by the year 2030 it will represent 20 percent of the U.S. population (51 million persons) (Plum, 1979). As the number of aged persons increases, dementia will demand an increasing share of the health care budget, health care work-hours, and hospital and nursing home beds. Responding to this challenge demands an integrated, comprehensive, and systematic approach to identification of dementing illnesses, differentiation of the many etiologies of dementia, and development of management programs.

ETIOLOGIES OF DEMENTIA

Table 8-1 presents the differential diagnosis of the dementia syndrome. Each major etiology of dementia is discussed and the distinguishing clinical features described. The relationship between the topography of central nervous system (CNS) involvement and the pattern of intellectural alteration is emphasized.

Alzheimer's Disease

Dementia of the Alzheimer type (DAT) almost invariably begins after the age of 50 and becomes increasingly common with advancing age. In 20 percent of cases the disease is inherited as an autosomal dominant condition, and in the remaining 80 percent there is an increased incidence of DAT among family members (Cook et al., 1979; Feldman et al., 1963; Pratt, 1970).

Dementia of the Alzheimer type progresses through three stages in a relatively orderly and consistent manner (Table 8-2) (Cummings and Benson, 1983; Lishman, 1978). In the first stage the patient has empty speech with few substantive words and a paucity of ideas. There may be an anomia on tests of naming, and the patient will have difficulty generating word lists (e.g., number of animals names produced in 1 minute). Memory, cognition, and visuospatial skills are also compromised in the early phases of the disease, but speech articulation and other motor functions remain normal. Patients usually are indifferent to their deficits, and EEG and computerized tomographic (CT) scans are unremarkable.

In the second stage of the disease all intellectual functions continue to deteriorate. Language is characterized by a fluent paraphasic output, impaired comprehension, and relatively preserved repetition (Cummings et al., 1985). Memory, for both recent and remote information, is severely impaired; visuospatial abilities are further compromised, and patients cannot find their way about or copy constructions; cognitive skills, including calculation and abstraction, are severely impaired. Apraxia and agnosia are present but difficult to demonstrate because of the patients' limited language and memory. Motor strength and coordination are normal, but the patients become markedly restless, wandering and pacing incessantly. There is usually theta-range slowing of the EEG, and the CT scan is normal or shows moderate diffuse cortical atrophy.

TABLE 8-1.   Differential Diagnosis of the Dementia Syndrome

Alzheimer's disease	Toxic and metabolic dementias
Pick's disease	Hydrocephalic dementias

Extrapyramidal syndromes with dementia
    Parkinson's disease
    Huntington's disease
    Wilson's disease
    Progressive supranuclear palsy
    Spinocerebellar degenerations
    Miscellaneous extrapyramidal syndromes
	Traumatic dementias
	Neoplastic dementias
	
	Myelin diseases with dementia
	Dementias associated with psychiatric disorders
	    Depression

Multi-infarct dementia	Schizophrenia Miscellaneous psychiatric disorders

Viral and other infectious dementias
    Jakob-Creutzfeldt's disease
    Syphilis
    Chronic meningitis
    Miscellaneous CNS infections	

In the final stage all intellectual functions are severely impaired, and the patients' cognitive abilities are largely untestable. Verbal output is reduced to echolalia, palilalia, or mutism. Sphincter control is lost, and the patient's limbs assume a rigid, flexed position. The EEG reveals delta-range slowing, and the CT scan demonstrates diffuse cerebral atrophy with ventricular dilatation and sulcal enlargement. Death results from aspiration pneumonia or urinary tract infection with sepsis.

The diagnosis of DAT is conventionally approached as a matter of exclusion based on the elimination of other more easily diagnosed causes of dementia. Negative laboratory evaluations and nonspecific physical findings, however, also characterize other types of dementia such as the dementia syndrome of depression, some insidiously progressive toxic and metabolic processes, and some vascular dementias. Diagnosis by exclusion results in the inclusion of all unrecognized dementias as DAT and renders DAT a nonspecific diagnosis. To ensure that the diagnosis of DAT is applied to a homogeneous group of patients suffering from the same illness, all patients identified as suffering from DAT should have clinical features and course similar to that described here. They should have an insidiously progressive clinical syndrome, including aphasia, amnesia, and visuospatial abnormalities, and motor, reflex and sensory function should be normal throughout most of the clinical course. The diagnosis of DAT should be viewed skeptically if the patient's clinical features or course deviate substantially from this pattern.

Pathologically, the brains of DAT patients are atrophic with ventricular and sulcal enlargement. Histological investigation reveals neuronal loss, senile plaques, and intracellular neurofibrillary tangles (Tomlinson, 1977). These changes are most abundant in the parietal and frontal association areas and in the hippo-

campus (Brun and Gustafson, 1978). Neurons in the latter region also exhibit numerous intracellular granulovacuolar changes (Tomlinson and Kitchner, 1972). Neurochemical analyses demonstrate a preferential loss of presynaptic cholinergic neurons in a similar topographic distribution (Bowen et al., 1976; Davies, 1978). Loss of cholinergic neurons from the nucleus basalis in the inferior medial forebrain area correlates with the loss of cholinergic innervation of the cerebral cortex (Whitehouse et al., 1982.)

The etiology of DAT is unknown, and attempts to treat the disease have not resulted in clinically significant improvement (Cummings and Benson, 1983).

Pick's Disease

Pick's disease, like DAT, affects primarily cortical structures. The two diseases are clinically similar, beginning in late middle life or later and progressing through a series of stages (Table 8-2) (Cummings, 1982). It may be difficult to distinguish the two disorders, but several clinical, radiological, and EEG features have differentiating value, particularly when the patient is observed in the early phases of the illness. Compared with DAT patients, Pick's disease victims have less memory, calculation, and visuospatial impairment and more extravagant personality alterations (Cummings and Benson, 1983; Lishman, 1978; Wechsler et al., 1982). Both diseases produce aphasia, but Pick's disease patients have a greater tendency to produce a stereotyped verbal output, repeating the same story or joke again and again (Mayer-Gross et al., 1937–1938). Features of the Klüver-Bucy syndrome (hyperorality, dietary changes, hypermetamorphosis, placidity, hypersexuality, sensory agnosia) may appear early in the course of Pick's disease, whereas they are confined to

TABLE 8-2. Characteristics of the Three Stages of Alzheimer's and Pick's Diseases

Stage	Alzheimer's disease	Pick's disease
Stage I		
Language	Anomia, empty speech	Anomia
Memory	Defective	Relatively spared
Visuospatial skills	Impaired	Relatively spared
Calculation	Impaired	Relatively spared
Personality	Indifferent	Disinhibited
Klüver-Bucy syndrome	Absent	Present
Motor system	Normal	Normal
EEG	Normal	Normal
CT Scan	Normal	Normal
Stage II		
Language	Fluent aphasia	Aphasia, stereotyped output
Memory	Severly impaired	Impaired
Visuospatial skills	Severely impaired	Impaired
Personality	Indifferent	Disinhibited
Motor system	Restlessness	Restless, stereotyped behavior
EEG	Slowing of background rhythms	Slowing of background rhythms or frontal-temporal slowing
CT Scan	Atrophy	Frontal and/or temporal atrophy
Stage III		
Intellectual function	Severely impaired	Severely impaired
Language	Palilalia, echolalia, or mutism	Echolalia, mutism
Sphincter control	Incontinence	Incontinence
EEG	Diffuse slowing	Diffuse of frontotemporal slowing
CT Scan	Diffuse atrophy	Frontal and/or temporal atrophy

the late stages of DAT (Cummings and Duchen, 1981; Lilly et al., 1983). The EEG and CT scan are normal in the initial stages of Pick's disease, but as the disease progresses, frontotemporal slowing may appear on the EEG, and focal frontal and/or temporal atrophy may be evident on the CT scan (Fig. 8-1) (Cummings and Duchen, 1981; McGeachie et al., 1979).

Pathologically, the brains of Pick disease patients have focal atrophy involving the frontal and/or anterior temporal lobes (Corsellis, 1976). The two characteristic histological changes are the presence of inflated neurons and neurons containing highly argyrophilic Pick bodies. Neuronal loss and a fibrillary gliosis of the subcortical white matter are also evident (Jervis, 1971). Neurochemical studies have found no selective involvement of specific transmitter systems (White et al., 1977).

Like DAT, the etiology of Pick's disease has not been determined, and treatment is directed at the control of aberrant behavior and prevention of secondary complications.

Extrapyramidal Syndromes with Dementias

Instrumental functions such as language, learning, visual perception, and praxis are mediated by cerebral cortex and are impaired by cerebral cortical diseases. Fundamental functions such as alertness, arousal, motivation, attention, and timing are mediated by subcortical structures and are disrupted by diseases affecting the basal ganglia, thalamus, and rostral brainstem (Albert, 1978; Cummings and Benson, 1984). *Subcortical dementia* refers to the pattern of intellectual defi-

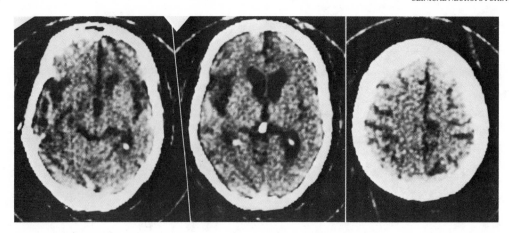

Figure 8-1. Computerized tomographic scan of a patient with Pick's disease demonstrating focal cortical atrophy affecting the temporal lobes. Reproduced from Cummings JL and Duchen LW. The Klüver-Bucy syndrome in Pick disease. *Neurology,* 1981, *31*, Figure 1. With permission of the publisher.

cits produced by diseases affecting subcortical structures and disrupting the functions they mediate. The cardinal features of subcortical dementia include psychomotor retardation, memory impairment, abnormal cognition, mood disturbances, and speech and motor system abnormalities (Table 8-3) (Albert et al., 1974; Cummings and Benson, 1984). These abnormalities contrast sharply with the aphasia, agnosia, apraxia, amnesia, and normal motor function characteristic of disorders involving primarily the cerebral cortex. Extrapyramidal syndromes with dementia manifest almost exclusively features of subcortical dysfunction, whereas conditions such as multi-infarct dementias, viral infections, trauma, neoplasms, and chronic toxic–metabolic disorders pro-

duce symptoms of both cortical and subcortical dysfunction. Extrapyramidal syndromes with subcortical dementia include Parkinson's disease, Huntington's disease, Wilson's disease, progressive supranuclear palsy, spinocerebellar degenerations, and a number of less common conditions such as Hallervorden-Spatz disease, idiopathic basal ganglia calcification, and familial choreoacanthocytosis (Albert et al., 1974; Cummings and Benson, 1983; Cummings et al., 1983).

Dementia is present in approximately 60 percent of patients with Parkinson's disease, and as many as 93 percent have deficits on specific neuropsychological tests (Cummings and Benson, 1984; Mayeux et al., 1981; Pirozzolo et al., 1982). The dementia correlates best

TABLE 8-3.   Distinguishing Features of Dementing Illnesses Affecting Primarily Cortical or Subcortical Structures

Clinical Characteristics	Cortical Dementia	Subcortical Dementia
Intellectual functions	Aphasia Amnesia Visuospatial disorder Poor abstraction Acalculia Apraxia Agnosia	Psychomotor retardation Forgetfulness Cognitive dilapidation Impaired insight Poor strategy formulation
Personality/Emotion	Indifference	Depression (rarely, mania)
Speech	Normal (until late)	Dysarthria
Motor System	Normal (until late)	Abnormal (parkinsonism, chroea, dystonia, etc.)
Anatomic involvement	Neocortical association areas and hippocampus	Thalamus, basal ganglia, rostral brainstem

with the presence of bradykinesia and is least associated with tremor. Pathologically, Parkinson's disease is characterized by loss of dopamine-containing cells in the substantia nigra and the ventral tegmental area (Javoy-Agid and Agid, 1980; Greenfield and Bosanquet, 1953). Modest improvement in the dementia of Parkinson's disease is noted when levodopa therapy is initiated (Halgin et al., 1977; Marsh et al., 1971; Meier and Martin, 1970).

Dementia is a uniform part of Huntington's disease and may be the initial manifestation preceding the appearance of chorea or other neuropsychiatric abnormalities (Cummings and Benson, 1983; McHugh and Folstein, 1975). Autopsy studies reveal profound cellular loss in the caudate and putamen and less marked atrophy of the thalamus (Corsellis, 1976). Neurochemical investigation demonstrates that γ-aminobutyric acid is preferentially depleted (Bird et al., 1973; Perry et al., 1973). Atrophy of the caudate may be visible on CT scans where the normal convex bulge of the caudate nucleus into the lateral wall of the frontal horn of the lateral ventricle disappears (Fig. 8-2) (Barr et al., 1978; Terrence et al., 1977).

Multi-infarct Dementia

Multiple vascular occlusions lead to tissue infarction with progressive disruption of brain function and eventual dementia. The characteristics of the dementia are highly variable and may include predominantly cortical features (aphasia, amnesia, agnosia, apraxia) or mainly subcortical symptoms (slowness, depression, forgetfulness, cognitive dilapidation) (Cummings and Benson, 1983). Combinations of cortical and subcortical characteristics are common, but some neurobehavioral features, including psychomotor retardation and emotional lability are present in most cases. Table 8-4 lists the principal historical and clinical features that aid in the identification of multi-infarct dementia (Hachinski et al., 1975).

Sustained hypertension leading to fibrinoid necrosis and occulusion of cerebral arterioles is the most com-

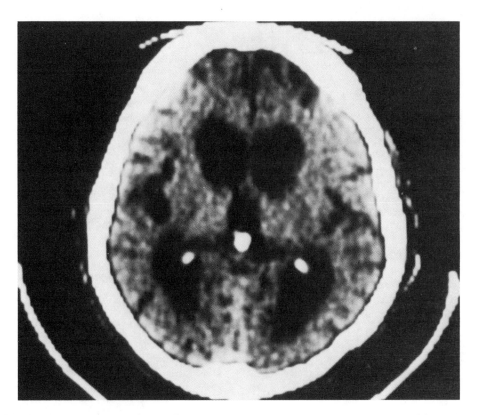

Figure 8-2. Computerized tomographic scan of a patient with Huntington's disease revealing atrophy of the caudate nuclei. Reproduced from Cummings JL and Benson DF. *Dementia: a clinical approach.* Boston, Butterworths Publishers, 1983, Figure 4-1. With permission of Butterworths Publishers.

TABLE 8-4.   Principal Characteristics of Multi-infarct
                    Dementia

History

　Abrupt onset
　Stepwise deterioration
　Fluctuating course
　Previous stroke or transient ischemic attacks
　Previous hypertension or other cardiovascular disease

Neurological examination

　Focal neurological deficits
　Pseudobulbar palsy (with dysarthria)

Mental status examination

　Dementia (cortical and/or subcortical features)
　Depression
　Emotional lability
　Relative preservation of personality

Laboratory assessment

　Focal slowing on EEG
　Lucent regions on CT scan

mon cause of vascular dementia. The infarctions (la-cunes) are concentrated in the thalamus, basal ganglia, and internal capsule near the base of the brain, and the most common form of multi-infarct dementia is known as the *lacunar state* (CM Fisher, 1965, 1969b). In Binswanger's disease, the infarctions preferentially involve the hemispheric white matter (Caplan and Schoene, 1978; De Reuck et al., 1980).

In addition to hypertension-related arteriosclerosis, a variety of other vascular disorders can produce multiple cerebral infarctions, including atherosclerosis of larger vessels, emboli from the heart or vessels of the neck, inflammatory conditions, and hematologic disorders (Cummings and Benson, 1983; Ferris and Levine, 1973; Levine and Swanson, 1969).

Infarctions are frequently visible on computerized tomograms of the head, but in some cases they may be too small to be visualized radiologically, and a normal scan does not preclude the diagnosis of vascular dementia. A scan similar to that seen in obstructive hydro-cephalus may be produced in multi-infarct dementia when concentration of the infarctions in the deep periventricular structures leads to ventricular dilation with little enlargement of the cortical sulci. Cisternography may be necessary in order to differentiate the two conditions (Benson et al., 1972). Electroencephalography may reveal multifocal slowing in cases of vascular dementia.

Treatment of multi-infarct dementia is directed at resolving the underlying condition. Dysarthria and aphasia may improve with speech and language therapy.

Dementias Produced by Viruses and Other Infectious Agents

Dementias may be produced by slow virus infections of the brain, bacterial encephalitis (syphilis, Whipple's disease), or chronic meningitis (tuberculous, fungal, parasitic) (Table 8-5).

Jakob-Creutzfeldt Disease

The Jakob-Creutzfeldt disease is a rapidly progressive viral infection of the nervous system that usually leads to death within 6 months of onset. The clinical features of the disease are diverse, and, early in the course, symptoms may affect function of the spinal cord, cerebellum, extrapyramidal system, or cerebral cortex. As the disease progresses, the virus spreads to involve the nervous system diffusely, and the patients eventually die in a vegetative state (Jones and Nevin, 1954; Kirschbaum, 1968; Masters and Richardson, 1978; Siedler and Malamud, 1963). Myoclonus is a prominent clinical finding but may not appear until late in the course in some patients. The EEG reveals periodic polyphasic sharp wave discharges superimposed on a slow background in a majority of cases (Burger et al., 1972; Chiofalo et al., 1980).

The Jakob-Creutzfeldt disease is produced by an unconventional slow virus that differs from conventional viral agents in its failure to stimulate an inflammatory or immune response, its invisibility to electron microscopy, and its unusual resistance to traditional physical and chemical disinfectant techniques (Gajdusek, 1977). Human-to-human transmission is very rare but has occurred as a result of corneal transplantations from an infected to an uninfected host and in cases where contaminated depth electrodes were used for recording in uninfected patients (Bernoulli et al., 1977; Duffy et al., 1974).

Pathologically the disease is characterized by hypertrophy of large fibrous astrocytes and by a spongiform appearance produced by vacuoles within astrocytes and neurons (Masters and Richardson, 1978). No effective treatment is available.

Other Viral Dementias

Other viral demetias include progressive multifocal leukoencephalopathy, paraneoplastic limbic encephalitis, subacute sclerosing panencephalitis, and progressive rubella panencephalitis. The latter two disorders are confined to children, adolescents, and young adults infected prenatally or in early life by rubeola or rubella viruses, respectively (Lorand et al., 1962; Osetowska and Torck, 1962; Weil et al., 1975).

Progressive multifocal leukoencephalopathy (PML)

is a slowly progressive papovavirus infection occurring almost exclusively in patients with chronic lympho-proliferative, myeloproliferative, or granulomatous diseases (Narayan et al., 1973; Richardson, 1970). There is a gradual accrual of focal neurological deficits, and dementia supervenes in the final stages. Pathologically, the brains have multiple demyelinated lesions with abnormal astrocytes, inclusion-containing oligodendrocytes, and inflammatory cells (Mancall, 1965). A few patients have improved with cytarabine therapy, whereas others have failed to respond, and no consistently effective therapy has been discovered (Bauer et al., 1973; Conomy et al., 1974).

Limbic encephalitis is a syndrome of progressive intellectual impairment occurring in patients with systemic neoplasms, particularly oatcell carcinoma of the lung (Brierley et al., 1960; Corsellis et al., 1968; Henson et al., 1965). Amnesia is the most prominent neurological deficit, and the maximal pathological changes are found in the hippocampi. At autopsy, alterations include inflammatory changes most consistent with a viral infection, although no agent has been consistently isolated.

Bacterial Infections Producing Dementia

Syphilitic general paresis is probably the best known example of a dementia syndrome produced by a bacterial infection of the brain. Although currently rare, general paresis once accounted for 10–30 percent of all mental hospital admissions. The disorder typically becomes manifest 15-30 years after the initial infection and is characterized by progressive intellectual impairment combined, in some cases, with psychosis (Bruetsch, 1959; Hahn et al., 1959). Facial and lingual tremors are common, and two-thirds of patients have pupillary abnormalities (Lishman, 1978). Pathologically, the *Treponema pallidum* organisms are most abundant in the frontal cortex, and 75 percent of patients improve with penicillin treatment (Hahn et al., 1959).

Whipple's disease is a rare bacterial meningo-encephalitis manifest by diarrhea and gastrointestinal malabsorption symptoms, lymphadenopathy, arthritis, anemia, and fever as well as neurological abnormalities, including dementia. If initiated early, antibiotic therapy may halt progression of the disease (Feurle et al., 1979; Romanul et al., 1977).

Chronic Meningitis

Chronic meningitis with dementia may be caused by syphilis, tuberculosis, fungi, or parasites. In addition to intellectual deterioration, affected patients manifest cranial nerve palsies, stiff neck, and headache. Focal neurological deficits may occur, and hydrocephalus may

TABLE 8-5.   Infectious Conditions Producing Dementia

Viral diseases

    Jakob-Creutzfeldt's disease
    Progressive multifocal leukoencephalopathy
    Paraneoplastic limbic encephalitis
    Subacute sclerosing panencephalitis
    Progressive rubella panencephalitis

Bacterial encephalitis

    Syphilis (general paresis)
    Whipple's disease

Chronic meningitis

    Bacterial
      Tuberculosis
      Syphilis (meningovascular form)
    Fungal
    Parasitic

be an acute or late complication. Early recognition and treatment reverses the deficits in most cases (Ellner and Bennett, 1976).

Toxic and Metabolic Dementias

Adequate intellectual and emotional function demands normal cellular metabolism with cells supplied sufficient amounts of appropriate metabolic ingredients free of toxins. Metabolic and toxic disturbances frequently produce intellectual disturbances, and in some cases the neurobehavioral alterations may overshadow systemic manifestations. When the mental state disturbance has an abrupt onset and short course, an acute confusional state is diagnosed; when the intellectual deterioration has a gradual onset and is insidiously progressive, persisting for weeks, months, or longer, the disorder is a dementia syndrome.

Like other dementias, toxic and metabolic dementias are most prevalent in the elderly population; 86 percent of individuals over age 65 suffer from one chronic illness, and 50 percent have two or more (Jarvik and Perl, 1981; Levenson and Hall, 1981). Many of these disorders are capable of compromising intellectual function. The high frequency of systemic illnesses also results in a high rate of drug consumption in the elderly. Those over age 65 comprise 11 percent of the population and use 25 percent of all prescribed pharmaceuticals. Almost 70 percent of elderly patients regularly use over-the-counter medication, as compared with 10 percent of the general adult population (Thompson et al., 1983). Furthermore, alterations in body mass, serum binding proteins, and drug metabolism render the elderly vulnerable to drug intoxication even when conventional doses are administered. The prevalence of

TABLE 8-6. Metabolic and Toxic Causes of Dementia

Metabolic disorders

  Hypoxia
    Cardiopulmonary disease or failure
    Anemia
  Uremia and dialysis dementia
  Hepatic encephalopathy
  Vitamin deficiencies

    B_{12}
    Folate
    Niacin

  Endocrine diseases
    Thyroid and parathyroid disorders
    Adrenal abnormalities

  Electrolyte disturbances
  Porphyria

Toxic Disorders

  Drugs
    Psychotropic agents
    Anticholinergic and antihypertensive agents
    Anticonvulsants
    Antineoplastic drugs
    Antibiotics
    Miscellaneous therapeutic agents
    Alcohol and drug abuse (glue sniffing, etc.)

  Metals
    Lead
    Mercury
    Manganese
    Arsenic
    Thallium

  Industrial Agents
    Organic solvents
    Organophosphate insecticides
    Carbon monoxide

chronic physical illness in the aged and the consumption of the drugs used to treat these disorders thus converge to produce an increased prevalence of metabolic and toxic dementias in older individuals. Recognition of these dementia syndromes is particularly important since most are treatable with partial or complete reversal of neuropsychological dysfunction.

Metabolic Disorders Causing Dementia

Table 8-6 lists the principal etiologies of chronic toxic and metabolic encephalopathies. Cerebral anoxia embarrasses cerebral metabolism and compromises intellectual function. The anoxia may be a product of cardiac failure, pulmonary disease, or severe anemia (Dalessio et al., 1965; Haruda et al., 1981; Krop et al., 1973; Lishman, 1978). Severe pulmonary disease with continuous oxygen deprivation and carbon dioxide retention produces a syndrome of confusion, headache, papilledema, tremor and twitching of the extremities, and evidence of cardiopulmonary decompensation (Austen et al., 1957; Bacchus, 1958; Bulger et al., 1966; Hamilton and Gross, 1963). Acute profound anoxia, as occurs with cardiopulmonary arrest, may produce a prominent postanoxic dementia syndrome (Norris and Chandrasekar, 1971; Richardson et al., 1959).

Patients with chronic renal failure may develop a uremic encephalopathy, and patients on dialysis are vulnerable to dialysis dementia. Uremia-related dementias are characterized by mental status changes, tremor, asterixis, and conspicuous slowing of the EEG (Ginn, 1975; Jacob et al., 1965; Raskin and Fishman, 1976; Shreiner, 1959). Dialysis dementia is a progressive fatal encephalopathy with intellectual deterioration, prominent dysarthria, and myoclonus (Alfrey et al., 1976; Baratz and Herzog, 1980; Lederman and Henry, 1978). The EEG in dialysis dementia reveals generalized slowing with intermittent bursts of polyspike complexes (Hughes and Schreeder, 1980). The occurrence of dialysis dementia appears to be related to the amount of aluminum in the dialysis solution, and the incidence has diminished with attention to the amount of parenteral aluminum received by dialysis patients (Dunea et al., 1978; Rozas et al., 1978).

Hepatic (portosystemic) encephalopathy is produced by advanced hepatic disease and shunting of portal venous blood into the general circulation. Clinically, the syndrome includes a chronic confusional state, tremor, asterixis, and evidence of hepatic dysfunction (Hoffman, 1981; Leavitt and Tyler, 1964; Sherlock et al., 1954). The EEG is generally slow, with bursts of delta-frequency triphasic waves (Silverman, 1962). Strict limitation of dietary protein and prevention of ammonia production by gastrointestinal flora through the use of neomycin and lactulose frequently result in an improved mental state (Conn, 1969; Welsh et al., 1974). A few patients with persistent hepatic encephalopathy develop an irreversible dementia syndrome and a choreiform movement disorder (Victor et al., 1965).

Vitamin deficiencies including lack of B_{12}, folate, or niacin produce dementia syndromes. Thiamine deficiency leads to the Wernicke–Korsakoff syndrome, an amnestic state with little impairment of other intellectual functions (Chapter 4). Vitamin B_{12} deficiency leads to dementia, myelopathy, peripheral neuropathy, optic neuropathy, and anemia. The dementia may be the predominant neurological abnormality and may precede blood and marrow changes (Strachan and Henderson, 1965). Folate deficiency may exist without concomitant neurological deficits but in some cases leads to a clinical syndrome, including a dementia closely resembling that of B_{12} deficiency (Strachan and Henderson, 1967). Lack of niacin produces a syndrome manifested by gastrointestinal tract lesions (gingivitis, glossitis, enteritis), diarrhea, dermatitis, and dementia (Jolliffe et al., 1940; Syndenstricker, 1943).

Endocrine disturbances are well-known causes of dementia. Hypothyroidism produces dementia, psychosis, neuropathy, and/or myopathy (Asher, 1949; Browning et al., 1954). Hyperthyroidism classically produces anxiety, restlessness, tachycardia, palpitations, and heat intolerance but in the elderly may present as a "simple" dementia syndrome with little systemic evidence of excessive thyroid activity (Arnold et al., 1974; Thomas et al., 1970). Hyperparathyroidism causes elevated serum calcium levels, dementia, weight loss, renal colic, abdominal pain, and bone and joint pain (Fitz and Hallmann, 1952; Gatewood et al., 1975; Karpati and Frame, 1964). In some cases, dementia may be the presenting manifestation. Hypoparathyroidism leads to basal ganglia calcification, dementia, and parkinsonism or choreoathetosis (Eraunt, 1974; Hossain, 1970; Muenter and Whisnant, 1968; Slyter, 1979). In both Cushing's and Addison's disease, reflecting excessive and inadequate adrenal function respectively, dementia is one manifestation of the clinical symptomatology (Cleghorn, 1951; Lishman, 1978; Starkman and Schteingart, 1981).

Toxic Conditions Causing Dementia

A wide variety of drugs have been associated with toxic dementia syndromes. Nearly any drug can produce intellectual compromise if administered in excessive amounts, but some can alter CNS function even in conventional dosages. The agents that have most often been implicated in drug-induced chronic confusional states are listed in Table 8-6. Psychotropic drugs, including neuroleptic agents, antidepressants, lithium, and minor tranquilizers are all capable of producing toxic dementias (Hollister, 1979; Shopsin et al., 1970; Van Putten et al., 1974). Anticholinergic agents used in the treatment of extrapyramidal and cardiac disorders and psychotropic agents with prominent anticholinergic activity impair central cholinergic activity and disturb intellectual function (Longo, 1966). Antihypertensive agents and anticonvulsants produce dementia syndromes when present in toxic amounts, and in some patients, dementia may be the only toxic manifestation (Adler, 1974; Ambrosetto et al., 1977; Cummings et al., 1980a,b; Lavin and Alexander, 1975; Trimble and Reynolds, 1976; Vallarta et al., 1974). Antibiotics, antineoplastic agents, digitalis, disulfiram, bromides, levodopa,

and many other agents may produce dementia syndromes in specific circumstances (Cummings and Benson, 1983).

In addition to iatrogenic dementias, chronic toxic encephalopathies occur commonly in multidrug abusers. In some cases the neuropsychological deficits remit with abstinence, but in others the dementia may be permanent. Electroencephalographic abnormalities often accompany the intellectual impairment (Grant and Judd, 1976; Grant et al., 1976).

Clinically significant dementia also occurs in approximately 3 percent of alcoholic patients, and careful neuropsychological testing reveals subtle intellectual deficits in up to 50 percent. The mental status impairments include disturbances of attention and abstraction, visuospatial alterations, and memory deficits (Carlen et al., 1981; Cutting, 1978; Lishman, 1981). The dementia syndrome includes many deficits beyond the restricted memory disturbance occurring in alcoholics with the Wernicke–Korsakoff syndrome, and alcoholic dementia is far more common than the Korsakoff state. The dementia is at least partially reversible with abstinence, and the atrophy visible on the CT scans of some alcoholics also reverses in many who remain abstinent (Carlen et al., 1978).

Metals (lead, mercury, manganese, arsenic, thallium) are highly toxic to the nervous system, and excessive exposure produces dementia and peripheral neuropathy (Goetz and Klawans, 1979; Graef, 1979; Vroom and Greer, 1972). Industrial and agricultural agents, including organic solvents (trichloroethylene, toluene, carbon tetrachloride, carbon disulfide), organophosphate insecticides, and carbon monoxide produce dementia in circumstances involving chronic excessive exposure (Allen, 1979; Cummings and Benson, 1983; Prockop, 1979; Metcalf and Holmes, 1969). As in other toxic and metabolic conditions, elimination of the exposure leads to symptomatic improvement in a majority of cases.

Hydrocephalic Dementias

Hydrocephalus refers to the presence of excessive cerebrospinal fluid (CSF) in the head and in essentially all cases entails ventricular enlargement with increased fluid within the ventricular cavities. Hydrocephalus can be the end result of several processes as shown in Table 8-7. In hydrocephalus ex vacuo, the ventricular dilatation is a product of tissue loss with no change in the dynamics of CSF flow (nonobstructive hydrocephalus). Obstructive hydrocephalus, on the other hand, occurs when there is a blockage of CSF pathways. The obstruction may be within the ventricular system or at the level of the outlet foramina, preventing the fluid from mov-

TABLE 8-7. Differential Diagnosis of Conditions Causing Hydrocephalus

Nonobstructive hydrocephalus
  Hydrocephalus ex vacuo
    (secondary to loss of cerebral tissue)

Obstructive hydrocephalus

  Noncommunicating

    Intraventricular blockade

      Aqueductal stenosis
      Ventricular masses

    Obstruction of ventricular outlet foramina

      Posterior fossa neoplasms
      Basilar meningitis
      Congenital malformations

  Communicating (normal-pressure hydrocephalus)

    Posttraumatic
    Posthemorrhagic
    Postinfectious
    Indiopathic
    Ectatic basilar artery

ing from within the ventricular system to the subarachnoid space (noncommunicating hydrocephalus), or it may be within the subarachnoid space, preventing absorption of the fluid by the pacchionian villi of the arachnoid granulations (communicating hydrocephalus). In the former, ventricular pressure is usually increased, whereas in communicating hydrocephalus the intracranial pressure often remains normal (normal-pressure hydrocephalus) (Benson, 1975; Benson et al., 1972).

The clinical characteristics of obstructive hydrocephalus include dementia, gait disturbance, and incontinence. Apathy, inattention, poor memory, and impaired judgement and abstraction are typical of hydrocephalic dementia (McHugh, 1964). The gait disturbance may have a predominantly ataxic, apraxic, or spastic quality, and the incontinence is usually a late feature (Messert and Baker, 1966; Yakovlev, 1947).

Intraventricular blockade in noncommunicating obstructive hydrocephalus may be produced by aqueductal stenosis or ventricular masses (neoplasms, hematomas, colloid systs). Obstruction of the outlet foramina can be caused by posterior fossa neoplasms, basilar meningitis, or congenital malformations. Absorption blockade in communicating hydrocephalus usually follows trauma with subarachnoid bleeding, subarachnoid hemorrhage from aneurysms or vascular malformations, or CNS infections (Adams et al., 1965; Benson, 1975; Cummings and Benson, 1983).

Determination of the type of hydrocephalus is made by a combination of CT scan and cisternographic findings. The CT scan reveals large ventricles in all cases of hydrocephalus. Patients with hydrocephalus ex vacuo usually have symmetrically dilated ventricles and enlarged cerebral sulci, whereas patients with obstructive hydrocephalus have ventricular enlargement out of proportion to the sulcal enlargement, the anterior portions of the ventricles are more enlarged than the posterior portions, and there may be periventricular edema (LeMay and Hochberg, 1979). Radioisotope flow studies in hydrocephalus ex vacuo show ventricular reflux of the tracer substance and normal flow over the cerebral convexities; in normal-pressure hydrocephalus (obstructive communicating hydrocephalus) there is ventricular reflux and blockage of flow over the convexities, and in noncommunicating hydrocephalus there is no ventricular reflux and normal flow over the convexities (Benson et al., 1970).

Of patients with obstructive hydrocephalus, 40–60 percent benefit from ventriculoperitoneal shunting with improved mental and motor function (Hughes et al., 1978; Udvarhelyi et al., 1975). The currently available laboratory tests do not predict which patients will improve with shunting, and any patient meeting clinical, radiological, and cisternographic criteria for obstructive hydrocephalus should be allowed the opportunity for improvement by shunting.

Traumatic Dementias

Cerebral trauma is the most common cause of dementia in young individuals and in western countries is usually a product of motor vehicle accidents (Alexander, 1982). The lesions may be primarily contusions of the cerebral gray matter or shearing lesions of the subcortical white matter (Courville, 1950; Lindenberg and Freytag, 1960; Strich, 1961). Amnesia and personality changes are common and reflect medial temporal and orbitofrontal damage, respectively. Aphasia, impaired concentration, poor abstracting abilities, and apraxia occur in some cases. The long-term prognosis for recovery is good in most cases, but intellectual restitution may take several years and may never be complete (Miller and Stern, 1965).

Subdural hematomas should be considered in any patient with mental status changes following trauma, and in the elderly the inciting traumatic event may be minimal (Perlmutter and Gables, 1961; Stuteville and Welch, 1958). Mental status alterations include fluctuating arousal, irritability, poor attention, and impaired memory. Focal neurological signs may be present. In most cases subdural blood collections are visible on CT scans, but they may become isodense with brain tissue and thus difficult to detect (Greenhouse and Barr, 1979; Jacobson and Farmer, 1979).

Dementia pugilistica is an uncommon dementia syndrome occurring in boxers who have sustained multiple episodes of cerebral trauma. The dementia begins late in the boxer's career or after retirement and gradually progresses. The intellectual impairment is combined with ataxia and extrapyramidal disturbances, and autopsy studies reveal neuronal loss, astrocytic proliferation, and prominent neurofibrillary tangles (Corsellis et al., 1973; Critchley, 1957; Mawdsley and Ferguson, 1963).

Neoplastic Dementias

Brain tumors produce dementia syndromes by causing local tissue destruction or compression, by compromising cerebral blood flow, by increasing intracranial pressure, and in some cases by obstructing CSF flow and producing hydrocephalus. Dementia is most common with tumors of the frontal lobe. Such tumors may impair judgment and abstraction and increase intracranial pressure without producing focal neurological disturbances (Direkze et al., 1971; A Fisher, 1969; Frazier, 1936; Sachs, 1950). Temporal lobe tumors, tumors of subcortical structures, and neoplastic meningitis may also produce dementia syndromes.

Myelin Diseases with Dementia

Multiple sclerosis may have a relatively benign clinical course with little intellectual impairment, or it may be an aggressive remitting and relapsing or chronically progressive disorder with profound neuropsychological deterioration (Bergin, 1957; Kahana et al., 1971; Koenig, 1968; Young et al., 1976). Nearly all patients with multiple sclerosis have eye movement disturbances, as well as motor, sensory, and reflex abnormalities. The CT scan may reveal periventricular cerebral lucencies, and the spinal fluid may contain an increased number of lymphocytes, elevated protein, or excessive gamma globulin content (Aita et al., 1978; Tourtellotte, 1970).

Metachromatic leukodystrophy and adrenoleukodystrophy are two rare inherited diseases of myelin metabolism that cause dementia in adults. Metachromatic leukodystrophy is a recessively inherited disorder manifesting dementia and peripheral neuropathy (Austin et al., 1968; Bosch and Hart, 1978; Muller et al., 1969). Adrenoleukodystrophy is an X-linked recessive disorder producing dementia and adrenal failure (Powell et al., 1975; Schaumburg et al., 1975).

Dementias Associated with Psychiatric Disorders

The dementia syndromes associated with psychiatric disorders have often been called *pseudodementias*, but the prefix "pseudo-" is inappropriate when dementia is defined as a clinical syndrome produced by

TABLE 8-8. Psychiatric Disorders Associated with Dementia Syndromes

Affective disorders
Depression
Mania
Schizophrenia
Hysteria
Conversion symptoms
Ganser syndrome
Miscellaneous
Anxiety
Obsessive–compulsive disorders
Malingering

a variety of diverse disorders. Patients with intellectual impairment associated with psychiatric disturbances meet the syndromic definition of dementia utilized here. Their potential treatability makes recognition of the dementia syndromes occurring with psychiatric disorders particularly important. Table 8-8 lists the psychiatric conditions that may compromise intellectual performance.

Depression

Depression is the most common psychiatric disorder that produces a syndrome of intellectual impairment. Follow-up studies of patients diagnosed as suffering from degenerative dementia have revealed that 30–50 percent do not undergo the expected neuropsychological deterioration and are eventually rediagnosed. The disorder most frequently misidentified as degenerative dementia is depression (Nott and Fleminger, 1975; Ron et al., 1979).

The dementia syndrome of depression occurs primarily in elderly individuals with manic–depressive illness, recurrent unipolar depression, or late-onset endogenous depression (Caine, 1981; Folstein and McHugh, 1978). Attention and memory deficits are ubiquitous in depressed patients of all ages, but intellectual impairment sufficient to produce a dementia syndrome is rare in young patients and occurs in at least 10 percent of aged depressed patients (Kay et al., 1955).

The dementia usually occurs in patients with retarded depressions manifesting both neurovegetative and neuromotor disturbances. They have a parkinsonianlike appearance with psychomotor retardation, bowed posture, and hypophonic speech. In addition, they suffer from insomnia, loss of appetite, constipation, and diminished libido. Mental status alterations characteristic of the dementia syndrome of depression include slowness of responses, lack of attention, poor memory, disorientation, impaired motivation, and disturbed ability to abstract and grasp the meaning of situations. Poor word-list generation and simplification of constructions are also common, and incomplete performances and "I don't know" and "I can't" responses are frequent. The patients may have mood-congruent hallucinations and delusions and ideas of reference (Caine, 1981; Folstein and McHugh, 1978; McAllister, 1983; McHugh and Folstein, 1979; Wells, 1979).

Laboratory studies of patients with the dementia syndrome of depression usually reveal cerebral atrophy on the CT scan, a positive dexamethasone suppression test (failure of suppression of endogenous cortisol secretion by administration of dexamethasone), and a normal EEG (Grunhaus et al., 1983; McAllister et al., 1982). Unfortunately, enlarged ventricles and sulci are common in normal elderly individuals as well as those with dementia, and abnormal dexamethasone suppression tests occur in many types of dementia without depression (Spar and Gerner, 1982). These tests do not effectively distinguish depressed patients from those with other causes of dementia.

In some cases, the diagnosis of depression-related dementia may depend on treatment responsiveness, and antidepressant therapy should be considered in any patient where depression may be producing or exacerbating a dementia syndrome. Heterocyclic antidepressants, monoamine oxidase (MAO) inhibitors, lithium, and electroconvulsive therapy have all been used successfully to treat the depression of patients with an associated dementia syndrome (Allen, 1982; Cowdry and Goodwin, 1981; Glass et al., 1981; Good, 1981).

Mania

Mania is a rare cause of dementia, but a few cases have been reported in which the disorganized, disinhibited behavior led to a dementia syndrome (Chiles and Cohen, 1979; Smith et al., 1976; Smith and Kiloh, 1981). Memory disturbances and disorientation are common in advanced stages of mania, but in most cases the associated hyperactivity, flight of ideas, pressured speech, and expansive grandiosity make the diagnosis obvious (Carlson and Goodwin, 1973). Improvement usually follows treatment with lithium, and many patients require a major tranquilizer to control the acute episode (Baldessarini and Lipinski, 1975). Elderly manic patients may develop confusional states in the course of manic episodes and respond more slowly to treatment (Chapter 7).

Schizophrenia

Intellectual impairment may occur in schizophrenia as part of an acute psychotic episode in the buffoonery syndrome when the patient manifests clowning, jocularity, and facetious responses or as an integral part of the schizophrenic disorder in a specific subpopulation of schizophrenic patients (Cummings and Benson, 1983; Lishman, 1978). The latter group is distinguished from schizophrenia without neuropsychological deterioration by ventricular enlargement on CT scan, a preponderance of negative schizophrenic symptoms (apathy, withdrawal, flat affect, anhedonia), poor premorbid adjustment, and poor response to treatment (Chapter 13) (Andreasen et al., 1982; Crow, 1980; Golden et al., 1980; Johnstone et al., 1978).

Hysteria

Dementia as a manifestation of an hysterical conversion reaction is rare. The hallmark of the syndrome is the marked contrast between the patient's relatively normal performance in unstructured circumstances and markedly impoverished performance in the testing situation (Kiloh, 1961; McEvoy and Wells, 1979). Whenever an hysterical conversion syndrome is identified, it must be borne in mind that the symptom complex is usually the harbinger of a neurological or major psychiatric disorder (Chapter 15) (Merskey and Buhrich, 1975; Slater, 1965; Stefansson et al., 1976).

Ganser Syndrome

The Ganser syndrome is considered by many to be a variant of hysterical dementia but has separate and unique clinical features. The most unusual and characteristic feature is the patient's penchant for replying to simple questions (e.g., "How many legs does a dog have?" "Where was the battle of Waterloo fought?") with ridiculous or approximate answers. In addition, the typical Ganser syndrome includes disturbances of consciousness, amnesia for the episode, hallucinations, and motor or sensory deficits similar to those found in conversion reactions (Enoch and Trethowan, 1979; Goldin and MacDonald, 1955; Tyndel, 1956; Weiner and Braiman, 1955; Whitlock, 1967). The disorder usually improves spontaneously, but in many cases an underlying metabolic or neurological disorder contributes to the symptomatology.

Miscellaneous Psychosyndromes with Dementia

In rare cases, severe anxiety, disabling obsessive–compulsive symptoms, or malingering may interrupt the patient's performance and create an appearance of dementia. Observation and response to treatment usually clarify the diagnosis.

DEMENTIA EVALUATION

The large number of potential causes of dementias make it impossible to construct a laboratory battery that would adequately screen for all causes of intellectual impairment. In addition, many syndromes (degenerative dementias, depression) lack pathognomonic laboratory features that would allow such identification. Instead, recognition of the different causes of dementia depends on integration of information from the clinical history, neurological and general physical examinations, and mental status assessment as well as from selected laboratory tests (Table 8-9). A thorough history will reveal any evidence of industrial exposure, drug ingestion, past physical illnesses or psychiatric disturbances, and any family history suggestive of an inherited neuromedical or psychiatric disability. A general physical examination may uncover evidence of a systemic or toxic disturbance that may be compromising intellectual function, and a neurological examination will provide evidence for focal, multifocal, or diffuse involvement of the CNS. The mental status assessment may be of great value in determining whether the pattern of intellectual deficits is most consistent with predominantly cortical dysfunction (Alzheimer's disease, Pick's disease), subcortical dysfunction (extrapyramidal syndromes, lacunar state), or mixed cortical and subcortical involvement (multi-infarct dementia, CNS infections, etc.) Mental status examination will also provide evidence for any psychiatric disturbance (depression, mania, schizophrenia) that may be etiologically relevant to the dementia syndrome.

A core group of laboratory studies should be obtained on all demented patients to evaluate for the most common systemic disorders responsible for dementia syndromes (Table 8-9). This elementary laboratory assessment includes a complete blood count; analyses of erythrocyte sedimentation rate (ESR), serum electrolytes, blood glucose, blood urea nitrogen, serum calcium and phosphorous levels, liver function and thyroid function tests, analyses of serum vitamin B_{12} and folate levels, and a serologic test for syphilis. A lumbar puncture should be performed whenever there is question of an infectious, inflammatory, or demyelinating disorder involving the CNS. Abnormalities revealed in the history, physical examination, neurological examination, mental status assessment, or preliminary laboratory studies will require confirmation and further definition by more extensive and specific laboratory tests.

The EEG is a valuable tool in the evaluation of the dementia patient (Cummings and Benson, 1983; Harner, 1975). Focal abnormalities are most consistent with localized disorders such as tumors, abscesses, subdural hematomas, or cerebral infarctions; diffuse slowing occurs in toxic and metabolic disorders and in advanced degenerative diseases; and normal records suggest a dementia syndrome of depression or an early degenerative disorder.

TABLE 8-9.   Evaluation of the Demented Patient

History
Physical examination
Neurological examination
Mental status examination
Laboratory assessment
Complete blood count, ESR determination
Electrolytes, blood glucose, blood urea nitrogen analyses
Serum calcium and phosphorus analyses
Liver function tests
Serum B_{12} and folate level determinations
Throid function tests
Serologic test for syphilis
Lumbar puncture
Electroencephalogram
Computerized tomogram of the head

Computerized tomography plays an important role in the dementia evaluation. Its greatest usefulness is in the delineation of focal lesions (infarcts, neoplasms, traumatic changes, subdural hematomas, abscesses) and hydrocephalus. Enlarged ventricles and cortical sulci are evident on the scans of many demented patients, but this atrophy correlates best with the patient's age, is a poor index of intellectual function, and cannot be used as evidence for the existence of a cortical degenerative process such as Alzheimer's disease (Huckman et al., 1975; Wells and Duncan, 1977). When hydrocephalus is demonstrated on the CT scan, cisternography may be necessary to determine whether the patient is a candidate for a ventriculoperitoneal shunt.

MANAGEMENT OF THE DEMENTIA PATIENT

Management of demented patients involves four separate objectives: (1) etiologic diagnosis and disease-specific management, (2) management of behaviors produced by the dementia, (3) prevention of secondary complications, and (4) support of the patient's family. This chapter has emphasized the need to identify the cause of the dementia syndrome in any patient with acquired intellectual impairment. Dementia cannot be appropriately managed when considered as a unitary syndrome of brain failure. Rather, dementia must be recognized to be a complex clinical syndrome produced by a multitude of different disease processes. Proper management depends on identifying the etiologic disorder and instituting disease-specific treatment. Thus control of hypertension or elimination of a source of emboli can halt the progression of multi-infarct dementia, shunting may reverse the deficits in hydrocephalic dementia, some infectious dementias can be treated with antibiotics, metabolic dementias respond to treatment of the underlying condition, toxic dementias usually resolve when harmful exposure is eliminated, and the dementia syndrome of depression responds to pharmocotherapy or electroconvulsive therapy (ECT). The dementia of Parkinson's disease improves with levodopa therapy, and the dementia of Wilson's disease may be prevented or reversed by the timely administration of penicillamine (Halgin et al., 1977; Marsh et al., 1971; Meier and Martin, 1970; Scheinberg and Sternlieb, 1960).

For many demented patients, however, no specific treatment is available (e.g., those suffering from Alzheimer's disease, Pick's disease, and other degenerative dementias), and it is not uncommon for patients with treatable illnesses to remain partially impaired even after appropriate therapy has been initiated. Treatment of these patients is directed at minimizing the disabling effects of the dementia and controlling unacceptable behaviors (Snyder and Harris, 1976). A safe, contained environment is necessary for DAT patients whose restless wandering and hyperoral behavior may lead to their getting lost or ingesting inappropriate items. Adequate hydration and nutrition must be maintained and social and sensory deprivation eliminated. Nocturnal confusion can be minimized by a nightlight, and a soft restraint may be necessary to keep the patient in bed; however, restraints should be used as sparingly as pos-

sible. Urinary infections and aspiration pneumonia must be guarded against, and, in the final stages when the patient is bed-bound, decubiti must be avoided by frequent turning and protective cushioning.

When drugs are necessary to gain control of unacceptable behavior, a major tranquilizer given in small doses should be utilized. Minor tranquilizers and soporific agents should be avoided since they tend to increase confusion in the intellectually compromised patient (Hier and Caplan, 1980). Depression may accompany many dementia syndromes, particularly extrapyramidal disorders and multi-infarct dementia, and can exacerbate any preexisting neuropsychological impairment. Treatment of the depression may reverse at least a portion of the mental status deficits. Anticoagulants, cerebral stimulants, and vasodilators have all been used in the treatment of dementia patients, but with limited success, and their role in the management of dementia is not established.

Attention must also be directed toward the family of the demented patient. Education is a primary goal: family members should be informed about the cause of the patient's changed behavior, any available treatments, and the patient's prognosis. In addition, provision of social supports such as home health aids and visiting nurses may allow the patient to be maintained in the home for an extended period of time. Legal advice is necessary to aid the family regarding estate disposition and conservatorship. Finally, psychotherapy, either with an individual therapist or through disease-oriented support groups, may provide insight into feelings of loss, grief, and guilt common among family members.

REFERENCES

Adams RD, Fisher CM, Hakim S, Ojemann RG, and Sweet WT. Symptomatic occult hydrocephalus with "normal" cerebrospinal fluid pressure. New Engl J Med, 1965, 273, 117–126.

Adler S. Methyldopa-induced decrease in mental activity. JAMA, 1974, 230, 1428–1429.

Aita JF, Bennett DR, Anderson RE, and Ziter F. Cranial CT appearance of acute multiple sclerosis. Neurology, 1978, 28, 251–255.

Albert ML. Subcortical dementia. In Katzman R, Terry RD, and Bick KL (Eds.): Alzheimer's disease: senile dementia and related disorders. New York, Raven Press, 1978, pp. 173–180.

Albert ML, Feldman RG, and Willis AL. The "subcortical dementia" of progressive supranuclear palsy. J Neurol Neurosurg Psychiat, 1974, 37, 121–130.

Alexander MP. Traumatic brain injury. In Benson DF and

Blumer D (Eds.): Psychiatric aspects of neurologic disease, Vol. 2. New York, Grune & Stratton, 1982, pp. 219–248.

Alfrey AC, Legendre GR, and Kaehny WD. The dialysis encephalopathy syndrome. Possible aluminum intoxication. New Engl J Med, 1976, 294, 184–188.

Allen N. Solvents and other industrial organic compounds. In Vinken PJ and Bruyn GW (Eds.): Intoxications of the nervous system, Part I, Vol. 36. Handbook of clinical neurology. New York, North-Holland Publishing Company, 1979, pp. 361–389.

Allen RM. Pseudodementia and ECT. Biol Psychiat, 1982, 17, 1435–1443.

Ambrosetto G, Tassinari CA, Baruzzi A, and Lugaresi E. Phenytoin encephalopathy as probable idiosyncratic reaction: case report. Epilepsia, 1977, 18, 405–408.

Andreasen NC, Olsen SA, Dennert JW, and Smith MR. Ventricular enlargement in schizophrenia: relationship to positive and negative symptoms. *Am J Psychiat*, 1982, *139*, 297–302.

Arnold BM, Casal G, and Higgins HP. Apathetic thyrotoxicosis. *Canad Med Assoc J*, 1974, *3*, 957–958.

Asher R. Myxoedematous madness. *Br Med J*, 1949, *2*, 555–562.

Austen FK, Carmichael MW, and Adams RD. Neurologic manifestations of chronic pulmonary insufficiency. *New Engl J Med*, 1957, *257*, 579–590.

Austin J, Armstrong D, Fouch S, Mitchell C, Stumpf D, Shearer L, and Briner O. Metachromatic leukodystophy (MLD). *Arch Neurol*, 1968, 225–240.

Bacchus H. Encephalopathy in pulmonary disease. *Arch Int Med*, 1958, *102*, 194–198.

Baldessarini RJ and Lipinski JF. Lithium salts: 1970–1975. *Ann Intern Med*, 1975, *83*, 527–533.

Baratz R and Herzog AG. The communication disorder in dialysis dementia: a case report. *Brain Lang*, 1980, *10*, 378–389.

Barr AN, Heinze WT, Dubben GD, Valvassori GE, and Sugar O. Bicaudate index in computerized tomography in Huntington disease and cerebral atrophy. *Neurology*, 1978, *28*, 1196–1200.

Bauer WR, Turel AP Jr, and Johnson KP. Progressive multifocal leukoencephalopathy and cytarabine. *JAMA*, 1973, *226*, 174–176.

Benson DF. The hydrocephalic dementias. In Benson DF and Blumer D (Eds.): *Psychiatric aspects of neurologic disease*. New York, Grune & Stratton, 1975, pp. 83–97.

Benson DF, LeMay M, Patten DH, and Rubens AB. Diagnosis of normal-pressure hydrocephalus. *New Engl J Med*, 1970, *283*, 609–615.

Benson DF, Patten DH, and LeMay M. Hydrocephalic dementia. In Harbert JC (Ed.): *Cisternography and hydrocephalus*. Springfield, Illinois, Charles C Thomas, Publisher, 1972, pp. 343–355.

Bergin JD. Rapidly progressing dementia in disseminated sclerosis. *J Neurol Neurosurg Psychiat*, 1957, *20*, 285–292.

Bernoulli C, Siegfried J, Baumgartner G, Regli F, Rabinowitz T, Gajdusek DG, and Gibbs CJ Jr. Danger of accidental person-to-person transmission of Creutzfeldt-Jakob disease by surgery. *Lancet*, 1977, *1*, 478–479.

Bird ED, Mackay AVP, Rayner CN, and Iversen LL. Reduced glutamic-acid–decarboxylase activity of the post-mortem brain in Huntington's chorea. *Lancet*, 1973, *1*, 1090–1092.

Bosch EP and Hart MN. Late adult-onset metachromatic leukodystrophy. *Arch Neurol*, 1978, *35*, 475–477.

Bowen DM, Smith CB, White P, and Davidson AN. Neurotransmitter-related enzymes and indices of hypoxia in senile dementia and other abiotrophies. *Brain*, 1976, *99*, 459–496.

Breutsch WL. Neurosyphilitic conditions. In Arieti S (Ed.): *American handbook of psychiatry*, New York, Basic Books, 1959, pp. 1003–1020.

Brierley JB, Corsellis JAN, Hierons R, and Nevin S. Subacute encephalitis of later adult life mainly affecting the limbic areas. *Brain*, 1960, *83*, 357–368.

Browning TB, Atkins RW, and Weiner H. Cerebral metabolic disturbances in hypothyroidism. *Arch Int Med*, 1954, *93*, 938–950.

Brun A and Gustafson L. Limbic lobe involvement in presenile dementia. *Arch Psychiat Nervenkr*, 1978, *226*, 79–93.

Bulger RJ, Schrier RW, Arend WP, and Swanson AG. Spinal-fluid acidosis and the diagnosis of pulmonary encephalopathy. *New Engl J Med*, 1966, *274*, 433–437.

Burger LJ, Rowan J, and Goldensohn ES, Creutzfeldt-Jakob disease. An electroencephalographic study. *Arch Neurol*, 1972, *26*, 428–433.

Caine ED. Pseudodementia. Current concepts and future directions. *Arch Gen Psychiat*, 1981, *38*, 1359–1364.

Caplan LR and Schoene WC. Clinical features of subcortical arteriosclerotic encephalopathy (Binswanger disease). *Neurology*, 1978, *28*, 1206–1215.

Carlen PL, Wilkinson A, Wortzman G, Holgate R, Cordingley J, Lee MA, Huszar L, Moddel G, Singh R, Kiraly L, and Rankin JG. Cerebral atrophy and functional deficits in alcoholics without clinically apparent liver disease. *Neurology*, 1981, *31*, 377–385.

Carlen PL, Wortzman G, Holgate RC, Wilkinson DA, and Rankin JG, Reversible atrophy in recently abstinent chronic alcoholics measured by computed tomography. *Science*, 1978, *200*, 1076–1078.

Carlson GA and Goodwin FK, The stages of mania. *Arch Gen Psychiat*, 1973, *28*, 221–228.

Chiles JA and Cohen D. Pseudodementia and mania. *J Nerv Ment Dis*, 1979, *167*, 357–358.

Chiofalo N, Fuentes A, and Galvez S. Serial EEG findings in 27 cases of Creutzfeldt-Jakob disease. *Arch Neurol*, 1980, *37*, 143–145.

Cleghorn RA. Adrenal cortical insufficiency: psychological and neurological observations. *Canad Med Assoc J*, 1951, *65*, 449–454.

Conn HO. A rational program for the management of hepatic coma. *Gastroenterology*, 1969, *57*, 715–723.

Conomy JP, Beard NS, Matsumoto M, and Roessmann U. Cytarabine treatment of progressive multifocal leukoencephalopathy. *JAMA*, 1974, *229*, 1313–1316.

Cook RH, Bard BE, and Austin JH. Studies in aging of the brain: IV. Familial Alzheimer disease: relation to transmissible dementia, aneuploidy, and microtubular defects. *Neurology*, 1979, *29*, 1402–1412.

Corsellis JAN. Aging and the dementias. In Blackwood W and Corsellis JAN (Eds.): *Greenfield's neuropathology*. London, Edward Arnold Publishers, 1976, pp. 796–848.

Corsellis JAN, Bruton CJ, and Freeman-Browne D. The aftermath of boxing. *Psychol Med*, 1973, *3*, 270–303.

Corsellis JAN, Goldberg GJ, and Norton AR. ''Limbic encephalitis'' and its association with carcinoma. *Brain*, 1968, *91*, 481–496.

Courville CB. The mechanism of coup-contrecoup injuries of the brain. *Bull Neurol Soc*, 1950, *15*, 72–86.

Cowdry RW and Goodwin FK. Dementia of bipolar illness: diganosis and response to lithium. *Am J Psychiat*, 1981, *138*, 1118–1119.

Critchley M. Medical aspects of boxing, particularly from a neurological standpoint. *Br Med J*, 1957, *1*, 357–362.

Crow TJ, Molecular pathology of schizophrenia: more than one disease process? *Br Med J*, 1980, *280*, 66–68.

Cummings JL. Cortical dementias. In Benson DF and Blumer D (Eds.): *Psychiatric aspects of neurologic disease*, Vol. 2. New York, Grune & Stratton, 1982, pp. 93–120.

Cummings JL and Benson DF. *Dementia: a clinical approach*. Boston, Butterworths, 1983.

Cummings JL and Benson DF. Subcortical dementia review of an emerging concept. *Arch Neurol*, 1984, *41*, 874–879.

Cummings JL, Benson DF, and LoVerme S Jr. Reversible dementia. *JAMA*, 1980a, *243*, 2434–2439.

Cummings JL, Benson DF, Hill MA, and Read S. Aphasia in dementia of the Alzheimer type. *Neurology*, 1985, *35*, 394–397.

Cummings JL and Duchen LW. The Klüver-Bucy syndrome in Pick disease. *Neurology*, 1981, *31*, 1415–1422.

Cummings JL, Gosenfeld LF, Houlihan JP, and McCaffrey T. Neuropsychiatric disturbances associated with idiopathic calcification of the basal ganglia. *Biol Psychiat*, 1983, *18*, 591–601.

Cummings J, Hebben NA, Obler L, and Leonard P. Nonaphasic misnaming and other neurobehavior features of an unusual toxic encephalopathy: case study *Cortex*, 1980b, *16*, 315–323.

Cutting J. The relationship between Korsakov's syndrome and alcoholic dementia. *Br J Psychiat*, 1978, *132*, 240–251.

Dalessio DJ, Benchimol A, and Dimond EG. Chronic encephalopathy related to heart block. *Neurology*, 1965, *15*, 449–503.

Davies P. Studies on the neurochemistry of central cholinergic systems in Alzheimer's disease. In Katzman R, Terry RD, and Bick KL (Eds.): *Alzheimer's disease: senile dementia and related disorders*. New York, Raven Press, 1978, pp. 453–468.

De Reuck J, Crevits L. De Coster W, Sieben G, and vander Eecken H. Pathogenesis of Binswanger chronic progressive subcortical encephalopathy. *Neurology*, 1980, *30*, 920–928.

Direkze M, Bayliss SG, and Cutting JC. Primary tumours of the frontal lobe. *Br J Clin Pract*, 1971, *25*, 207–213.

Duffy P, Wolf J, Collins G, DeVoe AG, Streeten B, and Cowen D. Possible person-to-person transmission of Creutzfeldt-Jakob disease. *New Engl J Med*, 1974, *290*, 692.

Dunea G, Mahurkar SD, Mandani B, and Smith EC. Role of aluminum in dialysis dementia. *Ann Int Med*, 1978, *88*, 502–504.

Ellner JJ and Bennett JE. Chronic meningitis. *Medicine*, 1976, *55*, 341–369.

Enoch MD and Trethowan WH. *Uncommon psychiatric syndromes*. 2nd ed. Bristol, John Wright and Sons Ltd., 1979.

Eraut D. Idiopathic hypoparathyroidism presenting as dementia. *Br Med J*, 1974, *1*, 429–430.

Feldman RG, Chandler KA, Levy II, and Glaser GH. Familial Alzheimer's disease. *Neurology*, 1963, *13*, 811–824.

Ferris EJ and Levine HL. Cerebral arteritis: a classification. *Radiology*, 1973, *109*, 327–341.

Feurle GE, Volk B, and Waldherr R. Cerebral Whipple's disease with negative jejunal histology. *New Engl J Med*, 1979, *300*, 907–908.

Fisher A. On meningioma presenting with dementia. *Proc Aust Assoc Neurol*, 1969a, *6*, 29–38.

Fisher CM. Lacunes: small, deep cerebral infarcts. *Neurology*, 1965, *15*, 774–784.

Fisher CM. The arterial lesions underlying lacunes. *Acta Neuropathol*, 1969, *12*, 1–15.

Fitz TE and Hallman BL. Mental changes associated with hyperparathyroidism. *Arch Int Med*, 1952, *89*, 547–551.

Folstein MF and McHugh PR. Dementia syndrome of depression. In Katzman R, Terry RD, and Bick KL (Eds.): *Alzheimer's disease: senile dementia and related disorders*. New York, Raven Press, 1978, pp. 87–93.

Frazier CH. Tumor involving the frontal lobe alone. *Arch Neurol Psychiat*, 1936, *35*, 525–571.

Gajdusek DC. Unconventional viruses and the origin and disappearance of kuru. *Science*, 1977, *197*, 943–960.

Gatewood JW, Organ CH Jr, and Mead BT. Mental changes associated with hyperthyroidism. *Am J Psychiat*, 1975, *132*, 129–132.

Ginn HE. Neurobehavioral dysfunction in uremia. *Kidney Internat*, 1975, *217* (Suppl. 2), S217–S221.

Glass RM, Uhlenhuth EH, Hartel FW, Matzas W, and Fischman MW. Cognitive dysfunction and imipramine in outpatient depressives. *Arch Gen Psychiat*, 1981, *38*, 1045–1051.

Goetz CG and Klawans HL. Neurologic aspects of other metals. In Vinken PJ and Bruyn GW (Eds.): *Intoxications of the nervous system*, Part I. Vol. 36, *Handbook of clinical neurology*. New York, North-Holland Publishing Company, 1979, pp. 319–345.

Golden CJ, Moses JA Jr, Zelazowski R, Graber B, Zatz LM, Horvath TB, and Berger PA. Cerebral ventricular size and neuropsychological impairment in young chronic schizophrenics. *Arch Gen Psychiat*, 1980, *37*, 619–623.

Goldin S and MacDonald JE. The Ganser state. *J Ment Sci*, 1955, *101*, 267–280.

Good MI. Pseudodementia and physical findings masking significant psychopathology. *Am J Psychiat*, 1981, *138*, 811–814.

Graef JW. Clinical aspects of lead poisoning. In Vinken PJ and Bruyn GW (Eds.): *Intoxications of the nervous system*, Part I, Vol 36, *Handbook of clinical neurology*. New York, North-Holland Publishing Company, 1979, pp. 1–34.

Grant I and Judd LL. Neuropsychological and EEG disturbances in polydrug users. *Am J Psychiat*, 1976, 133, 1039–1042.

Grant I, Mohns L, Miller M, and Reitan RM. A neuropsychological study of polydrug users. *Arch Gen Psychiat*, 1976, *33*, 973–978.

Greenfield JG and Bosanquet FD. The brain-stem lesions in parkinsonism. *J Neurol Neurosurg Psychiat*, 1953, *16*, 213–226.

Greenhouse AH and Barr JW. The bilateral isodense subdural hematoma on computerized tomographic scan. *Arch Neurol*, 1979, *36*, 305–307.

Grunhaus L, Dilsaver S, Greden JF, and Carroll BJ. Depressive pseudodementia: a suggested diagnostic profile. *Biol Psychiat*, 1983, *18*, 215–225.

Gunner-Svensson F and Jensen K. Frequency of mental disorders in old age. *Acta Psychiat Scand*, 1976, *53*, 283–297.

Hachinski VC, Iliff LD, Zilhka E, DuBoulay GH, McAllister VC, Marshall J, Russell RWR, and Symon L. Cerebral blood flow in dementia. *Arch Neurol*, 1975, *32*, 632–637.

Hahn RD, Webster B, Weickhardt G, Thomas E, Timberlake W, Solomon H, Stokes JH, Moore JE, Heyman A, Gammon G, Gleeson GA, Curtis AC, and Cutler JC. Penicillin treatment of general paresis (dementia paralytica). *Arch Neurol Psychiat*, 1959, *81*, 557–590.

Halgin R, Ricklan M, and Misiak H. Levodopa, parkinsonism, and recent memory. *J Nerv Ment Dis*, 1977, *164*, 268–272.

Hamilton JD and Gross NJ. Unusual neurological and cardiovascular complications of respiratory failure. *Br Med J*, 1963, *2*, 1092–1096.

Harner RN. EEG evaluation of the patient with dementia. In Benson DF and Blumer D (Eds.): *Psychiatric aspects of neurologic disease*. New York, Grune & Stratton, 1975, pp. 63–82.

Haruda F, Friedman JH, Ganti SR, Hoffman N, and Chutorian AM. Rapid resolution of organic mental syndrome in sickle cell anemia in response to exchange transfusion. *Neurology*, 1981, *31*, 1015–1016.

Henson RA, Hoffman HL, Urich H. Encephalomyelitis with carcinoma. *Brain*, 1965, *88*, 449–464.

Hier DB and Caplan LR. Drugs for senile dementia. *Drugs*, 1980, *30*, 74–80.

Hoffman NE. Gastrointestinal diseases presenting as psychiatric symptoms. In Levenson AJ and Hall RCW (Eds.): *Neuropsychiatric manifestations of physical disease in the elderly*. New York, Raven Press, 1981, pp. 49–57.

Hollister LE. Psychotherapeutic drugs. In Levenson AJ (Ed.): *Neuropsychiatric side effects of drugs in the elderly*. New York, Raven Press, 1979, pp. 79–88.

Hossain M. Neurological and psychiatric manifestations in idiopathic hypoparathyroidism: response to treatment. *J Neurol Neurosurg Psychiat*, 1970, *33*, 153–156.

Huckman MS, Fox J, and Topel J. The validity of criteria for the evaluation of cerebral atrophy by computed tomography. *Radiology*, 1975, *116*, 85–92.

Hughes CP, Siegel BA, Coxe WS, Gado MH, Grubb RL, Coleman RE, and Berg L. Adult idiopathic communicating hydrocephalus with and without shunting. *J Neurol Neurosurg Psychiat*, 1978, *41*, 961–971.

Hughes JR and Schreeder MT. EEG in dialysis encephalopathy. *Neurology*, 1980, *30*, 1148–1154.

Jacob JC, Gloor P. Elwan OH, Dossetor JB, and Pateras VR. Electroencephalographic changes in chronic renal failure. *Neurology*, 1965, *15*, 419–429.

Jacobson PL and Farmer TW. The ''hypernormal'' CT scan in dementia: bilateral isodense subdural hemotomas. *Neurology*, 1979, *29*, 1522–1524.

Javoy-Agid F and Agid Y. Is the mesocortical dopaminergic system involved in Parkinson disease? *Neurology*, 1980, *30*, 1326–1330.

Jarvik LF and Perl M. Overview of physiologic dysfunctions related to psychiatric problems in the elderly. In Levenson AJ and Hall RCW (Eds.): *Neuropsychiatric manifestations of physical disease in the elderly*. New York, Raven Press, 1981, pp. 1–15.

Jervis GA. Pick's disease. In Minkler J (Ed.): *Pathology of the nervous system*, Vol 2. New York, McGraw-Hill Book Company, 1971, pp. 1395–1401.

Johnstone EC, Crow TJ, Frith CD, Steven M, Kreel L, and Husband J. The dementia of dementia praecox. *Acta Psychiat Scand*, 1978, *57*, 305–324.

Jolliffe N, Bowman KM, Rosenblum LA, and Fein HD. Nicotinic acid deficiency encephalopathy. *JAMA*, 1940, *114*, 307–312.

Jones DP and Nevin S. Rapidly progressive cerebral degeneration (subacute vascular encephalopathy) with mental disorder, focal disturbances, and myoclonic epilepsy. *J Neurol Neurosurg Psychiat*, 1954, *17*, 148–159.

Kahana E, Leibowitz U, and Alter M. Cerebral multiple sclerosis. *Neurology* 1971, *21*, 1179–1185.

Karpati G and Frame B. Neuropsychiatric disorders in primary hyperparathyroidism. *Arch Neurol*, 1964, *10*, 387–397.

Kay DWK, Roth M, and Hopkins B. Affective disorders arising in the senium. *J Ment Sci*, 1955, *101*, 302–318.

Kiloh LG. Pseudo-dementia. *Acta Psychiat Scand*, 1961, *37*, 336–351.

Kirschbaum WR. *Jakob-Creutzfeldt disease*. New York, American Elsevier Publishing Company, 1968.

Koenig H. Dementia associated with the benign form of multiple sclerosis. *Trans Am Neurol Assoc.*, 1968, *93*, 227–228.

Krop HD, Block AJ, and Cohen E. Neuropsychiatric effects of continuous oxygen therapy in chronic obstructive pulmonary disease. *Chest*, 1973, *64*, 317–322.

Lavin P and Alexander CP. Dementia associated with clonidine therapy. *Br Med J*, 1975, *1*, 628.

Leavitt S and Tyler HR. Studies in asterixis. *Arch Neurol*, 1964, *10*, 360–368.

Lederman RJ and Henry CE. Progressive dialysis encephalopathy. *Ann Neurol*, 1978, *4*, 199–204.

LeMay M and Hochberg FH. Ventricular differences between hydrostatic hydrocephalus and hydrocephalus ex vacuo by computed tomography. *Neuroradiology*, 1979, *17*, 191–195.

Levenson AJ and Hall RCW (Eds.): *Neuropsychiatric manifestations of physical disease in the elderly*. New York, Raven Press, 1981.

Levine J and Swanson PD. Nonatherosclerotic causes of stroke. *Ann Intern Med*, 1969, *70*, 807–816.

Lilly R, Cummings JL, Benson DF, and Frankel M. The human Klüver-Bucy syndrome. *Neurology*, 1983, *33*, 1141–1145.

Lindenberg R and Freytag E. The mechanism of cerebral contusions. *Arch Pathol*, 1960, *69*, 440–469.

Lishman WA. *Organic psychiatry*. London, Blackwell Scientific Publishers, 1978.

Lishman WA. Cerebral disorder in alcoholism. Syndromes of impairment. *Brain*, 1981, *104*, 1–20.

Longo VG. Behavioral and electroencephalographic effects of

atropine and related compounds. *Pharm Rev,* 1966, *18,* 965–996.

Lorand B, Nagy T, and Tariska S. Subacute progressive panencephalitis. *World Neurol,* 1962, *3,* 376–394.

Mancall EL. Progressive multifocal leukoencephalopathy. *Neurology,* 1965, *15,* 693–699.

Marsh GG, Markham CM, and Ansel R. Levodopa's awakening effect on patients with parkinsonism. *J Neurol Neurosurg Psychiat,* 1971, *34,* 209–218.

Masters CL and Richardson EP Jr. Subacute spongiform encephalopathy (Creutzfeldt-Jakob disease). *Brain,* 1978, *101,* 333–344.

Mawdsley C and Ferguson FR. Neurological disease in boxers. *Lancet,* 1963, *2,* 795–801.

Mayer-Gross W, Critchley M, Greenfield JG, and Meyer A. Discussion on the presenile dementias: symptomatology, pathology, and differential diagnosis. *Proc Roy Soc Med,* 1937–1938; *31,* 1443–1454.

Mayeux R, Stern Y, Rosen J, and Leventhal J. Depression, intellectual impairment, and Parkinson disease. *Neurology,* 1981, *31,* 645–650.

McAllister TW. Overview: pseudodementia. *Am J Psychiat,* 1983, *140,* 528–533.

McAllister TW, Ferrell RB, Price TRP, and Neville MB. The dexamethasone suppression test in two patients with severe depressive pseudodementia. *Am J Psychiat,* 1982, *139,* 479–481.

McEvoy JP and Wells CE. Case studies in neuropsychiatry II: conversion pseudodementia. *J Clin Psychiat,* 1979, *40,* 447–449.

McGeachie RE, Fleming JO, Sharer LR, and Hyman RA. Diagnosis of Pick's disease by computed tomography. *J Comput Asst Tomog* 1979, *3,* 113–115.

McHugh PR. Occult Hydrocephalus. *Quart J Med,* 1964, *33,* 297–308.

McHugh PR and Folstein MF. Psychiatric syndromes of Huntington's chorea; a clinical and phenomenologic study. In Benson DF and Blumer D (Eds.): *Psychiatric aspects of neurologic disease.* New York, Grune & Stratton, 1975, pp. 267–285.

McHugh PR and Folstein MF. Psychopathology of dementia: implications for neuropathology. In Katzman R (Ed.): *Cogenital and acquired cognitive disorders.* New York, Raven Press, 1979, pp. 17–30.

Meier MJ and Martin WE. Intellectual changes associated with levodopa therapy. *JAMA,* 1970, *213,* 465–466.

Merskey H and Buhrich NA. Hysteria and organic brain disease. *Br J Med Psychol,* 1975, *48,* 359–366.

Messert B and Baker NH. Sydrome of progressive spastic ataxia and apraxia sssociated with occult hydrocephalus. *Neurology,* 1966, *16,* 440–452.

Metcalf DR and Holmes JH. EEG, psychological, and neurological alterations in humans with organophosphorus exposure. *Ann NY Acad Sci,* 1969, *160,* 357–365.

Miller H and Stern G. The long-term prognosis of severe head injury. *Lancet,* 1965, *1,* 225–229.

Mortimer JA, Schuman LM, and French LR, Epidemiology of dementing illness. In Mortimer JA and Schuman LM (Eds.): *The epidemiology of dementia.* New York, Oxford University Press, 1981, pp. 3–23.

Muenter MD and Whisnant JP. Basal ganglia calcification, hypoparathyroidism, and extrapyramidal motor manifestations. *Neurology,* 1968, *18,* 1075–1083.

Muller D, Pilz H. and Ter Muelen V. Studies on adult metachromatic leukodystrophy. Part 1. Clinical, morphological, and histochemical observations in two cases. *J Neurol Sci,* 1969, *9,* 567–584.

Naef RW, Berry RG, and Schlezinger NS. Neurologic aspects of porphyria. *Neurology,* 1959, *9,* 313–320.

Narayan O, Penney JB Jr, Johnson RT, Herndon RM, and Weiner LP. Etiology of progressive multifocal leukoencephalopathy. *New Engl J Med,* 1973, *289,* 1278–1282.

Nielsen J. Geronto-psychiatric period-prevalence investigation in a geographically delimited population. *Acta Psychiat Scand,* 1962, *38,* 307–330.

Norris JR and Chandrasekar S. Anoxic brain damage after cardiac resuscitation. *J Chron Dis,* 1971, *24,* 585–590.

Nott PN and Fleminger JJ. Presenile dementia: the difficulties of early diagnosis. *Acta Psychiat Scand,* 1975, *51,* 210–217.

Osetowska E and Torck P. Subacute sclerosing leukoencephalitis. *World Neurol,* 1962, *3,* 566–578.

Perlmutter I and Gables C. Subdural hematomia in older patients. *JAMA,* 1961, *176,* 212–214.

Perry TL, Hansen S, and Kloster M. Huntington's chorea, deficiency of gamma-aminobutyric acid in brain. *New Engl J Med,* 1973, *288,* 337–342.

Pirozzolo FJ, Hansch EC, Mortimer JA, Webster DA, and Kuskowski MA. Dementia in Parkinson's disease: a neuropsychological analysis. *Brain Cognit,* 1982, *1,* 71–83.

Plum F. Dementia: an approaching epidemic. *Nature,* 1979, *279,* 372–373.

Powell H, Tindall R, Schultz P, Paa D, O'Brien J, and Lampert P. Adrenoleukodystrophy, *Arch Neurol,* 1975, *32,* 250–260.

Pratt RTC. The genetics of Alzheimer's disease. In Wolstenholme GEW and O'Connor M (Eds.): *Alzheimer's disease and related conditions.* London, J and A Churchill, 1970, pp. 137–139.

Prockop L. Neurotoxic volatile substances. *Neurology,* 1979, *29,* 862–865.

Raskin NH and Fishman RA. Neurologic disorders in renal failure. *New Engl J Med,* 1976, *294,* 143–148, 204–210.

Richardson EP Jr. Progressive multifocal leukoencephalopathy. In Vinken PJ and Bruyn GW (Eds.): *Multiple sclerosis and other demyelinating diseases,* Vol. 9, *Handbook of clinical neurology.* New York, American Elsevier Publishing Company, 1970, pp. 485–499.

Richardson JC, Chambers RA, and Heywood PM. Encephalopathies of anoxia and hypoglycemia. *Arch Neurol,* 1959, *1,* 178–190.

Romanul FCA, Radvany J, and Rosales RK. Whipple's disease confined to the brain: a case studied clinically and pathologically. *J Neurol Neurosurg Psychiat,* 1977, *40,* 901–909.

Ron MA, Toone BK, Garralda ME, and Lishman WA. Diagnostic accuracy in pre-senile dementia. *Br J Psychiat,* 1979, *134,* 161–168.

Rozas VV, Port FK, and Rutt WM. Progressive dialysis encephalopathy from dialysate aluminum. *Arch Int Med,* 1978, *138,* 1375–1377.

Sachs E Jr. Meningiomas with dementia as the first presenting feature. *J Ment Sci,* 1950, *96,* 998–1007.

Schaumburg HH, Powers JM, Raine CS, Suzuki K, and Richardson EP Jr. Adrenoleukodystrophy. *Arch Neurol,* 1975, *32,* 577–591.

Scheinberg IH and Sternlieb I. The long term management of hepatolenticular degeneration (Wilson's disease). *Am J Med,* 1960, *29,* 316–333.

Schreiner GE. Mental and personality changes in the uremic syndrome. *Med Ann Dist Columbia,* 1959, *28,* 316–362.

Sherlock S, Summerskill WHJ, White LP, and Phear EA. Portal-systemic encephalopathy. *Lancet,* 1954, *2,* 453–457.

Shopsin B, Johnson G, and Gershon S. Neurotoxicity with lithium: differential drug responsiveness. *Internat Pharmacopsychiat,* 1970, *5,* 170–182.

Siedler H and Malamud N. Creutzfeldt-Jakob's disease. *J Neuropath Exp Neurol,* 1963, *22,* 381–402.

Silverman D. Some observations on the EEG in hepatic coma. *Electroenceph Clin Neurophysiol,* 1962, *14,* 53–59.

Slater E. Diagnosis of "hysteria." *Br Med J,* 1965, *1,* 1395–1399.

Slyter H. Idiopathic hypoparathyroidism presenting as dementia. *Neurology,* 1979, *29,* 393–394.

Smith JS and Kiloh LG. The investigation of dementia: results in 200 consecutive admissions. *Lancet,* 1981, *1,* 824–827.

Smith JS, Kiloh LG, Ratnavale GS, and Grant DA. The investigation of dementia. *Med J Aust,* 1976, *2,* 403–405.

Snyder BD and Harris S. Treatable aspects of the dementia syndrome. *J Am Geriat Soc,* 1976, *24,* 179–184.

Spar JE and Gerner R. Does the dexamethasone suppression test distinguish dementia from depression? *Am J Psychiat,* 1982, *139,* 238–240.

Starkman MN and Schteingart DE. Neuropsychiatric manifestations of patients with Cushing's syndrome. *Arch Int Med,* 1981, *141,* 215–219.

Stefansson JG, Messina JA, and Meyerowitz S. Hysterical neurosis, conversion type: clinical and epidemiological considerations. *Acta Psychiat Scand,* 1976, *53,* 119–138.

Strachan RW and Henderson JG. Psychiatric syndromes due to avitaminosis B$_{12}$ with normal blood and marrow. *Quart J Med,* 1965, *34,* 303–317.

Strachan RW and Henderson JG. Dementia and folate deficiency. *Quart J Med,* 1967, *36,* 189–204.

Strich SJ. Shearing of nerve fibers as a cause of brain damage due to head injury. *Lancet,* 1961, *2,* 443–448.

Stuteville P and Welch K. Subdural hematoma in the elderly person. *JAMA,* 1958, *168,* 1445–1449.

Sydenstricker VP. The neurological complications of malnutrition. Psychic manifestations of nicotinic acid deficiency. *Proc Roy Soc Med,* 1943, *36,* 169–171.

Terrence CF, Delaney JF, and Alberts MC. Computed tomography for Huntington's disease. *Neuroradiology,* 1977, *13,* 173–175.

Thomas FB, Mazzaferri EL, and Skillman TG. Apathetic thyrotoxicosis: a distinctive clinical and laboratory entity. *Ann Int Med,* 1970, *72,* 679–685.

Thompson TL II, Moran MG, and Nies AS. Psychotropic drug use in the elderly. *New Engl J Med,* 1983, *308,* 134–138, 194–199.

Tomlinson BE. The pathology of dementia. In Wells CE (Ed.): *Dementia,* 2nd ed. Philadelphia. FA Davis Company, 1977, pp. 113–153.

Tomlinson BE and Kitchner D. Granulovacuolar degeneration of hippocampal pyramidal cells. *J Pathol,* 1972, *106,* 165–185.

Tourtellotte WW. Cerebrospinal fluid in multiple sclerosis. In Vinken PJ and Bruyn GW (Eds.): *Multiple sclerosis and other demyelinating diseases,* Vol. 9, *Handbook of clinical neurology.* New York, American Elsevier Publishing Company, 1970, pp. 324–382.

Trimble MR and Reynolds EH. Anticonvulsant drugs and mental symptoms: a review. *Psychol Med,* 1976, *6,* 169–178.

Tyndel M. Some aspects of the Ganser state. *J Ment Sci,* 1956, *102,* 324–329.

Udvarhelyi GB, Wood JH, James AE Jr, and Bartelt D. Results and complications in 55 shunted patients with normal pressure hydrocephalus. *Surg Neurol,* 1975, *3,* 271–275.

Vallarta JM, Bell DB, and Reichert A. Progressive encephalopathy due to chronic hydantoin intoxication. *Am J Dis Childh,* 1974, *128,* 27–34.

Van Putten T, Multalipassi LR, and Malkin MD. Phenothiazine-induced decompensation. *Arch Gen Psychiat,* 1974, *30,* 102–105.

Victor M, Adams RD, and Cole M. The acquired (non-Wilsonian) type of chronic hepatocerebral degeneration. *Medicine,* 1965, *44,* 345–396.

Vroom FQ and Greer M. Mercury vapor intoxication. *Brain,* 1972, *95,* 305–318.

Wechsler AF, Verity M, Rosenschein S, Fried I, and Scheibel AB. Pick's disease. *Arch Neurol,* 1982, *39,* 87–90.

Weil ML, Itabashi HH, Cremer NE, Oshiro LS, Lennette EH, and Carnay L. Chronic progressive panencephalitis due to rubella virus simulating subacute sclerosing panencephalitis. *New Eng J Med,* 1975, *292,* 994–998.

Weiner H and Braiman A. The Ganser syndrome. *Am J Psychiat,* 1955, *111,* 767–773.

Wells CE. Pseudodementia. *Am J Psychiat,* 1979, *136,* 895–900.

Wells CE and Duncan GW. Danger of over-reliance on computerized cranial tomography. *Am J Psychiat,* 1977, *134,* 811–813.

Welsh JD, Cassidy D, Prigatano GP, and Gunn CG. Chronic hepatic encephalopathy treated with oral lactose in a patient with lactose malabsorption. *New Engl J Med,* 1974, *291,* 240–241.

White P, Goodhardt MJ, Keet JP, Hiley CR, Carrasco LH,

Williams IEI, and Bowen DM. Neocortical cholinergic neurons in elderly people. *Lancet*, 1977, *1*, 668–670.

Whitehouse PJ, Price DL, Struble RG, Clark AW, Coyle JT, and DeLong MR. Alzheimer's disease and senile dementia: loss of neurons in the basal forebrain. *Science*, 1982, *215*, 1237–1239.

Whitlock FA. The Ganser syndrome. *Br J Psychiat*, 1967, *113*, 19–29.

Yakovlev PI. Paraplegias of hydrocephalics (a clinical note and interpretation). *Am J Ment Def*, 1947, *51*, 561–576.

Young AC, Saunders J, and Ponsford JR. Mental change as an early feature of multiple sclerosis. *J Neurol Neurosurg Psychiat*, 1976, *39*, 1008–1013.

Chapter 9

Epilepsy: Ictal and Interictal Behavioral Alterations

The term "epilepsy" derives from Greek roots meaning to be seized by alien forces and refers to a brain condition manifest by recurrent seizures (Adams and Victor, 1977; Forster and Booker, 1975). Epilepsy is a common disorder, affecting approximately 1 percent of the population, and may involve individuals of any age. It is associated with an array of behavioral changes ranging from minor alterations of consciousness during a brief seizure to chronic schizophrenialike psychoses and affective disorders persisting in the interictal period. Some of the behaviors are a direct manifestation of the epileptic cerebral discharge, whereas others may be related to the existence of a lesion giving rise to both the epilepsy and the behavioral changes. The effects of chronic anticonvulsant therapy and the psychological consequences of suffering from an unpredictable socially disabling disease also contribute to the behavioral alterations of epileptic patients. This chapter describes the behavioral manifestations of epileptic seizures, the neuropsychiatric alterations occurring during the interictal period in patients with epilepsy, and the neuropsychiatric aspects of anticonvulsant medications.

Table 9-1 presents a classification of behavioral alterations occurring in epileptic patients. Ictal behaviors are produced by epileptic discharges within the cerebral hemispheres; postictal behaviors occur during the confusional period immediately following a seizure; and interictal behaviors are those that are manifest between seizures and become a more stable part of the behavior of the epileptic patient (Pond, 1957).

SEIZURES AND ICTAL BEHAVIORAL ALTERATIONS

Ictal Behavioral Phenomena

Table 9-2 presents a classification of seizures and lists the principal types of behavioral alteration occurring with each seizure type. Seizures are divided into partial forms that begin in localized areas in the cerebral cortex and primarily generalized forms that begin in subcortical structures and spread to involve both hemispheres simultaneously. Partial seizures are classified into elementary types that do not impair consciousness and complex types that are associated with impaired consciousness and incomplete recall of the seizure events. Partial seizures of either type may spread to involve both hemispheres·producing secondarily generalized convulsions. Primary generalized seizures include petit mal and grand mal seizures as well as a variety of atypical petit mal, myoclonic, clonic, tonic, and akinetic seizures. Simple partial seizures include focal motor seizures with or without a Jacksonian march, elementary sensory symptoms (unformed visual, auditory, and somatosensory hallucinations), autonomic symptoms (respiratory, cardiac, and gastrointestinal disturbances), and compound forms with combinations of these signs and symptoms (Commission on Classification and Terminology of the International League Against Epilepsy, 1981; Gastaut, 1970; Van Buren, 1958).

Complex partial seizures are manifest primarily by behavioral and experiential phenomena. These seizures are distinguished from simple partial seizures by impairment of consciousness, amnesia for the seizures, and the complex nature of the ictal events. The patient may remember the initial portions of the seizure, and these recalled experiences constitute the "aura" of the seizure. In most cases, the ictal experience or behavior is brief and stereotyped with little variation in symptomatology from one attack to another. Complex partial seizures have, in the past, been called *temporal lobe seizures* or *psychomotor seizures,* but the anatomic focus need not be located in the temporal lobe, and the associated phenomena are not limited to psychomotor automatisms. Complex partial seizures arise from lesions of the limbic system, and the associated seizure disorder could appropriately be called *limbic epilepsy* (Penry, 1975).

The behavioral characteristics of complex partial

TABLE 9-1.   Classification of Behavioral
             Alterations Occuring in
             Epileptic Patients

Ictal behavioral events

Postictal behavioral changes

Interictal neuropsychiatric alterations

   Personality changes
   Schizophrenialike psychoses
   Affective disturbances
   Dissociative disturbances

      Depersonalization
      Fugue states, poriomania
      Multiple personality

   Aggression
   Altered sexual behavior

TABLE 9-2.   Classification of Epileptic Seizure with Major
             Behavioral Alterations Occuring with Each
             Type of Seizure

Partial Seizures

   Simple partial seizures (consciousness not impaired)

      Motor signs
      Sensory symptoms
      Autonomic symptoms
      Compound forms
      Psychic symptoms without impairment of consciousness

   Complex partial seizures (consciousness impaired)

      Impaired consciousness only
      Intellectual symptomatology

         Aphasia
         Memory distortion

            Déjà vu, jamais vu
            Déjà entendu, jamais entendu
            Déjà penseé
         Cognitive alterations

            Dreamy state
            Depersonalization
            Forced thinking
            Thought blocking

      Affective Symptomatology (ictal emotions)

         Fear
         Depression
         Miscellaneous

            Pleasant experience
            Unpleasant experience
            Anxiety
            Embarrassment
            Anger

      Psychosensory symptomatology

         Illusions
         Hallucinations

      Psychomotor symptomatology

         Automatisms (Table 9-4)

      Compound forms

         Temporal lobe ''march''
         Ictal psychosis

   Partial seizures evolving to secondarily generalized
   seizures

Generalized seizures

   Absence seizures (petit mal)

      Brief absence attacks
      Stupor
      Ictal psychosis

   Atypical absense seizures
   Myoclonic seizures
   Clonic seizures
   Tonic seizures
   Tonic–clonic seizures (grand mal)
   Atonic seizures

Modified from: Commission on Classification and Terminology of the
International League Against Epilepsy. Proposal for revised clinical and
electroencephalographic classification of epileptic seizures. *Epilepsia*,
1981, *22*, 489–501. Gastaut H. Clinical and electroencephalographic
classification of epileptic seizures. *Epilepsia*, 1970, *11*, 102–113. With
permission.

seizures are extremely diverse. They represent fragments from the individual's complex repertoire of behavior and experience. The simplest type of complex partial seizure is interruption of consciousness without associated behavioral activity. These seizures are manifest by brief lapses of consciousness of which the individual may or may not be aware (Dreifuss, 1975). The brief absence attacks are frequently misdiagnosed as petit mal seizures, but, as shown in Table 9-3, the two similar seizure types can be distinguished by their clinical features, EEG characteristics and response to therapy.

Complex partial seizures can give rise to alterations of language, memory, cognition, emotion, sensation, or behavior. Aphasia can occur as a manifestation of seizure activity in the language dominant hemisphere and in some cases is the sole indication of the seizure. The aphasia may have either fluent or nonfluent characteristics (De Pesquet et al, 1976; Dinner et al., 1981; Hamilton and Matthews, 1979; Racy et al., 1980; Solomon, 1957; Wilson et al., 1983). Aphasia is a linguistic manifestation of epilepsy in the left hemisphere, whereas speech arrest or verbal automatisms may occur with epileptic disturbances in either hemisphere (Gilmore and Heilman, 1981; Serafetinides and Falconer, 1963; Vernea, 1974).

Memory distortions are also common constituents of complex partial seizures. *Déjà vu* refers to the sense

TABLE 9-3. Characteristics that Distinguish Complex Partial Seizures Manifested Solely by Impaired Consciousness and Petit Mal Seizures

Characteristic	Complex Partial Seizures	Petit Mal Seizures
Age of onset	Any age, rare in childhood	Childhood
Aura	Yes	No
Duration	Minutes	Seconds
Frequency	Few per day or less	May be many per day
Precipitants	No	Hyperventilation
Postictal confusion	Yes	No
EEG	Focal (usually temporal) spike or slowing	Generalized 3/second spike and wave pattern
Etiology	Acquired (trauma, neoplasm, anteriovenous malformation, etc.)	Inherited
Treatment	Phenytoin Carbamazepine Phenobarbital	Ethosuximide Sodium valproate

of having had a particular experience before and *jamais vu* to the absence of an appropriate sense of familiarity (Cole and Zangwill, 1963; Dreifuss, 1975; Mullan and Penfield, 1959). Occasionally, patients have the *déjà* or *jamais* feelings associated with specific thoughts, *déjà penseé* (Brickner and Stein, 1942), or with auditory experiences *(déjà entendu, jamais entendu)* (Dreifuss, 1975; Mullan and Penfield, 1959).

Cognitive manifestations of complex partial seizures include dreamy states, depersonalization, forced thinking, and thought blocking. Dreamy states and depersonalization are characterized by a sense of detachment and loss of contact with the environment or the self (Jackson, 1888–1889; Kenna and Sedman, 1965). *Thought blocking* refers to the sudden interruption of thinking, whereas *forced thinking* is characterized by the sudden intrusive appearance of a thought that may then be reiterated several times (Brickner et al., 1940; Gastaut, 1953; Hill and Mitchell, 1953; Karagulla and Robertson, 1955; Whitten, 1969).

A wide range of ictal emotional experiences have been described in complex partial seizures. The most common ictal emotion is fear, accounting for approximately 60 percent of all cases of seizure-related emotions (Daly, 1958; Henricksen, 1973; Macrae, 1954a,b; McLachlan and Blume, 1980; Strauss et al., 1982; Weil, 1959; Williams, 1956). The fear begins and ends abruptly and is usually associated with an epileptogenic lesion in the anterior or middle temporal region (Williams, 1956). Visceral symptoms commonly accompany ictal fear, as they do nonepileptic fear. Depression is the second most common ictal emotion and, unlike ictal fear, once initiated may persist for from several hours to several days. The epileptic focus is in the anterior or middle temporal lobe of either hemisphere (Daly, 1958;

Weil, 1955, 1956, 1959; Williams, 1956). In addition to these two common ictal emotions, a variety of other emotions have been recorded in a small number of patients, including euphoria, unpleasant feelings, anxiety, embarrassment, anger, or impending death (Daly, 1958; Devinsky et al., Greenberg et al., 1984; Weil, 1956, 1959; Williams, 1956). The most famous example of ictal euphoria involved the Russian novelist, Fyodor Dostoyevsky (Alajouanine, 1963; Geschwind, 1984). Speaking through the person of Prince Myshkin in *The Idiot*, Dostoyevsky wrote:*

> Among other things he fell to thinking that in his attacks of epilepsy there was a pause just before the fit itself . . . when suddenly in the midst of sadness, spiritual darkness, and a feeling of oppression, there were instants when it seemed his brain was on fire, and in an extraordinary surge all his vital forces would be intensified. The sense of life, the consciousness of self were multiplied tenfold in these moments, which lasted no longer than a flash of lightning. His mind and heart were flooded with extraordinary light; all torment, all doubt, all anxieties were relieved at once, resolved in a kind of lofty calm, full of serene, harmonious joy and hope, full of understanding and the knowledge of the ultimate cause of things. But these moments, these flashes were only the presage of that final second (never more than a second) with which the fit itself began.

Psychosensory symptoms accompanying complex partial seizures include illusions (distortions) and formed and unformed hallucinations involving auditory and vi-

---

*From Dostoyevsky F. *The idiot* (translated by Carlisle H and Carlisle O). New York, New American Library, 1969, p. 245.

TABLE 9-4.   Psychomotor Automatisms

Simple psychomotor automatisms

Incoordination	Chewing
Negativism	Swallowing
Staring	Spitting
Pushing	Lip Smacking
Groping	Rubbing
Searching	Plucking

Speech automatisms

Shouting .
Screaming
Verbal reiteration

Affective automatisms

Gelastic epilepsy (laughing)
Dacrystic or quiritarian epilepsy (crying)

Complex automatisms

Cursive epilepsy (running)	Masturbation
Drinking	Prolonged twilight states with automatisms
Undressing	

sual sensory modalities (Currie et al., 1971; Fischer-Williams et al., 1964; Karagula and Robertson, 1955; King and Marsan, 1977; Mundy-Castle, 1951; Russell and Whitty, 1955). The hallucinations are often recollections of events previously experienced by the patient. Visual illusions include macropsia (objects appearing too large), micropsia (objects appearing too small) and metamorphopsia (visual distortions).

Psychomotor automatisms are usually simple, perseverative, poorly executed, purposeless motor behaviors (Table 9-4). Typical examples are pushing, groping, chewing, swallowing, spitting, lip smacking, rubbing, and plucking (Geier et al., 1976, 1977; Gibbs et al., 1948; Hecker et al., 1972; Theodore et al., 1983). Automatisms preceded by an initial motionless stare originate in the temporal lobe, whereas automatisms without an intial state often originate from nontemporal limbic areas (Escueta et al., 1977, 1982). Speech automatisms include shouting, screaming, and verbal reiteration such as repeating a brief statememt over and over (Gibbs et al., 1948; Serafetinides and Falconer, 1963). Ictal automatisms involving expressions of affect, usually without an associated mood change, include epileptic laughter (gelastic seizures) and crying (dacrystic or quiritarian seizures) and alterations in facial expression (Ames and Enderstein, 1975; Chen and Forster, 1973; Daly and Mulder, 1957; Gumpert et al., 1970; Jacome et al., 1980; Lehtinen and Kivalo, 1965; Loiseau et al., 1971; Offen et al., 1976; Sethi and Rao, 1976; Strauss et al., 1983). More complex automatisms including running (cursive seizures), drinking, removal of clothing, and masturbation occur in rare cases (Chen and Forster, 1973; Hooshmand and Brawley, 1969; Remillard et al., 1981; Robertson and Fariello, 1979; Sethi and Rao, 1976; Sis-

ler et al., 1953; Spencer et al., 1983). Directed aggression in the course of seizures is extremely unusual, although injury may occur from poorly directed scratching and pushing or with agitated behavior during the postictal confusional period (Chapter 11) (Escueta et al., 1981). In some cases status epilepticus with prolonged psychomotor automatisms may occur. Such patients may have confusional behavior with automatisms persisting for up to several days (Belafsky et al., 1978; Engel et al., 1978; Escueta et al., 1974; Lugaresi et al., 1971; Markand et al., 1978; Mayeux and Lueders, 1978; Scott and Masland, 1953).

Any combination of the types of seizure described in the preceding paragraphs may occur together, and in some cases a temporal lobe "march" can be discerned with one symptom replaced by another as the seizure activity spreads within temporolimbic structures (Stevens, 1957). Partial complex seizures manifesting a combination of hallucinations, thought and memory disturbances, and psychomotor automatisms may produce an ictal psychosis resembling schizophrenia. The differential diagnosis of ictal psychosis must also include status epilepticus occurring in petit mal epilepsy. Although classical petit mal epilepsy is virtually confined to children and adolescents, petit mal status not infrequently involves adults and may present as an ictal psychosis or a period of prolonged confusional behavior (Andermann and Robb, 1972; Geier 1978; Niedermeyer and Khalifeh, 1965; Saper and Lossing, 1974; Schwartz and Scott, 1971; Weissberg 1975; Wells, 1975).

Complex automatisms can occur during the postictal confusional state immediately following a seizure as well as during the course of the seizure itself. When a complex partial or generalized seizure has terminated, the patient is left in a confusional state that may last from minutes to hours. In some cases, the initiating seizure may have been so brief as to go unnoticed. During the confused period the patient may talk or walk around but is usually disoriented and amnestic for both the ictal and postictal confusional period (Levin, 1952). It is often impossible to distinguish ictal and postictal behavioral activity.

Etiologies of Seizures

Identification of a seizure disorder should be followed by a careful search for the cause of the recurrent epileptic attacks. Table 9-5 presents the causes of complex partial seizures found in patients subjected to temporal lobe resection for seizure control (Currie et al., 1971; Engel et al., 1982a; Falconer et al., 1964; Malamud, 1966; Margerison and Corsellis, 1966). Mesial temporal sclerosis is the most common cause of complex partial seizures. The cause of this lesion is controversial: some believe the gliotic changes result from febrile convulsions of childhood (Falconer et al., 1964), whereas others have championed the idea that the lesion is a product of hippocampal deformation and injury sustained at the time of birth (Earle et al., 1953). Neoplasms—congenital hamartomas, gliomas and oligodendrogliomas—are the second most common lesion associated with complex partial seizures. The temporal lobe is also vulnerable to injury in the course of head trauma, and traumatic lesions are a common cause of complex partial seizures (Evans, 1962; Jennett, 1975; Walker, 1962). Vascular malformations, congenital cerebral malformations, and a variety of miscellaneous conditions including encephalitis, cerebral infarctions, abscesses, meningitis, and aneurysms account for the remaining cases (Aguilar and Rasmussen, 1960; Dodge et al., 1954, Kamrin, 1966).

Unlike complex partial seizures, elementary partial seizures are most likely to indicate the presence of a neoplasm (meningioma, astrocytoma, oligodendroglioma, glioblastoma, metastasis), although trauma, vascular malformations, and infections can also produce elementary seizures (Evans, 1962; Jennett, 1975; Sumi and Teasdall, 1963).

Most primary generalized seizures are genetically determined autosomal dominant disorders with variable penetrance (Metrakos and Metrakos, 1961), typically with onset in childhood or adolescence.

Diagnosis and Differential Diagnosis

The differential diagnosis of seizures includes disorders that lead to loss of consciousness similar to generalized epileptic convulsions and disorders that produce

TABLE 9-5.   Etiologies of Comples Partial Seizures

Etiology	Frequency (%)
Mesial temporal sclerosis	47–90
Tumors	9–18
Trauma	3–11
Vascular malformations	2–7
Cerebral malformations	0–15
None found	0–14
Micellaneous	0–16

Encephalitis
   Infarction
   Abscess
   Meningitis
   Aneurysm	

Ranges from Currie et al; 1971; Engel et al; 1982a; Falconer et al; 1964; Malamud, 1966; Margerison and Corsellis, 1966.

complex behaviors for which the patient is partially or completely amnestic, imitating complex partial seizures. The former are considered here (Table 9-6), and the latter are the subject of Chapter 10.

In addition to epilepsy, toxic and metabolic disorders sufficiently severe to disrupt cerebral function not uncommonly cause generalized convulsions. The most commom metabolic conditions producing convulsions are alcohol and drug withdrawal, hypoglycemia, hyponatremia, hypocalcemia, uremia, hepatic encephalopathy, anoxia, and porphyria (Earnest and Yarnell, 1976; Schmidt and Wilder, 1968; Trimble, 1981; Wolfe and Victor, 1969). Children under the age of 5 may have seizures induced by high fever (Hammill and Carter, 1966; Nelson and Ellenberg, 1976; Ouellette, 1974). Isoniazid, insulin, lidocaine, and psychotropic medications are among the most common drugs to induce seizures (Messing et al., 1984).

Events closely imitating epileptic seizures may also occur as conversion reactions. Although commonly called *pseudoseizures,* they are better identified as pseudoepileptic since it is the epileptic nature of the seizures that is "pseudo-," the motor activity itself is real (Gross, 1983; Krumholz and Neidermeyer, 1983). Pseudoepileptic seizures can usually be distinguished from epileptic seizures on the basis of clinical, EEG, neuroendocrinologic, and therapeutic observations (Table 9-7) (Desai et al., 1982; Ferriss, 1959; Gross, 1983; Johnson and Lewis, 1976; Riley and Brannon, 1980). Although no single clinical feature distinguishes the two, pseudoepileptic seizures often have a more gradual onset, less stereotyped body movements, less tongue biting, less micturition and defecation, less self-injury, little impairment of consciousness or postictal confusion, and a longer duration than epileptic seizures. Interictal EEGs are often of little value in distinguishing the two condi-

TABLE 9-6.   Differential Diagnosis of Generalized
Seizures

Seizures

   Epilepsy

   Toxic–metabolic seizures

      Drug-induced (psychotropic agents, lidocaine,
      isoniazid, etc.)
      Drug withdrawal (especially barbiturates, alcohol)
      Hypoglycemia
      Hyponatremia
      Hypocalcemia
      Uremia
      Hepatic Encephalopathy
      Anoxia
      Porphyria

   Febrile convulsions (in children)

Pseudoepileptic seizures

Nonseizure disturbances

   Syncope

      Cardiac dysfunction
      Postural hypotension
      Vasovagal attacks
      Breath-holding spells (in children)

   Transient ischemic attacks

   Migraine
   Narcolepsy

   Acute dystonic reactions

---

tions since they may be either normal or abnormal in both conditions. Ictal EEG recordings, however, are useful: the tracing obtained during a pseudoepileptic seizure will be no different from the interictal tracing, whereas that obtained during an epileptic seizure will reveal spike and wave discharges (Gulick et al., 1982; King et al., 1982; Luther et al., 1982). A new dimension that has recently been added to the differential diagnosis of pseudoepileptic and epileptic seizures involves the neuroendocrinologic changes accompanying some epileptic seizures. Prolactin levels are elevated five- to tenfold above baseline levels after most generalized seizures and complex partial seizures, whereas they are usually unaffected by pseudoepileptic seizures or simple partial seizures (Collins et al., 1983; Dana-Haeri et al., 1983; Pritchard et al., 1983; Trimble, 1978; Wyllie et al., 1984). Finally, reduction or elimination of anticonvulsants will exacerbate epileptic seizures but will have no effect on pseudoepileptic seizures. Pseudoepileptic seizures occur in up to 20 percent of epileptics, and significant neurological or psychiatric disease is not uncommon in patients manifesting pseudoepileptic seizures (Cohen and Suter, 1982; King

et al., 1982; Krumholz and Niedermeyer, 1983; Lesser et al., 1983; Luther et al., 1982; Ramani and Gumnit, 1982a; Ramani et al., 1980; Standage, 1975). The most common psychiatric disorder associated with pseudoepileptic seizures is depression, although they have also been observed in conjunction with a variety of personality disorders (Stewart et al., 1983).

Epileptic seizures must also be distinguished from a variety of nonseizure disturbances that produce loss of consciousness or cause behavioral alterations that imitate generalized seizures. Among these conditions are syncope, transient ischemic attacks, migraine, breath-holding spells (in children), narcolepsy, and acute generalized dystonic reactions (Angus and Simpson, 1970; Bickerstaff, 1961; Braham et al., 1981; Dreifuss, 1975; Haslam and Jameson, 1973; Lees and Watkins, 1963; Lombroso and Lerman, 1967; Parkes, 1982; Riley, 1982).

Epilepsy is a clinical diagnosis that depends on recognizing the characteristic features presented previously and excluding those conditions that may closely simulate epileptic seizures. The EEG may help considerably when abnormal; however, because EEG abnormalities may be undetectable by surface recordings of epileptic patients and tracings may be abnormal in individuals with no identifiable brain disease, it is definitive only when it reveals a paroxysmal spike and wave pattern coinciding temporally with discrete behavioral changes. Occasionally, an empirical trial of anticonvulsants will have to be undertaken in equivocal cases to help clarify the diagnosis. A CT scan will reveal most neoplasms, vascular malformations, infarctions, and abscesses associated with partial seizures but will be normal in a substantial number of epileptics.

The treatment of epilepsy is discussed in the final section of this chapter.

INTERICTAL BEHAVIORAL ALTERATIONS

The permanent alterations of behavior noted in patients with epilepsy are among the most controversial and poorly understood areas of contemporary neuropsychiatry. Such changes have been insisted on by some and denied with equal vehemence by others. Those who subscribe to the occurrence of interictal change in epileptics are divided as to whether the alterations are psychodynamic reactions to having an unpredictable and frightening disorder, are related to intermittent spiking in the brain, or are a product of a brain injury giving rise to both seizures and behavioral changes. The correlation of specific behavioral disturbances with specific types of seizure (complex partial or generalized) has also been questioned. This section presents the available in-

TABLE 9-7.   Characteristics Distinguishing Epileptic Seizures and Pseudoepileptic Seixures

Characteristic	Pseudoepileptic	Epileptic
Clinical features		
Onset	Often gradual	Abrupt
Body movements	Struggling, asynchronous	Rigidity, then tonic–clonic
Biting	Lips, arms, other areas	Tongue
Micturition	Rare	Common
Defecation	Rare	Occasional
Self-injury	Rare	Common
Postictal confusion	Absent	Present
Consciousness	Complete or partial retention	Lost
Duration	Several to many minutes	30 seconds to a few minutes
Initiation or termination by suggestion	Yes	No
EEG		
Interictal	± Abnormal	± Abnormal
Ictal	No change	Abnormal
Neuroendocrinology		
Prolactin	No change	Increase
Therapy		
Anticonvulsant withdrawal	No increase in seizures	Increase in seizures

Desai et al; 1982; Ferriss, 1959; Johnson and Lewis, 1976; Riley and Brannon, 1980.

formation with regard to personality alterations, schizophrenialike disorders, and affective changes in epileptic patients.

Prevalence of Behavioral Alterations Among Epileptic Patients

There is an increased occurrence of behavioral pathology and psychiatric disease among patients with epilepsy. This statement has been challenged, but the majority of epidemiologic studies indicate that epileptics are overrepresented in psychiatric populations and that behavioral alterations are found with unusual frequency in patients with epilepsy. Studies assessing the prevalence of behavioral changes among all epileptics suggest that 10–80 percent have behavioral alterations (Dominian et al., 1963; Pond and Bidwell, 1959;nb60; Ramani and Gumnit, 1982b; Rodin, 1978; Standage and Fenton, 1975). The prevalence of behavioral changes is also significantly greater among epileptics than among patients with other chronic debilitating illnesses, suggesting that the alterations cannot be explained entirely as psychological reactions to their disease (Rutter et al., 1970; Standage and Fenton, 1975). The prevalence varies with the type of epilepsy studied. Patients with elementary partial seizures have the lowest frequency of behavioral changes, occurring in 5–13 percent (Gibbs, 1951); 30–90 percent of patients with generalized seizures have associated behavioral alterations (Shukla et al., 1979; Small et al., 1966; Stevens, 1966, 1975); and similarly, 30–90 percent of patients with complex partial seizures have behavioral changes (Camfield et al., 1984; Gibbs, 1951; Lindsay et al., 1979; Shukla and Katiyar, 1980; Shukla et al., 1979; Small et al., 1966; Stevens, 1966, 1975). The findings vary with the population studied, the definitions of behavior change applied, and the care with which psychological alterations were sought. Cumulatively, the studies suggest that patients with simple partial seizures have the lowest rates of psychological alterations, whereas those with complex partial seizures have the highest rates and most severe types of behavioral change.

Personality Changes

The existence of an "epileptic personality" has been claimed since antiquity but has given rise to considerable controversy, and many questions remain unanswered (Temkin, 1971; Tizard, 1962; Trimble, 1983). Several of the personality alterations formerly ascribed to epileptics can now be recognized to be the consequences of recurrent uncontrolled seizures with repeated anoxic insults or head injuries, the result of treatment with potentially toxic agents such as bromides, and the effects of chronic institutionalization and social ostracism. Most of these factors have now been modified through appropriate use of anticonvulsant medications. Beyond these considerations, however, associations have been sought between specific personality alterations and the occurrence of complex partial seizures. Patients with temporal lobe epilepsy have been noted to be hyper-religious, hyposexual, circumstantial, viscous, and hypergraphic (Bear and Fedio, 1977; Bear et al., 1982; Fenton, 1981; Geschwind et al., 1980; Roberts et al., 1982; Waxman and Geschwind, 1974, 1975). These characteristics differentiate patients with temporal lobe epilepsy from normal controls and are among the most distinctive personality alterations that may occur in patients with epileptic disorders. The symptom complex, however, can also be seen in patients suffering from many other types of neuropsychiatric disturbance and is not pathognomonic of epilepsy (Bear and Fedio, 1977; Bear et al., 1982; Hermann and Riel, 1981; Mungas, 1982; Rodin and Schmaltz, 1984).

The major instrument used for personality assessment in the clinical setting is the Minnesota Multiphasic Personality Inventory (MMPI). Application of this tool to patients with temporal lobe epilepsy has yielded variable results, but epileptic patients have usually been found to have elevated paranoia and schizophrenia scale scores (Hermann et al., 1982; Trimble, 1983).

An increased incidence of dissociative experiences, fugue stages, and multiple personality among patients with temporal lobe epilepsy has also been suggested and is discussed in more detail in Chapter 10 (Mesulam, 1981; Schenk and Bear, 1981). Aggression in epileptics is addressed in Chapter 11, and alterations in sexual behavior are presented in Chapter 17.

Schizophrenialike Psychosis

The best documented neuropsychiatric complication of epilepsy is the schizophrenialike psychosis that may occur in patients with complex partial seizures (temporal lobe epilepsy). Psychosis occurs with increased frequency in all types of epilepsy, but a schizophrenialike disorder appears to be associated primarily with temporal lobe epilepsy (Perez and Trimble, 1980; Small et al., 1962; Stevens, 1966).

Hill (1935) was among the first to point out that some epileptic patients develop a chronic paranoid–hallucinatory psychosis that resembles idiopathic schizophrenia. Slater and Beard (1963) studied the occurrence of such psychoses among epileptics and confirmed Hill's observation that the two disorders occur together too frequently to be ascribed to chance. In their series,

the mean age of onset of psychosis was 29.8 years, and the mean duration of the epilepsy prior to the onset of the psychosis was 14 years. Most of the patients had paranoid delusions and auditory hallucinations, and approximately half had a formal thought disorder. There was no consistent relationship between the severity and course of the psychosis and the frequency of seizures. In several cases, in fact, the seizures had greatly diminished in frequency or ceased at the time the psychosis occurred. Over time, half of the patients had a chronic deteriorating psychotic course, 30 percent improved, and 20 percent had a fluctuating course. Slater and Beard (1963) also noted that the psychosis occurred specifically in patients with temporal lobe epilepsy. They observed that the patients had less flattening of affect than did those with idiopathic schizophrenia, and there was an increase in obsessional traits (pedantry, circumstantiality) in their personalities. The disorder was further distinguished from idiopathic schizophrenia by an absence of phychosis among family members and of schizoid traits in the premorbid personality of affected patients. More recent studies have refined, extended, and largely confirmed these original observations and have established the prevalence of the psychosis to be between 10 and 30 percent of patients with complex partial seizures (Bartlet, 1957; Bruens, 1971; Glaser, 1964; Kristensen and Sindrup, 1978; Kury and Cobb, 1964; Perez and Trimble, 1980; Rodin et al., 1957; Sherwin, 1981; Toone et al., 1982). Additional risk factors for the development of the psychosis include female gender, left-handedness, occurrence of both complex partial and generalized seizures, and onset of seizures during puberty (Rodin et al., 1976; Slater and Moran, 1969; Taylor, 1971, 1975).

The laterality of the lesion also appears to influence the occurrence of psychosis: it is significantly more common with left-sided than with right-sided seizure foci (Flor-Henry, 1969a,b, 1972; Sherwin, 1977, 1981; Sherwin et al., 1982). Within the temporal lobe, anterior and medial periamygdaloid foci have the highest correlation with the occurrence of the schizophrenialike illness (Gibbs, 1951; Kristensen and Sindrup, 1978).

In summary, temporal lobe epilepsy is associated with a schizophrenialike illness in 10–30 percent of patients. The psychosis is manifest by ideas of reference, delusions that frequently have a religious connotation, and auditory hallucinations. The patients have usually had long-standing epilepsy arising from foci in the left temporal lobe, and the seizure focus is most likely to be in the anterior or medial temporal region.

The interictal schizophrenialike psychosis must be distinguished from other causes of psychosis that may occur in epileptic patients, including ictal psychoses, postictal psychoses, and psychoses associated with metabolic disturbances such as anticonvulsant toxicity, anticonvulsant withdrawal, and anticonvulsant-induced folate deficiency (Table 9-8) (Adebimpe, 1977; Bruens, 1974; Dongier, 1959–1960; Ramani and Gumnit, 1982b; Reynolds, 1967; Sironi et al., 1979; Toone, 1981; Wells, 1975).

Epilepsy-related interictal psychosis does not respond to treatment with anticonvulsants and may require the use of neuroleptic agents. In some cases improved control of seizure activity may lead to an exacerbation of the interictal behavioral disturbances (Flor-Henry, 1983; Trimble, 1981a).

Affective Disorders

Depression is the most common reason for psychiatric hospitalization of epileptic patients (Betts, 1981; Perez and Trimble, 1980). Interictal depression must be distinguished from ictal and postictal depression and from anticonvulsant-induced mood alterations (Table 9-9) (Whitlock, 1982; Williams, 1956). Interictal depression may be a psychological reaction to having a chronic socially and occupationally disabling disorder, or it may be an interictal expression of the underlying disorder. The observation that the depression can either develop or worsen when there is a significant reduction in seizure frequency suggests that the depression is not exclusively a reaction phenomenon (Betts, 1981; Flor-Henry, 1969a). Recognition of depression among epileptics is particularly important because of the increased frequency of suicide and suicide attempts in this population (Gunn, 1973; Hawton et al., 1980; Mackay, 1979).

Differential Diagnosis of Interictal Behavioral Disturbances

Table 9-10 lists the major causes of behavioral alterations found in patients with epilepsy. First, the patient's seizures and behavioral changes may both be manifestations of a specific underlying lesion. For example, frontal lobe disturbances, some dementing disorders (e.g., Alzheimer's disease), aphasias, amnesic states, the Klüver-Bucy syndrome, and other behavioral alterations may be produced by CNS insults that also cause seizures. In such cases the seizures must be treated with anticonvulsants while a search for the underlying cause of the behavioral syndrome is sought.

The effects of anticonvulsants must also be considered in the epileptic whose behavior deteriorates. Toxic encephalopathies can be produced by all classes of anticonvulsants including barbiturates, benzodiazepines, hydantoins, valproate sodium, succinimides, and sulfonamides (Cummings and Benson, 1983; Reynolds and Travers, 1974; Rivinus, 1982; Trimble and Reynolds, 1976). In addition to these direct effects, anti-

TABLE 9-8. Causes of Psychosis in Epileptic Patients

Ictal Psychoses
Complex partial status epilepticus
Petit mal status epilepticus
Postictal psychosis
Interictal psychosis
Schizophrenialike psychoses
Forced normalization
Affective disorders with psychosis
Anticonvulsant-related psychoses
Anticonvulsant toxicity
Anticonvulsant withdrawal
Folate dificiency

convulsants may produce alterations such as anemia, folate deficiency, hepatotoxicity, and electrolyte imbalance that indirectly impair intellectual and emotional function.

Finally, ictal and interictal behavioral disturbances must be distinguished from the psychological reactions that can be anticipated in any group of patients suffering from a disorder such as epilepsy with its attendant social and occupational limitations.

Pathophysiology of Interictal Behavioral Alterations

Several pathophysiological mechanisms have been proposed to explain the development of interictal behavioral disturbances in patients with epilepsy. The main focus of investigation has been the relationship of the schizophrenialike psychosis to temporal lobe epilepsy. The principal hypotheses include subictal discharges, "hyperconnection" of affect and experience, limbic system dysfunction, seizure-induced alterations in dopamine metabolism, disruption of symbolic and linguistic mechanisms of the left hemisphere, abnormal REM sleep, folate deficiency, and psychological reactions. Subictal limbic system discharges have been proposed as the cause of the psychosis, and it has even been suggested that idiopathic schizophrenia results from con-

TABLE 9-9. Etiologies of Depression in Epilepsy

Psychological reaction to diagnosis and associated social and occupational limitations
Ictal depression
Postictal depression
Interictal affective disorder
Depression coexisting with interictal psychosis
Anticonvulsant-induced mood alterations

TABLE 9-10.   Differential Diagnosis of Behavioral Disturbances in Patients with Epilepsy

Behavior dependent on underlying condition

Behavioral changes produced by anticonvulsant medications

Direct effects
   Toxic encephalopathy

Indirect effects
   Anemia
   Hepatotoxicity
   Folate deficiency
   Electrolyte imbalance

Behavioral alterations determined by the personal and social reactions to the epileptic condition

Behavioral changes determined by existence and location of the epileptic focus

   Ictal behavioral alterations
   Postictal disturbances
   Interictal psychiatric disorders

tinuous subictal epileptic activity without overt seizures. As discussed earlier, the cognitive, affective psychosensory, and psychomotor expressions of complex partial seizures may closely simulate schizophrenic behavior and experience, and several investigators have observed electrical abnormalities in surface or depth-electrode EEG records of schizophrenic patients (Heath, 1958, 1962; Stevens and Livermore, 1982; Sem-Jacobsen et al., 1955). The lack of success in treating either idiopathic schizophrenia or the schizophrenialike psychosis of epilepsy with anticonvulsants and the occasional emergence of psychosis following surgical removal of an epileptic focus, however, suggest that the psychosis cannot be explained fully on the basis of continuous subictal electrical activity, and other explanations must be sought.

The hyperconnection theory proposes that the epileptic activity within the limbic system results in a suffusion of experience with emotional coloration, leading to emotional deepening and loss of reality testing (Bear, 1979; Bear et al., 1981; Waxman and Geschwind, 1975). Patients with ictal fear might be particularly susceptible, with the hyperconnection leading to paranoia and psychosis (Hermann and Chabria, 1980; Hermann et al., 1982).

Against the concept of hyperconnection is the observation that the frequency of seizures and the occurrence of psychosis are independent and sometimes inversely correlated. One would expect that psychosis and seizures would be correlated if both were the product of limbic epileptic activity. In addition, metabolic scans of patients with epilepsy reveal that the area of

the focus is hypometabolic during the interictal period (Bernardi et al., 1983; Engel et al., 1982b,c). The latter findings, along with the observations that schizophrenialike syndromes are not uncommon in patients with nonepileptic limbic system lesions, suggest that the location of the lesion may be at least as important as its epileptogenicity (Chapter 13) (Cummings, 1985, Malamud, 1967; Torrey and Peterson, 1974).

The emergence of the dopamine theory of schizophrenia led to attempts to relate the epileptic process to alterations in dopamine metabolism. Lamprecht (1977) and Trimble (1977) observed that dopamine blockade with neuroleptics increased the likelihood of seizures and improved psychosis, whereas dopaminergic agents raised the seizure threshold and aggravated psychosis. This inverse correlation suggested that dopaminergic alterations could be involved in the epileptic psychosis. A mechanism by which seizures could lead to dopamine changes has been described by Stevens and Livermore (1978), who found that, in experimental animals, long-standing seizure activity led to (kindled) alterations in the mesolimbic dopamine system and produced behavioral alterations. Differences in CSF catecholamine metabolite levels between epileptic patients with and without psychosis have been documented and lend further support to this hypothesis (Peters, 1979). A dopaminergic mechanism is far from established as the cause of psychosis in epilepsy but offers a promising means of synthesizing observations concerning idiopathic schizophrenia and schizophenialike disorders associated with seizures.

Other hypotheses that have been suggested include disruption of linguistic processes by the epileptic focus, a mechanism that would correlate with the prevalence of left-sided foci but leaves unexplained why language disturbances would produce psychosis (Ferguson et al., 1969; Sherwin et al., 1982). Sherwin (1977) hypothesized that the limbic lesions lead to REM sleep abnormalities that eventually "spill over" into the waking state as psychoses. Reynolds (1967, 1968) suggested that anticonvulsant-induced folate deficiency might be playing a role in the psychosis. Personality factors have also been implicated and may contribute to the anxiety and depression found in epileptic patients, but the lack of premorbid personality disturbances (Slater and Beard, 1963) and absence of a relationship between disruptive childhood environment and later development of psychosis (Lindsay et al., 1979) suggest that personality factors do not play a major role in the schizophrenialike psychosis. Several of the above mentioned mechanisms interacting with such host factors as age of onset of epilepsy, age at time of CNS insult, gender, lesion location, and seizure severity and type may play a role in determining which patients will and which will not become psychotic.

TABLE 9-11. Comparative Pharmacology of Major Anticonvulsants.

Anticonvulsant	Daily Adult Dosage (mg)	Therapeutic Serum Level (μg/ml)	Half-Life (hours)	Time to Reach Steady State
Phenytoin	200–400	10–20	18–30	4–6 days
Carbamazepine	800–1200	8–12	10–30	2–6 days
Phenobarbital	90–180	15–40	50–120	11–25 days
Primidone (25% metabolized to phenobarbital)	500–1500	5–12	3–12	16–60 hours
Valproic acid	1000–2500	50–100	8–15	40–75 hours
Ethosuximide	1500–2500	40–100	40–60	8–12 days

TREATMENT OF EPILEPSY

The management of epilepsy has traditionally focused on the control of seizures. Although this is an important aspect of epilepsy therapy, the prevalence of behavioral disorders among epileptic patients makes it imperative to consider all aspects of behavior when developing a therapeutic approach. Approximately 20 percent of all epileptics will also be treated with antidepressants or neuroleptics (Wilensky et al., 1981) and the influence of these agents on seizure control must be kept in mind. At the same time, anticonvulsants have neuropsychiatric side effects that may alter the patient's behavior, and these must also be considered in designing an optimal therapeutic regimen. Finally, when temporal lobectomy is considered for treatment of refractory epilepsy, the psychiatric and neuropsychological consequences of surgery require exploration.

Pharmacology of Anticonvulsants

Phenytoin

Table 9-11 presents the comparative pharmacology of the principal anticonvulsants currently utilized in the management of seizures. Phenytoin (Dilantin, manufactured by Parke-Davis) has been the treatment of choice for partial seizures and grand mal seizures, although in recent years carbamazepine has begun to replace phenytoin in some circumstances. The usual adult dosage is 200–400 mg/day given in one or two doses; the therapeutic serum level is 10–20 μg/ml; the drug half-life is 18–30 hours; and a stable serum level is achieved after 4–6 days (Kutt and Penry, 1974; Rall and Schliefer, 1980). Phenytoin may be administered orally or intravenously (IV) but should not be given intramuscularly (IM) because of its tendency to produce crystalline granulomas (Eadie, 1980). Intravenous phenytoin, administered at a rate of 50 mg/min or slower, is the most definitive therapy of status epilepticus, although IV diazepam may

be necessary to control seizure activity while the phenytoin is being administered (Browne, 1978).

The most common side effects produced by phenytoin are nystagmus (usually evident at a serum level of 20 μg/ml), ataxia (at 30 μg/ml), and lethargy at 40 μg/ml) (Kutt et al., 1964). In addition to these common symptoms of toxicity, less common side effects include rash, nausea, chronic encephalopathy, psychosis, cerebellar degeneration, ophthalmoplegia, peripheral neuropathy, pseudolymphoma, lupus erythematosus, hepatitis, folate deficiency and megaloblastic anemia, gingival hyperplasia, blood dyscrasias, hirsuitism, hypocalcemia, and osteomalacia (Ambrosetto et al., 1977; Eadie, 1980; Iivanainen et al., 1977; Baylis et al., 1971; Glaser, 1973; McDanal and Bolman, 1975; Selhorst et al., 1972; Spector et al., 1976; Vallarta et al., 1974). Phenytoin, in toxic concentrations, can also produce asterixis, ballismus, dystonia, and a choreic disorder with buccolingual dyskinesia similar to tardive dyskinesia (Chapter 12) (Ahmed et al., 1975; Chadwick et al., 1976; Chalhub et al., 1976; Kooiker and Sumi, 1974; Luhdorf and Lund, 1977; McLellan and Swash, 1974; Murphy and Goldstein, 1974; Opida et al., 1978; Shuttleworth et al., 1974). Recent studies suggest that even in therapeutic concentrations, phenytoin may produce subtle but measurable impairment of cognition, memory, concentration, and psychomotor speed (Thompson et al., 1981; Trimble, 1981b; Trimble and Richens, 1981; Trimble et al., 1982).

Drug interactions are very common with phenytoin. Agents capable of increasing serum concentrations and producing toxicity include isoniazid, dicoumarol, disulfiram, chloramphenicol, valproic acid, imipramine, chlorpromazine, phenylbutazone, propoxyphene, methylphenidate, digoxin, benzodiazepines, and ethosuximide (Bruni et al., 1980a; Hartshorn, 1975; Kutt, 1975; Perucca and Richens, 1977, 1980; Rall and Schleifer, 1980). The metabolism of phenytoin may be accelerated by carbamazepine, diazepam, clonazepam, folic acid, and ethanol, but the effect on the serum level is usually small. Phenobarbital may either increase or decrease serum phenytoin levels. Phenytoin tends to decrease tricyclic antidepressant and neuroleptic serum levels (Braithwaite et al., 1975; Forrest et al., 1970; Linnoila et al., 1980).

Carbamazepine

Like phenytoin, carbamazepine (Tegretol, manufactured by Geigy) is used in the treatment of partial seizures and grand mal seizures. It is administered orally in doses of 800–1200 mg/day; the therapeutic serum level is 8–12 μg/ml; the serum half-life is 10–30 hours; and a stable serum levels is achieved after 2–6 days (Table 9-11) (Kutt and Penry, 1974; Rall and Schleifer, 1980). Side effects of carbamazepine include nausea and vomiting, rash, nystagmus, ataxia, lethargy, ophthalmoplegia, orolingual dyskinesia, dystonia, and collagen disease (Crosley and Swender, 1979; Eadie, 1980; Joyce and Gunderson, 1980; Mullally, 1982; Simpson, 1966). Hematologic abnormalities can be induced by carbamazepine: approximately 2 percent of patients manifest reversible leukopenia or thrombocytopenia, and fatal aplastic anemia is a rare complication (Hart and Easton, 1982; Silverstein et al., 1983). Carbamazepine produces fewer cosmetically disfiguring effects (gum hyperplasia, hirsuitism) than does phenytoin. It also produces less cognitive blunting and may improve the intellectual and emotional status of treated patients (Dalby, 1971; Dodrill and Troupin, 1977; Trimble et al., 1982).

Few drug interactions occur with carbamazepine. Propoxyphene interferes with its catabolism, raising serum levels, whereas phenytoin, phenobarbital, and primidone accelerate metabolism and lower serum levels. Carbamazepine lowers phenytoin and coumadin serum concentrations and may produce small elevations in phenobarbital and primidone levels (Kutt, 1975; Massey, 1983; Perucca and Richens, 1980).

The use of carbamazepine in the treatment of depression and mania is discussed in Chapter 14.

Phenobarbital and Primidone

Phenobarbital (Luminal, manufactured by Winthrop) is used in the treatment of partial seizures and grand mal seizures. It can be administered IV or orally but is absorbed erratically from IM injections. The usual adult daily dosage is 90–180 mg, and a therapeutic serum level is 15–40 μg/ml. It is very slowly metabolized, has a half-life of 50–120 hours, and does not reach a serum steady state for 11–25 days (Kutt and Penry, 1974; Rall and Schleifer, 1980). Primidone (Mysoline, manufactured by Ayerst) is partially metab-

olized to phenobarbital and to phenylethylmalonomide and has side effects and a drug interaction profile similar to those of phenobarbital. Primidone is available only for oral administration. The usual adult daily dosage is 500–1500 mg; and the therapeutic serum level is 5–12 μg/ml. The half-life of primidone is 3–12 hours, and the drug reaches a steady state in the blood after 16–60 hours. Achievement of a steady state of the phenobarbital metabolite takes considerably longer (11–25 days).

The principal side effects of phenobarbital and primidone are lethargy and intellectual dulling, but the drugs may also produce nystagmus, ataxia, nausea, impotence, and rash. They may produce facial dyskinesia and asterixis (Chadwick et al., 1976; Eadie, 1980).

Phenobarbital induces hepatic microenzymes and accelerates the metabolism—lowering the serum levels—of many drugs, including benzodiazepines, neuroleptics, tricyclic antidepressants, corticosteroids, quinine, phenylbutazone, digitoxin, and quinidine (Ellenor et al., 1978; Forrest et al., 1970; Hartshorn, 1975; Linnoila et al., 1980; Perucca and Richens, 1980; Rivinus, 1982). Drugs that may interfere with phenobarbital metabolism and predispose to toxicity include phenytoin, sodium valproate, methylphenidate, dicoumarol, alcohol, benzodiazepines, chlorpropamide, quinine and quinidine, and tricyclic antidepressants (Bruni et al., 1980b; Hartshorn, 1975; Perucca and Richens, 1980; Rivinus, 1982). Thioradizine may accelerate phenobarbital metabolism and lead to diminished serum levels (Gay and Madsen, 1983).

Valproic Acid

Valproic acid (sodium valproate; Depakene, manufactured by Abbott) is used primarily in the treatment of petit mal seizures, but it is also efficacious in partial and grand mal seizures and is used when contraindications for phenytoin or carbamazepine are present or when adjunctive therapy is necessary for seizure control (Browne, 1980; Bruni and Albright, 1983). The drug is administered orally in doses of 1000–2500 mg daily, the therapeutic serum level is 50–100 μg/ml; the serum half-life is 8–15 hours; and it reaches a stable serum level after 40–75 hours.

The principal side effects of valproic acid include gastrointestinal disturbances, sedation, impaired coagulation, alopecia, tremor, hyperammonemia, red cell aplasia, and hepatotoxicity (Browne, 1980; Hyman et al., 1979; MacDougall, 1982; Rawat et al., 1981). The latter is potentially the most catastrophic effect and may be fatal (Suchy et al., 1979).

Drug interactions with valproic acid occur primarily with the other anticonvulsants. Administration of valproic acid concurrently with phenobarbital may increase phenobarbital levels by as much as 40 percent and produce lethargy or coma (Bruni et al., 1980a; Rall and Schleifer, 1980). Phenytoin levels may rise transiently and then decline when valproic acid is added to a stable phenytoin regimen (Bruni et al., 1980a,b; Freil et al., 1979).

Ethosuximide

Ethosuximide (Zarontin, manufactured by Parke-Davis) is the treatment of choice for petit mal seizures (Browne et al., 1975). It is administered orally in doses of 1500–2500 mg daily, the therapeutic serum level is 40–100 g/ml, the serum half-life is 40–60 hours; and it reaches a steady-state level in the serum after 8–12 days.

Side effects of ethosuximide include nausea and vomiting, euphoria, dizziness, photophobia, agitation, rash, blood dyscrasias, and dyskinesias (Kirschberg, 1975; Rall and Schleifer, 1980).

Other Anticonvulsants

In addition to the agents discussed in the preceding paragraphs, other anticonvulsants, including mephenytoin, trimethadione, diazepam, clonazepam, phenacemide, acetazolamide, and clorazepate, may be utilized when combination therapy is needed or when more conventional agents cannot be used.

Use of Psychotropic Agents in Epilepsy

The prevalence of behavioral disturbances among patients with epilepsy has its correlate in the frequency with which psychoactive drugs are prescribed for this population. Unfortunately, most of these agents have a tendency to exacerbate seizures, and their utilization in epileptics must be approached with caution. The administration of neuroleptics, tricyclic antidepressants, and lithium in epilepsy is presented here, and the pharmacology of these agents is discussed in Chapters 13 and 14.

Neuroleptics

Soon after the introduction of phenothiazines into clinical practice it was realized that these agents had a potential for exacerbating seizures in patients with epilepsy and of inducing convulsions in patients with no prior history of seizures (Fabisch, 1955; Kurtzke, 1957; Liddell and Retterstol, 1957; Lomas et al., 1955; Mendez et al., 1984; Schlichter et al., 1956; Vaughan et al., 1955; Voegele and May, 1957). In most patients the risk of seizure exacerbation or induction is low but is increased if there is a history of prior seizures or brain

TABLE 9-12. Relative Risk of Seizure Exacerbation by Agents Within Two Classes of Psychotropic Drugs

Neuroleptics	
Chlorpromazine	Highest risk
Perphenazine Thiothixene Haloperidol	Moderate risk
Thioridazine Fluphenazine Molindone	Lowest risk
Antidepressants	
Maprotiline Amitriptyline Nortriptyline	Highest risk
Trimipramine Protriptyline Imipramine Lithium	Moderate risk
Desipramine Doxepin Alprazolam MAOI[a]	Lowest risk

Itil and Soldatos, 1980; Mendez et al; 1984 in press.
[a]Monoamine oxidase inhibitor.

injury or if the neuroleptic doses or serum levels are unusually high (Logothetis, 1967; Remick and Fine, 1979; Rivera-Calimlin et al., 1973, 1976; Toone and Fenton, 1977). Not all neuroleptics are equally likely to produce seizures: chlorpromazine carries the highest risk; perphenazine, thiothixene, and haloperidol are moderately likely to induce seizures; and thioridazine, fluphenazine, and molindone are the least likely to cause seizure activity (Table 9-12) (Itil and Soldatos, 1980; Mendez et al., 1984; Olivier et al., 1982; Remick and Fine, 1979). Neuroleptic-induced seizures must be carefully distinguished from neuroleptic-induced generalized dystonic reactions. In the latter, consciousness is preserved.

Administration of neuroleptics results in the following EEG changes: slowing and increase in amplitude of nonepileptic tracings, exaggeration of any preexisting focal or generalized abnormality, augmentation of epileptiform discharges (Fabisch, 1957; Jorgensen and Wulff, 1958; Logothetis, 1967).

Antidepressants

Like neuroleptics, the antidepressants (tricyclic, tetracyclic) have a potential for precipitating seizures. Maprotiline is among the most likely to induce convulsions; amitriptyline and nortriptyline are also likely to cause seizures; trimipramine, protriptyline, imipramine, and lithium carry a moderate seizure risk; and doxepin, monoamine oxidase (MAO) inhibitors, alprazolam, and desipramine are least likely to result in seizure activity (Table 9-12) (Betts et al., 1968; Brown et al., 1973; Dallos and Healthfield, 1969; Hoffman and Wachsmuth, 1982; Holliday et al., 1982; Itil and Solderatos, 1980; Ives and Health, 1980; Lowry and Dunner, 1980; Luchins et al., 1894 Mendez et al., 1984, Molnar, 1983; Petti and Campbell, 1975; Schwartz and Swaminathan, 1982; Shepherd and Kerr, 1978; Trimble, 1980). In most cases the risk of precipitating seizures is small, and any exacerbation of the epilepsy can be managed by adjusting the anticonvulsant dosage. In some cases improved seizure control occurs following treatment with a tricyclic antidepressant agent, perhaps because of resolution of depression with regularization of diet and sleeping habits (Fromm et al., 1978; Ojemann et al., 1983). Monoamine oxidase inhibitors do not potentiate seizure activity and may even have anticonvulsant properties (Prockop et al., 1959).

Electroencephalographic effects of antidepressant drugs include activation of epileptiform abnormalities and production of theta-range slow-wave activity in normal subjects (Davison, 1965; Fink, 1959; Kiloh et al., 1961).

Lithium Carbonate

Lithium carbonate also has the potential for exacerbating seizure activity (Ghadirian and Lehmann, 1980; Moore, 1981; Jus et al., 1973; Solomon, 1979; Wharton, 1969). In most patients the effect is minor, and in some patients seizure control may even improve as the patient's mania subsides and eating and sleeping habits become normalized (Erwin et al., 1973).

Lithium has profound affects on the EEG, producing a disorganization and slowing of background rhythms, causing diffuse theta-range slowing, exaggerating focal abnormalities, and increasing epileptiform activity (Itil and Akpinar, 1971; James and Reilly, 1971; Johnson et al., 1970; Mayfield and Brown, 1966; Platman and Fieve, 1969).

Temporal Lobectomy

Patients whose seizures cannot be controlled by appropriate medications; who have an epileptic focus that is surgically accessible within the temporal lobe; and whose recurrent seizures are producing progressive impairment in social, emotional, and neuropsychological function may be candidates for temporal lobectomy. With carefully chosen candidates, surgery will produce complete seizure control in 50 percent of patients, and

an additional 25 percent will have a significant reduction in seizure frequency (Bengzon et al., 1968; Engel et al., 1975; Falconer and Serafetinides, 1963; Glaser, 1980; Penfield and Flanigin, 1950).

The response of the neuropsychiatric disorders associated with epilepsy has been much less favorable than the improvement in seizure control attained by surgery. In those with reduced seizure activity, personality and social functioning is improved and aggressiveness is reduced (Falconer, 1973; Falconer and Serafetinides, 1963; Hill et al., 1957; Taylor, 1972; Taylor and Falconer, 1968). Depression, however, is not uncommon in the postoperative period and may persist for up to 2 years (Falconer and Serafetinides, 1963; Hill et al., 1957). Ictal and postictal psychoses are reduced with improved seizure control, but the schizophrenialike interictal disorder is not significantly improved by surgery and may even emerge after lobectomy (Jensen and Larsen, 1979; Serafetinides and Falconer, 1962; Sherwin, 1981; Sherwin et al., 1982).

Neuropsychological investigation of patients subjected to temporal lobectomy reveals that their general cognitive function may improve with the diminished seizure frequency and reduced need for medication. Studies of memory function, however, demonstrate that verbal memory is impaired after temporal lobectomy of the left hemisphere, and perceptual memory may be disturbed after right temporal lobectomy (Milner, 1958, 1968; Novelly et al., 1984). These defects following unilateral surgery are usually mild in degree, but if both temporal lobes are removed or if one is removed and the contralateral lobe has a preexisting abnormality, a severe and permanent amnesia will be evident post–operatively (Milner et al., 1968; Penfield and Mathieson, 1979; Penfield and Milner, 1958; Scoville and Milner, 1957).

Social and Psychological Rehabilitation

In addition to efforts directed at seizure control and pharmacological management of affective and psychotic disorders, the successful rehabilitation of epileptic patients depends on effective social and psychological interventions designed to assist in finding housing and occupational situations that are prepared to consider their special needs. To accomplish this difficult task, rehabilitation programs must avoid focusing too narrowly on the convulsions. Although control of seizures is one important task, adequate care of the epileptic depends on recognizing that epilepsy is more than a seizure disorder; it is a complex neuropsychiatric condition with effects on the emotional, cognitive, and psychiatric functions of the victim. A rehabilitation program must take all these factors into consideration.

REFERENCES

Adams RD and Victor M. *Principles of neurology.* New York, McGraw-Hill Book Company, 1977.

Adebimpe VR. Complex partial seizures simulating schizophrenia. *JAMA,* 1977, *237,* 1339–1341.

Aquilar MJ and Rasmussen T. Role of encephalitis in pathogenesis of epilepsy. *Arch Neurol,* 1960, *2,* 663–676.

Ahmed S, Laidlaw J, Houghton GW, and Richens A. Involuntary movements caused by phenytoin intoxication in epileptic patients. *J Neurol Neurosurg Psychiat,* 1975, *38,* 225–231.

Alajouanine T. Dostoiewski's epilepsy. *Brain,* 1963, *86,* 209–218.

Ambrosetto G, Tassinari CA, Baruzzi A, and Lugaresi E. Phenytoin encephalopathy as probably idiosyncratic reaction: case report. *Epilepsia,* 1977, *18,* 405–408.

Ames FR and Enderstein O. Ictal laughter: a case report with clinical, cinefilm and EEG observations. *J Neurol Neurosurg Psychiat,* 1975, *38,* 11–17.

Andermann F and Robb JP. Absence status. A reappraised following review of thirty-eight patients. *Epilepsia,* 1972, *13,* 177–187.

Angus JWS and Simpson GM. Hysteria and drug-induced dystonia. *Acta Psychiat Scand,* 1970, Suppl. 212, 52–58.

Bartlet TEA. Chronic psychosis following epilepsy. *Am J Psychiat,* 1957, *114,* 338–343.

Baylis EM, Crowley JM, Preece JM, Sylvester PE, and Marks V. Influence of folic acid on blood-phenytoin levels. *Lancet,* 1971, *1,* 62–64.

Bear DM. Temporal-lobe epilepsy—a syndrome of sensory-limbic hyperconnection. *Cortex,* 1979, *15,* 357–384.

Bear DM and Fedio P. Quantitative analysis of interictal behavior in temporal lobe epilepsy. *Arch Neurol,* 1977, *34,* 454–467.

Bear D, Levin K, Blumer D, Chetham D, and Ryder J. Interictal behavior in hospitalized temporal lobe epileptics: relationship to idiopathic psychiatric syndromes. *J Neurol Neurosurg Psychiat,* 1982, *45,* 481–488.

Bear D, Schenk L, and Benson H. Increased autonomic responses to neutral and emotional stimuli in patients with temporal lobe epilepsy. *Am J Psychiat,* 1981, *138,* 843–845.

Belafsky MA, Carwille S, Miller P, Waddell G, Boxley-Johnson J, and Escueta AVD. Prolonged epileptic twilight states: continuous recordings with nasopharyngeal electrodes and videotape analysis. *Neurology,* 1978, *28,* 239–245.

Bengzon ARA, Rasmussen T, Gloor P, Dussault T, and Stephens M. Prognostic factors in the surgical treatment of temporal lobe epileptics. *Neurology,* 1968, *18,* 717–731.

Bernardi S, Trimble MR, Frackowiak RST, Wise RJS, and Jones T. An interictal study of partial epilepsy using positron emission tomography and the oxygen-15 inhalation technique. *J Neurol Neurosurg Psychiat,* 1983, *46,* 473–477.

Betts TA. Depression, anxiety, and epilepsy. In Reynolds EH and Trimble MR (Eds.): *Epilepsy and psychiatry.* New York, Churchill Livingston, 1981, pp. 60–71.

Betts TA, Kalra PL, Cooper R, and Jeavons PM. Epileptic fits as a possible side-effect of amitriptyline. *Lancet,* 1968, *1,* 390–392.

Bickerstaff ER. Impairment of consciousness in migraine. *Lancet,* 1961, *2,* 1057–1059.

Braham J, Hertzeanu H, Yahini JH, and Neufeld HN. Reflex cardiac arrest presenting as epilepsy. *Ann Neurol,* 1981, *10,* 277–278.

Braithwaite RA, Flanagen RJ, and Richens A. Steady-state plasma nortriptyline concentrations in epileptic patients. *Br J Clin Pharmacol,* 1975, *2,* 469–471.

Brickner RM, Rosner AA, and Munro R. Physiological aspects of the obsessive state. *Psychosom Med,* 1940, *2,* 369–383.

Brickner RM, and Stein A. Intellectual symptoms in temporal lobe lesions including *deja pensee. J Mount Sinai Hosp,* 1942, 9, 344–348.

Brown D, Winsberg BG, Bialer I, and Press M. Imipramine therapy and seizures: three children treated for hyperactive behavior disorder. *Am J Psychiat,* 1973, *130,* 210–212.

Browne TR. Drug therapy reviews: drug therapy of status epilepticus. *Am J Hosp Pharm,* 1978, *35,* 915–922.

Browne TR. Valproic acid. *New Engl J Med,* 1980, *302,* 661–666.

Browne TR, Dreifus FE, Dyken PR, Goode DJ, Perry JK, Porter RJ, White BG, and White PT. Ethosuximide in the treatment of absence (petit mal) seizures. *Neurology,* 1975, *25,* 515–524.

Bruens JH. Psychoses in epilepsy. *Psychiat Neurol Neurochir,* 1971, *75,* 175–192.

Bruens JH. Psychoses in epilepsy. In Vinken PJ and Bruyn GW (Eds.): *The epilepsies,* Vol. 15, *Handbook of clinical neurology.* New York, American Elsevier Publishing Company, 1974, pp. 593–610.

Bruni J and Albright P. Valproic acid therapy for complex partial seizures. *Arch Neurol,* 1983, *40,* 135–137.

Bruni J, Gallo JM, Lee CS, Perchalski RJ, and Wilder BJ. Interactions of valproic acid with phenytoin. *Neurology,* 1980a, *30,* 1233–1236.

Bruni J, Wilder BJ, Perchalski RJ, Hammond EJ, and Villarreal HJ. Valproic acid and plasma levels of phenobarbital. *Neurology,* 1980b, *30b,* 94–97.

Camfield PR, Gates R, Ronen G, Camfield C, Ferguson A, and Macdonald GW. Comparison of cognitive ability, personality profile and school success in epileptic children with pure right versus left temporal lobe EEG foci. *Ann Neurol,* 1984, *15,* 122–126.

Chadwick D, Reynolds EH, and Marsden CD. Anticonvulsant-produced dyskinesias: a comparison with dyskinesias induced by neuroleptics. *J Neurol Neurosurg Psychiat,* 1976, *39,* 1210–1218.

Chalhub EG, Devivo DC, and Volpe JJ. Phenytoin-induced dystonia and choreoathetosis in two retarded epileptic children. *Neurology,* 1976, *26,* 494–498.

Chen RC and Forster FM. Cursive epilepsy and gelastic epilepsy. *Neurology,* 1973, *23,* 1019–1029.

Cohen RJ and Suter C. Hysterical seizures: suggestion as a provocative EEG test. *Ann Neurol*, 1982, *11*, 391–395.

Cole M and Zangwill OL. *Deja vu* in temporal lobe epilepsy. *J Neurol Neurosurg Psychiat*, 1963, *26*, 37–38.

Collins WCJ, Lanigan O, and Callaghan N. Plasma prolactin concentrations following epileptic and pseudoseizures. *J Neurol Neurosurg Psychiat*, 1983, *46*, 505–508.

Commission on Classification and Terminology of the International League Against Epilepsy. Proposal for revised clinical and electroencephalographic classification of epileptic seizures. *Epilepsia*, 1981, *22*, 489–501.

Crosley CJ and Swender PT. Dystonia associated with carbamazepine administration: experience in brain-damaged children. *Pediatrics*, 1979, *63*, 612–615.

Cummings JL. Organic delusions: phenomenology, anatomical correlations, and review. *Br J Psychiat*, 1984, *46*, 184–197.

Cummings JL and Benson DF. *Dementia: a clinical approach.* Boston, Butterworths, 1983.

Currie S, Heathfield KWG, Henson RA, and Scott DF. Clinical course and prognosis of temporal lobe epilepsy. *Brain*, 1971, *94*, 173–190.

Dalby MA. Antiepileptic and psychotropic effects of carbamazepine (Tegretol®) in the treatment of psychomotor epilepsy. *Epilepsia*, 1971, *12*, 325–334.

Dallos V and Healthfield K. Iatrogenic epilepsy due to antidepressant drugs. *Br Med J*, 1969, *4*, 80–82.

Daly D. Ictal affect. *Am J Psychiat*, 1958, *115*, 97–108.

Daly DD and Mulder DW. Gelastic epilepsy. *Neurology*, 1957, *7*, 189–192.

Dana-Haeri J, Trimble MR, and Oxley J. Prolactin and gonodotrophin changes following generalized and partial seizures. *J Neurol Neurosurg Psychiat*, 1983, *46*, 331–335.

Davison K. EEG activation after intravenous amitriptyline. *Electroenceph Clin Neurophysiol*, 1965, *19*, 298–300.

De Pasquet EG, Gaudin ES, Bianchi A, and de Mendilaharsu SA. Prolonged and monosymptomatic dysphasic status epileptics. *Neurology*, 1976, *26*, 244–247.

Desai BT, Porter RJ, and Penry JK. Psychogenic seizures. *Arch Neurol*, 1982, *39*, 202–209.

Devinsky O, Hafler DA, and Victor J. Embarrassment as the aura of a complex partial seizure. *Neurology*, 1982, *32*, 1284–1285.

Dinner DS, Leuders H, Lederman R, and Gretter TE. Aphasic status epilepticus: a case report. *Neurology*, 1981, *31*, 888–890.

Dodge PR, Richardson EP Jr, and Victor M. Recurrent convulsive seizures as a sequel to cerebral infarctions: a clinical and pathological study. *Brain*, 1954, *77*, 610–638.

Dodrill C and Troupin AS. Psychotropic effects of carbamazepine in epilepsy: a double-blind comparison with phenytoin. *Neurology*, 1977, *27*, 1023–1028.

Dominian J, Serafetinides EA, and Dewhurst M. A follow-up study of acute-onset epilepsy. II. Psychiatric and social findings. *Br Med J*, 1963, *1*, 431–435.

Dongier S. Statistical study of clinical and electroencephalographic manifestations of 536 psychotic episodes occurring in 516 epileptics between clinical seizures. *Epilepsia*, 1959–1960, *1*, 117–142.

Dostoyevsky F. *The idiot* (translated by Carlisle H and Carlisle O). New York, New American Library, 1969.

Dreifuss FE. The differential diagnosis of partial seizures with complex symptomatology. *Adv Neurol*, 1975, *11*, 187–197.

Eadie MT. Unwanted effects of anticonvulsant drugs. In Tyrer JH (Ed.): *The treatment of epilepsy.* Philadelphia, JB Lippincott Company, 1980, pp. 129–160.

Earle KM, Baldwin M, and Penfield W. Incisural sclerosis and temporal lobe seizures produced by hippocampal herniation at birth. *Arch Neurol Psychiat*, 1953, *69*, 27–42.

Earnest MP and Yarnell PR. Seizure admissions to a city hospital: the role of alcohol. *Epilepsia*, 1976, *17*, 387–393.

Ellenor GL, Musa MN, and Beuthin FC. Phenobarbital–thioridazine interaction in man. *Res Commun Chem Path Pharmacol*, 1978, *21*, 185–188.

Engel J Jr, Brown WJ, Kuhl DE, Phelps ME, Mazziota JC, and Crandall PH. Pathological findings underlying focal temporal lobe hypometabolism in partial epilepsy. *Ann Neurol*, 1982a, *12*, 518–528.

Engel J Jr, Driver MV, and Falconer MA. Electrophysiological correlates of pathology and surgical results in temporal lobe epilepsy. *Brain*, 1975, *98*, 129–156.

Engel J Jr, Kuhl DE, Phelps ME, and Crandell PH. Comparative localization of epileptic foci in partial epilepsy by PCT and EEG. *Ann Neurol*, 1982b, *12*, 529–537.

Engel J Jr, Kuhl DE, Phelps ME, and Mazziotta JC. Interictal cerebral glucose metabolism in partial epilepsy and its relation to EEG changes. *Ann Neurol*, 1982c, *12*, 510–517.

Engel J Jr, Ludwig BI, and Fetell M. Prolonged partial complex status epilepticus: EEG and behavioral observations. *Neurology*, 1978, *28*, 863–869.

Erwin CW, Gerber CJ, Morrison SD, and James JF. Lithium carbonate and convulsive disorder. *Arch Gen Psychiat*, 1973, *28*, 646–648.

Escueta AVD, Bacsal FE, and Treiman DM. Complex partial seizures on closed-circuit television and EEG: a study of 691 attacks in 79 patients. *Ann Neurol*, 1982, *11*, 292–300.

Escueta AV, Boxley J, Stubbs N, Waddell G, and Wilson WA. Prolonged twilight state and automatisms: a case report. *Neurology*, 1974, *24*, 331–339.

Escueta AV, Kunze U, Waddell G, Boxley J, and Nadel A. Lapse of consciousness and automatisms in temporal lobe epilepsy: a videotape analysis. *Neurology*, 1977, *27*, 144–155.

Escueta AVD, Mattson RH, King L, Goldensohn ES, Spiegel H, Madsen J, Crandall P, Dreifuss F, and Porter RJ. The nature of aggression during epileptic seizures. *New Engl J Med*, 1981, *305*, 711–716.

Evans JH. Post-traumatic epilepsy. *Neurology*, 1962, *12*, 665–674.

Fabisch W. Chlorpromazine and epilepsy. *Lancet*, 1955, *1*, 1277.

Fabisch W. The effect of chlorpromazine on the electroencephalogram of epileptic patients. *J Neurol Neurosurg Psychiat*, 1957, *20*, 185–190.

Falconer MA. Reversibility by temporal-lobe resection of the behavioral abnormalities of temporal-lobe epilepsy. *New Engl J Med*, 1973, *289*, 451–455.

Falconer MA and Serafetinides EA. A follow-up study of surgery in temporal lobe epilepsy. *J Neurol Neurosurg Psychiat*, 1963, *26*, 154–165.

Falconer MA, Serafetinides EA, and Corsellis JAN. Etiology and pathogenesis of temporal lobe epilepsy. *Arch Neurol*, 1964, *10*, 233–248.

Fenton GW. Personality and behavioral disorders in adults with epilepsy. In Reynolds EH and Trimble MR (Eds.): *Epilepsy and psychiatry*. London, Churchill Livingston, 1981, pp. 77–91.

Ferguson SM, Rayport M, Gardner R, Kass W, Weiner H, and Reiser MF. Similarities in mental content of psychotic states, spontaneous seizures, dreams, and responses to electrical brain stimulation in patients with temporal lobe epilepsy. *Psychosom Med*, 1969, *31*, 479–498.

Ferriss GS. The recognition of nonepileptic seizures. *South Med J*, 1959, *52*, 1557–1567.

Fink M. Electroencephalographic and behavioral effects of tofranil. *Canad Psychiat Assoc*, 1959 (Suppl. 4), 161–171.

Fischer-Williams M, Bickford RG, and Whisnant JP. Occipito-parieto-temporal seizure discharge with visual hallucinations and aphasia. *Epilepsia*, 1964, *5*, 279–292.

Flor-Henry P. Schizophrenia-like reactions and affective psychoses associated with temporal lobe epilepsy: etiological factors. *Am J Psychiat*, 1969a, *126*, 400–404.

Flor-Henry P. Psychosis and temporal lobe epilepsy. *Epilepsia*, 1969b, *10*, 363–395.

Flor-Henry P. Ictal and interictal psychiatric manifestations in epilepsy: specific or nonspecific? *Epilepsia*, 1972, *13*, 773–783.

Flor-Henry P. Determinants of psychosis in epilepsy: laterality and forced normalization. *Biol Psychiat*, 1983, *18*, 1045–1057.

Forrest FM, Forrest IS, and Serra MT. Modification of chlorpromazine metabolism by some other drugs frequently administered to psychiatric patients, *Biol Psychiat*, 1970, *2*, 53–58.

Forster FM and Booker HE. The epilepsies and convulsive disorders. In Baker A and Baker HL (Eds.): *Clinical neurology*. New York, Harper and Row, 1975, Chapter 24, pp. 1–45.

Friel PN, Leal KW, and Wilensky AT. Valproic acid-phenytoin interaction. *Ther Drug Monitor*, 1979, *1*, 243–248.

Fromm GH, Wessel HB, Glass JD, Alvin JD, and Van Horn G. Imipramine in absence and myoclonic-astatic seizures. *Neurology*, 1978, *28*, 953–957.

Gastaut H. So-called "psychomotor" and "temporal" epilepsy: A critical study. *Epilepsia*, 1953, *2*, 59–76.

Gastaut H. Clinical and electroencephalographic classification of epileptic seizures. *Epilepsia*, 1970, *11*, 102–113.

Gay PE and Madsen JA. Interaction between phenobarbital and thioridazine. *Neurology*, 1983, *33*, 1631–1632.

Geier S. Prolonged psychic epileptic seizures: a study of the absence status. *Epilepsia*, 1978, *19*, 431–445.

Geier S, Bancaud J, Talairach J, Bonis A, Enjelvin M, and Hossard-Bonchard H. Automatisms during frontal lobe epileptic seizures. *Brain*, 1976, *99*, 447–458.

Geier S, Bancaud J, Talairach J, Bonis A, Szikla G, and Enjelvin M. The seizures of frontal lobe epilepsy. *Neurology*, 1977, *27*, 951–958.

Geschwind N. Dostoievsky's epilepsy. In Bulmer D (Ed.): *Psychiatric aspects of epilepsy*. Washington, D.C., American Psychiatric Press, 1984, pp. 325–334.

Geschwind N, Shader RI, Bear D, North B, Levin K, and Chetham D. Behavioral changes with temporal lobe epilepsy: assessment and treatment. *J Clin Psychiat*, 1980, *41*, 89–95.

Ghadirian AM and Lehmann HE. Neurological side effects of lithium: organic brain syndrome, seizures, extrapyramidal side effects and EEG changes. *Comp Psychiat*, 1980, *21*, 327–335.

Gibbs EL, Gibbs FA, and Fuster B. Psychomotor epilepsy. *Arch Neurol Psychiat*, 1948, *60*, 331–339.

Gibbs FA. Ictal and non-ictal psychiatric disorders in temporal lobe epilepsy. *J Nerv Ment Dis*, 1951, *113*, 522–528.

Gilmore RL and Heilman KM. Speech arrest in partial seizures: evidence of an associated language disorder. *Neurology*, 1981, *31*, 1016–1019.

Glaser GH. The problem of psychosis in psychomotor temporal lobe epileptics. *Epilepsia*, 1964, *5*, 271–278.

Glaser GH. Diphenylhydantoin. Toxicity. In Woodbury DM, Penry JK, and Schmidt RP (Eds.): *Antiepileptic drugs*. New York, Raven Press, 1973, pp. 219–226.

Glaser GH. Treatment of intractable temporal lobe–limbic epilepsy (complex partial seizures) by temporal lobectomy. *Ann Neurol*, 1980, *8*, 455–459.

Greenberg DB, Hochberg FH, and Murray GB. The theme of death in complex partial seizures. *Am J Psychiat*, 1984, *141*, 1587–1589.

Gross M. The clinical diagnosis of psychogenic seizures. In Gross M (Ed.): *Pseudoepilepsy*. Lexington, Massachusetts, Lexington Books, 1983, pp. 79–96.

Gulick TA, Spinks IP, and King DW. Pseudoseizures: ictal phenomena. *Neurology*, 1982, *32*, 24–29.

Gumpert J, Hansotia, P, and Upton A. Gelastic epilepsy. *J Neurol Neurosurg Psychiat*, 1970, *33*, 479–483.

Gunn J. Affective and suicidal symptoms in epileptic prisoners. *Psychol Med*, 1973, *3*, 108–114.

Hamilton NG and Matthews T. Aphasia: the sole manifestation of focal status epilepticus. *Neurology*, 1979, *29*, 745–748.

Hammill JF and Carter S. Febrile convulsions. *New Engl J Med*, 1966, *274*, 563–565.

Hart RG and Easton JD. Carbamazepine and hematological monitoring. *Ann Neurol*, 1982, *11*, 309–312.

Hartshorn EA. Interactions of CNS drugs: psychotherapeutic agents—the antipsychotic drugs. *Drug Intel Clin Pharmacol*, 1975, *9*, 536–550.

Haslam RHA and Jameson D. Cardiac standstill simulating repeated epileptic attacks. *JAMA*, 1973, *224*, 887–889.

Hawton K, Fagg J, and Marsack P. Association between epilepsy and attempted suicide. *J Neurol Neurosurg Psychiat*, 1980, *43*, 168–170.

Heath RG. Correlation of electrical recordings from cortical and subcortical regions of the brain with abnormal behavior in human subjects. *Confin Neurol*, 1958, *13*, 305–315.

Health RG. Common characteristics of epilepsy and schizophrenia: clinical observation and depth electrode studies. *Am J Psychiat*, 1962, *118*, 1013–1026.

Hecker A, Andermann F, and Rodin EA. Spitting automatisms in temporal lobe seizures. *Epilepsia*, 1972, *13*, 767–772.

Henriksen GF. Status epilepticus partialis with fear as clinical expression. *Epilepsia*, 1973, *14*, 39–46.

Hermann BP, Dikmen S, Schwartz MS, and Kearnes WE. Interictal psychopathology in patients with ictal fear: a quantitative investigation. *Neurology*, 1982, *32*, 7–11.

Hermann BP and Chabria S. Interictal psychopathology in patients with ictal fear. Examples of sensory-limbic hyperconnection? *Arch Neurol*, 1980, *37*, 667–668.

Hermann BP and Riel P. Interictal personality and behavior traits in temporal lobe and generalized epilepsy. *Cortex*, 1981, *17*, 125–128.

Hill D. Psychiatric disorders of epilepsy. *Med Press*, 1953, *229*, 473–475.

Hill D and Mitchell W. Epileptic anamnesis. *Folia Psychiat*, 1953, *56*, 718–725.

Hill D, Pond DA, Mitchell W, and Falconer MA. Personality changes following temporal lobectomy for epilepsy. *J Ment Sci*, 1957, *103*, 18–27.

Hoffman BF and Wachsmuth R. Maprotiline and seizures. *J Clin Psychiat*, 1982, *43*, 117–118.

Holliday W, Brasfield KH Jr, and Powers B. Grand mal seizures induced by maprotiline. *Am J Psychiat*, 1982, *139*, 673–674.

Hooshmand H and Brawley BW. Temporal lobe seizures and exhibitionism. *Neurology*, 1969, *19*, 1119–1124.

Hyman NM, Dennis PD, and Sinclair KGA. Tremor due to sodium valproate. *Neurology*, 1979, *29*, 1177–1180.

Iivanainen M, Viukari M, and Helle E-P. Cerebellar atrophy in phenytoin-treated mentally retarded epileptics. *Epilepsia*, 1977, *18*, 375–386.

Itil TM and Akpinar S. Lithium effect on human electroencephalogram. *Clin Electroenceph*, 1971, *2*, 89–102.

Itil TM and Soldatos C. Epileptogenic side effects of psychotropic drugs. *JAMA*, 1980, *244*, 1460–1463.

Ives T and Heath R. Amitriptyline-induced tonic-clonic seizures in the mentally retarded. *Drug Intel Clin Pharmacol*, 1980, *14*, 378.

Jackson JH. On a particular variety of epilepsy ("intellectual aura"), one case with symptoms of organic brain disease. *Brain*, 1888–1889, *11*, 179–207.

Jacome DE, McLain W Jr, and Fitzgerald R. Postural reflex gelastic seizures. *Arch Neurol*, 1980, *37*, 249–251.

James JF and Reilly E. The electroencephalographic recording of short- and long-term lithium effect. *South Med J*, 1971, *64*, 1322–1327.

Jennett B. *Epilepsy after non-missile head injuries*, 2nd ed. London, William Heinemann Medical Books Ltd., 1975.

Jensen I and Larsen JK. Mental aspects of temporal lobe epilepsy. Follow-up of 74 patients after resection of a temporal lobe. *J Neurol Neurosurg Psychiat*, 1979, *42*, 256–265.

Johnson G, Maccario M, Gershon S, and Korein J. The effects of lithium on electroencephalogram, behavior and serum electrolytes. *J Nerv Ment Dis*, 1970, *151*, 273–289.

Johnson SM and Lewis JA. The hysterical seizure. *Am J EEG Technol*, 1976, *16*, 23–29.

Jorgensen RS and Wulff MH. The effect of orally administered chlorpromazine on the electroencephalogram of man. *Electroenceph Clin Neurophysiol*, 1958, *10*, 325–329.

Joyce RP and Gunderson CH. Carbamazepine-induced orofacial dyskinesia. *Neurology*, 1980, *30*, 1333–1334.

Jus A, Villenueve A, Gautier J, Pires N, Cote JM, Jus K, Villenueve R, and Perron D. Some remarks on the influence of lithium carbonate on patients with temporal epilepsy. *Internat J Clin Pharmacol Ther Toxicol*, 1973, *7*, 67–74.

Kamrin RP. Temporal lobe epilepsy caused by unruptured middle cerebral artery aneurysms. *Arch Neurol*, 1966, *14*, 421–427.

Karagulla S and Robertson EE. Psychical phenomena in temporal lobe epilepsy and the psychoses. *Br Med J*, 1955, *1*, 748–752.

Kenna TC and Sedman G. Depersonalization in temporal lobe epilepsy and the organic psychoses. *Br J Psychiat*, 1965, *111*, 293–299.

Kiloh LG, Davison K, and Osselton JW. An electroencephalographic study of the analeptic effects of imipramine. *Electroenceph Clin Neurophysiol*, 1961, *13*, 216–223.

King DW, Gallagher BB, Murvin AJ, Smith DB, Marcus DJ, Horthage LC, and Ward LC III. Pseudoseizures: diagnostic evaluation. *Neurology*, 1982, *32*, 18–23.

King DW and Marsan CA. Clinical features and ictal patterns in epileptic patients with EEG temporal lobe foci. *Ann Neurol*, 1977, *2*, 138–147.

Kirschberg GJ. Dyskinesia—an unusual reaction to ethosuximide. *Arch Neurol*, 1975, *32*, 137–138.

Kooiker JC and Sumi SM. Movement disorder as a manifestation of diphenylhydantoin intoxication. *Neurology*, 1974 *24*, 68–71.

Kristensen O and Sindrup EH. Psychomotor epilepsy and psychosis. I. Physical aspects. *Acta Neurol Scand*, 1978, *57*, 361–369.

Krumholz A and Niedermeyer E. Psychogenic seizures: a clinical study with follow up data. *Neurology*, 1983, *33*, 498–502.

Kurtzke TF. Seizures with promazine. *J Nerv Ment Dis*, 1957, *125*, 119–125.

Kury G and Cobb S. Epileptic dementia resembling schizophrenia: clinico-pathological report of a case. *J Nerv Ment Dis*, 1964, *138*, 340–347.

Kutt H. Interactions of antiepileptic drugs. *Epilepsia*, 1975, *16*, 393–402.

Kutt H and Penry JK. Usefulness of blood levels of antiepileptic drugs. *Arch Neurol*, 1974, *31*, 283–288.

Kutt H, Winters W, Kokenge R, and McDowell F. Diphenylhydantoin metabolism, blood levels and toxicity. *Arch Neurol*, 1964, *11*, 642–648.

Lamprecht F. Epilepsy and schizophrenia: a neurochemical bridge. *J Neurol Transmis*, 1977, *40*, 159–170.

Lees F and Watkins SM. Loss of consciousness in migraine. *Lancet*, 1963, *2*, 647–650.

Lehtinen L and Kivalo A. Laughter epilepsy. *Acta Neurol Scand*, 1965, *41*, 255–261.

Lesser RP, Leuders H, and Dinner DS. Evidence for epilepsy is rare in patients with psychogenic seizures. *Neurology*, 1983, *33*, 502–504.

Levin S. Epileptic clouded states. *J Nerv Ment Dis*, 1952, *116*, 215–225.

Liddell DW and Retterstol N. The occurrence of epileptic fits in leucotomized patients receiving chlorpromazine therapy. *J Neurol Neurosurg Psychiat*, 1957, *20*, 105–107.

Lindsay J, Ounsted C, and Richards P. Long-term outcome in children with temporal lobe seizures. III. Psychiatric aspects in childhood and adult life. *Develop Med Child Neurol*, 1979, *21*, 630–636.

Linnoila M, Viukari M, Vaisanen K, and Auvinen J. Effect of anticonvulsants on plasma haloperidol and thioridazine levels. *Am J Psychiat*, 1980, *137*, 819–821.

Logothetis J. Spontaneous epileptic seizures and electroencephalographic changes in the course of phenothiazine therapy. *Neurology*, 1967, *17*, 869–877.

Loiseau P, Cohadon F, and Cohadon S. Gelastic epilepsy. A review and report of five cases. *Epilepsia*, 1971, *12*, 313–323.

Lomas J, Boardman RH, and Markowe M. Complications of chlorpromazine therapy in 800 mental-hospital patients. *Lancet*, 1955, *1*, 1144–1147.

Lombroso CT and Lerman P. Breathholding spells (cyanotic and pallid infantile syncope). *Pediatrics*, 1967, *39*, 563–579.

Lowry MR and Dunner FJ. Seizures during tricyclic therapy. *Am J Psychiat*, 1980, *137*, 1461–1462.

Luchins DR, Oliver AP, and Wyatt RJ. Seizures with antidepressants: an in vitro technique to assess relative risk. *Epilepsia*, 1984, *25*, 25–32.

Lugaresi E, Pazzaglia P, and Tassinari CA. Differentiation of "absence status" and "temporal lobe status." *Epilepsia*, 1971, *12*, 77–87.

Luhdorf K, and Lund M. Phenytoin-induced hyperkinesia, *Epilepsia*, 1977, *18*, 409–415.

Luther JS, McNamara JO, Carwile S, Miller P, and Hope V. Pseudoepileptic seizures: methods and video analysis to aid diagnosis. *Ann Neurol*, 1982, *92*, 458–462.

MacDougall LG. Pure red cell aplasia associated with sodium valproate therapy. *JAMA*, 1982, *247*, 53–54.

Mackay A. Self-poisoning—a complication of epilepsy. *Br J Psychiat*, 1979, *134*, 277–282.

Macrae D. Isolated fear. A temporal lobe aura. *Neurology*, 1954a, *4*, 497–505.

Macrae D. On the nature of fear, with reference to its occurrence in epilepsy. *J Nerv Ment Dis*, 1954b, *120*, 385–393.

Malamud N. The epileptogenic focus in temporal lobe epilepsy from a pathological standpoint. *Arch Neurol*, 1966, *14*, 190–195.

Malamud N. Psychiatric disorder with intracranial tumors of limbic system. *Arch Neurol*, 1967, *17*, 113–123.

Margerison JH and Corsellis JAN. Epilepsy and the temporal lobes. *Brain*, 1966, *89*, 499–530.

Markand ON, Wheeler GL, and Pollack SL. Complex partial status epilepticus (psychomotor status). *Neurology*, 1978, *28*, 189–196.

Massey EW. Effect of carbamazepine on coumadin metabolism. *Ann Neurol*, 1983, *13*, 691–692.

Mayeux R and Leuders H. Complex partial status epilepticus: case report and proposal for diagnostic criteria. *Neurology*, 1978, *28*, 957–961.

Mayfield D and Brown RG. The clinical laboratory and electroencephalographic effects of lithium. *J Psychiat Res*, 1966, *4*, 207–219.

McDanal CE Jr and Bolman WM. Delayed idiosyncratic psychosis with diphenylhydantoin. *JAMA*, 1975, *231*, 1063.

MaLachlan RS and Blume WT. Isolated fear in complex partial status epilepticus. *Ann Neurol*, 1980, *8*, 639–641.

McLellan DL and Swash M. Choreo-athetosis and encephalopathy induced by phenytoin. *Br Med J*, 1974, *2*, 204–205.

Mendez MF, Cummings JL, and Benson DF. The use of psychotropic drugs in epilepsy. *Psychosomatics*, 1984, *25*, 883–894.

Messing RO, Clossan RG, and Simon RP. Drug-induced seizures: a 10-year experience. *Neurology*, 1984, *34*, 1582–1586.

Mesulam MM. Dissociative states with abnormal temporal lobe EEG. *Arch Neurol*, 1981, *38*, 176–181.

Metrakos K and Metrakos JD. Genetics of convulsive disorders II. Genetic and electroencephalographic studies in centrencephalic epilepsy. *Neurology*, 1961, *11*, 474–483.

Milner B. Psychological defects produced by temporal lobe excision. *Assoc Res Nerv Ment Dis*, 1958, *36*, 244–257.

Milner B. Visual recognition and recall after right temporal-lobe excision in man. *Neuropsychologia*, 1968, *6*, 191–209.

Milner B, Corkin S, and Teuber H-L. Further analysis of the hippocampal amnesia syndrome: 14-year follow-up study of H.M. *Neuropsychologia*, 1968, *6*, 215–234.

Molnar G. Seizures associated with high maprotiline serum concentrations. *Canad J Psychiat*, 1983,; t0328, 555–556.

Moore DP. A case of petit mal epilepsy aggravated by lithium. *Am J Psychiat*, 1981, *138*, 690–691.

Mullally WJ. Carbamazepine-induced ophthalmoplegia. *Arch Neurol*, 1982, *39*, 64.

Mullan S and Penfield W. Illusions of comparative interpretation and emotion. *Arch Neurol Psychiat*, 1959, *81*, 269–284.

Mundy-Castle AC. A case in which visual hallucinations related to past experience was evoked by photic stimulation. *Electroenceph Clin Neurophysiol*, 1951, *3*, 353–356.

Mungas D. Interictal behavior abnormality in temporal lobe epilepsy. A specific syndrome or nonspecific psychopathology? *Arch Gen Psychiat*, 1982, *39*, 108–111.

Murphy MJ and Goldstein MN. Diphenylhydantoin-induced asterixis. *JAMA*, 1974, *229*, 538–540.

Nelson KB and Ellenberg JH. Predictors of epilepsy in children who have experienced febrile seizure. *New Engl J Med*, 1976, *295*, 1029–1033.

Niedermeyer E and Khalifeh R. Petit mal status ("spike-wave stupor"). *Epilepsia*, 1965, *6*, 250–262.

Novelly RA, Augustine EA, Mattson RH, Glaser GH, Williamson PD, Spencer DD, and Spencer SS. Selective memory improvement and impairment in temporal lobectomy for epilepsy. *Ann Neurol*, 1984, *15*, 64–67.

Offen ML, Davidoff RA, Troost BT, and Richey ET. Dacrystic epilepsy. *J Neurol Neurosurg Psychiat*, 1976, *39*, 829–834.

Ojemann LM, Friel PN, Trejo WJ, and Dudley DL. Effect of doxepin on seizure frequency in depressed epileptic patients. *Neurology*, 1983, *33*, 646–648.

Oliver AP, Luchins DJ, and Wyatt RJ. Neuroleptic-induced seizures. *Arch Gen Psychiat*, 1982, *39*, 206–209.

Opida CL, Korthals JK, and Somasundaram M. Bilateral ballismus in phenytoin intoxication. *Ann Neurol*, 1978, *3*, 186.

Ouellette EM. The child who convulses with fever. *Ped Clin N Am*, 1974, *21*, 467–481.

Parkes JD. Narcolepsy. In Riley TL and Roy A (Eds.): *Pseudoseizures*. Baltimore, Williams & Wilkins, 1982, pp. 62–82.

Penfield W and Flanigin H. Surgical therapy of temporal lobe seizures. *Arch Neurol Psychiat*, 1950, *64*, 491–500.

Penfield W and Mathieson G. Memory. Autopsy findings and comments on the role of hippocampus in experiential recall. *Arch Neurol*, 1974, *31*, 145–154.

Penfield W and Milner B. Memory deficit produced by bilateral lesions in the hippocampal zone. *Arch Neurol Psychiat*, 1958, *79*, 475–497.

Penry JK. Perspectives in complex partial seizures. *Adv Neurol*, 1975, *11*, 1–11.

Perez MM and Trimble MR. Epileptic psychosis—diagnostic comparison with process schizophrenia. *Br J Psychiat*, 1980, *137*, 245–249.

Perucca E and Richens A. Interaction between phenytoin and imipramine. *Br J Clin Pharmacol*, 1977, *4*, 485–486.

Perucca E and Richins A. Anticonvulsant drug interactions. In Tyrer JH (Ed.): *The treatment of epilepsy*. Philadelphia, LB Lippincott Company, 1980, pp. 95–128.

Peters JG. Dopamine, noradrenaline and serotonin spinal fluid metabolities in temporal lobe epileptic patients with schizophrenic symptomatology. *Eur Neurol*, 1979, *18*, 15–18.

Petti TA and Campbell M. Imipramine and seizures. *Am J Psychiat*, 1975, *132*, 538–540.

Platman SR and Fieve RR. The effect of lithium carbonate on the electroencephalogram of patients with affective disorders. *Br J Psychiat*, 1969, *115*, 1185–1188.

Pond DA. Psychiatric aspects of epilepsy. *J Ind Med Prof*, 1957, *3*, 1141–1151.

Pond DA and Bidwell BH. A survey of epilepsy in fourteen general practices. II. Social and psychological aspects. *Epilepsia*, 1959–1960, *1*, 285–299.

Pritchard PB III, Wannamaker BB, Sagel J, Nair R, and DeVillier C. Endocrine function following complex partial seizures. *Ann Neurol*, 1983, *14*, 27–32.

Prockop DJ, Shore PA and Brodie BB. Anticonvulsant properties of monoamine oxidase inhibitors. *Ann NY Acad Sci*, 1959, *80*, 643–651.

Racy A, Osborn MA, Vern BA, and Molinari GF. Epileptic aphasia. First onset of prolonged monosymptomatic status epilepticus in adults. *Arch Neurol*, 1980, *37*, 419–422.

Rall TW and Schleifer LS. Drugs effetive in the therapy of the epilepsies. In Gilman AG, Goodman LS, and Gilman A (Eds.): *The pharmacological basis of therapeutics*, 6th ed. New York, Macmillan Publishing Company, 1980, pp. 448–474.

Ramani V and Gumnit RJ. Management of hysterical seizures in epileptic patients. *Arch Neurol*, 1982a, *39*, 78–81.

Ramani V and Gumnit PJ. Intensive monitoring in interictal psychosis in epilepsy. *Ann Neurol*, 1982b, *11*, 613–622.

Ramani SV, Quesney LF, Olson D, and Gumnit RJ. Diagnosis of hysterical seizures in epileptic patients. *Am J Psychiat*, 1980, *137*, 705–709.

Rawat S, Borkowski WJ Jr, and Swick HM. Valproic acid and secondary hyperammonemia. *Neurology*, 1981, *31*, 1173–1174.

Remick RA and Fine SH. Antipsychotic drugs and seizures. *J Clin Psychiat*, 1979, *40*, 78–80.

Remillard GM, Andermann F, Gloor P, Olivier A, and Martin JB. Water drinking as ictal behavior in complex partial seizures. *Neurology*, 1981, *31*, 117–124.

Reynolds EH. Schizophrenia-like psychoses of epilepsy and disturbances of folate and vitamin B_{12} metabolism induced by anticonvulsant drugs. *Br J Psychiat*, 1967, *113*, 911–919.

Reynolds EH. Epilepsy and schizophrenia. *Lancet*, 1968, *1*, 398–401.

Reynolds EH and Travers RD. Serum anticonvulsant concentrations in epileptic patients with mental symptoms. *Br J Psychiat*, 1974, *124*, 440–445.

Riley TL. Syncope and hyperventilation. In Riley TL and Roy A (Eds.): *Pseudoseizures*. Baltimore, Williams & Wilkins, 1982, pp. 34–61.

Riley TL and Brannon WL Jr. Recognition of pseudoseizures. *J Fam Pract*, 1980, *10*, 213–220.

Rivera-Calimlim L, Castaneda L, and Lasagna L. Effects of mode of management on plasma chlorpromazine in psychiatry patients. *Clin Pharmacol Ther*, 1973, *14*, 978–986.

Rivera-Calimlim L, Nasrallah H, Strauss J, and Lasagna L. Clinical response and plasma levels: effects of dose, dosage schedules, and drug interactions, on plasma chlorpromazine levels. *Am J Psychiat*, 1976, *133*, 646–652.

Rivinus TM. Psychiatric effects of the anticonvulsant regimens. *J Clin Psychopharm*, 1982, *2*, 165–191.

Roberts JKA, Robertson MM, and Trimble MR. The lateralizing significance of hypergraphia in temporal lobe epilepsy. *J Neurol Neurosurg Psychiat*, 1982, *45*, 131–138.

Robertson WC and Fariello RG. Eating epilepsy associated with deep forebrain glioma. *Ann Neurol*, 1979, *6*, 271–273.

Rodin EA. Psychiatric disorders associated with epilepsy. *Psychiat Clin N Am*, 1978, *1*, 101–115.

Rodin EA, De Jong RN, Waggoner RW, and Bagchi BK. Relationship between certain forms of psychomotor epilepsy and "schizophrenia." *Arch Neurol Psychiat*, 1957, *77*, 449–463.

Rodin EA, Katz M, and Lennox K. Differences between patients with temporal lobe seizures and those with other forms of epileptic attacks. *Epilepsia*, 1976, *17*, 313–320.

Rodin E and Schmaltz S. The Bear-Fedio personality inventory and temporal lobe epilepsy. *Neurology*, 1984, *34*, 591–596.

Russell RW and Whitty CWM. Studies in traumatic epilepsy.

3. Visual fits. *J Neurol Neurosurg Psychiat*, 1955, *18*, 79–96.

Rutter M, Graham P, and Yule W. *A neuropsychiatric study in childhood*. Philadelphia, JB Lippincott, 1970.

Saper JR and Lossing JH. Prolonged trance-like stupor in epilepsy. *Arch Int Med*, 1974, *134*, 1079–1082.

Schenk L and Bear D. Multiple personality and related dissociative phenomena in patients with temporal lobe epilepsy. *Am J Psychiat*, 1981, *138*, 1311–1316.

Schlicther W, Bristow ME, Schultz S, and Henderson AL. Seizures occurring during intensive chlorpromazine therapy. *Canad Med Assoc J*, 1956, *74*, 364–366.

Schmidt RP and Wilder RJ. *Epilepsy*. Philadelphia, FA Davis Company, 1968.

Schwartz L and Swaminathan S. Maprotiline hydrochloride and convulsions: a case report. *Am J Psychiat*, 1982, *139*, 244–245.

Schwartz MS and Scott DF. Isolated petit-mal status presenting de novo in middle age. *Lancet*, 1971, *2*, 1399–1401.

Scott JS and Masland RL. Occurrence of "continuous symptoms" in epilepsy patients. *Neurology*, 1953, *3*, 297–301.

Scoville WB and Milner B. Loss of recent memory after bilateral hippocampal lesions. *J Neurol Neurosurg Psychiat*, 1957, *20*, 11–21.

Selhorst JB, Kaufman B, and Howitz SJ. Diphenylhydantoin-induced cerebellar degeneration. *Arch Neurol*, 1972, *27*, 453–456.

Sem-Jacobsen CW, Peterson MC, Lararte JA, Dodge HW Jr, and Holman CB. Intercerebral electrographic recordings from psychotic patients during hallucinations and agitation. *Am J Psychiat*, 1955, *112*, 278–288.

Serafetinides EA and Falconer MA. The effects of temporal lobectomy in epileptic patients with psychosis. *J Ment Sci*, 1962, *108*, 584–593.

Serafetinides EA and Falconer MA. Speech disturbances in temporal lobe seizures: a study of 100 epileptic patients submitted to anterior temporal lobectomy. *Brain*, 1963, *86*, 333–346.

Sethi PK and Rao S. Gelastic, quiritarian, and cursive epilepsy. *J Neurol Neurosurg Psychiat*, 1976, *39*, 823–828.

Shepherd GAA and Kerr F. Maprotiline hydrochloride and grand-mal seizures. *Br Med J*, 1978, *1*, 1523.

Sherwin I. Clinical and EEG aspects of temporal lobe epilepsy with behavior disorder, the role of cerebral dominance. *McLean Hosp J*, 1977 (Special Issue), 40–50.

Sherwin I. Psychosis associated with epilepsy: significance of laterality of the epileptogenic lesion. *J Neurol Neurosurg Psychiat*, 1981, *44*, 83–85.

Sherwin I, Peron-Magnan P, Bancaud J, Bonis A, and Talairach J. Prevalence of psychosis in epilepsy as a function of the laterality of the epileptogenic lesion. *Arch Neurol*, 1982, *39*, 621–625.

Shukla GD and Katiyar BC. Psychiatric disorders in temporal lobe epilepsy: the laterality effect. *Br J Psychiat*, 1980, *137*, 181–182.

Shukla GD, Srivastava ON, Katiyar BG, Joshi V, and Mohan PK. Psychiatric manifestations in temporal lobe epilepsy: a controlled study. *Br J Psychiat*, 1979, *135*, 411–417.

Shuttleworth E, Wise G, and Paulson G. Choreoathetosis and diphenylhydantoin intoxication. *JAMA*, 1974, *230*, 1170–1171.

Silverstein FS, Bower L, and Johnston MV. Hematological monitoring during therapy with carbamazepine in children. *Ann Neurol*, 1983, *13*, 685–686.

Simpson JR. "Collaegen disease" due to carbamazepine (tegretol). *Br Med J*, 1966, *2*, 1434.

Sironi UA, Franzini A, Ravagnate L, and Marossero F. Interictal acute psychoses in temporal lobe epilepsy during withdrawal of anticonvulsant therapy. *J Neurol Neurosurg Psychiat*, 1979, *42*, 724–730.

Sisler GC, Levy LL, and Roseman F. Epilepsia cursiva. *Arch Neurol Psychiat*, 1953, *69*, 73–79.

Slater E and Beard AW. The schizophrenia-like psychoses of epilepsy. Psychiatric aspects. *Br J Psychiat*, 1963, *109*, 95–150.

Slater F and Moran PAR. The Schizophrenia-like psychosis of epilepsy: relation between ages of onset. *Br J Psychiat*, 1969, *115*, 599–600.

Small JG, Milstein V, and Stevens JR. Are psychomotor epileptics different? *Arch Neurol*, 1962, *7*, 187–194.

Small JG, Small IF, Hayden MP. Further psychiatric investigations of patients with temporal and nontemporal lobe epilepsy. *Am J Psychiat*, 1966, *123*, 303–310.

Solomon A. An unusual receptive aphasia as a manifestation of temporal-lobe epilepsy. *New Engl J Med*, 1957, *235*, 313–317.

Solomon JG. Seizures during lithium-amitriptyline therapy. *Postgrad Med*, 1979, *66*, 145–148.

Spector RH, Davidoff RA, and Schwartzman RJ. Phenytoin-induced ophthalmoplegia. *Neurology*, 1976, *26*, 1031–1034.

Spencer SS, Spencer DD, Williamson PD, and Mattson RH. Sexual automatisms in complex partial seizures. *Neurology*, 1983, *33*, 527–533.

Standage KF. The etiology of hysterical seizures. *Canad Psychiat Assoc J*, 1975, *20*, 67–73.

Standage KF and Fenton GW. Psychiatric symptom profiles of patients with epilepsy: a controlled investigation. *Psychol Med*, 1975, *5*, 152–160.

Stevens JR. The "march" of temporal lobe epilepsy. *Arch Neurol Psychiat*, 1957, *77*, 227–236.

Stevens JR. Psychiatric implications of psychomotor epilepsy. *Arch Gen Psychiat*, 1966, *14*, 461–171.

Stevens JR. Interictal clinical manifestations of complex partial seizures. *Adv Neurol*, 1975, *11*, 85–107.

Stevens JR and Livermore A Jr. Kindling of the mesolimbic dopamine system: animal model of psychosis. *Neurology*, 1978, *28*, 36–46.

Stevens JR and Livermore A. telemetered EEG in schizophrenia: spectral analysis during abnormal behaviour episodes. *J Neurol Neurosurg Psychiat*, 1982, *45*, 385–395.

Stewart RS, Lovitt R, and Stewart RM. Psychopathology associated with hysterical seizures. In Gross M (Ed.): *Pseudoepilepsy*, Lexington, Massachusetts, Lexington Books, 1983, pp. 97–108.

Strauss E, Risser A, and Jones MW. Fear responses in patients with epilepsy. *Arch Neurol*, 1982, *39*, 626–630.

116

CLINICAL NEUROPSYCHIATRY

Strauss E, Wada J, and Kosaka B. Spontaneous facial expressions occurring at onset of focal seizure activity. *Arch Neurol*, 1983, *40*, 545–547.

Suchy FJ, Balistreri WF, Buchino JJ, Sondheimer JM, Bates SR, Kearns GL, Stull JD, and Bone KE. Acute hepatic failure associated with the use of sodium valproate. *New Engl J Med*, 1979, *300*, 962–966.

Sumi SM and Teasdall RD. Focal seizures. A review of 150 cases. *Neurology*, 1963, *13*, 582–586.

Taylor DC. Ontogenesis of chronic epileptic psychosis: a re-analysis. *Psychol Med*, 1971, *1*, 247–253.

Taylor DC. Mental state and temporal lobe epilepsy. A correlative account of 100 patients treated surgically. *Epilepsia*, 1972, *13*, 727–765.

Taylor DC. Factors influencing the occurrence of schizophrenia-like psychosis in patients with temporal lobe epilepsy. *Psychol Med*, 1975, *5*, 249–254.

Taylor DC and Falconer MA. Clinical, socio-economic, and psychological changes after temporal lobectomy for epilepsy. *Br J Psychiat*, 1968, *114*, 1247–1261.

Temkin O. *The falling sickness*, 2nd ed. Baltimore, Johns Hopkins Press, 1971.

Theodore WH, Porter RJ, and Penry JK. Complex partial seizures: clinical characteristics and differential diagnosis. *Neurology*, 1983, *33*, 1115–1121.

Thompson P, Huppert FA, and Trimble M. Phenytoin and cognitive function: effects on normal volunteers and implications for epilepsy. *Br J Clin Psychol*, 1981, *20*, 155–162.

Tizard B. The personality of epileptics: a discussion of the evidence. *Psychol Bull*, 1962, *59*, 196–210.

Toone B. Psychoses of epilepsy. In Reynolds EH and Trimble MR (Eds.): *Epilepsy and psychiatry*. London, Churchill Livingston, 1981, pp. 113–137.

Toone BK and Fenton GW. Epileptic seizures induced by psychotropic drugs. *Psychol Med*, 1977, *7*, 265–270.

Toone BK, Garralda ME, and Ron MA. The psychosis of epilepsy and functional psychoses: a clinical and phenomenological comparison. *Br J Psychiat*, 1982, *141*, 256–261.

Torrey EF and Peterson MR. Schizophrenia and the limbic system. *Lancet*, 1974, *2*, 942–946.

Trimble MR. The relationship between epilepsy and schizophrenia: a biochemical hypothesis. *Biol Psychiat*, 1977, *12*, 299–304.

Trimble MR. Serum prolactin in epilepsy and hysteria. *Br Med J*, 1978, *4*, 1682.

Trimble MR. New antidepressant drugs and the seizure threshold. *Neuropharmacology*, 1980, *19*, 1227–1228.

Trimble MR. *Neuropsychiatry*. New York, John Wiley & Sons, 1981a.

Trimble MR. Anticonvulsant drugs, behavior, and cognitive abilities. *Cur Develop Psychopharm*, 1981b, *6*, 56–91.

Trimble MR. Personality disturbances in epilepsy. *Neurology*, 1983, *33*, 1332–1334.

Trimble MR and Reynolds EH. Anticonvulsant drugs and mental symptoms: a review. *Psychol Med*, 1976, *6*, 169–178.

Trimble MR and Richens A. Psychotropic effects of anticonvulsant drugs. *Adv Hum Psychopharm*, 1981, *2*, 183–202.

Trimble MR, Thompson P, and Corbett J. Anticonvulsant drugs, cognitive function, and behavior. In Sandler M (Ed.): *Psychopharmacology of anticonvulsants*. New York, Oxford University Press, 1982, pp. 106–121.

Vallarta JM, Bell DB, and Reichert A. Progressive encephalopathy due to chronic hydantoin intoxication. *Am J Dis Childh*, 1974, *128*, 27–34.

Van Buren JM. Some autonomic concomitants of ictal automatism. *Brain*, 1958, *81*, 505–528.

Vaughan GF, Leiberman DM, and Cook LC. Chlorpromazine in psychiatry. *Lancet*, 1955, *1*, 1083–1087.

Vernea JJ. Partial status epilepticus with speech arrest. *Proc Aust Assoc Neurol*, 1974, *11*, 223–228.

Voegele GE and May PH. Epileptiform seizures under promazine therapy: occurrence in two cases without history of former seizures. *Am J Psychiat*, 1957, *113*, 655–656.

Walker AE. Post-traumatic epilepsy. *World Neurol*, 1962, *3*, 185–194.

Waxman SG and Geschwind N. Hypergraphia in temporal lobe epilepsy. *Neurology*, 1974, *24*, 629–636.

Waxman SG and Geschwind N. The interictal behavior syndrome of temporal lobe epilepsy. *Arch Gen Psychiat*, 1975, *32*, 1580–1586.

Weil AA. Depressive reactions associated with temporal lobe–uncinate seizures. *J Nerv Ment Dis*, 1955, *121*, 505–510.

Weil AA. Ictal depression and anxiety in temporal lobe disorders. *Am J Psychiat*, 1956, *113*, 149–157.

Weil AA. ictal emotions occurring in temporal lobe dysfunction. *Arch Neurol*, 1959, *1*, 87–97.

Weissberg MP. A case of petit-mal status: a diagnostic dilemma. *Am J Psychiat*, 1975, *132*, 1200–1201.

Wells CE. Transient ictal psychosis. *Arch Gen Psychiat*, 1975, *32*, 1201–1203.

Wharton RN. Grand mal seizures with lithium treatment. *Am J Psychiat*, 1969, *125*, 1446.

Whitlock FA. *Symptomatic affective disorders*. New York, Academic Press, 1982.

Whitten JR. Psychical seizures. *Am J Psychiat*, 1969, *126*, 560–565.

Wilensky AJ, Leal KW, Dudley DL, and Friel PN. Characteristics of psychotropic drug use in an epilepsy center population. *Epilepsia*, 1981, *22*, 247.

Williams D. The structure of emotions reflected in epileptic experiences. *Brain*, 1956, *79*, 29–67.

Wilson A, Petty R, Penry A, and Rose FC. Paroxysmal language disturbance in an epileptic treated with clobazam. *Neurology*, 1983, *33*, 652–654.

Wolfe SM and Victor M. The relationship of hypomagnesemia and alkalosis to alcohol withdrawal symptoms. *Ann NY Acad Sci*, 1969, *161*, 973–984.

Wyllie E, Lüders H, MacMillan TP, and Gupta M. Serum prolactin levels after epileptic seizures. *Neurology*, 1984, *34*, 1601–1604.

Chapter 10

Dissociative States, Depersonalization, Multiple Personality, and Episodic Memory Lapses

The patient who complains of periods of unrecallable behavior presents one of the most complex and perplexing of neurobehavioral problems. When examined, such a patient may appear completely normal but memory for the period in question may be completely absent or, at best, incomplete. The clinician thus has few clues with which to construct a tentative diagnosis and formulate an evaluation. Often, the differential diagnosis is limited to epilepsy and psychogenic amnesia—an impoverished list that does not reflect the wide variety of neurological, toxic, and idiopathic disorders that may become manifest as periods of unrecalled behavior. This chapter presents the differential diagnosis of dissociative states and episodic memory loss. The first portion of the discussion describes fugues and periodic lapses of memory, and the second portion describes the related phenomenon of depersonalization. When violence is prominent during the unrecallable period, the differential diagnosis will overlap with the entities considered in Chapter 11.

FUGUE STATES, EPISODIC MEMORY LAPSES, AND MULTIPLE PERSONALITY

Terminological confusion surrounds the group of disorders that present with episodic periods of unrecalled behavior. They might all be termed *fugue states,* but "fugue" often carries a psychogenic or functional connotation that is inappropriate for many of the disorders to be discussed. The descriptive phrase "episodic memory lapse" is utilized here. Phenomenologically, three types of episode are observed: the first is a true amnesia in which the patient is unable to learn during the period, asks the same questions again and again, and has a limited retrograde amnesia in addition to the ongoing anterograde amnesia. Included in this category are transient global amnesia and postconcussion amne-

sia. The second type of episode includes periods of confusion in which the patient's behavior is disorganized and purposeless. Postictal confusional states, brief toxic and metabolic encephalopathies, and somnambulism are included in this group. The third category includes periods of behavior that are fully integrated and coherent but cannot be remembered at a later time. The behavior may be consistent with the patient's usual personality as in alcoholic blackouts, or the patient may assume a completely different personality as in the multiple personality syndromes.

There have been few studies examining the relative prevalence of disorders presenting as fugue states or memory lapses. Table 10-1 presents the results of several such studies. Each investigation is subject to collection biases and varying standards of diagnosis, but collectively they give an idea of the relative frequency and spectrum of disorders that may produce episodic memory lapses. It can be seen that a majority of cases are associated with neurological diseases, depression, malingering, and personality disorders.

Table 10-2 lists the principal disorders that may manifest episodic amnesias or fugue states. The characteristics of the principal etiologies are discussed in the following sections.

Neurological Disorders

Neurological disorders are among the most common causes of episodic alterations in behavior that cannot be recalled, and the evaluation of any patient with periodic memory lapses must include a careful search for central nervous system (CNS) disturbances. Epilepsy is the most frequent neurological condition, producing intermittent memory loss; however, migraine, transient global amnesia, and postconcussion amnesia must also be considered.

TABLE 10-1. Relative Frequency (in percent) of Disorders Presenting with Transient Memory Lapses

Diagnosis	Stengel %	Wilson et al %	Berrington %	Kennedy and Neville %	Croft et al %	Total %
Epilepsy	17	5	—	12	18	10
Alcohol-related	—	10	—	—	—	2
Miscellaneous neuromedical (encephalitis, trauma, etc.)	6	10	—	43	72	28
Manic–depressive illness	22	—	—	—	—	3
Depresion	39	—	16	7	—	13
Schizophrenia	8	12	4	3	—	5
Hysteria	6	8	16	—	—	5
Miscellaneous psychiatric	3	7	—	8	10	6
Malingering	—	47	—	7	—	13
Personality disorder	—	—	64	20	—	16
Total	100[b]	100[c]	100[d]	100[e]	100[f]	100[g]

Epilepsy

The diagnosis of epilepsy is not difficult if the patient manifests a classic convulsion (Chapter 9). In some cases, however, the patient may be amnesic for any aura preceding the ictus and may manifest psychomotor automatisms during the ictal or postictal period without a generalized convulsion. In such cases, diagnostic confusion may arise, but there are several clues to the ictal nature of these events. Seizures begin abruptly in a stereotyped manner and end suddenly, although there is usually a variable period of postictal confusion. The patient is often fatigued after the seizure, and postictal headache is common. Seizures are also typically brief, frequently lasting only a few minutes, although episodes lasting for up to 2 days have been reported (Markand et al., 1978). Most importantly, behavior during the seizure or in the postictal state is simple and stereotyped, lacking complexity and purpose. The patient is either partially responsive or unresponsive to external stimuli. Most patients manifesting such periods of episodic behavior have a history of previous generalized seizures or of a predisposing brain injury. Patients presenting with prolonged automatic behavior may have either complex partial or petit mal status epilepticus (Chapter 9) (Ballenger et al., 1983; Belafsky et al., 1978; Engel et al., 1978; Escueta et al., 1974; Goldensohn and Gold, 1960; Saper and Lossing, 1974; Schwartz and Scott, 1971; Wells, 1975).

Two additional epilepsy-related conditions must be considered in the differential diagnosis of memory lapses: poriomania and multiple personality. *Poriomania* refers to unrecallable prolonged ambulatory behavior in epileptic patients. Mayeux and colleagues (1979) reported

three cases and reviewed 20 additional cases reported in the literature. All patients had episodes of unrecallable behavior lasting for several hours to several days, all had abnormal EEGs, and all were depressed. The patients accomplished highly complex tasks during the unrecalled period (e.g., drove many miles), and it is unlikely that the episodes represented status epilepticus. Rather, the behavior is more likely to have occurred during a period of retrograde or postictal amnesia or between recurrent ictal episodes. As discussed later, depression is a common setting for fugue states, but the beneficial response of poriomania to the administration of anticonvulsants suggests a close relationship to seizure activity.

An association between multiple personality and epilepsy has also been suggested. In their review of 17 reported cases of multiple personality, Sutcliffe and Jones (1962) found that five had epileptic manifestations. Similarly, several other series of patients with complex partial seizures reveal an excessive number with multiple personality, possession states, and other dissociative disorders (Glaser, 1978; Mesulam, 1981; Schenk and Bear, 1981). Multiple personality is unlikely to be an ictal manifestation per se and is more likely an expression of the complex interictal behavioral changes that can occur in patients with temporal lobe epilepsy (Chapter 9). Multiple personality is discussed in more detail in the sections that follow.

Migraine

Migraine may produce recurrent episodes of automatic behavior that cannot be remembered by the patient. The behavior is usually poorly integrated, lacks

TABLE 10-2. Etiologies of Periodic Memory Lapses

Neurological disorders	Metabolic conditions
Epilepsy	Uremia
Migraine	Hypoglycemia
Transient global amnesia	Hypertensive encephalopathy
Postconcussion amnesia	Porphyria
Toxic and metabolic disorders	Sleep disorders
Toxic disturbances	Somnambulism
Alcoholic blackouts	Narcolepsy
Barbiturates	Other hypersomnias
Phencyclidine	Idiopathic neuropsychiatric disorders
LSD	
Steroids	Psychogenic amnesia
	Psychogenic fugue
	Multiple personality
	Ganser syndrome

goal direction, and persists for less than an hour. The automatisms occur during the initial part of the attack; are usually preceded by visual distortions, hallucinations, vertigo, numbness, or other migrainous phenomena; and are followed by a prominent unilateral throbbing headache. Complete loss of consciousness may occasionally occur during the height of the attack. Acute confusional migraine is more common in children but can occur in any age group (Bickerstaff, 1961; Ehyai and Fenichel, 1978; Lees and Watkins, 1963; Moersch, 1924). Differentiation between migraine and epilepsy can be difficult. A postepisode headache that is unilateral, throbbing, and associated with photophobia and nausea is more characteristic of migraine. Electroencephalographic alterations are common in migraine but usually consist of excessive theta-range slowing rather than epileptic abnormalities (Camp and Wolff, 1961; Hockaday and Whitty, 1969; Slater, 1968). If attacks of confusional migraine occur frequently, prophylactic therapy with propranolol, imipramine, or methysergide may provide relief.

Transient Global Amnesia

Transient global amnesia is a true amnesia manifested by disturbances of new learning in the absence of significant alterations of remote memory, cognition, or personality (Chapter 4) (Benson, 1978). The amnesia begins abruptly and is manifest by difficulty in learning new information or remembering what is said. The same questions are asked repeatedly. The memory alteration includes a retrograde amnesia extending back in time over several weeks or months as well as the anterograde learning deficit. Transient global amnesia usually lasts for less than 24 hours, and the anterograde portion shrinks to within a few minutes of onset of the amnesic period when the episode terminates (Heathfield et al., 1973; Rowan and Protass, 1979; Shuping et al., 1980; Shuttleworth and Morris, 1966; Steinmetz and Vroom, 1972). Most cases of transient global amnesia appear to represent transient ischemic attacks, but other causes include migraine, cerebral angiography, intoxication with sedatives, cerebral neoplasms, and seizures. Precipitating factors have included sexual intercourse, sudden alterations in body temperature, highly emotional circumstances, and pain (Caplan et al., 1981; Cochran et al., 1982; Fisher, 1982; Gilbert and Benson, 1972; Lisak and Zimmerman, 1977; Mathew and Meyer, 1974; Mayeux, 1979; Shuping et al., 1980; Shuttleworth and Wise, 1973). Transient global amnesia can be distinguished from psychogenic amnesia by the retention of personal identity, the character of the retrograde amnesia, and the patient's emotional upset regarding the amnesia (Evans, 1966).

Postconcussion Amnesia

Amnesia is a frequent consequence of trauma and is associated with medial temporal injury (Chapter 4). Brief periods of amnesia lasting for minutes to a few days may follow cerebral concussion. During the amnesic period the patient may accomplish complex activities and appear to behave normally. The onset of the amnesia is associated with a blow to the head, but loss of consciousness may not necessarily occur. The most dramatic cases of postconcussion amnesia have been recorded in boxers (Critchley, 1957; Sercl and Jaros, 1962; Spillane, 1962). Winterstein (1937) described several such cases, including one boxer who was amnesic for a period of several hours between the fourth round of a match and his return home later that evening. During the unrecalled period he completed and won the fight, washed and dressed, collected his money, bought train tickets for himself and three friends, and traveled home. Gene Tunney, former heavy-weight champion of the world, had a similar episode in association with a training bout while preparing for his second fight with Jack Dempsy, and the experience significantly influenced his decision to retire from the ring (Martland, 1928). The amnesia includes both a retrograde period preceding the concussion and a longer anterograde period following the concussion-producing blow. The victim will not recall being struck, therefore, and, unless external trauma is obvious, the etiology of the amnesic episode may not be obvious.

Toxic and Metabolic Disorders

Alcoholic blackouts are the most common amnesic episodes associated with systemic intoxication. During the blackout period the patient appears normal in actions and in conversation and may complete elaborate activities. When sobriety is recovered, usually the following morning after a period of sleep, the actions of the previous evening cannot be recalled. Alcoholic blackouts occur in 30–40 percent of alcoholics, usually following periods of heavy alcoholic intake (Goodwin et al., 1969). Experimental studies show that alcoholics experiencing blackouts have difficulty with recent memory and new learning during the period of acute intoxication.

Other pharmacological agents that have been associated with amnesic episodes with automatic behavior include barbiturates, phencyclidine, LSD, and steroids (Akhtar and Brenner, 1979).

Virtually any of the causes of acute confusional states presented in Chapter 7 can produce periods of unrecallable behavior. Among the more common conditions associated with amnesic episodes are uremia, hypoglycemia, hypertensive encephalopathy, and porphyria (Akhtar and Brenner, 1979). Behavior during the confusional period is usually poorly coordinated, perseverative, and disorganized.

Sleep Disorders

Unrecallable behavior may occur with a variety of sleep –wakefulness disorders. The automatic behavior may occur during the period of sleep in the case of som-

nambulism or during apparently wakeful periods in narcolepsy and other sleep disturbances. Somnambulism (sleep walking) occurs in 1–6 percent of the population, is more common in children than adults, and affects more males than females. In 25 percent of cases there is a family history of sleep walking. Somnambulism may last for only a few seconds, with the patient simply sitting upright in bed, or it may last up to an hour and include modestly complex behavior such as walking around objects, dressing, and opening doors. Coordination is generally poor, however, and movements are stiff and clumsy. The somnambulist's eyes are open, and efforts to communicate may elicit slurred or mumbled responses. There is complete amnesia for the episode (Anders and Weinstein, 1972; Kales and Kales, 1974; Williams et al., 1982). Kleitman (1963) cited an example of a man who walked along a window ledge 12 stories above the ground and returned to bed without awakening. Somnambulism usually occurs within the first 3 hours of going to sleep when the patient is in a transition period between slow-wave sleep (Stage III or IV) and rapid-eye-movement (REM) sleep. On EEG, the somnambulistic period is preceded by rhythmic, paroxysmal, low-frequency, delta-range slow wave bursts (Anders and Weinstein, 1972; Broughton, 1966). Frequent somnambulistic episodes may improve with agents such as benzodiazepines that suppress slow-wave sleep (Anders and Weinstein, 1972).

Automatic behavior may also occur in narcolepsy and other hypersomnias. Patients may perform complex behaviors such as walking or driving without mishap. The patients are completely amnesic for the episodes and are surprised by their behavior when normal consciousness is resumed. The amnesic episodes have no definite relationship to attacks of sleep but have been attributed to the occurrence of multiple microepisodes of disrupted consciousness (Guilleminault et al., 1975a,b; Roth, 1980).

Idiopathic Neuropsychiatric Disorders

Idiopathic neuropsychiatric syndromes in which periodic memory lapses are prominent include psychogenic amnesia, psychogenic fugues, multiple personality, and the Ganser syndrome (Table 10-2).

Psychogenic Amnesia

The essential criteria for the diagnosis of psychogenic amnesia are a sudden inability to recall important personal information and lack of any identifiable neurological cause of the memory disturbance. The amnesia may be *circumscribed,* encompassing a relatively brief period of time; *selective,* in which some details are remembered whereas others are forgotten; *generalized,* in which the individual's entire life and identity are included; and *continuous,* beginning at a specific point in time and continuing into the present (*Diagnostic and statistical manual of mental disorders,* 1980). Behavior during the forgotten period is usually integrated and organized despite the memory loss. The amnesia usually begins and ends abruptly, and its onset is related to emotionally stressful events or circumstances. Psychogenic amnesia differs from amnesia associated with identifiable neurological and systemic disorders by the absence of the typical anterograde and retrograde aspects of the memory loss, lack of evidence of somatic illness, and frequent loss of personal identity (Abeles and Schilder, 1935; Kanzer, 1939; Pincus, 1982).

Psychogenic amnesia is a conversion syndrome occurring at times of stress in patients predisposed by an underlying psychiatric or neurological disorder. Depression is the most common predisposing condition, but psychogenic amnesia also occurs in patients with mania, schizophrenia, and personality disorders (Abeles and Schilder, 1935; Croft et al., 1973; Kennedy and Neville, 1957; Wilson et al., 1950). Malingering also accounts for a portion of cases (Kennedy and Neville, 1957).

Psychogenic Fugues

Psychogenic fugues are characterized by sudden unexpected travel away from one's home or customary place of work with inability to recall one's past, complete or partial assumption of a new identity, and absence of a neurological disorder sufficient to explain the disorder. The fugue may last for a few hours or several months, and the behavior may vary from brief purposeless travel to assumption of a new identity and new occupation (*Diagnostic and statistical manual of mental disorders,* 1980). The behavior is more purposeful and integrated than that occurring in patients with psychogenic amnesia, but the new identity is less complete and does not alternate with the original as in multiple personality. As in the case of psychogenic amnesia, affective disorder is the most common condition predisposing to psychogenic fugue (Stengel, 1941, 1943). Psychogenic fugue is also more likely to occur in certain personality disorders, including histrionic, compulsive, schizoid, avoidant, and borderline personalities (Millon, 1981). As noted earlier, similar fuguelike behavior may occur in epilepsy (Mayeux et al., 1979; Mohan et al., 1975; Zlotlow, 1968). In a study comparing epilepsy and psychogenic fugues, Roy (1977) found that the latter had a later onset, happened more frequently, and occurred in patients with concurrent affective symptoms and a history of previous psychiatric disturbances.

Multiple Personality

The criteria for the diagnosis of multiple personality include the existence within the individual of two or more distinct personalities, each of which is dominant at a particular time. The personality that is dominant determines the individual's behavior at that time, and each personality is complex and integrated with its own unique behavior patterns and social relationships (*Diagnostic and statistical manual of mental disorders,* 1980; Greaves, 1980). The original personality is usually completely amnestic for the behavior of any other subpersonalities, but when more than one subpersonality is present, each may be aware of the others to varying degrees. All the personalities are aware of discontinuities in their experience with "lost" periods of unrecallable time. The individual personalities are usually discrepant, displaying types of behavior unlike that of the original host personality. The subpersonalities may report being of the opposite sex, of a different race or age, or from a different sociocultural background from that of the original. The subpersonalities usually act in accordance with an age younger than that of the host pesonality (Abse, 1982; Cutler and Reed, 1975; *Diagnostic and statistical manual of mental diseases,* 1980; Greaves, 1980; Taylor and Martin, 1944).

Table 10-3 presents some signs of multiplicity that can be utilized by the clinician to deduce the presence of alternate personalities. The patients are aware of lapses of time, and observers may report behavior foreign to and unrecalled by the patient. During the time lapses, the patients may call themselves by different names or refer to themselves in the third person. They may discover writings, drawings, or purchases among their personal effects that are not recognized and cannot be accounted for. In therapy, a patient may use the word "we" in a plural rather than editorial sense, and alternate personalities may be elicited by hypnosis or during an amytal interview. The patients frequently complain of headaches, and they may report hearing voices that originate from within and are not identified as separate (*Diagnostic and statistical manual of mental disorders,* 1980; Greaves, 1980).

In addition to the behavioral changes exhibited by the alternate personalities, they may also manifest changes in pain sensitivity, galvanic skin responses, EEG pattern, evoked response patterns, and even handedness (Coons et al., 1982; Ischlondsky, 1955; Larmore et al., 1977; Ludwig et al., 1972; Schenk and Bear, 1981; Thigpen and Cleckley, 1954). The EEG alterations present in the subpersonalities reflect changes in alertness, arousal, concentration, and muscle tension (Coons et al., 1982; Ludwig et al., 1972).

The origin of this complex behavioral syndrome

TABLE 10-3.   Signs of Multiplicity

1.   Reports of time distortions, lapses, and discontinuities

2.   Being told of behavioral episodes by others that are not remembered by the patient

3.   Being recognized by others or called by another name by people whom the patient does not recognize

4.   Notable changes in the patient's behavior reported by a reliable observer; the patient may call himself by a different name or refer to himself in the third person

5.   Other personalities are elicited under hypnosis or during amytal interviews

6.   Use of the word "we" in the course of an interview

7.   Discovery of writings, drawings, or other productions or objects (identification cards, clothing, etc.) among the patient's personal belongings which are not recognized or cannot be accounted for

8.   Headaches

9.   Hearing voices originating from within and not identified as separate

10.   History of severe emotional or physical trauma as a child (usually before the age of five years)

Adapted from Greaves GB. Multiple personality 165 years after Mary Reynolds. *J Nerv Ment Dis, 1980, 168, p. 584*. Copyright 1980, The Williams & Wilkins Company, Baltimore. With permission.

is obscure and controversial. Severe emotional or physical trauma in childhood provides a significant developmental contribution to the occurrence of multiple personality. Many of the patients have been subjected to extreme disciplinary actions, physical deprivation, emotional distress, or sexual abuses that amount to torture (Abse, 1982; Greaves, 1980). Neurophysiological disturbances also appear to play a role in a significant number of patients. Epilepsy has been noted in up to 25 percent of patients with multiple personality, and even larger percentages have a history of brain injury (Coons et al., 1982; Horton and Miller, 1972; Mesulam, 1981; Schenk and Bear, 1981; Sutcliff and Jones, 1962). Schenk and Bear (1981) noted that one-third of patients with complex partial seizures had dissociative phenomena, including classic multiple personality, a marked tendency to describe themselves as having more than one personality but without amnesia for the actions of the alternate, or ascription of their intense emotional feelings to a foreign presence such as a demon. Multiple personality and other dissociative experiences bear no obvious relationship to the seizures of patients with complex partial epilepsy and are most likely related to the interictal behavioral alterations noted in these patients (Chapter 9).

Ganser's Syndrome

The Ganser syndrome was presented in Chapter 8 as one of the "pseudodementias" but deserves brief reconsideration here since it manifests episodic unrecallable behavior. Considered by most to be an hysterical dementia whose occurrence is facilitated by the presence of CNS dysfunction, the principal features of Ganser syndromes are hallucinations, prominent sensory changes of an hysterical type, alterations of consciousness with amnesia for the episode, and verbal responses that are either illogical or "near misses" (Goldin and Macdonald, 1955; May et al., 1960; Tyndel, 1956; Weiner and Braiman, 1955; Whitlock, 1967). Although described by Wertham as an "hysterical pseudo-stupidity which occurs almost exclusively in jails and in old fashioned German textbooks," the Ganser syndrome has occurred in association with toxic confusional states, head injuries, alcoholic dementias, general paresis, postpartum psychoses, schizophrenia, depression, hysteria, and as a manifestation of malingering (Whitlock, 1967). The hallmark of the syndrome is the illogical or approximate answers to even simple questions. Recovery from the syndrome is abrupt, and the patient is amnesic for the period encompassing the Ganser behavior.

DEPERSONALIZATION

Depersonalization refers to a subjective experience of estrangement involving the self, the body, or the environment. There is often a feeling of loss of ability to experience emotion, a lack of will or a feeling that one is an automaton, complaints of diminished concentration and memory, and a disturbance of the perception of time. The patient may feel as if in a dream. Derealization is frequently present with a feeling of loss of reality of the external world; alteration in the perceived shape, size, or color of external objects; or perception of people as dead or mechanical. The depersonalization experience may be brief, lasting for only a few seconds, or more prolonged, persisting for several months (Ackner, 1954a,b; *Diagnostic and statistical manual of mental disorders,* 1980; Saperstein, 1949; Shorvon, 1946).

TABLE 10-4.   Etiologies of Depersonalization

Neurological disorders	Idiopathic psychiatric disorders
Epilepsy	Schizophrenia
Migraine	Depression
Brain tumors	Mania
Cerebrovascular disease	Hysteria
Cerebral trauma	Anxiety
Encephalitis	Obsessive–compulsive disorders
General paresis	Personality disorders
Alzheimer's disease	Phobic–anxiety depersonalization syndrome
Huntington's disease	
Spinocerebellar degeneration	"Normal" subjects
	Exhaustion
Toxic and metabolic disorders	Boredom; sensory deprivation
	Emotional shock
Hypoglycemia	
Hypoparathyroidism	Hemidepersonalization
Carbon monoxide poisoning	
Mescalin intoxication	Lateralized (usually right parietal) focal brain lesion
Botulism	
Hyperventilation	
Hypothyroidism	

Ackner (1954b), Kenna and Sedman (1965); Mayer-Gross, (1935); Saperstein (1949); and Shorvon (1946).

Depersonalization, like other dissociative experiences, is a behavioral syndrome that may be produced by neurological, systemic, and idiopathic psychiatric disorders (Table 10-4). Depersonalization may also occur in neuropsychiatrically normal individuals subjected to severe exhaustion, boredom and sensory deprivation, or emotional trauma.

The principal neurological disorder producing depersonalization is temporal lope epilepsy. Experiences common in complex partial seizures, including "dreamy state," micropsia, macropsia, déjà vu, jamais vu, metamorphopsia, and anxiety also occur in idiopathic depersonalization syndromes and may complicate diagnostic efforts (Brickner and Stein, 1942; Cole and Zangwill, 1963; Jackson, 1888–1889; Kenna and Sedman, 1965; Remick and Wada, 1979). The two syndromes can usually be distinguished by the occurrence in the epileptic patient of brief and stereotyped depersonalization experiences, generalized seizures, epileptiform EEG abnormalities, and a predisposing CNS disease. Harper and Roth (1962; Roth and Harper, 1962) compared the experiences of patients with complex partial seizures with those of patients with the phobic–anxiety–depersonalization syndrome and found that the latter were more likely to have emotional precipitants, occurred more frequently (at least daily), resolved more slowly, lacked postictal confusion, had an earlier age of onset, and were more likely to have involved patients from families with psychiatric illness. The phobic–anxiety–depersonalization patients also had more depression, persistent anxiety, irrational fears, phobias, and hypochondriacal

symptoms. There was no single symptom that discriminated the two syndromes.

Other neurological disorders that have produced depersonalization include migraine, brain tumors, cerebrovascular disease, cerebral trauma, encephalitis, general paresis, degenerative dementias, and extrapyramidal disturbances. Toxic and metabolic conditions associated with depersonalization include hypoglycemia, hypoparathyroidism, hypothyroidism, hyperventilation, botulism, carbon monoxide intoxication, and mescalin ingestion (Table 10-4) (Ackner, 1954b; Kenna and Sedman, 1965; Mayer-Gross, 1935; Saperstein, 1949; Shorvon, 1946).

Depersonalization also occurs in a wide variety of idiopathic psychiatric disturbances, including schizophrenia, depression, mania, hysteria, anxiety syndromes, obsessive–compulsive disorders, and personality disorders (Table 10-4). Depersonalization usually occurs early in the course of schizophrenic, manic, and depressive episodes and disappears as the disorders progress to more advanced stages (Saperstein, 1949).

Hemidepersonalization refers to the unique experience of some patients with focal brain disease in which they come to view the affected side as unreal, of distorted size or shape, or as belonging to someone else. The syndrome is one manifestation of anosognosia and occurs primarily in patients with parietal lobe lesions of the right hemisphere (Critchley, 1953; Cutting, 1978; Weinstein and Kahn, 1950).

Depersonalization must be distinguished from delusions where one believes that either oneself or the world is changed and from hallucinations where one has an actual visual perception of one's own body (Christodoulou, 1978a,b; Damas-Mora et al., 1980; Dewhurst and Pearson, 1955; Lhermitte, 1951). The experience of depersonalization has an "as if" quality in which one acknowledges that it is as if the world is unreal or as if one is outside one's own body. These experiences may simulate the delusional syndrome of subjective doubles or autoscopic hallucinations, but the depersonalized patient is usually aware that it is the experience of the self or external reality that is altered, and not the self or external reality per se.

EVALUATION AND DIAGNOSIS

The wide range of potential etiologies dictates that the evaluation of the patient with episodic memory lapses or dissociative experiences must include a thorough appraisal of neurological, systemic, and idiopathic psychiatric disorders.

Neurological evaluation includes computerized tomography of the head and electroencephalography. Epilepsy is one of the most prominent disorders entering the differential diagnosis of dissociative experiences, and adequate EEG investigation should include nasopharyngeal electrodes and multiple recordings or continuous monitoring on telemetry. Neuroendocrinologic testing has added a useful dimension to the identification of complex partial seizures. The latter produce transient increases in serum prolactin levels, whereas nonictal experiences cause no change in prolactin levels. The level must be determined within 20–30 minutes of termination of the experience to detect the seizure-induced elevation (Collins et al., 1983; Dana-Haeri et al., 1983; Pritchard et al., 1983; Trimble, 1978). Systemic and toxic conditions producing depersonalization must be detected by appropriate laboratory studies. Some psychiatric illnesses producing depersonalization— schizophrenia, mania, and depression—may be obvious on clinical examination. Additional useful information in the investigation of dissociative states and multiple personality may be gained through hypnosis or an Amytal interview.

REFERENCES

Abeles M and Schilder P. Psychogenic loss of personal identity. *Arch Neurol Psychiat*, 1935, *34*, 587–604.

Abse W. Multiple personality. In Roy A (Ed.): *Hysteria*. New York, John Wiley & Sons, 1982, 165–184.

Ackner B. Depersonalization. I. Aetiology and phenomenology. *J Ment Sci*, 1954a, *100*, 838–853.

Ackner B. Depersonalization. II. Clinical syndromes. *J Ment Sci*, 1954b, *100*, 854–872.

Akhtar S and Brenner I. Differential diagnosis of fugue-like states. *J Clin Psychiat*, 1979, *40*, 381–385.

Anders TF and Weinstein P. Sleep and its disorders in infants and children: a review. *Pediatrics*, 1972, *50*, 312–324.

Ballenger CE III, King DW, and Gallagher BB. Partial complex status epilepticus. *Neurology*, 1983, *33*, 1545–1552.

Belafsky MA, Carwille S, Miller P, Waddell G, Boxley-Johnson J, and Delgado-Escueta AV. Prolonged epileptic twilight states: continuous recordings with nasopharyngeal electrodes and videotape analysis. *Neurology*, 1978, *28*, 239–245.

Benson DF. Amnesia. *South Med J*, 1978, *71*, 1221–1228.

Berrington WP, Liddell DW, and Foulds GA. A re-evaluation of the fugue. *J Ment Sci*, 1956, *102*, 280–286.

Bickerstaff ER. Impairment of consciousness in migraine. *Lancet*, 1961, *2*, 1057–1059.

Brickner RM and Stein A. Intellectual symptoms in temporal lobe lesions including "deja penseé." *J Mt Sinai Hosp*, 1942, *9*, 344–348.

Broughton RJ. Sleep disorders: disorders of arousal? *Science*, 1966, *159*, 1070–1078.

Camp WA and Wolff HG. Studies on headache. Electroencephalographic abnormalities in patients with vascular headache of the migraine type. *Arch Neurol*, 1961, *4*, 475–485.

Caplan L, Chedru F, Lhermitte F, and Mayman C. Transient global amnesia and migraine. *Neurology*, 1981, *31*, 1167–1170.

Christodoulou GN. Course and prognosis of the syndrome of doubles. *J Nerv Ment Dis*, 1978a, *166*, 68–72.

Christodoulou GN. Syndrome of subjective doubles. *Am J Psychiat*, 1978b, *135*, 249–251.

Cochran JW, Morrell F, Huckman MS, and Cochran EJ. Transient global amnesia after cerebral angiography. *Arch Neurol*, 1982, *39*, 593–594.

Cole M and Zangwill OL. Deja vu in temporal lobe epilepsy. *J Neurol Neurosurg Psychiat*, 1963, *26*, 37–38.

Collins WCJ, Lanigan O, and Callaghan N. Plasma prolactin concentrations following epileptic and pseudoseizures. *J Neurol Neurosurg Psychiat*, 1983, *46*, 505–508.

Coons PM, Multstein V, and Marley C. EEG studies of two multiple personalities and a control. *Arch Gen Psychiat*, 1982, *39*, 823–825.

Critchley M. *The parietal lobes*. New York, Hafner Press, 1953.

Critchley M. Medical aspects of boxing, particularly from a neurological standpoint. *Br Med J*, 1957, *1*, 357–362.

Croft PB, Heathfield KWG, and Swash M. Differential diagnosis of transient amnesia. *Br Med J*, 1973, *4*, 593–596.

Cutler B and Reed J. Multiple personality. A single case study with a 15 year follow-up. *Psychol Med*, 1975, *5*, 18–26.

Cutting J. Study of anosognosia. *J Neurol Neurosurg Psychiat,* 1978, *41,* 548–555.

Damas-Mora JMR, Jenner FA, and Eacott SE. On heautoscopy or the phenomenon of the double: case presentation and review of the literature. *Br J Med Psychol,* 1980, *53,* 75–83.

Dana-Haeri J, Trimble MR, and Oxley J. Prolactin and gonadotrophin changes following generalized and partial seizures. *J Neurol Neurosurg Psychiat,* 1983, *46,* 331–335.

Dewhurst K and Pearson J. Visual hallucinations of the self in organic disease. *J Neurol Neurosurg Psychiat,* 1955, *18,* 53–57.

Diagnostic and statistical manual of mental disorders, 3rd ed. Washington, D.C., American Psychiatric Association, 1980.

Ehyai A and Fenichel GM. The natural history of acute, confusional migraine. *Arch Neurol,* 1978, *35,* 368–369.

Engel J Jr, Ludwig BI, and Fetell M. Prolonged partial complex status epilepticus: EEG and behavioral observations. *Neurology,* 1978, *28,* 863–869.

Escueta AV, Boxley J, Stubbs N, Waddell G, and Wilson WA. Prolonged twilight state and automatisms: a case report. *Neurology,* 1974, *24,* 331–339.

Evans JH. Transient loss of memory, an organic mental symptom. *Brain,* 1966, *89,* 539–548.

Fisher CM. Transient global amnesia. Precipitating activities and other observations. *Arch Neurol,* 1982, *39,* 605–608.

Gilbert JJ and Benson DF. Transient global amnesia: report of two cases with definite etiologies. *J Nerv Ment Dis,* 1972, *154,* 461–464.

Glaser GH. Epilepsy, hysteria, and "possession." *J Nerv Ment Dis,* 1978, *166,* 268–274.

Goldensohn ES and Gold AP. Prolonged behavioral disturbances as ictal phenomena. *Neurology,* 1960, *10,* 1–9.

Goldin S and Macdonald JE. The Ganser state. *J Ment Sci,* 1955, *101,* 267–280.

Goodwin DW, Crane JB, and Guze SB. Alcoholic "blackouts": a review and clinical study of 100 alcoholics. *Am J Psychiat,* 1969, *126,* 191–198.

Greaves GB. Multiple personality 165 years after Mary Reynolds. *J Nerv Ment Dis,* 1980, *168,* 577–596.

Guilleminault C, Billiard M, Montplaisir J, and Dement WC. Altered states of consciousness in disorders of daytime sleepiness. *J Neurol Sci,* 1975a, *26,* 377–393.

Guilleminault C, Phillips R, and Dement WC. A syndrome of hypersomnia with automatic behavior. *Electroenceph Clin Neurophysiol,* 1975b, *38,* 403–413.

Harper M and Roth M. Temporal lobe epilepsy and the phobic anxiety–depersonalization syndrome. Part I: a comparative study. *Comp Psychiat,* 1962, *3,* 129–151.

Heathfield KWG, Croff PB, and Swash M. The syndrome of transient global amnesia. *Brain,* 1973, *96,* 729–736.

Hockaday JM and Whitty CWM. Factors determining the electroencephalogram in migraine: a study of 560 patients, according to clinical type of migraine. *Brain,* 1969, *92,* 769–788.

Horton P and Miller D. The etiology of multiple personality. *Comp Psychiat,* 1972, *13,* 151–159.

Ischlondsky ND. The inhibitory process in the cerebro-physiological laboratory and in the clinic. *J Nerv Ment Dis,* 1955, *121,* 5–18.

Jackson JH. On a particular variety of epilepsy ("intellectual aura"), one case with symptoms of organic brain disease. *Brain,* 1888–1889, *11,* 179–207.

Kales A and Kales JD. Sleep disorders. Recent findings in the diagnosis and treatment of disturbed sleep. *New Engl J Med,* 1974, *290,* 487–499.

Kanzer M. Amnesia: a statistical study. *Am J Psychiat,* 1939, *96,* 711–716.

Kenna JC and Sedman G. Depersonalization in temporal lobe epilepsy and the organic psychoses. *Br J Psychiat,* 1965, *111,* 293–299.

Kennedy A and Neville J. Sudden loss of memory. *Br Med J,* 1957, *2,* 428–433.

Kleitman N. *Sleep and wakefulness.* Chicago, University of Chicago Press, 1963.

Larmore K, Ludwig AM, and Cain RL. Multiple personality—an objective case study. *Br J Psychiat,* 1977, *131,* 35–40.

Lees F and Watkins SM. Loss of consciousness in migraine. *Lancet,* 1963, *2,* 647–650.

Lhermitte J. Visual hallucination of the self. *Br Med J,* 1951, *1,* 431–434.

Lisak RP and Zimmerman RA. Transient global amnesia due to a dominant hemisphere tumor. *Arch Neurol,* 1977, *34,* 317–318.

Ludwig AM, Brandsma JM, Wilbur CB, Bendfeldt F, and Jameson DH. The objective study of a multiple personality. *Arch Gen Psychiat,* 1972, *26,* 298–310.

Markand ON, Wheeler GL, and Pollack SL. Complex partial status epilepticus (psychomotor status). *Neurology,* 1978, *28,* 189–196.

Martland HS. Punch drunk. *JAMA,* 1928, *91,* 1103–1107.

Mathew NT and Meyer JS. Pathogenesis and natural history of transient global amnesia. *Stroke,* 1974, *5,* 303–311.

May RH, Voegele GE, and Paolino AF. The Ganser syndrome: a report of three cases. *J Nerv Ment Dis,* 1960, *130,* 331–339.

Mayer-Gross W. On depersonalization. *Br J Med Psychol,* 1935, *15,* 103–122.

Mayeux R. Sexual intercourse and transient global amnesia. *New Engl J Med,* 1979, *300,* 864.

Mayeux R, Alexander MP, Benson DF, Brandt J, and Rosen J. Poriomania. *Neurology,* 1979, *29,* 1616–1619.

Mesulam M-M. Dissociative states with abnormal temporal lobe EEG. *Arch Neurol,* 1981, *38,* 176–181.

Millon T. *Disorders of personality.* DSM III: Axis III. New York, John Wiley & Sons, 1981.

Moersch FP. Psychic manifestations in migraine. *Am J Psychiat,* 1924, *80,* 697–716.

Mohan KJ and Nagaswami S. A case of limbic system dysfunction with hypersexuality and fugue state. *Dis Nerv Syst,* 1975, *36,* 621–624.

Pincus J. Hysteria presenting to the neurologist. In Roy A (Ed.): *Hysteria.* New York, John Wiley & Sons, 1982, pp. 131–143.

Pritchard PB III, Wannamaker BB, Sagel J, Nair R, and DeVillier C. Endocrine function following complex partial seizures. *Ann Neurol,* 1983, *14,* 27–32.

Remick RA and Wada JA. Complex partial and pseudoseizure disorders. *Am J Psychiat*, 1979, *136*, 320–323.

Roth B. *Narcolepsy and hypersomnia*. New York, S. Karger, 1980.

Roth M and Harper M. Temporal lobe epilepsy and the phobic anxiety–depersonalization syndrome. Part II: practical and theoretical considerations. *Comp Psychiat*, 1962, *3*, 215–226.

Rowan AJ and Protass LM. Transient global amnesia: clinical and electroencephalographic findings in 10 cases. *Neurology*, 1979, *29*, 869–872.

Roy A. Nonconvulsive psychogenic attacks investigated for temporal lobe epilepsy. *Comp Psychiat*, 1977, *18*, 591–593.

Saper JR and Lossing JH. Prolonged trance-like stupor in epilepsy. *Arch Int Med*, 1974, *134*, 1079–1082.

Saperstein JL. On the phenomena of depersonalization. *J Nerv Ment Dis*, 1949, *110*, 236–251.

Schenk L and Bear D. Multiple personality and related dissociative phenomena in patients with temporal lobe epilepsy. *Am J Psychiat*, 1981, *138*, 1311–1316.

Schwartz MS and Scott DF. Isolated petit-mal status presenting de novo in middle age. *Lancet*, 1971, *2*, 1399–1401.

Sercl M and Jaros O. The mechanisms of cerebral concussion in boxing and their consequences. *World Neurol*, 1962, *3*, 351–358.

Shorvon HJ. The depersonalization syndrome. *Proc Roy Soc Med*, 1946, *39*, 779–792.

Shuping JR, Rollinson RD, and Toole JF. Transient global amnesia. *Ann Neurol*, 1980, *7*, 281–285.

Shuping JR, Toole JF, and Alexander E Jr. Transient global amnesia due to glioma of the dominant hemisphere. *Neurology*, 1980, *30*, 88–90.

Shuttleworth EC and Morris CE. The transient global amnesia syndrome. *Arch Neurol*, 1966, *15*, 515–520.

Shuttleworth EC and Wise GR. Transient global amnesia due to arterial embolism. *Arch Neurol*, 1973, *29*, 340–342.

Slater KH. Some clinical and EEG findings in patients with migraine. *Brain*, 1968, *91*, 85–98.

Spillane JD. Five boxers. *Br Med J*, 1962, *2*, 1205–1210.

Steinmetz EF and Vroom FQ. Transient global amnesia. *Neurology*, 1972, *22*, 1193–1200.

Stengel E. On the etiology of the fugue states. *J Ment Sci*, 1941, *87*, 572–599.

Stengel E. Further studies on pathological wandering (fugues with the impulse to wander). *J Ment Sci*, 1943, *89*, 224–241.

Sutcliffe JP and Jones J. Personal identity, multiple personality, and hypnosis. *Internat J Clin Exp Hypnos*, 1962, *10*, 231–269.

Tamerin JS, Weiner S, Poppen R, Steinglisi P, and Mendelson JH. Alcohol and memory: amnesia and short-term memory function during experimentally induced intoxication. *Am J Psychiat*, 1971, *127*, 1659–1664.

Taylor WS and Martin MF. Multiple personality. *J Abnorm Soc Psychol*, 1944, *39*, 281–300.

Thigpen CH and Cleckley H. A case of multiple personality. *J Abnorm Soc Psychol*, 1954, *49*, 135–151.

Trimble MR. Serum prolactin in epilepsy and hysteria. *Br Med J*, 1978, *2*, 1682.

Tyndel M. Some aspects of the Ganser state. *J Ment Sci*, 1956, *102*, 324–329.

Weiner H and Braiman A. The Ganser syndrome. *Am J Psychiat*, 1955, *111*, 767–773.

Weinstein EA and Kahn RL. The syndrome of anosognosia. *Arch Neurol Psychiat*, 1950, *64*, 772–791.

Wells CE. Transient ictal psychosis. *Arch Gen Psychiat*, 1975, *32*, 1201–1203.

Whitlock FA. The Ganser syndrome. *Br J Psychiat*, 1967, *113*, 19–29.

Williams RL, Derman S, and Karacan I. Disorders of excessive sleep and the parasomnias. In Zales MR (Ed.): *Eating, sleeping, and sexuality. Treatment of disorders of basic life functions*. New York, Bruner-Mazel, 1982, pp. 150–185.

Wilson G, Rupp C, and Wilson WW. Amnesia. *Am J Psychiat*, 1950, *106*, 481–485.

Winterstein CE. Head injuries attributable to boxing. *Lancet*, 1937, *2*, 719–720.

Zlotlow M. Temporal lobe "spike focus" associated with confusion, complete amnesia and fugues in a paranoid schizophrenic. *Psychiat Quart*, 1968, *42*, 738–748.

Chapter 11

Violence and Aggression

No widely accepted definitions of violence or aggression have been devised. For purposes of this chapter, violence is defined as overtly threatened or accomplished application of force resulting in personal injury or destruction of property or the use of threat of injury to compel action against one's will (Roberts et al., 1981; Wolfgang, 1981). Aggression is a wider concept that includes violence and also encompasses self-protective behavior where physical force or the threat of force is utilized to satisfy vital needs or to protect one's physical or psychological integrity (Valzelli, 1981). Violence has socially sanctioned forms such as capital punishment, a parent spanking a child, injury during the course of arrest for antisocial activity, and killing during military operations. It also has illegitimate forms such as assault, battery, rape, and murder (Wolfgang, 1981). This chapter reviews the role of neuropsychiatric factors in the etiology of unsanctioned violent behavior and provides a differential diagnosis of neurological disorders to be considered in the violent individual.

An acceptable definition of violence has been difficult to formulate partly because violence is not a unitary concept. Violence is not a diagnosis or even a clinical syndrome in the usual sense; it is a complex behavior and as such is not likely to have a single determinant. Genetic, social, educational, cultural, economic, neurological, metabolic, and situational factors frequently interact and reinforce each other to produce violent behavior. An individual from a lower socioeconomic background thus may grow up in a violent household sustaining brain injury from child abuse and later commit violent acts while intoxicated. Which factors are most important in this caldron of contributing ingredients? In most cases it will be impossible to do more than identify the final precipitating circumstances.

The importance of seeking neurological components in violent behavior is twofold: (1) neurological factors can easily be overlooked in a psychologically minded milieu where clinicians are attuned to the influence of early childhood experiences on adult behavior; and (2) detection of neurological factors may offer treat-

ment alternatives that will go unexplored if the brain disorder is undiscovered.

Animal models have been widely utilized to investigate the neurobiologic basis of aggressive behavior. These studies have been particularly useful in delineating anatomic regions of the brain most likely to be involved in mediating violent behavior and have identified the limbic system as the most important anatomic substrate of violence and aggression (Valzelli, 1981). The greater extent of intraspecies violence and interindividual cruelty among humans, however, clearly separates human behavior from that of other animals and limits the applicability of animal research to the understanding of human violence. For that reason, the results of animal experimentation are cited only sparingly in this discussion.

Two general approaches have been used to study the neurology of human violence. In the first, violent offenders have been investigated to determine whether they have evidence of neurological dysfunction that might have contributed to their violent behavior. In the second, violent behavior ensuing in the course of known neurological disorders is observed and studied. The results of each of these approaches are reviewed, and the latter is further divided into violent behavior directed at others and violent self-destructive behavior. Finally, an approach to evaluation and treatment of the violent individual is outlined.

NEUROLOGICAL ABNORMALITIES IN VIOLENT CRIMINALS

EEG Abnormalities

The most thoroughly studied parameter of neurological dysfunction in violent individuals is the EEG. Table 11-1 presents the results of 14 studies assessing EEG abnormalities in prison inmates and patients with antisocial behavior. One striking finding is the consistency with which investigators have found an increased

TABLE 11-1. Percentage of Abnormal EEGs Among Subjects Incarcerated for Various Types of Crime or Diagnosed as Antisocial Personality Disorder Because of Criminal Conduct

Investigators (year)	Behavioral Disorder	Percentage with Abnormal EEGs
Krynicki (1978)	Assaultive adolescent, habitual	57.1
	Assaultive adolescent, solitary	0
Okasha et al. (1975)	Murderers, in prison	43.5
	Murderers, in mental hospitals	56.7
Harper et al. (1972)	Psychopathic personality	
	Under 25 years old	61.6
	Over 25 years old	40.0
Williams (1969)	Violence, habitual	65
	Violence, solitary	24.4
Sayed et al. (1969)	Murderers	
	Psychopathic personality	50
	Psychotic	78
Small (1966)	All felons	34
	Theft	39
	Assult	33
	Murder	47
	Sex crime	27
Arthurs and Cahoon (1964)	Psychopathic personality	44
Gibbens et al. (1959)	Psychopathic personality	41
Levy and Kennard (1953)	Prison inmates	30
	Violent crimes	30
	Nonviolent crimes	30
Hill (1952)	Psychopathic personality	50
Hill and Pond (1952)	Murders	48
Stafford-Clark and Taylor (1949)	Murders	
	Committed incidentally	9.1
	Motivated	25
	Motiveless	73.5
	Sexually related	50
Silverman (1944)	Federal prisoners	
	Psychopathic personality	51.9
	Psychotic	23.8
	Neurological disorder	66.7
Hill (1944)	Psychopathic personality	65

frequency of EEG changes in violent populations. Of the studies shown in Table 11-1, the only two groups that showed no increase in the prevalence of EEG abnormalities were adolescents who had committed a single violent offense (Krynicki, 1978) and individuals who had committed murders as an incidental act during the course of some other activity (Stafford-Clark and Taylor, 1949). All other antisocial and criminal populations studied had EEG abnormalities in 24–78 percent of individuals. Electroencephalographic changes were found to be more common in subjects who had committed violent acts than in those with nonviolent crimes and were

more frequent in those with repeated violence than those with isolated violent acts (Krynicki, 1978; Small, 1966; Williams, 1969). When the violence had no apparent motive, there was also an increased chance of finding an EEG abnormality compared to violence that had been provoked (Stafford-Clark and Taylor, 1949; Williams, 1969).

Several types of EEG abnormalities have been found in violent offenders: generalized slowing, focal slowing, and epileptiform abnormalities (Arthurs and Cahoon, 1964; Hill, 1952; Okasha et al., 1975; Sayed et al., 1969; Small, 1966; Stafford-Clark and Taylor,

1949; Williams, 1969). No specific relationship was found between the type of EEG abnormality and characteristics of the crime, but Williams (1969) noted that when focal abnormalities were present they were most likely to be located in the temporal and frontal lobes. Interpretation of these findings is fraught with difficulty. A small percentage of the patients (0–15 percent) have epilepsy. As discussed later in this chapter, violence as an ictal event is rare, and it is unlikely that many of the violent acts are ictal in nature. The EEG alterations may reflect non-epileptic CNS changes relevant to the violent behavior. The presence of lesions within the limbic system can lead to personality alterations that may in turn lead to antisocial behavior (Devinsky and Bear, 1984; Serafetinides, 1965). Head trauma also produces frontal and temporal lesions, reduces the threshold of impulsive behavior and violence, and may be reflected in EEG abnormalities. Despite the difficulty in drawing direct inferences from these data, the EEG findings indicate that brain dysfunction is common among violent offenders and that in many cases the limbic system is the site of neurological abnormality.

Neuropsychological Assessment

Neuropsychological testing of criminal subjects has produced variable results, but there is a tendency for such patients to perform more poorly than matched control subjects (Lewis et al., 1979; Yeudall et al., 1982). Performance on tests assessing frontal lobe function is often preferentially compromised (Pontius and Yudowitz, 1980).

Neurological Abnormalities

Examination of violent delinquents and patients with impulsive character disorders reveals an increased incidence of neurological soft signs indicative of non-localizing neurological dysfunction (Lewis et al., 1979; Quitkin et al., 1976). One study also revealed an increased frequency of subjective experiences suggestive of limbic dysfunction (Lewis, 1976).

NEUROPSYCHIATRIC DISORDERS WITH VIOLENT BEHAVIOR

Various neuropsychiatric disorders have been associated with violent behavior (Table 11-2). Most of the attention has focused on the possible association between epilepsy and violence, but a number of other disorders have produced violence and must be considered in the differential diagnosis of violent behavior.

Epilepsy

Behavioral disturbances occurring in epileptic patients may occur during the ictal, postictal, and interictal period (Chapter 9). Likewise, violence may occur during any of these periods, and any violent act committed by epileptic patients must be considered in relation to this behavioral framework.

Many unresolved areas of controversy exist regarding the relationship of epilepsy to criminal behavior and violence (Kligman and Goldberg, 1975). The principal questions include: Is violence more common among epileptics than nonepileptics? Can violence occur as an ictal manifestation? Does violence occur with abnormal frequency during the interictal period in epileptics? If so, what are the determinants of interictal violence? Is violence more common with one type of epilepsy (e.g., temporal lobe epilepsy) than another (e.g., idiopathic epilepsy)? Unambiguous answers to these questions are not yet available, but tentative conclusions can be drawn from existing information.

The question regarding the prevalence of violent behavior among epileptics has been approached by investigating the frequency of violent acts in populations of epileptics (such as those attending seizure clinics) or determining the frequency of epilepsy among violent individuals. Although studies of the first type demonstrate that violence is uncommon in epilepsy, the latter technique has generally yielded results suggesting that epilepsy is two to four times more common among prison inmates than in the general population (Gunn, 1977a; Gunn and Bonn, 1971; Whitman et al., 1984).

If violence and antisocial behavior are more common among epileptics, do they occur during the ictal, postictal, or interictal period? This question has been the subject of heated debate. Rare cases of serious offenses, including murder, have been reported to have occurred during epileptic seizures or at least during a seizure-related amnesic period that could have been in either the ictal or immediate postictal period (Gunn, 1978; Gunn and Fenton, 1971; Knox, 1968; Pincus, 1980; Saint-Hilaire et al., 1980; Stevenson, 1963; Walker, 1961). Despite occasional reports of ictal violence, recordings of epileptic patients during ictal periods have shown that behavioral activity occurring as part of a seizure is usually brief, stereotyped, undirected, and poorly organized and unlikely to account for goal-directed violence (Ashford et al., 1980; Marsh, 1978; Delgado-Escueta et al., 1981; Ramani and Gumnit, 1981; Rodin, 1973). The current consensus suggests that although interpersonal injury could occur during an epileptic attack manifest by psychomotor automatisms, such activity is unpremeditated, usually poorly structured, and easily redirected. The greatest danger is dur-

TABLE 11-2.   Neuropsychiatric Differential Diagnosis of Violent Behavior

Epilepsy	Attention-deficit disorder in adults
Ictal	XYY genotype (?)
Postical	
Interictal	Idiopathic psychiatric disorders
	Nonpsychotic disturbances
Episodic dyscontrol syndrome	Personality disorders
Frontal lobe syndromes	Antisocial personality
Traumatic injuries	Borderline personality
Neoplasms	Paranoid personality
Degenerative dementias	Explosive disorders
Mental retardation	Intermittent
Hypothalamic–limbic rage syndrome	Isolated
Metabolic disorders	Paraphilia
Acute confusional states	Sexual sadism
Endocrine dysfunction	Childhood disorders
Premenstrual state	Conduct disorder
Testosterone excess	
Toxic disorders	Psychotic disturbances
Ethanol	Mania
Phencyclidene, LSD, barbiturates, etc.	Schizophrenia
	Paranoid disorders
Neurological delusional syndromes	Depression

ing the postictal confusional period when the actions of others may be misinterpreted and a more organized attack may occur.

If aggression is increased in epilepsy and is rare during ictal episodes, when does the violence occur? As noted, violence may occur during the postictal confusional period, but most episodes of violence appear to occur during the interictal period and are related to behavioral and psychiatric alterations occurring interictally (Chapter 9) (Devinsky and Bear, 1984; Fenton and Udwin, 1965; Hermann et al., 1980; Taylor, 1969). Although a few investigators have found equal rates of violence among patients with generalized and temporal lobe epilepsy, most have found violence to be more common among patients with the latter (Ounsted, 1969; Serafetinides, 1965; Stevens and Hermann, 1981). Furthermore, Serafetinides's (1965) finding that violence is significantly more common among patients with left than right temporal lesions emphasizes the potential importance of anatomic factors in determining the occurrence of violence in the interictal period.

Several interpretations have been offered for the observations concerning interictal violence in epileptics. Stevens and Hermann (1981) suggest that basal forebrain damage gives rise to both the seizures and the behavioral alterations and that the two consequences are behaviorally independent. Similarly, Treiman and Delgado-Escueta (1983) point out that interictal violence is most common in young, intellectually impaired men with histories of psychiatric abnormalities and long-standing, severe epilepsy. In such cases the associated neurological and psychiatric abnormalities may be responsible for the violent behavior. Serafetinides (1965) and Taylor (1969) hypothesize that the violence is learned behavior occurring in response to the adverse educational and social circumstances of the epileptic. Lewis et al. (1982) suggest that the violence is associated with paranoid and hallucinatory symptoms occurring in the epileptic and is a product of the psychosis occasionally associated with epilepsy. It seems likely that all these factors as well as others (anticonvulsant intoxication, economic and cultural influences) play varying roles in each epileptic patient manifesting aggressive behavior.

Episodic Dyscontrol Syndrome

The episodic dyscontrol syndrome was described in 1970 by Mark and Ervin as a constellation of behaviors including: (1) a history of physical assault, especially wife and child beating; (2) pathologic intoxication (violent behavior following ingestion of small amounts of alcohol); (3) impulsive sexual behavior, often including sexual assault; and (4) a history of many traffic violations and automobile accidents stemming from impulsive and reckless driving (Mark and Ervin, 1970). They cited a number of patients with temporal lobe epilepsy with the symptom complex and argued that the dyscontrol syndrome was a product of limbic system dysfunction and that many of the patients manifesting the syndrome improved markedly when treated with anticonvulsants. Similarly, Monroe (1970) suggested that episodic disinhibition of action with violent behavior could be a product of epilepsy or of "epileptoid" loss of control of instinctual drives or impulses. He proposed that there was a continuum of increasing dynamic and diminishing neurological determinants of violence as one moved from epilepsy through instinct and impulse dyscontrol to acting out. The principal feature that distinguishes patients with episodic dyscontrol from patients with sociopathic personality disorders is that the violent activity is isolated and infrequent, not in conjunction with an overall pattern of malevolence.

Despite these contributions, the nosologic validity of the episodic dyscontrol syndrome as a distinct diagnostic entity is open to question. As discussed previously, violent activity is uncommon as an ictal manifestation in epileptics, and the violence of those with episodic dyscontrol syndrome is likely to be an ictal manifestation in only a very small percentage of cases. In addition, in many patients with episodic dyscontrol, social and environmental factors play an important part in determining or triggering the violence (Bach-y-Rita et al., 1971; Rickler, 1982). The episodic dyscontrol syndrome thus might be viewed as a nonspecific syndrome of violence with many possible contributing etiologic factors. The more primitive and disorganized and the more distinctly episodic the behavior is, the more likely it is that acquired neurological factors are playing a significant role (Elliot, 1976). Occasionally, recognition of the syndrome will lead to the discovery of previously undiagnosed epilepsy, and in some cases where epilepsy is equivocally present, an empirical trial with anticonvulsants may be warranted.

Frontal Lobe Syndromes

Explosive violence may be a component of the behavioral change that follows damage to the frontal lobe (Chapter 6) (Alexander, 1982). Violent behavior may either accompany orbitofrontal injury, where it is a manifestation of disinhibition and lack of the usual restraints on antisocial impulses, or may occur with dorsolateral injuries, where the apathetic state is interrupted by brief outbursts of violence in response to trivial irritations. Attacks of explosive rage that follow head trauma are more likely to be a product of the frontal lobe damage than commonly accompanies traumatic head injury (Hooper et al., 1945; Johnson, 1969). Frontal lobe involvement is also common in dementia and mental retardation and may account for the occasional acts of violence or aggressive behavior reported in these syndromes.

Neuropsychologic investigations of criminals have revealed a subgroup with deficits consistent with frontal lobe dysfunction (Pontius and Yudowitz, 1980). This finding suggests that in some cases of idopathic violent behavior, occult frontal lobe dysfunction secondary to head trauma or delayed maturation may be a contributing factor.

Hypothalamic–Limbic Rage Syndromes

The violence associated with orbitofrontal injury can be partially attributed to involvement of limbic structures and disruption of the role of the limbic system in emotional modulation. Similarly, involvement of limbic structures of the hypothalamus by a variety of pathological processes has also produced intermittent rage behavior. The violence usually occurs in response to provocation, but the stimulus may be minimal. The rage behavior is often combined with amnesia, hyperphagia, and other evidence of hypothalamic dysfunction. In most cases the syndrome results from neoplastic invasion of the the hypothalamus (Haugh and Markesberry, 1983; Reeves and Plum, 1969).

The importance of the role played by hypothalamic structures in violent behavior is also attested to by the success of hypothalamotomy in the treatment of some types of violent behavior (Schvarcz et al., 1972).

Metabolic Disorders

Metabolic factors contribute to violent behavior in two general circumstances: acute confusional states and disorders of endocrine function. Acute confusional states are reviewed in Chapter 7, and violence can be a manifestation of any of the metabolic disturbances discussed there. The violence is usually poorly organized and undirected when it is a manifestation of confusion and impaired judgment but may result in serious injury. Hill and colleagues (1943) recorded a case of matricide occurring during a hypoglycemic episode.

Two types of endocrine alteration have been shown to contribute to violent behavior: 1) perimenstrual states, and 2) elevated testosterone levels. D'Orban and Dalton (1980) found that 44 percent of 50 women charged with violent crimes committed their offenses during the perimenstrual period and that there was a significant lack of offenses during the ovulation and postovulation phases of the menstrual cycle. Morton et al. (1953) found that in their female prisoners, 79 percent of violent crimes were committed during the week preceding menstruation or during the menstrual period.

Although results have not always been consistent,

several studies have revealed correlations between measures of aggression and serum testosterone levels (Schiavi et al., 1984; Sheard, 1979). Significantly elevated levels have been found in violent rapists and prisoners with histories of violent and aggressive crimes (Kreuz and Rose, 1972; Rada et al., 1976). The levels of testosterone were rarely beyond the range of normal; as a group, violent offenders had significantly higher levels than did nonviolent offenders. Similarly, testosterone levels in violent females were also elevated when compared with control populations (Ehlers et al., 1980). The principal role of endocrine factors appears to be to lower the threshold for, and thus increase the likelihood of, violence in predisposed individuals, although prolonged exposure to elevated testosterone levels may have effects on personality development as well.

Toxic Disorders

Alcohol is the intoxicant most commonly used by individuals involved in violent crime. Violence may occur during a period of intoxication with impaired judgment, during an alcoholic blackout (Chapter 10) for which the patient is amnesic, or as part of the syndrome of pathological intoxication. In the latter, chaotic disturbed behavior, often with violent outbursts, occurs following ingestion of small amounts of alcohol. The patient is completely or partially amnesic for the period of the aberrant behavior, and delusions, hallucinations, anxiety, or fear may occur during the episode (Bach-y-Rita et al., 1970). In some cases, alcohol withdrawal may be an activating agent for preexisting epileptic abnormalities, and the ensuing violence may be ictal or postictal in origin (Thompson, 1963).

Among the many other intoxicants used, violence is particularly likely with phencyclidine (PCP) ingestion but may also occur after use of LSD, psilocybin, stimulants, anticholinergics and sedative–hypnotics (Cohen, 1977; Cohen and Ditman, 1963; Di Sclafani et al., 1981; Klepfisz and Racy, 1973). Violence has also been reported as a manifestation of neuroleptic-induced akathisia (Keckich, 1978).

Neurological Delusional Syndromes

Delusions are a frequent manifestation of neurological disease. In dementing illnesses they are simple, loosely held, and transient, whereas in diseases affecting subcortical structures they tend to be more elaborate, rigid, and chronic (Chapter 13) (Cummings, 1985; Davison and Bagley, 1969). Paranoid ideation and persecutory fears are the most common manifestations of delusional thought, and action on delusional beliefs leading to violent activity is an unfortunate but frequent prod-

uct of persecutory delusions (Cummings, 1985; Petrie et al., 1982; Rabins et al., 1982).

Attention-Deficit Disorder in Adults

Attention-deficit disorder in children is manifest by attentional impairment, impulsivity, and nearly constant restless activity while awake (*Diagnostic and statistical manual of mental disorders*, 1980). Follow-up studies of these children as they reach adolescence and adulthood reveal that an unusually large number are involved in delinquent behavior or develop sociopathic or explosive personality disturbances (Hogenson, 1974; Mendleson et al., 1971; Morrison and Minkoff, 1975; Virkkunen and Nuutila, 1976; Wender et al., 1981). Physical hyperactivity rarely persists beyond childhood, but attentional disturbances continue, and behavioral improvement may follow administration of stimulants even in the adult patient.

Depression and low self-esteem resulting from the poor academic performance and poor social adjustment of hyperactive children are usually invoked as the explanations for sociopathic behavior, but a neurobiologic contribution from the underlying brain disturbance also seems likely.

XYY Genotype

Surveys of criminal populations revealed an increased incidence of inmates with an XYY genotype and led to the suggestion that XYY individuals were more likely to be violent and aggressive than were individuals with normal karyotypes (Hook, 1973). Further studies, however, have failed to confirm the suggestion that XYY patients are at increased risk for violent behavior or suggest that the risk is minimal (Editorial, 1974; Schiavi et al., 1984; Shah, 1976). Genotype XYY individuals do not have elevated testosterone levels (Schiavi et al., 1984), but they tend to be of lower intelligence and to be more mentally immature and impulsive, factors that may contribute to aggressive activity (Nielsen and Christensen, 1974). Until more information is obtained, the possible role of the XYY genotype is determining violent behavior remains unresolved.

Idiopathic Psychiatric Disorders

A number of idiopathic psychiatric disorders can give rise to violent behavior. They can usefully be divided into psychotic disorders in which the aggression is in response to a delusional belief and those that are nonpsychotic. Among the latter, personality disorders account for the majority of violent actions, but violence may be a manifestation of intermittent or isolated explosive disorders, sexual sadism, or childhood conduct disorders (*Diagnostic and statistical manual of mental disorders*, 1980; Millon, 1981). The personality disturbance most likely to produce repeated violence as a habitual behavioral style is the antisocial personality. Such personalities are characterized by the onset before age 15 of a disorder that, when fully evident, includes the inability to sustain a job, failure to adhere to the law and social norms of behavior, inability to provide consistent parenting or maintain enduring close personal relationships, irritability and aggressiveness, failure to honor financial obligations, and lack of forethought, poor judgment, and recklessness (Chapter 15) (*Diagnostic and statistical manual of mental disorders*, 1980). The antisocial personality pattern is most marked in late adolescence and early adulthood and tends to be ameliorated with age (Crafts, 1969). In addition to the antisocial personality, violence is not uncommon among individuals with borderline and paranoid personality disorders (*Diagnostic and statistical manual of mental disorders*, 1980; Millon, 1981; Thornton and Pray, 1973).

Explosive disorders are disturbances of impulse control in which an individual has a discrete episode of aggressiveness with property destruction or assault. There is an absence of generalized impulsivity, aggressiveness, or sociopathic behavior between episodes. The violence is usually out of proportion to the precipitating stimulus and may occur more than once (intermittent explosive disorder) or be confined to a single episode (isolated explosive disorder) (*Diagnostic and statistical manual of mental disorders*, 1980). This behavior is similar to the episodic dyscontrol syndrome, and explosive patients must be carefully evaluated for neurological determinants of their behavior.

Violence may also be a product of certain disturbances of sexual behavior, particularly sexual sadism. Sadism is a paraphilic disturbance in which sexual excitement is achieved by humiliating or injuring either a nonconsenting or a consenting partner (Chapter 17) (*Diagnostic and statistical manual of mental disorders*, 1980; Glasser, 1979).

Violence is not a common consequence of psychosis, and few psychotic individuals commit acts of violence (Gunn, 1977b; Guze et al., 1969). Under specific circumstances, however, psychotic ideation, particularly paranoid thinking, can lead to organized acts of aggression directed at presumed persecutors. Such actions may occur in any of the psychoses but have been found most commonly among patients with schizophrenia, women felons with affective disorders, and geriatric patients with late-onset paranoid delusional disorders (Good, 1978; Petrie et al., 1982). The importance of recognizing the psychotic origin of violent behavior stems from the read-

iness with which some of these disorders respond to neuroleptic medication.

NEUROPSYCHIATRIC DISORDERS WITH SELF-DESTRUCTIVE BEHAVIOR

Self-destructive behavior may occur along with violence directed at others in any of the syndromes presented in the preceding sections (Bach-y-Rita, 1974). In a few disorders, however, self-inflicted injury may occur as a prominent or even as the dominant behavioral disorder (Table 11-3). In children with mental retardation or autism, self-injury may occur in the course of head banging or other bizarre activities. In the Lesch-Nyhan syndrome (an X-linked disease characterized by overproduction of uric acid, deficiency of hypoxanthine-guanine phosphoribosyl-transferase, mental retardation, spasticity, and choreoathetosis) the afflicted children engage in self-mutilative behavior and are generally aggressive (Lloyd et al., 1981; Nyhan, 1968). The aggression often appears to be one manifestation of a compulsive disorder. Likewise, self-harm may occur as a result of some of the irresistible compulsive urges that occur in some patients with Gilles de la Tourette syndrome (Shapiro et al., 1978). Gilles de la Tourette patients with significant ocular trauma sustained as a result of compulsive striking of the eyes have been observed (Frankel and Cummings, 1984). Another neurological syndrome in which self-injury may be prominent is choreoacanthocytosis. This syndrome is manifest by a choreiform disorder resembling Huntington's disease, and studies of peripheral blood reveal a significant number of acanthocytes among red blood cells. Tongue and lip biting is often an early and prominent expression of the choreic syndrome (Sakai et al., 1981).

Idiopathic psychiatric disorders that may produce conspicuous self-injury behaviors include borderline personality, obsessive–compulsive disorders with self-mutilation rituals, schizophrenia, and depression (*Diagnostic and statistical manual of mental disorders*, 1980; Millon, 1981).

EVALUATION OF THE VIOLENT INDIVIDUAL

The most important principle involved in the evaluation of the violent individual is that violent behavior is rarely the result of a single circumstance (Bach-y-Rita and Veno, 1974; Bach-y-Rita et al., 1971). Rather, violent behavior is the result of neurological, toxic, characterological, social, and situational factors that conspire at a point in time to produce a violent act. An adequate evaluation and any hope of successful treat-

TABLE 11-3.   Neuropsychiatric Disorders with Self-
mutilative Behavior

Neurological disorders

  Mental retardation
  Autism
  Lesch-Nyhan syndrome
  Gilles de la Tourette syndrome
  Choreoacanthocytosis

Idiopathic psychiatric disorders

  Borderline personality disorder
  Schizophrenia
  Depression
  Obsessive–Compulsive disorder

ment thus depend on a thorough investigation of all possible contributing elements. The psychiatric interview will assess childhood, social, occupational, and educational experiences as well as determining current behaviors indicative of psychosis, affective disorder, character disorder, or other psychiatric disturbance. The neurological history should include inquiries regarding birth trauma, head injury, encephalitis, meningitis, systemic illnesses, drug or alcohol ingestion, and any evidence of seizurelike phenomena. The bedside mental status examination (Chapter 2) may help in identifying frontal lobe dysfunction, and formal neuropsychological assessment will determine the intellectual capacity of the patient. The elementary physical and neurological examinations will help in identifying systemic diseases or focal neurological deficits. In cases where violence has occurred as an isolated, ego-alien act or cannot be completely recalled by the patient, an EEG should be obtained to search for epileptiform abnormalities. Nasopharyngeal or sphenoidal electrodes and sleep deprivation prior to obtaining the recording may increase the likelihood of discovering an existing EEG abnormality. Computerized tomographic scans are an integral part of the evaluation on any patient with findings suggestive of brain disease. Laboratory assays of urine and blood may help in identifying metabolic disorders or the presence of toxic substances. In some cases, even after completion of a thorough evaluation, there is insufficient evidence to establish a definitive diagnosis or to determine the relative importance of factors contributing to the violent behavior. In these patients, empirical trials of the treatments discussed in the next section may aid not only in controlling the aggression, but also in determining its etiology.

TREATMENT OF THE VIOLENT INDIVIDUAL

Whereas many violent individuals are remanded to the criminal justice system and managed through incarceration and involuntary vocational rehabilitation, oth-

ers are referred to the mental health establishment for pharmacotherapy, behavior modification, psychotherapy, or, rarely, psychosurgery. Violence is a behavioral complex, not a single distinctive diagnostic entity; therefore, any treatment attempt must be individualized, and most treatment regimens are multifaceted. When an underlying disease process (systemic illness producing a confusional state, epilepsy, schizophrenia) is detected, treatment can be directed toward resolving the specific etiologic condition. In many cases, however, the cause of the violence will not be straightforward and treatment may involve any of a number of pharmacologic agents as well as behavioral therapy and/or psychotherapy (Lion, 1975).

Pharmacotherapy

Table 11-4 summarizes the pharmacological agents commonly used in the treatment of violent individuals and lists the principal disorders in which they have been utilized with some success.

Anticonvulsants

The rare cases in which violence is an ictal manifestation are obviously best managed by reducing the number of seizures. Since ictal violence occurs almost exclusively in complex partial seizures, the anticonvulsants most likely to be successful are carbamazepine or phenytoin (Chapter 9). Phenobarbital sometimes produces irritability and disinhibition and may increase the likelihood of violence in the epileptic. Violence occurring in the postictal confusional state will also be decreased if the number of seizures can be limited.

Anticonvulsants have also been used successfully in the management of the episodic dyscontrol syndrome. Carbamazepine and phenytoin have both been reported to decrease the number of violent outbursts (Maletzky and Klotter, 1974; Tunks and Dermer, 1977).

Anticonvulsants may also ameliorate the chronic aggressiveness and outbursts of violence occuring in some chronically pyschotic patients (Garbutt and Loosen, 1983; Monroe, 1975).

Propranolol

Propranolol, a beta-adrenergic receptor blocking agent, has been noted to decrease belligerent behavior as well as rage attacks in posttraumatic states, Alzheimer's disease, mental retardation, and schizophrenia (Elliot, 1977; Petrie and Ban, 1981; Ratey et al., 1983; Yudofsky et al., 1981, 1984). Dosages necessary for the control of violence have been in the range of 100–500 mg/day. The drug should be used with caution in those with a history of congestive heart failure, asthma, diabetes, or depression.

TABLE 11-4. Pharmacologic Agents Used in Treatment of Violent Behavior

Agents	Violent Disorders
Anticonvulsants: carbamazepine, phenytoin	Epilepsy (ictal, postictal); episodic dyscontrol syndrome; paroxysmal rage behavior
Propranolol	Neurological disorders (posttraumatic encephalopathy, mental retardation, etc.) with unprovoked violence
Lithium	Personality disorders with violence; recurrent unprovoked violence; mania with violence
Methylphenidate	Antisocial personality disorders (with history of attention-deficit syndrome)
Antiandrogens	Sexual violence; intractable violence in males
Progesterone	Premenstrual violence
Minor tranquilizers	Anxiety-related irritability and aggression (occasional paradoxical reaction reported)
Neuroleptics	Psychosis-related violence
Antidepressants	Depression-related violence

Lithium

Lithium, well known for its efficacy in treating mania, has also been utilized with success in the management of violence in aggressive criminals, character disorders, and children manifesting explosive anger and hostility (DeLong, 1978; Lena, 1979; Rifkin et al., 1972; Tupin et al., 1973). In some patients the violence may be an atypical manifestation of an underlying affective disorder, whereas in others the lithium appears to act independently of its antimanic effect. Dosages have been the same as those used in the treatment of manic–depressive illness (Chapter 14).

Methylphenidate

Attention-deficit disorder, as noted earlier, may persist into adulthood and predispose to antisocial personality disorders with violent behavior. Prescribing stimulants to this population entails a significant risk of abuse of the drugs, but in some cases improvement in behavior and reduction of violence have followed administration of methylphenidate or amphetamines (Rickler, 1982; Stringer and Josef, 1983). In closely controlled circumstances, stimulant administration may be a viable therapeutic alternative for adults with persistent or acquired attention-deficit disorders.

Hormonal Agents

Antiandrogenic agents such as medroxyprogesterone acetate and cyproterone acetate diminish sexual preoccupations in the paraphilias and improve self-control of aggressive sexual impulses (Berlin and Meinecke, 1981). These agents have also been reported to diminish interictal violence in temporal lobe epileptics and in patients exhibiting idiopathic chronic assaultiveness (Blumer and Migeon, 1975; Matthews, 1979). In the latter conditions, aberrant sexual impulses are not necessarily present, and the antiviolence potential of antiandrogens does not appear to be specific for sexually related aggressiveness.

Progesterone has been used to limit premenstrual aggression (Rickler, 1982).

Minor Tranquilizers

The use of minor tranquilizers in the management of aggression is controversial. Like alcohol, minor tranquilizers have the potential for disinhibiting antisocial impulses, and, indeed, paradoxical rage reactions and increased hostility have occasionally been reported following administration of anxiolytics (Bond and Lader, 1979; Gardos et al., 1968; Lion et al., 1975; Rosenbaum et al., 1984). Most investigators, however, have noted an improvement in aggressive impulses with minor tranquilizers (Azcorate, 1975; Bond and Lader, 1979; Monroe and Wise, 1965).

Neuroleptics and Antidepressants

Neuroleptic agents and antidepressants have a role in the treatment of violence when the aggression is the result of psychosis or depression (Gunn, 1979; Itil and Wadud, 1975).

Behavioral Therapy

The potential excesses of behavioral conditioning in the treatment of violent individuals have been dramatically portrayed by Anthony Burgess in his novel,

A Clockwork Orange (1963). When properly used, however, behavioral therapies can increase the patient's repertoire of adaptive skills, allow increased control of maladaptive responses, and decrease the number of violent outbursts (Liberman et al., 1981). In selected cases, behavior therapy can offer an important therapeutic dimension to the treatment and management of violent patients.

Psychosurgery

Psychosurgery is now rarely used in treatment of aggressive behavior but may be considered in some extreme cases where aggression is unmanageable and all other treatment modalities have failed. The two procedures that have relatively high success rates in the amelioration of violent behavior are bilateral amygdalotomy and posterior hypothalamotomy (Hitchcock and Cairns, 1973; Kiloh et al., 1974; Sano et al., 1970; Schvarcz et al., 1972; Small et al., 1977; Vaernet and Madsen, 1970).

REFERENCES

Alexander MP. Episodic behaviors due to neurologic disorders other than epilepsy. In Riley TL and Roy A (Eds.): *Pseudoseizures*. Baltimore, Williams and Wilkins, 1982, pp. 83–110.

Arthurs RGS and Cahoon EB. A clinical and electroencephalographic survey of psychopathic personality. *Am J Psychiat*, 1964, *120*, 875–877.

Ashford JW, Schulz SC, and Walsh GO. Violent automatism in a partial complex seizure. *Arch Neurol*, 1980, *39*, 120–122.

Azcarate CL. Minor tranquilizers in the treatment of aggression. *J Nerv Ment Dis*, 1975, *160*, 100–107.

Bach-y-Rita G. Habitual violence and self-mutilation. *Am J Psychiat*, 1974, *131*, 1018–1020.

Bach-y-Rita G, Lion JR, Climent CE, and Ervin FR. Episodic dyscontrol: a study of 130 violent patients. *Am J Psychiat*, 1971, *127*, 1473–1478.

Bach-y-Rita G, Lion JR, and Ervin FR. Pathological intoxication: clinical and electroencephalographic studies. *Am J Psychiat*, 1970, *127*, 698–703.

Bach-y-Rita G and Veno A. Habitual violence: a profile of 62 men. *Am J Psychiat*, 1974, *131*, 1015–1017.

Berlin FS and Meinecke CF. Treatment of sex offenders with antiandrogenic medication: conceptualization, review of treatment modalities, and preliminary findings. *Am J Psychiat*, 1981, *138*, 601–607.

Blumer D and Migeon C. Hormone and hormonal agents in the treatment of aggression. *J Nerv Ment Dis*, 1975, *160*, 127–137.

Bond A and Lader M. Benzodiazapines and aggression. In Sandler M (Ed.): *Psychopharmacology of aggression*. New York, Raven Press, 1979, pp. 173–182.

Burgess A. *A Clockwork Orange*. New York, Ballantine Books, 1963.

Cohen S. Angel dust. *JAMA*, 1977, *238*, 515–516.

Cohen S and Ditman KS. Prolonged adverse reactions to lysergic acid diethylamide. *Arch Gen Psychiat*, 1963, *8*, 475–480.

Craft M. The natural history of psychopathic disorders. *Br J Psychiat*, 1969, *115*, 39–44.

Cummings JL. Organic delusions: phenomenology, anatomical correlations, and review. *Br J Psychiat*, 1985, *146*, 184–197.

Davison K and Bagley CR. Schizophrenia-like psychoses associated with organic disorder of the central nervous system: a review of the literature. *Br J Psychiat*, 1969, Special Issue No. 4, 113–184.

Delgado-Escueta A, Mattson RH, King L, Goldensohn ES, Spiegel H, Madsen J, Crandall P, Driefuss F, and Porter RJ. The nature of aggression during epileptic seizures. *New Engl J Med*, 1981, *305*, 711–716.

DeLong GR. Lithium carbonate treatment of select behavior disorders in children suggesting manic-depressive illness. *J Pediat*, 1978, *93*, 689–694.

Devinsky O and Bear D. Varieties of aggressive behavior in temporal lobe epilepsy. *Am J Psychiat*, 1984, *141*, 651–656.

Diagnostic and statistical manual of mental disorders, 3rd ed. Washington, D.C., American Psychiatric Association, 1980.

Di Sclafani A II, Hall RCW, and Gardner ER. Drug-induced psychosis: emergency diagnosis and management. *Psychosomatics*, 1981, *22*, 845–855.

D'Orban PT and Dalton J. Violent crime and the menstrual cycle. *Psychol Med*, 1980, *10*, 353–359.

Editorial. What becomes of the XYY male? *Lancet*, 1974, *2*, 1297–1298.

Ehlers CL, Rickler KC, and Hovey JE. A possible relationship between plasma testosterone and aggressive behavior in a female outpatient population. In Girgis M and Kiloh LG (Eds.): *Limbic epilepsy and the dyscontrol syndrome*. New York, Elsevier-North Holland Biomedical Press, 1980, pp. 183–194.

Elliott FA. The dyscontrol syndrome. *Practitioner*, 1976, *217*, 51–60.

Elliott FA. Propranolol for the control of belligerent behavior following acute brain damage. *Ann Neurol*, 1977, *1*, 489–491.

Fenton GW and Udwin EL. Homicide, temporal lobe epilepsy and depression: a case report. *Br J Psychiat*, 1965, *111*, 304–306.

Frankel M and Cummings JL. Neuro-ophthalmic abnormalities in Tourette syndrome: anatomic and functional implications. *Neurology*, 1984, *34*, 359–361.

Garbutt JC and Loosen PT. Is carbamazepine helpful in paroxysmal behavior disorders? *Am J Psychiat*, 1983, *140*, 1363–1364.

Gardos G, DiMascio A, Salzman C, and Shader RI. Differential actions of chlordiazepoxide and oxazepam on hostility. *Arch Gen Psychiat*, 1968, *18*, 757–760.

Gibbens TCN, Pond DA, and Stafford-Clark D. A follow-up study of criminal psychopaths. *J Ment Sci*, 1959, *105*, 108–115.

Glasser M. Some aspects of the role of aggression in the perversions. In Rosen I (Ed.): *Sexual Deviation*, 2nd ed. New York, Oxford University Press, 1979, pp. 278–305.

Good MI. Primary affective disorder, aggression, and criminality. *Arch Gen Psychiat*, 1978, *35*, 954–960.

Gunn J. *Epileptics in Prison*. New York, Academic Press, 1977a.

Gunn J. Criminal behavior and mental disorder. *Br J Psychiat*, 1977b, *130*, 317–329.

Gunn J. Epileptic homicide: a case report. *Br J Psychiat*, 1978, 510–513.

Gunn J. Drugs in the violence clinic. In Sandler M (Ed.): *Psychopharmacology of Aggression*. New York, Raven Press, 1979, pp. 183–195.

Gunn J and Bonn J. Criminality and violence in epileptic patients. *Br J Psychiat*, 1971, *118*, 337–343.

Gunn J and Fenton G. Epilepsy, automatism, and crime. *Lancet*, 1971, *1*, 1173–1176.

Guze SB, Goodwin DW, and Crane JB. Criminality and psychiatric disorders. *Arch Gen Psychiat*, 1969, *20*, 583–591.

Harper MA, Morris M, and Bleyerveld J. The significance of an abnormal EEG in psychopathic personalities. *Aust New Zeal J Psychiat*, 1972, *6*, 215–224.

Haugh RM and Markesberry WR. Hypothalamic astrocytoma. Syndrome of hyperphagia, obesity, and disturbances of behavior and endocrine and autonomic function. *Arch Neurol*, 1983, *40*, 560–563.

Hermann BP, Schwartz MS, Whitman S, and Karrus WE. Aggression and epilepsy: seizure type comparisons and high-risk variables. *Epilepsia*, 1980, *22*, 691–698.

Hill D. Cerebral dysrhythmia: its significance in aggressive behavior. *Proc Roy Soc Med*, 1944, *37*, 317–328.

Hill D. EEG in episodic psychotic and psychopathic behavior. *Electroenceph Clin Neurophysiol*, 1952, *4*, 419–442.

Hill D and Pond DA. Reflections on one hundred capital cases submitted to electroencephalography. *J Ment Sci*, 1952, *98*, 23–43.

Hill D, Sargent W, and Heppenstall ME. A case of matricide. *Lancet*, 1943, *1*, 526–527.

Hitchcock E and Cairns V. Amygdalotomy. *Postgrad Med J*, 1973, *49*, 894–904.

Hogenson DI. Reading failure and juvenile delinquency. *Bull Orton Soc*, 1974, *24*, 164–169.

Hook EB. Behavioral implications of the human XYY genotype. *Science*, 1973, *179*, 139–150.

Hooper RS, McGregor JM, and Nathan PW. Explosive rage following head injury. *J Ment Sci*, 1945, *91*, 458–471.

Itil TM and Wadud A. Treatment of human aggression with major tranquilizers, antidepressants, and newer psychotropic drugs. *J Nerv Ment Dis*, 1975, *160*, 83–99.

Johnson J. Organic psychosyndromes due to boxing. *Br J Psychiat*, 1969, *115*, 45–53.

Keckich WA. Neuroleptics. Violence as a manifestation of akathisia. *JAMA*, 1978, *240*, 2185.

Kiloh LG, Gye RS, Rushworth RG, Bell DS, and White RT. Stereotactic amygdaloidotomy for aggressive behavior. *J Neurol Neurosurg Psychiat*, 1974, *37*, 437–444.

Klepfisz A and Racy J. Homicide and LSD. *JAMA*, 1973, *223*, 429–430.

Kligman D and Goldberg DA. Temporal lobe epilepsy and aggression. *J Nerv Ment Dis*, 1975, *160*, 324–341.

Knox SJ. Epileptic automatism and violence. *Med Sci Law*, 1968, *8*, 96–104.

Kreuz LE and Rose RM. Assessment of aggressive behavior and plasma testosterone in a young criminal population. *Psychosom Med*, 1972, *34*, 321–332.

Krynicki VE. Cerebral dysfunction in repetitively assaultive adolescents. *J Nerv Ment Dis*, 1978, *166*, 59–67.

Lena B. Lithium therapy in hyperaggressive behavior in adolescence. In Sandler M (Ed.): *Psychopharmacology of aggression*. New York, Raven Press, 1979, pp. 197–203.

Levy S and Kennard M. A study of the electroencephalogram as related to personality structure in a group of inmates of a state penitentiary. *Am J Psychiat*, 1953, *109*, 832–839.

Lewis DO. Delinquency, psychomotor epileptic symptoms, and paranoid ideation: a triad. *Am J Psychiat*, 1976, *133*, 1395–1398.

Lewis DO, Pincus TH, Shanok SS, and Glaser GH. Psychomotor epilepsy and violence in a group of incarcerated adolescent boys. *Am J Psychiat*, 1982, *139*, 882–887.

Lewis DO, Shanock SS, Pincus JH, and Glaser GH. Violent juvenile delinquents. *J Am Acad Child Psychiat*, 1979, *18*, 307–319.

Liberman RO, Marshall BD Jr, and Burke KL. Drugs and environmental interventions for aggressive psychiatric patients. In Stuart RB (Ed.): *Violent behavior: social learning approaches to prediction, management, and treatment*. New York, Brunner-Mazel, 1981, pp. 227–264.

Lion JR. Conceptual issues in the use of drugs for the treatment of aggression in man. *J Nerv Ment Dis*, 1975, *160*, 76–82.

Lion JR, Azcarate CL, and Koepke HH. "Paradoxical rage reactions" during psychotropic medication. *Dis Nerv Syst*, 1975, *36*, 557–558.

Lloyd KG, Hornykiewicz O, Davidson L, Shamak K, Farley I, Goldstein M, Shibuya M, Kelley WN, and Fox IH. Biochemical evidence of the dysfunction of brain neurotransmitters in the Lesch-Nyhan syndrome. *New Engl J Med*, 1981, *305*, 1106–1111.

Maletzky BM and Klotter J. Episodic dyscontrol: a controlled replication. *Dis Nerv Syst*, 1974, *37*, 175–179.

Mark VH and Ervin FR. *Violence and the brain*. New York, Harper and Row, 1970.

Marsh GG. Neuropsychological syndrome in a patient with episodic howling and violent motor behavior. *J Neurol Neurosurg Psychiat*, 1978, *91*, 366–369.

Matthews R. Testosterone levels in aggressive offenders. In

Sandler M (Ed.): *Psychopharmacology of aggression*. New York, Raven Press, 1979, pp. 123–130.

Mendelson W, Johnson N, and Stewart MA. Hyperactive children as teenagers: a follow-up study. *J Nerv Ment Dis*, 1971, *153*, 273–279.

Millon T. *Disorders of personality. DSM-III: Axs II*. New York, John Wiley & Sons, 1981.

Monroe RR. *Episodic behavioral disorders*. Cambridge, Massachusetts, Harvard University Press, 1970.

Monroe RR. Anticonvulsants in the treatment of aggression. *J Nerv Ment Dis*, 1975, *160*, 119–126.

Monroe RR and Wise SP III. Combined phenothiazine, chlordiazepoxide and primidone therapy for uncontrolled psychotic patients. *Am J Psychiat*, 1965, *122*, 694–698.

Morrison JR and Minkoff K. Explosive personality as a sequel to the hyperactive-child syndrome. *Comp Psychiat*, 1978, *16*, 343–348.

Morton JH, Additon H, Addison RG, Hunt L, and Sullivan JJ. A clinical study of premenstrual tension. *Am J Obstet Gynecol*, 1953, *65*, 1182–1191.

Nielsen J and Christensen AL. Thirty-five males with double Y chromosomes. *Psychol Med*, 1974, *4*, 28–37.

Nyhan WL. Summary of clinical findings. *Fed Proc*, 1968, *27*, 1034–1041.

Okasha A, Sadek A, and Moneim SA. Psychosocial and electroencephalographic studies of Egyptian murderers. *Br J Psychiat*, 1975, *126*, 34–40.

Ounsted C. Aggression and epilepsy. Rage in children with temporal lobe epilepsy. *J Psychosomat Res*, 1969, *13*, 237–242.

Petrie WM and Ban TA. Propranolol in organic agitation. *Lancet*, 1981, *1*, 324.

Petrie WM, Lawson EC, and Hollender MH. Violence in geriatric patients. *JAMA*, 1982, *248*, 443–444.

Pincus JH. Can violence be a manifestation of epilepsy? *Neurology*, 1980, *30*, 304–307.

Pontius AA and Yudowitz BS. Frontal lobe system dysfunction in some criminal actions as shown in the narratives test. *J Nerv Ment Dis*, 1980, *168*, 111–117.

Quitkin F, Rifkin A, and Klein DF. Neurologic soft signs in schizophrenia and character disorders. *Arch Gen Psychiat*, 1976, *33*, 845–853.

Rabins PV, Mace NL, and Lucas MJ. The impact of dementia on the family. *JAMA*, 1982, *248*, 333–335.

Rada RT, Laws DR, and Kellner R. Plasma testosterone levels in the rapist. *Psychosom Med*, 1976, *38*, 257–268.

Ramani V and Gumnit RJ. Intensive monitoring of epileptic patients with a history of episodic aggression. *Arch Neurol*, 1981, *38*, 570–571.

Ratey JJ, Morrill R, and Oxenkrug G. Use of propranolol for provoked and unprovoked episodes of rage. *Am J Psychiat*, 1983, *140*, 1356–1357.

Reeves AG and Plum F. Hyperphagia, rage, and dementia accompanying a ventromedial hypothalamic neoplasm. *Arch Neurol*, 1969, *20*, 616–624.

Rickler KC. Episodic dyscontrol. In Benson DF and Blumer D (Eds.): *Psychiatric aspects of neurologic disease*, Vol. 2. New York, Grune & Stratton, 1982, pp. 49–72.

Rifkin A, Quitkin F, Carrillo C, Blumberg AG, and Klein DF. Lithium carbonate in emotionally unstable character disorder. *Arch Gen Psychiat*, 1972, *27*, 519–523.

Roberts TK, Mock LAT, and Johnstone EE. Psychological aspects of the etiology of violence. In Hays JR, Roberts TK, and Solway KS (Eds.): *Violence and the violent individual*. New York, SP Medical and Scientific Books, 1981, pp. 9–33.

Rodin EA. Psychomotor epilepsy and aggressive behavior. *Arch Gen Psychiat*, 1973, *28*, 210–213.

Rosenbaum JF, Woods SW, Groves JE, and Klerman GL. Emergence of hostility during alprazolam treatment. *Am J Psychiat*, 1984, *141*, 792–793.

Saint-Hilaire JM, Gilbert M, Bouvier G, and Barbeau A. Epilepsy and aggression: two cases with depth electrode studies. In Robb P. (Ed.): *Epilepsy undated: causes and treatment*. Chicago, Year Book Medical Publishers, 1980, pp. 145–176.

Sakai T, Mawatari S, Iwashita H, Goto I, and Kuroiwa T. Choreoacanthocytosis. Clues to clinical diagnosis. *Arch Neurol*, 1981, *38*, 335–338.

Sano K, Mayanagi Y, Sekino H, Ogashiwa M, and Ishijima B. Results of stimulation and destruction of the posterior hypothalamus in man. *J Neurosurg*, 1970, *33*, 689–707.

Sayed VZA, Lewis SA, and Brittain RP. An electroencephalographic and psychiatric study of thirty-two insane murderers. *Br J Psychiat*, 1969, *115*, 1115–1124.

Schiavi RC, Theilgaard A, Owen DR, and White D. Sex chromosomes anomalies, hormones, and aggressivity. *Arch Gen Psychiat*, 1984, *41*, 93–99.

Schvarcz JR, Driollet R, Rios E, and Betti O. Stereotactic hypothalamotomy for behavior disorders. *J Neurol Neurosurg Psychiat*, 1972, *35*, 356–359.

Serafetinides EA. Aggressiveness in temporal lobe epileptics and its relation to cerebral dysfunction and environmental factors. *Epilepsia*, 1965, *6*, 33–42.

Shah SA. The 47, XYY chromosomal abnormality: a critical appraisal with respect to antisocial and violent behavior. In Smith WL and Kling A (Eds.): *Issues in brain/behavior control*. New York, Spectrum Publications, 1976, pp. 49–67.

Shapiro AK, Shapiro ES, Bruun RD, and Sweet RD. *Gilles de la Tourette syndrome*. New York, Raven Press, 1978.

Sheard MH. Testosterone and aggression. In Sandler M (Ed.): *Psychopharmacology of aggression*. New York, Raven Press, 1979, pp. 111–121.

Silverman D. The electroencephalogram of criminals. *Arch Neurol Psychiat*, 1944, *52*, 38–42.

Small JG. The organic dimension of crime. *Arch Gen Psychiat*, 1966, *15*, 82–89.

Small IF, Heimburger RF, Small TG, Milstein V, and Moor DF. Followup of stereotopic amygdalotomy for seizure and behavior disorders. *Biol Psychiat*, 1977, *12*, 401–411.

Stafford-Clark D and Taylor FH. Clinical and electroencephalographic studies of prisoners charged with murder. *J Neurol Neurosurg Psychiat*, 1949, *12*, 325–330.

Stevens JR and Hermann BP. Temporal lobe epilepsy, psychopathology, and violence: the state of the evidence. *Neurology*, 1981, *31*, 1127–1132.

Stevenson HG. Psychomotor epilepsy associated with criminal behavior. *Med J Aust*, 1963, *1*, 784–785.

Stringer AY and Josef NC. Methylphenidate in the treatment of aggression in two patients with antisocial personality disorder. *Am J Psychiat*, 1983, *140*, 1365–1366.

Taylor DC. Aggression and epilepsy. *J Psychosomat Res*, 1969 *13*, 229–236.

Thompson GN. The electroencephalogram in acute pathological alcoholic intoxication. *Bull LA Neurol Soc*, 1963, *28*, 217–224.

Thornton WE and Pray BJ. The portrait of a murderer. *Dis Nerv Syst*, 1973, *36*, 176–178.

Trieman DM and Delgado-Escueta AV. Violence and epilepsy: a critical review. In Pedley TA and Meldrum BJ (Eds.): *Recent advances in epilepsy*. New York, Churchill Livingston, 1983, pp. 179–209.

Tunks ER and Dermer SW. Carbamazepine in the dyscontrol syndrome associated with limbic system dysfunction. *J Nerv Ment Dis*, 1977, *164*, 56–63.

Tupin JP, Smith DB, Clanon TL, Kim LI, Nugent A, and Groupe A. The long-term use of lithium in aggressive prisoners. *Comp Psychiat*, 1973, *14*, 311–317.

Vaernet K and Madsen A. Stereotaxic amygdalotomy and basofrontal tractomy in psychotics with aggressive behavior. *J Neurol Neurosurg Psychiat*, 1970, *33*, 858–863.

Valzelli L. *Psychobiology of aggression and violence*. New York, Raven Press, 1981.

Virkkunen M and Nuutila A. Specific reading retardation, hyperactive child syndrome, and juvenile delinquency. *Acta Psychiat Scand*, 1976, *54*, 25–28.

Walker AE. Murder or epilepsy? *J Nerv Ment Dis*, 1961, *133*, 430–437.

Wender PH, Reimherr FW, and Wood DR. Attention deficit disorder ("minimal brain dysfunction") in adults. *Arch Gen Psychiat*, 1981, *38*, 449–456.

Whitman S, Coleman TE, Patmon C, Desai BT, Cohen R, and King LN. Epilepsy in prison: elevated prevalence and no relationship to violence. *Neurology*, 1984, *34*, 775–782.

Williams D. Neural factors related to habitual aggression. *Brain*, 1969, *92*, 503–520.

Wolfgang ME. Sociocultural overview of criminal violence. In Hays JR, Roberts TK, and Solway KS (Eds.): *Violence and the violent individual*. New York, SP Medical and Scientific Books, 1981, pp. 97–115.

Yeudall LT, From-Auch D, and Davies P. Neuropsychological impairment of persistent delinquency. *J Nerv Ment Dis*, 1982, *170*, 257–265.

Yudofsky SC, Stevens L, Silver J, Barsa J, and Williams D. Propranolol in the treatment of rage and violent behavior associated with Korsakoff's psychosis. *Am J Psychiat*, 1984, *141*, 114–115.

Yudofsky S, Williams D, and Gorman J. Propranolol in the treatment of rage and violent behavior in patients with chronic brain syndromes. *Am J Psychiat*, 1981, *138*, 218–220.

Chapter 12

Neuropsychiatric Aspects of Movement Disorders

This chapter addresses three general topics concerning the relationship between mental function and motility. Movement abnormalities that occur as part of the clinical symptomatology of idiopathic psychiatric disorders such as schizophrenia, affective disorders, obsessive–compulsive disorders, and anxiety are presented first, followed by discussion of movement disorders produced by psychotropic medications—tremor, parkinsonism, akathisia, acute dystonic reactions, and tardive dyskinesia. Finally, the psychiatric disturbances associated with primary movement disorders such as Huntington's disease, Parkinson's disease, Wilson's disease, spinocerebellar degenerations, idiopathic basal ganglia calcification, and Gilles de la Tourette syndrome are described. The principal theme developed in the chapter is that disorders of motility and disturbances of mental function are both expressions of a single underlying neuropathological process, and observations concerning movement, cognition, and emotional state all provide important diagnostic information.

MOVEMENT ABNORMALITIES IN IDIOPATHIC PSYCHIATRIC DISTURBANCES

Psychiatric diagnostic habits have tended to underemphasize the relevance of motor system abnormalities and to depend more on the patient's verbal representations of thoughts and experiences. This approach sacrifices the opportunity to use nonverbal motoric information in disease recognition. The disturbances of motility that may be observed in schizophrenia, mania, depression, obsessive–compulsive disorders, and anxiety are described here.

Schizophrenia

The symptomatology of schizophrenia and schizophrenialike disorders is presented in Chapter 13, and the discussion in the present chapter focuses only on the movement abnormalities associated with these psychoses. Motor system abnormalities found in schizophrenia include neurological "soft signs," neuroophthalmic abnormalities, and catatonic disturbances. Soft signs are nonlocalizing deviations in motor or sensory function usually associated with intrauterine or early-life brain insults. They are common in children with learning disabilities but are also found with increased frequency in schizophrenia and some personality disorders (Fish, 1977; Peters et al., 1975; Quitkin et al., 1976). Soft signs observed in schizophrenic patients include posturing of the upper extremities when the patient is asked to walk on heels or toes, lack of balance when hopping on either foot, clumsiness when walking or running, slow execution of fine finger movements (rapidly touching forefinger to thumb), mirror movements of the resting limb when asked to perform rapid alternating movements (pronation–supination of the hand, rapid tapping of the foot) with the contralateral limb, extinguishing the distal stimulus of the face–hand test, ataxia when asked to tandem walk, and articulatory imprecision when performing rapid mouth and tongue movements (la-la-la, te-te-te) or repeating "tongue twisters" (Quitkin et al., 1976). Soft signs are not present in all schizophrenics but tend to be more common in those with negative symptoms (withdrawal, affective flattening, alogia, avolition, anhedonia, attentional impairment, less prominent hallucinations and delusions). They are also correlate with ventricular enlargement on computerized tomographic scans, greater neuropsychological impairment, poor premorbid adjustment, poor response to neuroleptics, and poor prognosis (Andreasen and Olsen, 1982; Fish, 1977).

Neuroophthalmic abnormalities in schizophrenia include staring, deviation of gaze away from the examiner, increased blinking in acute psychotic episodes, decreased blinking in chronic psychoses, darting horizontal eye movements, and wide dilation or squeezed closure of the palpebral fissures (Marsden et al., 1975; Stevens, 1978).

Catatonia refers to a wide range of movement abnormalities that can be observed in the course of schizophrenia. The prevalence of catatonia in schizophrenia is impossible to estimate since catatonic features are poorly recognized and inconsistently sought on examination. Table 12-1 presents a classification of catatonia. The movements can conveniently be divided into those that occur spontaneously and those that occur in response to the clinician when the patient is being examined or interviewed (Hamilton, 1976). The former include various forms of stereotypy, mannerisms, fixed postures, stupor, and furor. *Stereotypy* refers to movements that are not goal directed and are carried out in a uniform manner, whereas mannerisms are goal-directed activities performed in a bizarre or exaggerated way (unusual ways of smoking, eating, etc.). A list of stereotypies observed in schizophrenia is presented in Table 12-2. Stereotyped movements may involve the nose, mouth, tongue, face, head and neck, limbs, and trunk (Jones, 1965; Marsden et al., 1975; Slater and Roth, 1977). These movements can be difficult to distinguish from tardive dyskinesia (Owens et al., 1982), but they usually appear more purposeful, do not have the motor characteristics of tardive dyskinesia described below, and were described by Bleuler (1950) and Kraepelin (1971) long before neuroleptic agents were introduced into clinical practice. In addition to mannerisms and stereotypies, schizophrenic patients may spontaneously adopt bizarre postures, become completely unresponsive (catatonic stupor), or develop short periods of intense physical excitement and agitation (catatonic furor) (Joyston-Bechol, 1966; Slater and Roth, 1977; Strauss and Griffith, 1955). These extreme forms of catatonia have become much less frequent since the discovery and widespread utilization of neuroleptic agents.

On examination, the schizophrenic patient may exhibit a diverse array of catatonic features. Automatic or involuntary obedience may be manifest as waxy flexibility (plastic increase in tone with a tendency to maintain unusual postures induced by the clinician), echolalia, echopraxia (imitation of the examiner's postures and movements), *mitmachen* (abnormal cooperation and passivity with slow return of the limb from an induced to a resting posture), *mitgehen* (the patient can be propelled simply by the light touch of the examiner), and speech-prompt responses (the patient immediately answers all questions even if the response is bizarre and unrelated to the question) (Hamilton, 1976; Taylor, 1981). Oppositional catatonic behaviors include negativism and aversion (the patient refuses to cooperate and faces away from the examiner), mutism, and gegenhalten (resistance to passive body movements).

Catatonia is by no means unique to schizophrenia and is, in fact, more common in nonschizophrenic than

TABLE 12-1. Classification of Catatonia

Abnormal spontaneous movements

  Stereotypy
  Mannerisms
  Bizarre postures
  Stupor
  Catatonic excitement (furor)

Abnormal induced movements

  Automatic obedience

    Waxy flexibility
    Echolalia
    Echopraxia
    Mitmachen
    Mitgehen
    Speech-prompt catatonia

  Opposition

    Negativism, aversion
    Mutism
    Gegenhalten

Data derived from Hamilton (1976).

schizophrenic disorders. In a study of 55 consecutive cases of catatonia admitted to a municipal hospital, Abrams and Taylor (1976) found that only 7 percent had schizophrenia, 62 percent were manic, 9 percent were depressed, 11 percent had neurological illnesses, and 5 percent had "reactive" psychoses. Table 12-3 presents the differential diagnosis of catatonia. Neurological disorders producing catatonia include diseases affecting the subcortical structures, the limbic system, or the frontal lobes. Basal ganglia disturbances causing catatonia include postencephalitic parkinsonism and bilateral lesions of the globus pallidus (Gelenberg, 1976a). The limbic system disease most commonly producing catatonic behavior is herpes encephalitis. The viral infection leads to destruction of the medial temporal lobes and is probably responsible for most cases of "fatal catatonia" (Kim and Perlstein, 1970; Misra and Hay, 1971; Penn et al., 1972; Raskin and Frank, 1974; Wilson, 1976). Other limbic system lesions with catatonia include neoplasms, temporal lobe infarction, and subacute sclerosing panencephalitis (Gelenberg, 1976a; Koehler and Jakumeit, 1976; Sours, 1962). Diencephalic disorders presenting with catatonic features have included thalamotomy (performed for relief of parkinsonism), traumatic hemorrhage, cortical venous thrombosis, Wernicke's encephalopathy, and neoplasms (Gangadhar et al., 1983; Gelenberg, 1976a; Newmann, 1955; Sternbach and Yager, 1981). Frontal lobe disturbances with catatonia include rupture of anterior cerebral artery aneurysms, traumatic contusions, frontal lobe arteriovenous malformations, frontal neoplasms, and general paresis of the insane (syphilis) (Belfer and d'Autremont, 1971; Gel-

TABLE 12-2.   Abnormal Movements Observed in Schizophrenia

Eyes

  Opening wide, squeezing shut, abnormal blinking, rapid lateral glances, staring, gaze deviation away from examiner

Nose

  Wrinkling, sniffing, flaring naris

Mouth and jaw

  Pouting (schnauzkrampf), lip smacking, grinning, grimacing, biting, chewing

Tongue

  Protrusion, licking, clicking

Face

  Wrinkling forehead

Head and neck

  Torsion movements, hyperextension, shaking, nodding

Extremities

  Picking, pulling, handling, twisting, kneading, grasping, tapping, rubbing, intertwining fingers, wringing hands, folding hands, spreading fingers, flinging arms

Trunk and whole body

  Shoulder shrugging, contortionist movements, backarching, rocking, shuffling, hopping, turning, skipping, running, excessive leg lifting, marionettelike movements

Data from Jones (1965), Marsden et al. (1975), and Stevens (1978).

enberg, 1976a; Herman et al., 1942; Thompson, 1970). Seizure-related confusional states may also include catatonic behavior (Gomez et al., 1982; Herman et al., 1942).

A wide variety of systemic disorders and metabolic disturbances have been reported to produce catatonia. Among the metabolic conditions causing catatonia are diabetic ketoacidosis, hyperparathyroidism with hypercalcemia, pellagra, acute intermittent porphyria, homocystinuria, glomerulonephritis, hepatic encephalopathy, thrombotic thrombocytopenic purpura, and systemic lupus erythematosus (Gelenberg, 1976a; Hockaday et al., 1966; Jaffe, 1967; Mac and Pardo, 1983; Read, 1983). Toxic agents producing catatonic behavior include organic fluorides, illuminating gas, mescaline, ethyl alcohol, chronic amphetamine intoxication, phencyclidine, glutethimide withdrawal, disulfiram, aspirin intoxication, and exogenous cortisone (Campbell et al., 1983; Gelenberg, 1976a; Herman et al., 1942; Reisberg, 1978; Schwab and Barrow, 1964). Neuroleptic agents are now among the most common agents producing catatonic behavior, and the catatonia may be either one manifestation of the neuroleptic malignant syndrome or may be part of an acute extrapyramidal reaction with parkinsonism (Brenner and Rheuban, 1978; Gelenberg and Mandel, 1977; McAllister, 1978; Weinberger and Kelly, 1977; Weinberger and Wyatt, 1978).

Idiopathic psychiatric disturbances manifesting catatonia include schizophrenia, mania, depression, and pe-

riodic catatonia (Abrams and Taylor, 1976, 1977). Catatonic schizophrenia represents at least 5 percent of all cases of schizophrenia, and the presence of catatonic features has been associated with a poor prognosis for the disorder (Guggenheim and Babigan, 1974; Yarden and Discipio, 1971). Catatonic features are not uncommon in the manic phase of manic–depressive illness and may also occur in the depressed phase (Kahlbaum, 1973; Kirby, 1913; Taylor and Abrams, 1977). Catatonic excitement is more likely to be associated with mania than the retarded, mute, negativistic, or akinetic type of catatonia (Morrison, 1973). Periodic catatonia is a variant of manic–depressive illness in which the clinical course is dominated by alternating catatonic excitement and catatonic stupor. The disorder responds well to lithium therapy (Gjessing, 1974; Gjessing and Gjessing, 1961; Petursson, 1976; Sovner and McHugh, 1974; Wald and Lerner, 1978).

Mania

The motility alterations of mania are hyperactivity, pressured speech with fast talking and intrusiveness, increased speech volume, inability to remain still, abrupt movements, and threatening, assaultive, or dominating behavior (Carpenter and Stevens, 1980; Marsden et al., 1975). The movements are well coordinated. The motility alterations progress as the mania increases and represent the motoric counterpart of the increasing mental

TABLE 12-3. Differential Diagnosis of Catatonia

Neurological disorders

    Basal ganglia disturbances

        Postencephalitic parkinsonism
        Globus pallidus lesions (bilateral)

    Limbic system disorders

        Viral encephalitis
        Temporal lobe infarction
        Neoplasms
        Subacute sclerosing panencephalitis

    Diencephalic lesions

        Thalamotomy for parkinsonism
        Traumatic hemorrhage
        Wernicke's encephalopathy
        Neoplasm

    Frontal lobe disorders
        Anterior cerebral artery aneurysm
        Traumatic contusion
        Arteriovenous malformation
        General paresis
        Neoplasms
        Cortical venous thrombosis

    Epilepsy

Systemic and metabolic disturbances

    Diabetic ketoacidosis
    Hypercalcemia (hyperparathyroidism)
    Pellagra
    Porphyria
    Homocystinuria
    Glomerulonephritis
    Hepatic encephalopathy
    Thrombotic thrombocytopenic purpura
    Systemic lupus erythematosus

Toxic agents and drug reactions

    Organic fluorides
    Illuminating gas
    Mescaline
    Ethyl alcohol
    Chronic amphetamine intoxication
    Phencyclidine
    Glutethimide withdrawal
    Disulfiram
    Aspirin intoxication
    Cortisone
    Neuroleptic administration

        Neuroleptic malignant syndrome
        Neuroleptic-induced catatonia

Idiopathic psychiatric disorders

    Schizophrenia
    Mania
    Depression
    Periodic catatonia

Data from Gelenberg (1976a) and Stoudemire (1982).

overactivity (Carlson and Goodwin, 1973; Weiss et al., 1974). As noted in the preceding section, catatonic features are present in as many as 25 percent of manic patients.

Depression

The movement disorder associated with retarded depression may be difficult to distinguish from a primary extrapyramidal disorder. Psychomotor retardation with akinesia is prominent, the patient assumes a flexed posture with bent knees and bowed head, and there is an unchanging facial expression (Marsden et al., 1975; Schwartz et al., 1976). Voice changes also resemble those of extrapyramidal disorders: the patient speaks softly in a monotone and there is an increase in speech pause time (Alpert, 1981; Greden et al., 1981). Tone changes are modest or nonexistent and tremor is absent.

Anxiety

Anxious patients also have motility disturbances. The eyebrows are raised, and there is deepening of the furrows of the forehead and widening of the palpebral fissures. The mouth is often held slightly open, the body is rigidly upright, and when the patient is seated the knees are pressed together. Respiratory movements are fast and shallow, perspiration is increased, and the pupils are dilated (Leff and Isaacs, 1981). Pacing is common.

Obsessive–Compulsive Disorder

The compulsions and rituals of obsessive–compulsive disorders impose unique alterations on the patient's motility and behavior. The patient is unable to resist cleaning, avoiding certain objects or circumstances, repeating specific acts, checking, counting, or pursuing other involuntary activities (Stern and Cobb, 1978). Patients may have to touch themselves, others, or specific things in the environment, or a rigid order may be imposed on the sequence of any activity. Trivial acts that would normally take minutes may require hours to perform because of the ritualistic embellishment, checking, and repeating. (The relationship of obsessions and compulsions to Gilles de la Tourette syndrome and other movement disorders is discussed later.)

MOVEMENT DISORDERS PRODUCED BY PSYCHOTROPIC DRUGS

Movement disorders produced by psychotropic drugs administered to behaviorally disturbed patients are now among the most common motility abnormalities

TABLE 12-4. Movement Disorders Produced by Psychotropic Agents

Early onset
Acute dystonic reactions
Parkinsonism
Rabbit syndrome
Tremor
Akathisia
Miscellaneous unusual drug-induced movement disorders
Myoclonus
Choreoathetosis
Ataxia
Late onset
Tardive dyskinesia

observed. A clinically useful classification is to divide such disorders into those that begin soon after the drug is administered—acute dystonic reactions, parkinsonism, tremor, and akathisia—and those such as the various forms of tardive dyskinesia that do not appear until after the patient has been medicated for months or years (Table 12-4).

Acute Dystonic Reactions

Acute dystonic reactions occur in approximately two percent of patients receiving neuroleptic medications (Ayd, 1961; Marsden and Jenner, 1980). They usually appear within 48–72 hours of initiating therapy or increasing the dose and tend to have their onset at a time when serum drug concentrations are falling (Garver et al., 1976). Dystonic reactions are more common in younger patients than older and occur more in men than in women (Ayd, 1961; Swett, 1975). They may occur with any of the classes of neuroleptic agents (phenothiazines, butyrophenones, thioxanthenes) but are most common with the high-potency agents (Ayd, 1961).

The head and neck are most commonly affected. Involuntary spasm of the tongue may lead to tongue protrusion or retraction, making talking and swallowing difficult. The masseter muscles may forcibly contract, producing trismus, and facial grimacing is common. Torticollis and oculogyric crises are also frequent. Occasionally the trunk and legs are involved, producing torsion postures and bizarre gaits. In some cases the entire body may assume an opisthotonic posture (Food and Drug Administration Task Force, 1973; Gupta and Lovejoy, 1967). Acute dystonic reactions are not infrequently misdiagnosed as tetany, hysteria, or seizures. They respond promptly to treatment with anticholinergic agents.

Dystonic reactions produced by neuroleptic agents must be distinguished from idiopathic, hereditary, and acquired dystonias in patients coincidently receiving these drugs for behavioral disturbances (Fahn and El-

dridge, 1976). Table 12-5 presents the differential diagnosis of dystonic disorders.

Parkinsonism

Parkinsonism occurs in 20–40 percent of patients treated with neuroleptic agents, is more common in women than men, occurs more commonly in older patients, usually develops within the first 3 months of treatment, and is more common with high-potency drugs (Ayd, 1961; Hausner, 1983; Marsden and Jenner, 1980). The increased occurrence of drug-induced parkinsonism in patients with a family history of parkinsonism, the parallels between the age incidence of Parkinson's disease and drug-induced parkinsonism, and the identification at autopsy of a partially depleted cell population in the substantia nigra of patients with drug-induced parkinsonism all suggest that many individuals manifesting the drug-induced disorder are predisposed by preexisting biochemical or morphological abnormalities in the extrapyramidal system (Marsden and Jenner, 1980; Myrianthopoulos et al., 1962; Rajput et al., 1982).

The entire parkinsonian syndrome, including akinesia, rigidity, postural abnormalities, and tremor, may be produced by neuroleptic agents, but akinesia is the earliest, most common, and frequently the only manifestation of the drug-induced state (Marsden et al., 1975). Akinesia accounts for the masked, expressionless face, loss of associated movements with drooling and diminished arm swing, slow initiation of motor activity, soft and monotonous speech, and slow micrographic handwriting (Angus and Simpson, 1970; Hall et al., 1956; Hoffman, 1981; Marsden et al., 1975). Alteration in script size can be a useful index of parkinsonian symptomatology. Comparison of the patient's current signature with previous signatures on credit cards or licenses, writing dictated or spontaneous sentences, or having the patient produce repeating loops or sequences such as the alphabet or digits (Fig. 12-1) will reveal the micrographia. Rigidity of the limbs, neck, and trunk follows the onset of the akinesia and is not the cause of the motor slowing and loss of associated movements. In some cases, a low-frequency (4–6-Hz), large-amplitude, resting tremor occurs, but tremor is the least common manifestation of drug-induced parkinsonism (Hausner, 1983; Marsden et al., 1975).

Drug-induced parkinsonism usually improves within a few days following initiation of anticholinergic therapy (McGeer et al., 1961; Sheppard and Merlis, 1967). Amantadine hydrochloride has also proved useful in the treatment of akinesia and may avoid complications associated with the administration of anticholinergic agents (confusion, blurred vision, dry mouth, urinary retention, bowel hypomotility, and fecal impaction). Most patients become symptom free within a few weeks of discontinuing the neuroleptic, but in a few cases the parkinsonism may persist for several months or even up to a year (Marsden and Jenner, 1980).

Although neuroleptic agents are the psychotropic agents most commonly responsible for drug-induced parkinsonism, lithium has been reported to produce cogwheel rigidity in a variable number of patients, and a few patients have developed a parkinsonian syndrome indistinguishable from that produced by neuroleptics (Apte and Langston, 1983; Asnis et al., 1979; Branchey et al., 1976; Kane et al., 1978; Lang, 1984; Reches et al., 1981; Shopsin and Gershon, 1975; Tyrer et al., 1980).

Drug-induced parkinsonism must be distinguished from other causes of akinesia and rigidity, including idiopathic and postencephalitic Parkinson's disease, other degenerative extrapyramidal syndromes, nonpsychotropic drug-induced states, lacunar states, endocrine disorders, hydrocephalus, basal ganglia neoplasms, and depression (Table 12-6).

Rabbit Syndrome

The "rabbit" syndrome is an uncommon drug-induced extrapyramidal syndrome in which the patient makes rapid, perioral chewinglike movements similar to those made by rabbits. The movements occur along a vertical axis at a frequency of 5 Hz and involve the oral and masticatory muscles and usually spare the tongue (Todd et al., 1983; Villeneuve, 1972). The syndrome most closely resembles a limited expression of a parkinsonian tremor and responds well to anticholinergic therapy. The rabbit syndrome is often misidentified as tardive dyskinesia, but the two can be distinguished by the faster, more regular movements of the rabbit syndrome and by its tendency to spare the tongue.

Tremor

Tremor is a common product of many disturbances affecting the central nevous system (CNS). There are four major varieties of tremor, and each must be distinguished to allow correct clinical management (Table 12-7). Parkinsonian tremors are large-amplitude, low-frequency resting tremors that accompany Parkinson's disease and other extrapyramidal syndromes and occasionally occur in parkinsonian syndromes produced by neuroleptic agents or lithium. Physiological tremors are small-amplitude, high-frequency action tremors that occur during activity and disappear at rest. They may occur normally in states of anxiety and fatigue and may be abnormally exaggerated by a variety of drugs, toxins, and metabolic disturbances. Essential tremors share

TABLE 12-5.   Differential Diagnosis of Dystonia

Primary

  Hereditary

    Dystonia musculorum deformans (autosomal dominant, autosomal, recessive, and x-linked recessive varieties)
    Dystonia with marked diurnal variation
    Familial paroxysmal choreoathetosis
    Hereditary nonprogressive chorea of early onset
    Familial benign chorea with intention tremor

  Nonhereditary

    Generalized dystonia
    Segmental dystonia (two adjacent body parts affected)
    Focal dystonia
      Torticollis
      Writer's cramp
      Oromandibular dystonia (Meige's syndrome)
      Spasmodic dysphonia

Secondary

  Associated with other extrapyramidal syndromes

    Parkinson's disease
    Wilson's disease
    Huntington's disease
    Hallervorden-Spatz disease
    Juvenile neuronal ceroidlipofuscinosis
    Dystonia with assorted associated inherited abnormalities (deafness, paraplegia, cataracts, nasal malformation)

  Produced by identified environmental causes

    Prenatal birth injury
    Encephalitis
    Postencephalitis
    Head trauma
    Stroke
    Neoplasm
    Drugs—manganese, carbon monoxide, phenothiazines

Reproduced from Fahn S and Eldridge R. Definition of dystonia and classification of the dystonic states. *Adv Neurol*, 1976, *14*, 1–5, Table 1. With permission.

the same amplitude and frequency characteristics of physiological tremors but occur on a sporadic, familial, or "senile" basis. Archimedes' loops (Fig. 12-2) provide a graphic method of assessing and following action tremors. The patient is asked to draw a spiral similar to the model drawn by the examiner and then a second spiral inside the lines drawn by the examiner. The tremor is present in both spirals drawn by the patient, and the second task is more demanding and usually produces an exaggeration of the abnormal movements. In most cases the action tremors are most apparent in the nondominant hand. Cerebellar tremors are also action (intention) tremors. They are of low frequency and increase in amplitude as the target is approached (crescendo

1 2 3 4 5 6 7 8 9 10 11 12 13 14 15 16 17 18 19 2

Figure 12-1.   Drug-induced micrographia with progressive diminution in digit size.

amplitude). Cerebellar tremors are produced by degenerative, demyelinating, toxic, and traumatic disorders of the cerebellum and midbrain (Fahn, 1972; Jankovic and Fahn, 1980; Rondot et al., 1978).

Table 12-8 presents the etiologies of the four major types of tremor. Among psychotropic agents, neuroleptic drugs and lithium may produce parkinsonian-type resting tremors, and heterocyclic antidepressants (tricyclic and tetracyclic) and lithium commonly cause action tremors (Rondot et al., 1978). An action tremor that may be disabling occurs in up to 60 percent of patients treated with lithium and appears to be more common in older patients and in those receiving combinations of lithium and neuroleptics (Bech et al., 1979; Bone et al., 1980; Pullinger and Tyrer, 1983; Van Putten, 1978; Vestergaard et al., 1980). Lithium-induced action tremors can be successfully treated with beta-blocking agents such as propranolol and metoprolol (Gaby et al., 1983; Kirk et al., 1973; Lapierre, 1976).

Akathisia

Akathisia refers to the subjective need to keep in constant motion. The patients cannot sit or stand still and have a drive to pace and fidget. It is among the most common reactions to neuroleptic agents, occurring in approximately 20 percent of patients. In its mild form the patients tap their feet and shift their weight when seated; when severe, they cannot remain seated, stamp their feet, and pace restlessly (Food and Drug Administration Task Force, 1973; Marsden et al., 1975). The syndrome usually begins within 3 months of initiating neuroleptic medication and is somewhat more frequent in women than in men. It has little age predilection (Ayd, 1961). Akathisia is usually an early-onset disorder that improves with anticholinergic therapy, but it has also been reported as a manifestation of tardive dyskinesia and may then be worsened by anticholinergic agents. Subacute akathisia responding poorly to an-

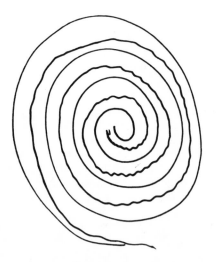
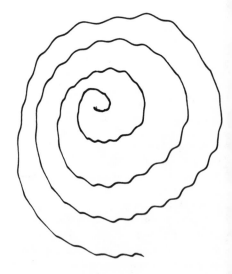

Figure 12-2.   Archimedes' loops demonstrating action tremor. The examiner provides a model (**A**) that is copied by the patient (**B**), the patient is then asked to draw a second spiral between the lines of the examiner's model (**A**).

ticholinergic drugs may improve when propranolol is administered concurrently with or instead of the anticholinergic agents (Lipinski et al., 1984). Akathisia must be distinguished from the restless-legs syndrome, which is characterized by peculiar creeping or crawling sensations in the lower legs (Ekbom, 1960).

Miscellaneous Drug-Induced Movement Disorders

Myoclonus

Myoclonus is a relatively rare side effect of psychotropic drug administration but has been reported as a consequence of both lithium and heterocyclic antidepressant therapy. The myoclonic jerking may occur at rest but is most apparent during motor activity and is primarily an action or intention myoclonus (Lippmann et al., 1977; Rosen and Stevens, 1983). The myoclonus disappears when the offending agents are discontinued.

Choreoathetosis

Choreoathetosis (nontardive dyskinesia type) has been induced by a variety of psychotropic agents, including tricyclic antidepressants, methylphenidate, carbamazepine, pemoline, methadone, and lithium (Burks et al., 1974; Extein, 1978; Joyce and Gunderson, 1980; Singh et al., 1983; Wasserman and Yahr, 1980; Weiner et al., 1978b; Zorumski and Bakris, 1983).

Ataxia

Lithium may produce an ataxic cerebellar syndrome as well as myoclonus, a parkinsonian syndrome, and choreoathetosis. Ataxia, unlike the other movement disorders, usually follows a period of acute lithium toxicity and may be permanent (Apte and Langston, 1983; Donaldson and Cunningham, 1983). In some patients, toxicity may occur with lithium levels in the usual therapeutic range.

Tardive Dyskinesia

The discovery of the dramatic amelioration of psychotic symptoms by dopamine-blocking neurologic agents revolutionized the care of the mentally ill and allowed many to leave the twilight world of disordered thought, hallucinations, and paranoia to enter a more useful, productive, and satisfying life. Within 10 years of their introduction and widespread use, however, it was recognized that these potent agents achieved their miraculous results by inducing alterations in cerebral function that had their own untoward consequences. Specifically, the use of neuroleptics causes a wide

TABLE 12-6. Differential Diagnosis of Parkinsonism

Degenerative disorders

  Paralysis agitans (idiopathic Parkinson's disease)
  Progressive supranuclear palsy
  Striatonigral degeneration
  Shy-Drager syndrome
  Guamanian ALS-Parkinsonism–dementia complex
  Huntington's disease (rigid variant)
  Wilson's disease
  Idiopathic basal ganglia calcification (Fahr's syndrome)
  Hallervorden-Spatz syndrome
  Olivopontocerebellar atrophy

Toxic agents

  Neuroleptics (phenothiazines, butyrophenones, thioxanthenes, etc.)
  Lithium
  Reserpine
  Methyldopa
  Manganese
  Organophosphates
  Cyanide
  Carbon disulfide
  Mercury
  Carbon monoxide

Infectious illnesses and postinfectious disorders

  Postencephalitic Parkinson's disease (von Economo encephalitis)
  Other viral encephalitides
  Jakob-Creutzfeldt disease

Vascular disorders

  Lacunar state (arteriosclerotic parkinsonism)

Metabolic conditions

  Hypoparathyroidism
  Hypothyroidism
  Taurine deficiency

Miscellaneous neurological conditions

  Normal-pressure hydrocephalus
  Basal ganglia neoplasms
  Dementia pugilistica
  Posttraumatic encephalopathy

Idiopathic psychiatric syndromes

  Depression with psychomotor retardation
  Schizophrenia with catatonia

Reproduced from Cummings JL and Benson DF. *Dementia: a clinical approach.* Boston, Butterworths, 1983, table 4-3. With permission from Butterworths Publishers.

variety of extrapyramidal syndromes, including early-onset dystonias, akathisia, and parkinsonism, and late-onset dyskinesias (Crane, 1968, 1973; Hunter et al.,

TABLE 12-7. Classification of Tremors

Tremor	Action Characteristic	Amplitude	Frequency	Etiology
Physiological	Action	Small	High (8–12 Hz)	Anxiety, fatigue, toxic–metabolic disorders
Essential	Action	Small	High (8–12 Hz)[a]	Senile, hereditary, sporadic
Parkinsonian	Resting	Large	Low (4–6 Hz)	Parkinsonian syndromes
Cerebellar	Action	Crescendo[b]	Low	Cerebellar or midbrain disease

[a]Essential tremor slows with increasing age and may eventually assume the frequency of a parkinsonian tremor (Marshall, 1961).
[b]The amplitude of cerebellar tremor increases as the target is approached (hence the name ''intention'' tremor).

TABLE 12-8. Etiologies of Tremor

Physiological tremor (normal and accentuated)

Psychotropic agents: lithium, tricyclic antidepressants, phenothiazines, butyrophenones
Nonpsychotropic drugs: epinephrine, isoproterenol, metaproterenol, terbutaline, xanthine (coffee, tea), theophylline, levodopa, amphetamines, thyroid hormone, hypoglycemic agents, adrenocorticosteroids, valproate sodium
Endocrine: thyrotoxicosis, hypoglycemia, pheochromocytoma
Stress-induced: anxiety, fright, fatigue, cold-shivering
Metabolic disorders: uremia, hepatic encephalopathy, anoxia
Miscellaneous agents and conditions: alcohol or sedative withdrawal, mercury, lead, arsenic, bismuth, carbon monoxide, methyl bromide, monosodium glutamate

Essential tremor

Autosomal dominant, senile, sporadic
With Charcot-Marie-Tooth disease (Roussy-Lévy syndrome)
With other movement disorders: parkinsonism, torsion dystonia, torticollis, writer's cramp, hereditary nonprogressive chorea

Cerebellar tremor

Cerebellar degenerations
Multiple sclerosis
Wilson's disease
With hereditary sensory neuropathy (Déjerine-Sottas disease)
Drugs and toxins: lithium, phenytoin, barbiturates, alcohol, mercury, 5-fluorouracil
Midbrain lesions (''rubral'' tremor)

Parkinsonian tremor (See Table 12-6)

Parkinson's disease
   Idiopathic
   Postencephalitic
Other degenerative extrapyramidal syndromes
Toxic and metabolic parkinsonian syndromes

Modified from data of Jankovic and Fahn (1980) and Young (1982).

1964; Schmidt and Jarcho, 1966; Uhrbrand and Faurbye, 1960). Whereas the former were easily treated and disappeared in the drug-free state, the latter were often permanent and irreversible. The late-onset tardive dyskinesias have been the subject of increasing concern, and the threat of their occurrence is now the major limiting factor in the use of neuroleptic drugs.

Prevalence and Risk Factors

Tardive dyskinesia has been found in from 7–56 percent of patients with extended exposure to neuroleptic medications (Brandon et al., 1971; Chouinard et al., 1979; Fann et al., 1972; Jeste and Wyatt, 1982; Kane and Smith, 1982; Mukherjee et al., 1982; Tepper and Haas, 1979), with an approximate mean prevalence of

15–20 percent among at-risk patients. This far exceeds the rate of spontaneous movements of similar types seen in the mentally ill prior to the introduction of neuroleptics (Barnes et al., 1983; Crane, 1973; Mettler and Crandell, 1959). A cumulative exposure of at least 3 months is necessary for the occurrence of tardive dyskinesia, and most patients will have had 2 years of neuroleptic administration before dyskinetic movements appear (Jeste and Wyatt, 1982). Interrupted exposure or drug-free holidays do not appear to diminish the risk (Jeste et al., 1979a). Tardive dyskinesia may follow exposure to any of the classes of dopamine blocking agents, including phenothiazines, butyrophenones, thioxanthenes, substituted benzamides (e.g., sulpiride), dibenzoxazepines (e.g. loxapine, amoxapine), dihydroindolones (e.g. molindone), and diphenylbutylpiperidines (e.g., penfluridol) (Lapierre and Anderson, 1983; Schooler and Kane, 1982; Thornton and Stahl, 1984). The relative risk of developing tardive dyskinesia with different neuroleptics has not been definitely determined, although a higher incidence with high potency agents (i.e., fluphenazine) and lower incidence with thioridazine has been suggested (Borison et al., 1983; Jeste and Wyatt, 1982; Mukherjee et al., 1982). Preliminary studies have revealed higher serum neuroleptic levels among patients with tardive dyskinesia—an observation that might explain why patients treated with apparently similar oral dosages develop dyskinesia at different rates (Jeste et al., 1979b).

In addition to the neuroleptic exposure, a number of host variables influence the occurrence of tardive dyskinesia. Increasing age has the highest correlation with increasing prevalence of tardive dyskinesia. It is three times more common in patients over the age of 40 and shows a progressive increase in frequency from ages 40 to 70 (Chouinard et al., 1979; Kane and Smith, 1982; Mukherjee et al., 1982; Smith and Baldessarini, 1980; Tepper and Haas, 1979). Patients over the age of 40 are also less likely to experience remission of symptoms when neuroleptics are discontinued (Smith and Baldessarini, 1980). Several studies have revealed an increase prevalence of tardive dyskinesia among female patients (Brandon et al., 1971; Chouinard et al., 1979; Kane and Smith, 1982; Mukherjee et al., 1982; Smith and Baldessarini, 1980; Tepper and Haas, 1979).

The occurrence of other extrapyramidal effects as a possible predictor of tardive dyskinesia has been examined, with inconclusive results. A few investigators have suggested that drug-induced parkinsonism occurs more frequently among patients eventually developing tardive dyskinesia, but proof that it represents a risk factor or effectively predicts the occurrence of tardive dyskinesia is lacking (Crane, 1972; Jeste and Wyatt, 1982; Mukherjee et al., 1982).

The interaction of tardive dyskinesia and primary psychiatric illness has also been examined. Although more schizophrenics suffer from tardive dyskinesia than any other diagnostic group, they also receive more treatment with neuroleptics and are, therefore, at greater risk for the disorder. Several studies have found an increased prevalence among patients with affective disorders (Davis et al., 1976; Rosenbaum et al., 1977; Yassa et al., 1984). During the course of bipolar affective disorders, tardive dyskinesia is most prominent during the depressed phase and may disappear in manic periods (Cutler et al., 1981; Weiner and Werner, 1982). Tardive dyskinesia has also been reported among nonpsychotic patients treated with neuroleptics for anxiety disorders and other illnesses (Klawans et al., 1974). Evidence suggesting that tardive dyskinesia is more common among brain-damaged individuals or those exposed to somatic therapies—insulin shock therapy, electroshock therapy, and prefrontal leukotomy—has been inconsistent (Jeste and Wyatt, 1982; Yassa et al., 1984).

Phenomenology and Clinical Variants

The most common expression of tardive dyskinesia is the bucco-lingual masticatory syndrome in which the patient has continuous movements of the mouth, jaw, and tongue. The tongue protrudes, twists, and curls inside the mouth and out with movements known as "fly catcher tongue" and "bon-bon sign" (distention of the cheek by tongue movements, making it appear that one has a candy bon-bon in one's mouth). There are opening, closing, and lateral chewing movements of the jaw, combined with a variety of pouting and sucking movements of the lips (Hunter et al., 1964; Marsden et al., 1975). Hypertrophy of the tongue and masseter muscles may be evident. In the classical dyskinesia syndrome, the upper face is largely spared and the movement disorder is confined to the lower facial musculature.

The second most common body areas to be involved by the dyskinesias are the hand and truncal–respiratory muscles. The hands exhibit choreoathetotic movements with twisting, flexion–extension, and spreading movements of the fingers that are most apparent when the patient is walking or engaged in other activities that do not involve the hands. Involvement of the abdominal musculature is frequent and produces irregularities of respiratory rate, rhythm, and amplitude that interrupt the normal breathing pattern as well as speech (Faheem et al., 1982; Jackson et al., 1980; Weiner et al., 1978a). Involvement of the feet is not uncommon but is less frequent than involvement of the mouth, hands, and trunk. The foot movements consist of flexion–extension of the ankles and dorsiflexion of the toes (Marsden et al.,

TABLE 12-9.   Characteristics of Typical Tardive
                        Dyskinesia

Distribution:	buccolingual > hands > truncal–respiratory > feet distal limbs > proximal limbs lower face > upper face

Resting movements

Movements can usually be volitionally suppressed
    temporarily

Movements are suppressed by action

Movements are increased by distraction

Patients are largely unaware of the movements

1975). Limb movements are bilateral but not necessarily symmetrical (Myslobodsky et al., 1984; Wilson et
al., 1984).

Elderly patients frequently manifest the bucco-
linguo-masticatory syndrome in isolation, whereas young
individuals are more likely to have truncal involvement
and combined dystonia and dyskinesia (Jeste and Wyatt,
1982; McLean and Casey, 1978; Tarsy et al., 1977).

A number of phenomenological characteristics help
to distinguish tardive dyskinesia from other choreiform
movement disorders (Table 12-9). The typical distribution of the movements has already been emphasized.
The movements are largely resting movements that can
be volitionally suppressed and are also suppressed by
activity of the involved part. If asked, therefore, the patient can usually voluntarily eliminate the movements
for brief periods of time, and if required to perform activities with the involved muscles (protrude the tongue,
write, etc.), the movements can also be dampened or
eliminated. Distraction of the patient's attention tends
to increase the movements. Bucco-lingual movements
are often most apparent when the patient is doing constructions during the mental status examination, and hand
movements are most obvious when the patient is walking or talking.

In addition to the classical dyskinesia syndrome, a

TABLE 12-10.   Clinical Varieties of Tardive Dyskinesia

Classical tardive dyskinesia

  Buccolinguomasticatory syndrome
  Truncal-respiratory and distal limb movements

Variants of tardive dyskinesia

  Tardive dystonia
  Tardive ballismus
  Tardive myoclonus
  Tardive akathisia
  Tardive Tourette syndrome
  Tardive Meige syndrome
  Tardive dyskinesia with concomitant drug-induced
      parkinsonism

number of less common variants have also been observed
(Table 12-10). Tardive dystonia is among the most frequently observed variants of tardive dyskinesia. The dystonic posture tends to involve the jaw (oromandibular
dystonia) or neck (torticollis, retrocollis, anterocollis)
and in younger patients may involve the trunk and limbs.
The syndrome must be distinguished from idiopathic dystonias (by the history of neuroleptic exposure and absence of a family history of dystonia) and from disorders
with secondary dystonic manifestations such as Huntington's disease, Parkinson's disease, the Hallervorden-
Spatz syndrome, Wilson's disease, and acquired CNS
insults (Table 12-5) (Angle and McIntire, 1968; Burke
et al., 1982; Fahn and Eldridge, 1976; Tarsy et al.,
1977).

In some cases the dyskinetic movements are more
proximal in character and may then assume a ballistic
character with rapid, large-amplitude flinging actions.
Myoclonic jerks may also occur in the tardive dyskin-
esic syndrome, frequently in conjunction with other dyskinetic symptoms (Marsden et al., 1975). In addition
to the tardive ballismus and myoclonus, tardive akathisia is not uncommon. The syndrome has all the characteristics of akathisia described previously for the
early-onset disorder. There is subjective restlessness with
an inability to sit quietly. Tardive akathisia begins after
months or years of neuroleptic therapy and unlike the
early-onset disorder is not improved and may even be
worsened by anticholinergic agents (Braude and Barnes,
1983; Kruse, 1960; Weiner and Luby, 1983).

The Gilles de la Tourette syndrome is a complex
neuropsychiatric illness that begins between age 2 and
15 years and is manifest by a waxing and waning repertoire of somatic tics and involuntary vocalizations (Shapiro et al., 1978). Tardive Tourette syndrome is a similar
disorder that begins after exposure to neuroleptic agents.
Involuntary somatic tics and vocalizations must be present in order to establish the diagnosis. The Gilles de la
Tourette symptoms may be the only manifestations of
the dyskinesia syndrome or may coexist with classical
dyskinesias (DeVeaugh-Geiss, 1980; Fogg and Pakkenberg, 1980; Klawans et al., 1978; Mueller and Aminoff, 1982; Singer, 1981).

Meige's syndrome (discussed below) is a disorder
characterized by the spontaneous occurrence of blepharospasm and oromandibular dystonia. The same symptoms have been recorded in some patients exposed to
chronic neuroleptic therapy (Glazer et al., 1983; Weiner
et al., 1981). Tardive Meige syndrome differs from classical tardive dyskinesia in that there is prominent involvement of the upper as well as the lower face.

All these syndromes are hyperkinesias varying in
speed from slow dystonias through classical dyskinesias to more rapid tic and myoclonic syndromes. The

hyperkinetic movements are irregular derangements of normal movements with anomalous contraction of muscle groups. These movements differ from tremor where there is a regular alteration of agonist and antogonist contraction, and tremor is one type of hyperkinesia that does not occur as a symptom of tardive dyskinesia.

Tardive dyskinesia may coexist with drug-induced parkinsonism, and then the dyskinetic syndrome will be complicated by bradykinesia, rigidity, and/or resting tremor (Crane, 1972; De Fraites et al., 1977; Fann and Lake, 1974; Gerlach, 1977; Richardson and Craig, 1982).

Diagnosis, Pathology, and Pathophysiology

The diagnosis of tardive dyskinesia has three criteria: (1) a history of at least 3 months of cumulative neuroleptic exposure, (2) identification of one of the dyskinesia syndromes described earlier, and (3) no other conditions or circumstances that could account for the abnormal movements (Gardos et al., 1978; Schooler and Kane, 1982).

Laboratory investigations are of little use in the diagnosis. Computerized tomographic scan studies of patients with tardive dyskinesia have been unrevealing (Brainin et al., 1983; Gelenberg, 1976b). Electroencephalographic studies have suggested an increased incidence of the β-mitten pattern (combinations of a sharp transient followed by a slow wave during deep sleep), but the significance and consistency of this finding has not been determined (Wegner et al., 1979). Cerebrospinal fluid (CSF) studies may show elevated levels of noradrenalin (Jeste et al., 1984), but the finding is not diagnostic.

Autopsy studies of patients with tardive dyskinesia have yielded conflicting results. Some investigators have found a diminished number of cells in the substantia nigra along with gliosis in the midbrain and brainstem, whereas others have failed to identify any significant alterations (Christensen et al., 1970; Hunter et al., 1968).

The pathophysiology of tardive dyskinesia remains obscure, but there is considerable evidence of neuroleptic-induced dopamine receptor hypersensitivity resulting in the extrapyramidal overactivity (Gerlach et al., 1974; Marsden et al., 1975; Tarsy and Baldessarini, 1977).

Course, Prognosis, and Treatment

Once initiated, tardive dyskinesia is not inevitably progressive. In fact, many dyskinesias remain stably restricted to a few body areas despite continued neuroleptic therapy (Gardos and Cole, 1983; Jeste and Wyatt, 1982; Wegner and Kane, 1982). In some cases, however, dyskinesias may progress and become life-threatening, particularly when they involve the upper throat and produce repeated retching and dysphagia (Casey and Rabins, 1978; Moss and Green, 1982). It is currently impossible to determine which syndromes will progress, although severe tardive dyskinesias have often had a rapidly developing malignant course (Gardos and Cole, 1983).

Despite its relatively benign nature in most cases, its unpredictability makes it important to limit the risk of tardive dyskinesia as much as possible. Prevention, or limitation of risk of developing tardive dyskinesia, is the first important element of any management program. The use of neuroleptics should be avoided except when specific indications exist, and when they are necessary their dosages should be as small as possible (Kane et al., 1983). Once dyskinetic movements appear, the need for neuroleptic therapy should be reevaluated. If neuroleptics are discontinued, approximately 30 percent of the dyskinesias will disappear within 2 years, although transient worsening may occur immediately after neuroleptic withdrawal (Jeste and Wyatt, 1982). In most cases, however, continued treatment with neuroleptics will be necessary and management of the dyskinesia will have to occur concomitantly with neuroleptic therapy. As long as the dyskinesia is mild, no treatment may be necessary. When treatment is needed, a variety of treatment strategies are available (Berger and Rexroth, 1980; Jeste and Wyatt, 1982; Klawans, 1973; Mackay and Sheppard, 1979). Increasing the dosage of neuroleptics is among the most effective forms of intervention and may be necessary in life-threatening situations but carries the risk of a subsequent reemergence of the dyskinetic symptoms. Among nonneuroleptics, dopamine depleting agents such as reserpine and tetrabenazine are the most efficacious agents available, producing improvement in up to two-thirds of cases (Jankovic, 1982; Kazamatsuri et al., 1972, 1973; Klawans et al., 1980; Kobayashi, 1977). Cholinergic agents (lecithin, choline) have also had ameliorating effects on some cases of tardive dyskinesia (Gelenberg et al., 1979; Growdon et al., 1977; Jackson et al., 1981). In addition, a large number of other drugs have been used with variable success, including lithium, propranolol, metoclopramide, clonazepam, phenobarbital, baclofen, and low-dose apomorphine and bromocriptine (Bobruff et al., 1981; Chaudry et al., 1982; Jeste et al., 1983; Karp et al., 1981; Korsgaard, 1976; Reda et al., 1974; Tolosa, 1978).

Anticholinergic medications worsen dyskinetic movements, and any patient receiving anticholinergic antiparkinsonian agents together with neuroleptics should have the anticholinergic dosage discontinued or adjusted downward until parkinsonian symptoms begin to appear (Good, 1981; Kiloh et al., 1973; Klawans and Rubovits, 1974).

TABLE 12-11.   Nonneuroleptic Causes of Orofacial
                            Dyskinesia

Drug-induced dyskinesia (nonneuroleptic agents)

   Levodopa
   Amphetamines
   Methylphenidate
   Fenfluramine
   Amantadine
   Metoclopramide
   Methyldopa
   Anticholinergic agents
   Tricyclic antidepressants
   Antihistamine agents
   Anticonvulsants (phenytoin, phenobarbital,
     carbamazepine)
   Benzodiazepines
   Antimalarial agents (chloroquine, amodiaquine)
   Lithium (may aggravate existing dyskinesia)
   Baclofen withdrawal

Extrapyramidal disorders

   Huntington's disease
   Wilson's disease
   Idiopathic basal ganglia calcification
   Meige's syndrome
   Idiopathic orofacial dyskinesia in the elderly
   Edentulous dyskinesia
   Withdrawal dyskinesia

Data from Ashcroft et al, 1965; Beitman, 1978; Birket-Smith, 1974;
Chadwick et al., 1976; Crews and Carpenter, 1977; Fann et al.,
1976; Granacher 1981; Jankovic, 1981; Jeste and Wyatt 1982; Joyce
and Gunderson, 1980; Kaplan and Murkofsky, 1978; Kirubakaran
et al., 1984; Osifo, 1979; Thach et al, 1975.

Differential Diagnosis

   Table 12-11 lists the drugs and conditions that can
produce orofacial dyskinesia and must be considered in
the differential diagnosis of tardive dyskinesia. Nonneuroleptic drug-induced disturbances are particularly important since most are readily reversible with discontinuation of the offending agents. In addition to these drug-
induced orofacial disorders, extrapyramidal syndromes
can also cause prominent facial motor disturbances that
closely resemble tardive dyskinesia, and spontaneous
dyskinesias appear in 6–16 percent of elderly and edentulous individuals who have no history of neuroleptic
exposure (Klawans and Barr, 1982; Koller, 1983; Varga
et al., 1982). Tardive dyskinesia must also be distinguished from withdrawal dyskinesia, a transient (duration less than 2 weeks) dyskinesia appearing after abrupt
discontinuation of neuroleptic agents.

   Tardive dyskinesia is a choreic syndrome and must
also be distinguished from disorders due to generalized
chorea. Table 12-12 presents the differential diagnosis

of neurologic, inflammatory, and toxic–metabolic causes
of chorea.

PSYCHIATRIC DISTURBANCES IN EXTRA-PYRAMIDAL DISEASES

   To complete this exposition of the relationship
between motor and mental functions, this section briefly
summarizes the psychiatric disturbances that commonly
accompany diseases of the extrapyramidal system (Table 12-13). The dementia that accompanies many extrapyramidal syndromes was discussed in Chapter 8 and
is not presented here.

Huntington's Disease

   George Huntington's original insightful observation that patients with Huntington's disease have an
increased rate of suicide has been amply confirmed
and extended. Dewhurst et al. (1969), in an extensive
study, found that a majority of Huntington's disease patients suffered from affective disturbances at some time
during the course of the illness, and these disturbances
constituted the principal reason for hospital admission
in 20 percent of cases. Both mania and depression have
been observed in association with Huntington's disease,
making it unlikely that the affective alterations are reactive in nature (Dewhurst et al., 1969; Folstein et al.,
1979; McHugh and Folstein, 1975).

   A schizophrenialike illness with prominent hallucinations and delusions also occurs with increased incidence among Huntington's disease patients (Caine
and Shoulson, 1983; Garron, 1973; McHugh and Folstein, 1975; Rosenbaum, 1941). Treatment of both
the schizophrenialike illness and affective disorders in
Huntington's disease is accomplished by use of the
same therapeutic modalities used in idiopathic psychiatric disorders.

Parkinson's Disease

   Idiopathic Parkinson's disease (paralysis agitans)
has an associated depression in 40–70 percent of cases
(Brown and Wilson, 1972; Celesia and Wanamaker,
1972; Jackson et al., 1923; Mindham, 1970). This
prevalence significantly exceeds that found in patients
with other illnesses and similar degrees of disability
such as paraplegics, medically ill patients, and patients
with mixed neurological and orthopedic disorders (Horn,
1974; Robins, 1976; Warburton, 1967). This excessive
rate of depression and the lack of improvement in depression despite considerable motoric improvement
following treatment with levodopa suggest that the

TABLE 12-12.   Differential Diagnosis of Chorea

Extrapyramidal diseases	Metabolic disorders
Huntington's disease	Hypoglycemia
Wilson's disease	Hypernatremia
Idiopathic basal ganglia calcification	Uremia
Benign familial chorea	Hepatocerebral degeneration
Choreoacanthocytosis	
Ataxia–telangiectasia	Drug-induced chorea
Spino–cerebellar degeneration	Tardive dyskinesia
Hallervorden-Spatz syndrome	Levodopa
Dystonia musculorum deformans	Amphetamines
	Tricyclic antidepressants
Infectious and inflammatory diseases	Isoniazid
Systemic lupus erythematosus	Lithium
General paresis (neurosyphilis)	Antihistamines
Viral encephalitides	Methylphenidate
Sydenham's chorea	Mercury
	Methadone
Endocrine conditions	Phenytoin
Hyperthyroidism	Ethosuximide
Hypoparathyroidism	Carbamazepine
Pregnancy (chorea gravidarum)	
Oral contraceptive administration	Miscellaneous
	Posthemiplegic choreoathetosis
	Postanoxic (including choreoathetotic cerebral palsy)
	Kernicterus
	Neoplasms
	Subdural hematomas

Reproduced from Cummings JL and Benson DF. *Dementia: a clinical approach*. Boston, Butterworths, 1983, Table 4-1. With permission from Butterworths Publishers.

depression is not reactive in origin, but is a reflection of the subcortical dysfunction of the Parkinson's disease (Mindham et al., 1976). The depression responds well to treatment with tricyclic antidepressants or electroconvulsive therapy (Anderson et al., 1980; Asnis, 1977; Laitinen, 1969; Lebensohn and Jenkins, 1975; Strang, 1965).

Postencephalitic Parkinson's disease was a permanent parkinsonian state that followed the 1919–1926 epidemic of von Economo's encephalitis. Postencephalitic Parkinson's disease has been associated with a remarkable number and diversity of psychopathological disorders, including depression, mania, a schizophrenialike psychosis, and obsessive–compulsive disorders (Bromberg, 1930; Fairweather, 1947; Jelliffe, 1929; Menninger, 1926; Sacks, 1976; Schilder, 1938). Most of those afflicted with postencephalitic Parkinson's disease have now died, and the disorder is currently uncommon, although sporadic cases continue to occur. Despite its rarity, postencephalitic Parkinson's disease with its many neuropsychiatric complications has tremendous importance in the history of the understanding of brain–behavior relationships. Appearing, as it did, simulta-

neously with the appearance and growing popularity of Freud's (1920) introduction of psychoanalysis, von Economo's encephalitis provided an undeniable link between brain disease and behavioral disturbances at a time when analytic explanations were increasingly invoked as causally deterministic of aberrant behavior.

Progressive Supranuclear Palsy

The tetrad of symptoms characterizing progressive supranuclear palsy is comprised of axial rigidity, supranuclear gaze palsy, pseudobulbar palsy, and mild dementia. In addition, depression is a not infrequent finding in the early and middle stages of the disease (Albert et al., 1974; Jackson et al., 1983; Kvale, 1982; Janati and Appel, 1984).

Wilson's Disease

Wilson's disease manifests a spectrum of associated psychopathological disorders similar to that of Huntington's disease and postencephalitic parkinsonism. Mania, depression, and a schizophrenialike illness

TABLE 12-13.   Psychiatric Disorders Occurring with Extrapyramidal Diseases

Extrapyramidal Disease	Psychiatric Disorder
Huntington's disease	Depression
	Mania
	Schizophrenialike psychosis
	Dementia
Parkinson's disease	
Idiopathic	Depression
	Dementia
Postencephalitic	Depression
	Mania
	Schizophrenialike psychosis
	Obsessive–compulsive disorder
	Dementia
Progressive supranuclear palsy	Dementia
	Depression
Wilson's disease	Depression
	Mania
	Schizophrenialike illness
	Dementia
Idiopathic basal ganglia calcification	Schizophrenialike psychosis
	Dementia
Meige's syndrome	Depression
	Obsessive–compulsive disorder
Spinocerebellar degeneration	Depression
	Schizophrenialike illness
	Dementia
Gilles de la Tourette syndrome	Obsessive–compulsive illness
	Hyperactivity

with hallucinations and delusions have all occurred in association with this inherited metabolic disorder, impacting primarily on the basal ganglia (Beard, 1959; Gysin and Cooke, 1950; Jackson and Immerman, 1919; Pandey et al., 1981; Scheinberg and Sternlieb, 1984).

Idiopathic Basal Ganglia Calcification

Idiopathic basal ganglia calcification (Fahr's disease) is an idiopathic extrapyramidal syndrome manifested by motor system abnormalities; neuropsychiatric disturbances; and extensive calcific deposits in the basal ganglia, thalamus, and cerebellar nuclei. Two clinical variants of the disorder have been described: a subcortical dementia and extrapyramidal movement disorder that has its onset around age 50 years, and a schizophrenialike illness that begins in the third or fourth decade (Bruyn et al., 1964; Cummings et al., 1983; Francis, 1979; Kalamboukis and Molling, 1962; Kasanin and Crank, 1935). The psychotic form of the disease eventually evolves to include the progressive de-

mentia and motor abnormalities, characteristic of the later-onset variety.

Meige's Syndrome

Meige's syndrome (also known as *Brueghel's syndrome*) is an idiopathic orofacial dystonia manifest by spontaneous blepharospasm, oromandibular dystonia, or both. In some cases the disorder progresses to involve the neck, upper limbs, or respiratory muscles (Marsden, 1976; Tolosa, 1981; Tolosa and Klawans, 1979). Depression has been noted in 25–40 percent of victims of the disease, and an association with obsessive–compulsive features has also been observed (Ashizawa et al., 1980; Jankovic and Ford, 1983; Tolosa, 1981). Meige's syndrome must be distinguished from the other causes of blepharospasm listed in Table 12-14.

Spinocerebellar Degenerations

The spinocerebellar degenerations are a heterogeneous group of disorders with variable degeneration of the spinal cord, cerebellum, and brainstem. In some

TABLE 12-14. Differential Diagnosis of Blinking and Blepharospasm

Extrapyramidal disorders

Meige's syndrome
Parkinson's disease
Huntington's disease
Wilson's disease
Gilles de la Tourette syndrome
Tic syndromes (non-Gilles de la Tourette)
Progressive supranuclear palsy
Dystonia musculorum deformans
Idiopathic basal ganglia calcification
Rheumatic chorea

Drug-induced

Antipsychotic agents
    Tardive dyskinesia (tardive Meige syndrome)
    Acute dyskinesia (accompanying oculogyric crises)
Antiemetic agents
Antihistamine agents
Levodopa
Bromocriptine
Phenytoin
Carbamazepine
Phenobarbital

Miscellaneous

Acquired midbrain disease

    Brainstem stroke
    Encephalitis
    Multiple sclerosis

Hemifacial spasm
Facial nerve aberrant regeneration (following Bell's palsy)
Myokymia (with multiple sclerosis)
Myotonia
Tetany
Tetanus
Ocular irritation
Central dazzle (painless photophobia with thalamic
    infarction)
Pseudobulbar palsy
Tic douloureux
Seizures (petit mal, complex partial)
Conversion reaction
Schizophrenia

Data from Frankel and Cummings (1984), Henderson (1956), and Jankovic et al (1982).

TABLE 12-15. Classification of Primary Tic Syndromes

Transient tic of childhood

Multiple tic of childhood or adolescence

Invariant tic beginning in childhood (single or multiple tics)

Invariant tic beginning in adulthood (usually single)

Gilles de la Tourette syndrome

    Classic type
    With other extrapyramidal features

        Dystonia
        Choreoathetosis

    With neuropsychiatric complications

        Hyperactivity
        Obsessive–compulsive disorder

is sometimes accompanied by a schizophrenialike illness labeled "Friedreich's psychosis" (Davies, 1949; Shepherd, 1955).

Gilles da la Tourette Syndrome

The Gilles de la Tourette syndrome is a chronic multiple tic syndrome characterized by multiple somatic tics and involuntary vocalizations beginning between the ages of 2 and 15 years and exhibiting a life-long waxing and waning course (Shapiro et al., 1978). There is no compromise of intellect in Gilles de la Tourette syndrome, but there is significant increase in the prevalence of obsessive–compulsive disorder and of hyperactivity in childhood (Chapter 15) (Corbett et al., 1969; Fernando, 1967; Montgomery et al., 1982; Morphew and Sim, 1969; Nee et al., 1980, 1982; Shapiro et al., 1978).

Gilles de la Tourette syndrome must be distinguished from a variety of other tic syndromes (Table 12-15) and from myoclonus. Tics are differentiated from myoclonus by their stereotyped distribution, sometimes complex character, suppression by neuroleptic agents, and susceptibility to temporary volitional control. Non-Gilles de la Tourette tic syndromes include transient tics of childhood that remit within 1 year, multiple tics of childhood or adolescence that may persist for several years but remit during the adolescent period, invariant tic syndromes (single or multiple) of childhood that begin early in life and continue unchanged throughout life, and invariant tic syndromes of adulthood that are usually characterized by a single tic beginning after adolescence and persisting throughout life (Shapiro and Shapiro, 1977).

cases, pathological changes extend to involve the basal ganglia, thalamus, and/or subthalamic structures. A number of patients have manifested depression or psychosis during the course of the illness (Chandler and Begin, 1956; Richards et al., 1974). Friedreich's ataxia

REFERENCES

Abrams R and Taylor MA. Catatonia. A prospective clinical study. *Arch Gen Psychiat*, 1976, *33*, 579–581.

Abrams R and Taylor MA. Catatonia: prediction of response to somatic treatments. *Am J Psychiat*, 1977, *134*, 78–80.

Albert ML, Feldman RG, and Willis AL. The "subcortical dementia" of progressive supranuclear palsy. *J Neurol Neurosurg Psychiat*, 1974, *37*, 121–130.

Alpert M. Speech and disturbances of affect. In Darby JK (Ed).: *Speech evaluation in psychiatry.* New York, Grune & Stratton, 1981, pp. 359–367.

Anderson J, Aabro E, Gulman N, Hjelmsted A, and Pederson HE. Anti-depressive treatment in Parkinson's disease. *Acta Neurol Scand*, 1980, *62*, 210–219.

Andreasen NC and Olsen S. Negative *v* positive schizophrenia. *Arch Gen Psychiat*, 1982, *39*, 789–794.

Angle CR and McIntire MS. Persistent dystonia in a brain-damaged child after ingestion of phenothiazine. *J Pediat*, 1968, *73*, 124–126.

Angus JWS and Simpson GM. Handwriting changes and response to drugs—a controlled study. *Acta Psychiat Scand*, 1970, Suppl. 212, 28–37.

Apte SN and Langston JW. Permanent neurological deficits due to lithium toxicity. *Ann Neurol*, 1983, *13*, 453–455.

Ashcroft GW, Eccleston D, and Waddell JL. Recognition of amphetamine addicts. *Br Med J*, 1965, *1*, 57.

Ashizawa T, Patten BM, and Jankovic J. Meige's syndrome. *South Med J*, 1980, *73*, 863–866.

Asnis G. Parkinson's disease, depression, and ECT: a review and case study. *Am J Psychiat*, 1977, *134*, 191–194.

Asnis GM, Asnis D, Dunner DL, and Fieve RR. Cogwheel rigidity during chronic lithium therapy. *Am J Psychiat*, 1979, *136*, 1225–1226.

Ayd FJ Jr. A survey of drug-induced extrapyramidal reactions. *JAMA*, 1961, *175*, 1054–1060.

Barnes TRE, Rossor M, and Trauer T. A comparison of purposeless movements in psychiatric patients treated with antipsychotic drugs and normal individuals. *J Neurol Neurosurg Psychiat*, 1983, *46*, 540–546.

Beard AW. The association of hepatolenticular degeneration with schizophrenia. *Acta Psychiat Neurol*, 1959, *34*, 411–428.

Bech P, Thomsen J, Prytz S, Vendsborg PB, Zilstorff K, and Rafaelsen OJ. The profile and severity of lithium-induced side effects in mentally healthy subjects. *Neuropsychobiology*, 1979, *5*, 160–166.

Beitman BD. Tardive dyskinesia reinduced by lithium carbonate. *Am J Psychiat*, 1978, *135*, 1229–1230.

Belfer ML and d'Autremont CC. Catatonia-like symptomatology. *Arch Gen Psychiat*, 1971, *24*, 119–120.

Berger PA and Rexroth K. Tardive dyskinesia: clinical, biological, and pharmacological perspectives. *Schiz Bull*, 1980, *6*, 102–116.

Birket-Smith E. Abnormal involuntary movements induced by anticholinergic therapy. *Acta Neurol Scand*, 1974, *50*, 801–811.

Bleuler E. *Dementia praecox or the group of schizophrenias* (translated by Zinkin J). New York, International Universities Press, 1950.

Bobruff A, Gardos G, Tarsy D, Rapkin RM, Cole JO, and Moore P. Clonazepam and phenobarbital in tardive dyskinesia. *Am J Psychiat*, 1981, *138*, 189–193.

Bone S, Roose SP, Dunner DL, and Fieve RR. Incidence of side effects in patients on long-term lithium therapy. *Am J Psychiat*, 1980, *137*, 103–104.

Borison RL, Hitri A, Blowers AJ, and Diamond BI. Antipsychotic drug action: clinical, biochemical, and pharmacological evidence for site specificity of action. *Clin Neuropharmacol*, 1983, *6*, 137–150.

Brainin M, Reisner TH, and Zeitlhofer J. Tardive dyskinesia: clinical correlation with computed tomography in patients aged less than 60 years. *J Neurol Neurosurg Psychiat*, 1983, *46*, 1037–1040.

Branchey MH, Charles J, and Simpson GM. Extrapyramidal side effects in lithium maintenance therapy. *Am J Psychiat*, 1976, *133*, 444–445.

Brandon S, McClelland HA, and Protheroe C. A study of facial dyskinesia in a mental hospital population. *Br J Psychiat*, 1971, *118*, 171–184.

Braude WM and Barnes TRE. Late-onset akathisia—an indicant of covert dyskinesia: two case reports. *Am J Psychiat*, 1983, *140*, 611–612.

Brenner I and Rheuban WJ. The catatonic dilemma. *Am J Psychiat*, 1978, *135*, 1242–1243.

Bromberg W. Mental states in chronic encephalitis. *Psychiat Quart*, 1930, *4*, 537–566.

Brown GL and Wilson WP. Parkinsonism and depression. *South Med J*, 1972, *65*, 540–545.

Bruyn GW, Bots GthAM, and Staal A. Familial bilateral vascular calcification in the central nervous system. *Psychiat Neurol Neurochir*, 1964, *67*, 342–346.

Burke RE, Fahn S, Jankovic J, Marsden CD, Lang AE, Gollomp S, and Ilson J. Tardive dystonia: late-onset and persistent dystonia caused by antipsychotic drugs. *Neurology*, 1982, *32*, 1335–1346.

Burks JS, Walker JE, Rumack BH, and Ott JE. Tricyclic antidepressant poisoning. Reversal of coma, choreoathetosis, and myoclonus by physostigmine. *JAMA*, 1974, *230*, 1405–1407.

Caine ED and Shoulson I. Psychiatric syndromes in Huntington's disease. *Am J Psychiat*, 1983, *140*, 728–733.

Campbell R, Schaffer CB, and Tupin J. Catatonia associated with glutethimide withdrawal. *J Clin Psychiat*, 1983, *44*, 32–33.

Carlson GA and Goodwin FK. The stages of mania. *Arch Gen Psychiat*, 1973, *28*, 221–228.

Carpenter WT Jr and Stephens JH. The diagnosis of mania. In Belmaker RH and van Pragg HM (Eds.): *Mania: An evolving concept.* Lancaster, England, MTP Press, 1980, pp. 7–24.

Casey DE and Rabins P. Tardive dyskinesia as a life-threatening illness. *Am J Psychiat*, 1978, *135*, 486–488.

Celesia GG and Wanamaker WM. Psychiatric disturbances in Parkinson's disease. *Dis Nerv Syst*, 1972, *33*, 577–583.

Chadwick D, Reynolds EH, and Marsden CD. Anticonvulsant-induced dyskinesias: a comparison with dyskinesias induced by neuroleptics. *J Neurol Neurosurg Psychiat*, 1976, *39*, 1210–1218.

Chandler JH and Begin J. Hereditary cerebellar ataxia. Olivopontocerebellar type. *Neurology*, 1956, *6*, 187–195.

Chaudhry R, Radonjic D, and Waters B. Efficacy of propranolol in a patient with tardive dyskinesia and extrapyramidal syndrome. *Am J Psychiat*, 1982, *139*, 674–676.

Chouinard G, Annable L, Ross-Chouinard A, and Nestorus JN. Factors related to tardive dyskinesia. *Am J Psychiat*, 1979, *136*, 79–83.

Christensen E, Moller JE, and Faurbye A. Neuropathological investigation of 28 brains from patients with dyskinesia. *Acta Psychiat Scand*, 1970, *46*, 14–23.

Corbett JA, Matthews AM, Connell PH, and Shapiro DA. Tics and Gilles de la Tourette syndrome: a follow-up study and critical review. *Br J Psychiat*, 1969, *115*, 1229–1241.

Crane GE. Dyskinesia and neuroleptics. *Arch Gen Psychiat*, 1968, *19*, 700–703.

Crane GE. Pseudoparkinsonism and tardive dyskinesia. *Arch Neurol*, 1972, *27*, 426–430.

Crane GE. Persistent dyskinesia. *Br J Psychiat*, 1973, *122*, 395–405.

Crews EL and Carpenter AE. Lithium-induced aggravation of tardive dyskinesia. *Am J Psychiat*, 1977, *134*, 933.

Cummings JL and Benson DF. *Dementia: a clinical approach.* Boston, Butterworths, 1983.

Cummings JL, Gosenfeld LF, Houlihan JP, and McCaffrey T. Neuropsychiatric disturbances associated with idiopathic calcification of the basal ganglia. *Biol Psychiat*, 1983, *18*, 591–601.

Cutler NR, Post RM, Rey AC, and Bunney WE Jr. Depression-dependent dyskinesias in two cases of manic–depressive illness. *New Engl J Med*, 1981, *304*, 1088–1089.

Davies DL. Psychiatric changes associated with Friedreich's ataxia. *J Neurol Neurosurg Psychiat*, 1949, *12*, 246–250.

Davis KL, Berger PA, and Hollister LE. Tardive dyskinesia and depressive illness. *Psychopharmacol Commun*, 1976, *2*, 125–130.

De Fraites EG Jr, Davis KL, and Berger PA. Coexisting tardive dyskinesia and parkinsonism: a case report. *Biol Psychiat*, 1977, *12*, 267–272.

DeVeaugh-Geiss J. Tardive Tourette syndrome. *Neurology*, 1980, *30*, 562–563.

Dewhurst K, Oliver J, Trick KLK, and McKnight AL. Neuropsychiatric aspects of Huntington's disease. *Confin Neurol*, 1969, *31*, 258–268.

Donaldson J MacG and Cunningham J. Persisting neurologic sequelae of lithium carbonate therapy. *Arch Neurol*, 1983, *40*, 747–751.

Ekbom KA. Restless legs syndrome. *Neurology*, 1960, *10*, 868–873.

Extein I. Methylphenidate-induced choreoathetosis. *Am J Psychiat*, 1978, *135*, 252–253.

Faheem AD, Brightwell DR, Burton GC, and Struss A. Respiratory dyskinesia and dysarthria from prolonged neuroleptic use: tardive dyskinesia? *Am J Psychiat*, 1982, *139*, 517–518.

Fahn S. Differential diagnosis of tremors. *Med Clin N Am*, 1972, *56*, 1363–1375.

Fahn S and Eldridge R. Definition of dystonia and classification of the dystonic states. *Adv Neurol*, 1976, *14*, 1–5.

Fairweather DS. Psychiatric aspects of the post-encephalitic syndrome. *J Ment Sci*, 1947, *93*, 201–254.

Fann WE, Davis JM, and Janowsky DS. The prevalence of tardive dyskinesia in mental hospital patients. *Dis Nerv Syst*, 1972, *33*, 182–186.

Fann WE and Lake R. On the coexistence of parkinsonism and tardive dyskinesia. *Dis Nerv Syst*, 1974, *35*, 324–326.

Fann WE, Sullivan JL, and Richman BW. Dyskinesias associated with tricyclic antidepressants. *Br J Psychiat*, 1976, *128*, 490–493.

Fernando SJM. Gilles de la Tourette's syndrome. *Br J Psychiat*, 1967, *113*, 607–617.

Fish B. Neurobiologic antecedents of schizophrenia in children. *Arch Gen Psychiat*, 1977, *34*, 1297–1313.

Fogg R and Pakkenberg H. Theoretical and clinical aspects of the Tourette syndrome (chronic multiple tic). *J Neurol Transmission*, 1980, Suppl. 16, 211–215.

Folstein SE, Folstein MF, and McHugh PR. Psychiatric syndromes in Huntington's disease. *Adv Neurol*, 1979, *23*, 281–289.

Food and Drug Administration Task Force. Neurologic syndromes associated with antipsychotic-drug use. *New Engl J Med*, 1973, *289*, 20–23.

Francis AF. Familial basal ganglia calcification and schizophreniform psychosis. *Br J Psychiat*, 1979, *135*, 360–362.

Frankel M and Cummings JL. Neuro-ophthalmic abnormalities in Gilles de la Tourette syndrome: functional and anatomic implications. *Neurology*, 1984, *34*, 359–361.

Freud S. *A general introduction to psychoanalysis* (translated by Riviere J). New York, Liverwright Publishing Corporation, 1920.

Gaby NS, Lefkowitz DS, and Israel JR. Treatment of lithium tremor with metoprolol. *Am J Psychiat*, 1983, *140*, 593–595.

Gangadhar BN, Keshavan MS, Goswami U, and Rao TV. Cortical venous thrombosis presenting as catatonia: a clinicopathologic report. *J Clin Psychiat*, 1983, *44*, 109–110.

Gardos G and Cole JO. The prognosis of tardive dyskinesia. *J Clin Psychiat*, 1983, *44*, 177–179.

Gardos G, Cole JO, and Tarsey D. Withdrawal syndromes associated with antipsychotic drugs. *Am J Psychiat*, 1978, *135*, 1321–1324.

Garron DC. Huntington's disease and schizophrenia. *Adv Neurol*, 1973, *1*, 729–734.

Garver DL, Davis JM, Dekirmenjian H, Tones FD, Casper R, and Haraszti J. Pharmacokinetics of red blood cell phenothiazine and clinical effects. Acute dystonic reaction. *Arch Gen Psychiat*, 1976, *33*, 862–866.

Gelenberg AJ. The catatonic syndrome. *Lancet*, 1976a, *1*, 1339–1341.

Gelenberg AJ. Computerized tomography in patients with tardive dyskinesia. *Am J Psychiat*, 1976b, *133*, 578–579.

Gelenberg AJ, Doller-Wojcik JC, and Growdon JH. Choline

and lecithin in the treatment of tardive dyskinesia: preliminary results from a pilot study. *Am J Psychiat*, 1979, *136*, 772–776.

Gelenberg AJ and Mandel MR. Catatonic reactions to high-potency neuroleptic drugs. *Arch Gen Psychiat*, 1977, *34*, 947–950.

Gerlach J. The relationship between parkinsonism and tardive dyskinesia. *Am J Psychiat*, 1977, *134*, 781–784.

Gerlach J, Reisby N, and Raudrup A. Dopaminergic hypersensitivity and cholinergic hypofuction in the pathophysiology of tardive dyskinesia. *Psychopharmacologia*, 1974, *34*, 21–35.

Gjessing LR. A review of periodic catatonia. *Biol Psychiat*, 1974, *8*, 23–45.

Gjessing R and Gjessing L. Some main trends in the clinical aspects of periodic catatonia. *Acta Psychiat Scand*, 1961, *37*, 1–13.

Glazer WM, Moore DC, Hansen TC, and Brenner LM. Meige syndrome and tardive dyskinesia. *Am J Psychiat*, 1983, *140*, 798–799.

Gomez EA, Comstock BS, and Rosario A. Organic versus functional etiology in catatonia: case report. *J Clin Psychiat*, 1982, *43*, 200–201.

Good MI. Reversibility of long-term tardive dyskinesia associated with antiparkinsonian medication: a case report. *Am J Psychiat*, 1981, *138*, 1112–1113.

Granacher RP. Differential diagnosis of tardive dyskinesia: an overview. *Am J Psychiat*, 1981, *138*, 1288–1297.

Greden JF, Albala AA, Smokler IA, Gardner R, and Carroll BJ. Speech pause time: a marker of psychomotor retardation among endogenous depressives. *Biol Psychiat*, 1981, *16*, 851–859.

Growdon JH, Hirsch MJ, Wurtman RJ, and Wiener W. Oral choline administration to patients with tardive dyskinesia. *New Engl J Med*, 1977, *297*, 524–527.

Gupta JM and Lovejoy FH Jr. Acute phenothiazine toxicity in children: a five-year study. *Pediatrics*, 1967, *39*, 771–774.

Guggenheim FG and Babigan HM. Catatonic schizophrenia: epidemiology and clinical course. *J Nerv Ment Dis*, 1974, *158*, 291–305.

Gysin WM and Cooke ET. Unusual mental symptoms in a case of hepatolenticular degeneration. *Dis Nerv Syst*, 1950, *28*, 305–309.

Hall RA, Jackson RB, and Swain JM. Neurotoxic reactions resulting from chlorpromazine administration. *JAMA*, 1956, *161*, 214–218.

Hamilton M. *Fish's schizophrenia*, 2nd ed. Bristol, England, John Wright and Sons, 1976.

Hausner RS. Neuroleptic-induced parkinsonism and Parkinson's disease: differential diagnosis and treatment. *J Clin Psychiat*, 1983, *44*, 13–16.

Henderson JW. Essential blepharospasm. *Trans Am Ophthalmol Soc*, 1956, *54*, 453–520.

Herman M, Harpham D, and Rosenblum M. Nonschizophrenic catatonic states. *NY State J Med*, 1942, *42*, 624–627.

Hockaday TDR, Keynes WM, and McKenzie JK. Catatonic stupor in elderly woman with hyperparathyroidism. *Br Med J*, 1966, *1*, 85–87.

Hoffman DF. The diagnosis and treatment of neuroleptic-induced parkinsonism. *Hosp Commun Psychiat*, 1981, *32*, 110–114.

Horn S. Some psychological factors in parkinsonism. *J Neurol Neurosurg Psychiat*, 1974, *37*, 27–31.

Hunter R, Blackwood W, Smith MC, and Cummings JN. Neuropathological findings in three cases of persistent dyskinesia following phenothiazine medication. *J Neurol Sci*, 1968, *7*, 263–273.

Hunter R, Earl CJ, and Thornicroft S. An apparently irreversible syndrome of abnormal movements following phenothiazine medication. *Proc Roy Soc Med*, 1964, *57*, 758–762.

Jackson IV, Davis LG, Cohen RK, and Nuttall EA. Lecithin administration in tardive dyskinesia: clinical and biomedical correlates. *Biol Psychiat*, 1981, *16*, 85–90.

Jackson IV, Volavka J, James B, and Reker D. The respiratory components of tardive dyskinesia. *Biol Psychiat*, 1980, *15*, 485–487.

Jackson JA, Free GBM, and Pike HV. The psychic manifestations in paralysis agitans. *Arch Neurol Psychiat*, 1923, *10*, 680–684.

Jackson JA and Immerman SL. A case of pseudosclerosis associated with a psychosis. *J Nerv Ment Dis*, 1919, *49*, 5–13.

Jackson JA, Jankovic J, and Ford J. Progressive supranuclear palsy: clinical features and response to treatment in 16 patients. *Ann Neurol*, 1983, *13*, 273–278.

Jaffe N. Catatonia and hepatic dysfunction. *Dis Nerv Syst*, 1967, *28*, 606–608.

Janati A and Appel AR. Psychiatric aspects of progressive supranuclear palsy. *J Nerv Ment Dis*, 1984, *172*, 85–89.

Jankovic J. Drug-induced and other orofacial–cervical dyskinesias. *Ann Int Med*, 1981, *94*, 788–793.

Jankovic J. Treatment of hyperkinetic movement disorders with tetrabenazine: a double-blind crossover study. *Ann Neurol*, 1982, *11*, 41–47.

Jankovic J and Fahn S. Physiologic and pathologic tremors. Diagnosis, mechanism, and management. *Ann Int Med*, 1980, *93*, 460–465.

Jankovic J and Ford J. Blepharospasm and orofacial–cervical dystonia: clinical and pharmacological findings in 100 patients. *Ann Neurol*, 1983, *13*, 402–411.

Jankovic J, Havins WE, and Wilkins RB. Blinking and blepharospasm. *JAMA*, 1982, *248*, 3160–3164.

Jelliffe SE. Oculogyric crises as compulsion phenomena in postencephalitis: their occurrence, phenomenology, and meaning. *J Nerv Ment Dis*, 1929, *69*, 59–68, 165–184, 278–297, 415–426, 531–551, 666–679.

Jeste DV, Cutler NR, Kaufman CA, and Karoum F. Low-dose apomorphine and bromocriptine in neuroleptic-induced movement disorders. *Biol Psychiat*, 1983, *18*, 1085–1091.

Jeste DV, Doongaji DR, and Linnoila M. Elevated cerebrospinal fluid noradrenalin in tardive dyskinesia. *Br J Psychiat*, 1984, *144*, 177–180.

Jeste DV, Potkin SG, Sinha S, Feder S, and Wyatt RJ. Tardive dyskinesia—reversible and persistent. *Arch Gen Psychiat*, 1979a, *36*, 585–590.

Jeste DV, Rosenblatt JE, Wagner RL, and Wyatt RJ. High serum neuroleptic levels in tardive dyskinesia? *New Engl J Med*, 1979b, *301*, 1184.

Jeste DV and Wyatt RJ. *Understanding and treating tardive dyskinesia*. New York, Guilford Press, 1982.

Jones IH. Observations on schizophrenic stereotypies. *Comp Psychiat*, 1965, *6*, 323–335.

Joyce RP and Gunderson CH. Carbamazepine-induced orofacial dyskinesia. *Neurology*, 1980, *30*, 1333–1334.

Joyston-Bechol MP. The clinical features and outcome of stupor. *Br J Psychiat*, 1966, *112*, 967–981.

Kahlbaum KL. *Catatonia*. (Translated by Levij Y and Pridau T). Baltimore, Johns Hopkins University Press, 1973.

Kalamboukis Z and Molling P. Symmetrical calcification of the brain in the predominance in the basal ganglia and cerebellum. *J Neuropathol Exp Neurol*, 1962, *21*, 364–371.

Kane J, Rifkin A, Quitkin F, and Klein DF. Extrapyramidal side effects with lithium treatment. *Am J Psychiat*, 1978, *135*, 851–853.

Kane JM, Rifkin A, Woerner M, Reardon G, Sarantakos S, Schiebel D, and Ramos-Lorenzi J. Low-dose neuroleptic treatment of outpatient schizophrenics. I. Preliminary results for relapse rates. *Arch Gen Psychiat*, 1983, *40*, 893–896.

Kane JM and Smith JM. Tardive dyskinesia. Prevalence and risk factors, 1959 to 1979. *Arch Gen Psychiat*, 1982, *39*, 473–481.

Kaplan SR and Murkofsky C. Oral–buccal dyskinesia symptoms associated with low-dose benzodiazepine treatment. *Am J Psychiat*, 1978, *135*, 1558–1559.

Karp JM, Perkel MS, Hersh T, and McKinney AS. Metoclopramide treatment of tardive dyskinesia. *JAMA*, 1981, *246*, 1934–1935.

Kasanin J and Crank RP. A case of extensive calcification in the brain. *Arch Neurol Psychiat*, 1935, *34*, 164–178.

Kazamatsuri H, Chien C-P, and Cole JO. Treatment of tardive dyskinesia. I. Clinical efficacy of a dopamine-depleting agent, tetrabenazine. *Arch Gen Psychiat*, 1972, *27*, 95–99.

Kazamatsuri H, Chien C-P, and Cole JO. Long-term treatment of tardive dyskinesia with haloperidol and tetrabenazine. *Am J Psychiat*, 1973, *130*, 479–483.

Kiloh LG, Smith JS, and Williams SE. Antiparkinson drugs as casual agents in tardive dyskinesia. *Med J Aust*, 1973, *2*, 591–593.

Kim CH and Perlstein MA. Encephalitis with catatonic schizophrenic symptoms. *Ill Med J*, 1970, *138*, 503–507.

Kirby GH. The catatonic syndrome and its relation to manic-depressive insanity. *J Nerv Ment Dis*, 1913, *40*, 694–704.

Kirk L, Baastrup PC, and Schou M. Propranolol treatment of lithium-induced tremor. *Lancet*, 1973, *2*, 1086–1087.

Kirubakaran V, Mayfield D, and Rengachary S. Dyskinesia and psychosis in a patient following baclofen withdrawal. *Am J Psychiat*, 1984, *141*, 692–693.

Klawans HL Jr. The pharmacology of tardive dyskinesia. *Am J Psychiat*, 1973, *130*, 82–86.

Klawans HL and Barr A. Prevalence of spontaneous lingual-facial-buccal dyskinesias in the elderly. *Neurology*, 1982, *32*, 558–559.

Klawans HL, Bergen D, Bruyn GW, and Paulson GW. Neuroleptic-induced tardive dyskinesias in nonpsychotic patients. *Arch Neurol*, 1974, *30*, 338–339.

Klawans HL, Falk DK, Nausieda PA, and Weiner WJ. Gilles de la Tourette syndrome after long-term chlorpromazine therapy. *Neurology*, 1978, *28*, 1064–1068.

Klawans HL, Goetz CG, and Perlik S. Tardive dyskinesia: review and update. *Am J Psychiat*, 1980, *137*, 900–908.

Klawans HL and Rubovits R. Effect of cholinergic and anticholinergic agents on tardive dyskinesia. *J Neurol Neurosurg Psychiat*, 1974, *37*, 941–947.

Kobayashi RM. Drug therapy of tardive dyskinesia. *New Engl J Med*, 1977, *296*, 257–260.

Koehler K and Jakumeit U. Subacute sclerosing panencephalitis presenting as Leonhard's speech-prompt catatonia. *Br J Psychiat*, 1976, *129*, 29–31.

Koller WC. Edentulous orodyskinesia. *Ann Neurol*, 1983, *13*, 97–99.

Korsgaard S. Baclofen (Lioresal) in the treatment of neuroleptic-induced tardive dyskinesia. *Acta Psychiat Scand*, 1976, *54*, 17–24.

Kraepelin E. *Dementia praecox and paraphrenia* (translated by Barclay RM). Huntington, New York, Robert E Krieger Publishing Company, 1971.

Kruse W. Persistent muscular restlessness after phenothiazine treatment: report of 3 cases. *Am J Psychiat*, 1960, *117*, 152–157.

Kvale JN. Amitriptyline in the management of progressive supranuclear palsy. *Arch Neurol*, 1982, *39*, 387–388.

Laitenen L. Desipramine in treatment of Parkinson's disease. *Acta Neurol Scand*, 1969, *45*, 109–113.

Lang AE. Lithium and parkinsonism. *Ann Neurol*, 1984, *15*, 214.

Lapierre YD. Control of lithium tremor with propranolol. *Can Med Assoc J*, 1976, *114*, 619–624.

Lapierre YD and Anderson K. Dyskinesia associated with amoxapine antidepressant therapy: a case report. *Am J Psychiat*, 1983, *140*, 493–494.

Lebensohn ZM and Jenkins RB. Improvement of parkinsonism in depressed patients treated with ECT. *Am J Psychiat*, 1975, *132*, 283–285.

Leff JP and Isaacs AD. *Psychiatric examination in clinical practice*, 2nd ed. London, Blackwell Scientific Publications, 1981.

Lipinski JR Jr, Zubenko GS, Cohen BM, and Barreira PJ. Propronolol in the treatment of neuroleptic-induced akathisia. *Am J Psychiat*, 1984, *141*, 412–415.

Lippmann S, Moskovitz R, and O'Tuama L. Tricyclic-induced myoclonus. *Am J Psychiat*, 1977, *134*, 90–91.

Mac DS and Pardo MP. Systemic lupus erythematosis and catatonia: a case report. *J Clin Psychiat*, 1983, *44*, 155–156.

Mackay AVP and Sheppard GP. Pharmacotherapeutic trials in tardive dyskinesia. *Br J Psychiat*, 1979, *135*, 489–499.

Marsden CD. Blepharospasm–oromandibular dystonia syndrome (Brueghel's syndrome). *J Neurol Neurosurg Psychiat*, 1976, *39*, 1204–1209.

Marsden CD and Jenner P. The pathophysiology of extrapyramidal side-effects of neuroleptic drugs. *Psychol Med*, 1980, *10*, 55–72.

Marsden CD, Tarsy D, and Baldessarini RJ. Spontaneous and drug-induced movement disorders in psychotic patients. In Benson DF and Blumer D (Eds.): *Psychiatric aspects of neurologic disease*. New York, Grune & Stratton, 1975, pp. 219–265.

Marshall J. The effect of ageing upon physiological tremor. *J Neurol Neurosurg Psychiat*, 1961, *24*, 14–17.

McAllister RG Jr. Fever, tachycardia, and hypertension with acute catatonic schizophrenia. *Arch Int Med*, 1978, *138*, 1154–1156.

McGeer PL, Boulding JE, Gibson WC, and Foulkes RG. Drug-induced extrapyramidal reactions. *JAMA*, 1961, *177*, 665–670.

McHugh PR and Folstein MF. Psychiatric syndromes of Huntington's chorea: a clinical and phenomenologic study. In Benson DF and Blumer D (Eds.): *Psychiatric aspects of neurologic disease*. New York, Grune & Stratton, 1975, pp. 267–285.

McLean P and Casey DE. Tardive dyskinesia in an adolescent. *Am J Psychiat*, 1978, *135*, 969–971.

Menninger KA. Influenza and schizophrenia. *Am J Psychiat*, 1926, *82*, 469–529.

Mettler FA and Crandell A. Neurologic disorders in psychiatric institutions. *J Nerv Ment Dis*, 1959, *128*, 148–159.

Mindham RHS. Psychiatric symptoms in parkinsonism. *J Neurol Neurosurg Psychiat*, 1970, *33*, 188–191.

Mindham RHS, Marsden CD, and Parkes JD. Psychiatric symptoms during L-dopa therapy for Parkinson's disease and their relationship to physical disability. *Psychol Med*, 1976, *6*, 23–33.

Misra PC and Hay GG. Encephalitis presenting as acute schizophrenia. *Br Med J*, 1971, *1*, 532–533.

Montgomery MA, Clayton PJ, and Friedhoff AJ. Psychiatric illness in Tourette syndrome patients and first-degree relatives. In Friedhoff AJ and Chase TN (Eds.): *Gilles de la Tourette syndrome*. New York, Raven Press, 1982, pp. 335–339.

Morphew JA and Sim M. Gilles de la Tourette's syndrome: a clinical and psychopathological study. *Br J Med Psychol*, 1969, *42*, 293–301.

Morrison JR. Catatonia. Retarded and excited types. *Arch Gen Psychiat*, 1973, *28*, 39–41.

Moss HB and Green A. Neuroleptic-associated dysphagia confirmed by esophageal manometry. *Am J Psychiat*, 1982, *139*, 515–516.

Mueller J and Aminoff MJ. Tourette-like syndrome after long-term neuroleptic treatment. *Br J Psychiat*, 1982, *141*, 191–193.

Mukherjee S, Rosen AM, Cardenas C, Varia V, and Olarte S. Tardive dyskinesia in psychiatric outpatients. *Arch Gen Psychiat*, 1982, *39*, 466–469.

Myrianthopoulos NC, Kurland AA, and Kurland LT. Hereditary predisposition in drug-induced parkinsonism. *Arch Neurol*, 1962, *6*, 5–9.

Myslobodsky MS, Holden T, and Sandler R. Asymmetry of abnormal involuntary movements: a prevalence study. *Biol Psychiat*, 1984, *19*, 623–628.

Nee LE, Caine ED, Polinski RJ, Eldridge R, and Ebert MH. Gilles de la Tourette syndrome: clinical and family study of 50 cases. *Ann Neurol*, 1980, *7*, 41–49.

Nee LE, Polinsky RJ, and Ebert MH. Tourette syndrome: clinical and family studies. In Friedhoff AJ and Chase TN (Eds.): *Gilles de la Tourette syndrome*. New York, Raven Press, 1982, pp. 291–295.

Newmann MA. Periventricular diffuse pinealoma. Report of a case with clinical features of catatonic schizophrenia. *J Nerv Ment Dis*, 1955, *121*, 193–204.

Osifo NG. Drug-related transient dyskinesia. *Clin Pharm Ther*, 1979, *25*, 767–771.

Owens DGC, Johnstone EC, and Frith CD. Spontaneous involuntary disorders of movement. *Arch Gen Psychiat*, 1982, *39*, 452–461.

Pandey RS, Sreenivas KN, Patil NM, and Swamy NS. Dopamine β-hydroxylase inhibition in a patient with Wilson's disease and manic symptoms. *Am J Psychiat*, 1981, *138*, 1628–1629.

Penn H, Racy J, Lapham L, Mandel M, and Sandt J. Catatonic behavior, viral encephalopathy, and death. *Arch Gen Psychiat*, 1972, *27*, 758–761.

Peters JE, Romine JS, and Dykman RA. A special neurological examination of children with learning disabilities. *Dev Med Child Neurol*, 1975, *17*, 63–78.

Petursson H. Lithium treatment of a patient with periodic catatonia. *Acta Psychiat Scand*, 1976, *54*, 248–253.

Pullinger S and Tyrer P. Acute lithium-induced tremor. *Br J Psychiat*, 1983, *143*, 40–41.

Quitkin F, Rifkin A, and Klein DF. Neurologic soft signs in schizophrenia and character disorders. *Arch Gen Psychiat*, 1976, *33*, 845–853.

Rajput AH, Rozdilsky B, Hornykiewicz O, Shannak K, Lee T, and Seeman P. Reversible drug-induced parkinsonism. Clinicopathologic study of two cases. *Arch Neurol*, 1982, *39*, 644–646.

Raskin DE and Frank SW. Herpes encephalitis with catatonic stupor. *Arch Gen Psychiat*, 1974, *31*, 544–546.

Read SL. Catatonia in thrombotic thrombocytopenic purpura: case report. *J Clin Psychiat*, 1983, *44*, 343–344.

Reches A, Tietler J, and Lavy S. Parkinsonism due to lithium carbonate poisoning. *Arch Neurol*, 1981, *38*, 471.

Reda FA, Scanlan JM, Kemp K, and Escobar JI. Treatment of tardive dyskinesia with lithium carbonate. *New Engl J Med*, 1974, *291*, 850.

Reisberg B. Catatonia associated with disulfiram therapy. *J Nerv Ment Dis*, 1978, *166*, 607–609.

Richards F II, Cooper MR, Pearce LA, Cowan RJ, and Spurr CL. Familial spinocerebellar degeneration, hemolytic anemia, and glutathione deficiency. *Arch Int Med*, 1974, *134*, 534–537.

Richardson MA and Craig TJ. The coexistence of parkinsonism-like symptoms and tardive dyskinesia. *Am J Psychiat*, 1982, *139*, 341–343.

Robins AH. Depression in patients with parkinsonism. *Br J Psychiat*, 1976, *128*, 141–145.

Rondot P, Jedynak CP, and Ferrey G. Pathological tremors: nosological correlates. *Progr Clin Neurophysiol*, 1978, *5*, 95–113.

Rosen PB and Stevens R. Action myoclonus in lithium toxicity. *Ann Neurol*, 1983, *13*, 221–222.

Rosenbaum AH, Niven RG, Hanson NP, and Swanson DW. Tardive dyskinesia: relationship with a primary affective disorder. *Dis Nerv Syst*, 1977, *38*, 423–427.

Rosenbaum D. Psychosis with Huntington's chorea. *Psychiat Quart*, 1941, *15*, 93–99.

Sacks O. *Awakenings*. New York, Vantage Books, 1976.

Scheinberg IH and Sternlieb I. *Wilson's disease*. Philadelphia, WB Saunders Company, 1984.

Schilder P. The organic background of obsessions and compulsions. *Am J Psychiat*, 1938, *94*, 1397–1413.

Schmidt WR and Jarcho LW. Persistent dyskinesias following phenothiazine therapy. *Arch Neurol*, 1966, *14*, 369–377.

Schooler NR and Kane JM. Research diagnoses for tardive dyskinesia. *Arch Gen Psychiat*, 1982, *39*, 486–487.

Schwab JJ and Barrow MV. A reaction to organic fluorides simulating classical catatonia. *Am J Psychiat*, 1964, *120*, 1196–1197.

Schwartz GE, Fair PL, Salt P, Mandel MR, and Klerman GL. Facial expression and imagery in depression: an electromyographic study. *Psychosom Med*, 1976, *38*, 337–347.

Shapiro AK and Shapiro E. Subcategorizing Gilles de la Tourette's syndrome. *Am J Psychiat*, 1977, *134*, 818–819.

Shapiro AK, Shapiro ES, Bruun RD, and Sweet RD. *Gilles de la Tourette syndrome*. New York, Raven Press, 1978.

Shepherd M. Report of a family suffering from Friedreich's disease, peroneal muscular atrophy, and schizophrenia. *J Neurol Neurosurg Psychiat*, 1955, *18*, 297–304.

Sheppard C and Merlis S. Drug-induced extrapyramidal symptoms: their incidence and treatment. *Am J Psychiat*, 1967, *123*, 886–889.

Shopsin B and Gershon S. Cogwheel rigidity related to lithium maintenace. *Am J Psychiat*, 1975, *132*, 536–538.

Singer WD. Transient Gilles de la Tourette syndrome after chronic neuroleptic withdrawal. *Dev Med Child Neurol*, 1981, *23*, 518–521.

Singh BK, Singh A, and Chusid E. Chorea in long-term use of pemoline. *Ann Neurol*, 1983, *13*, 218.

Slater E and Roth M. *Mayer-Gross, Slater and Roth: Clinical Psychiatry*, 3rd ed. London, Bailliere Tindall, 1977.

Smith JM and Baldessarini RJ. Changes in prevalence, severity, and recovery in tardive dyskinesia with age. *Arch Gen Psychiat*, 1980, *37*, 1368–1373.

Sours JA. Akinetic mutism simulating catatonic schizophrenia. *Am J Psychiat*, 1962, *119*, 451–455.

Sovner RD and McHugh PR. Lithium in the treatment of periodic catatonia: a case report. *J Nerv Ment Dis*, 1974, *158*, 214–221.

Stern RS and Cobb JP. Phenomenology of obsessive–compulsive neurosis. *Br J Psychiat*, 1978, *132*, 233–239.

Sternbach H and Yager J. Catatonia in the presence of midbrain and brainstem abnormalities. *J Clin Psychiat*, 1981, *42*, 352–353.

Stevens JR. Disturbances of ocular movements and blinking in schizophrenia. *J Neurol Neurosurg Psychiat*, 1978, *40*, 1024–1030.

Stoudemire A. The differential diagnosis of catatonic states. *Psychosomatics*, 1982, *23*, 245–252.

Strang RR. Imipramine in treatment of parkinsonism: a double-blind placebo study. *Br Med J*, 1965, *2*, 33–34.

Strauss EW and Griffith RM. Pseudo-reversibility in catatonic stupor. *Am J Psychiat*, 1955, *111*, 680–685.

Swett C Jr. Drug-induced dystonia. *Am J Psychiat*, 1975, *132*, 532–534.

Tarsy D and Baldessarini RJ. The pathophysiologic basis of tardive dyskinesia. *Biol Psychiat*, 1977, *12*, 431–450.

Tarsy D, Granacher R, and Bralower M. Tardive dyskinesia in young adults. *Am J Psychiat*, 1977, *134*, 1032–1034.

Taylor MA. *The neuropsychiatric mental status examination*. New York, SP Medical and Scientific Books, 1981.

Taylor MA and Abrams R. Catatonia. Prevalence and importance in the manic phase of manic–depressive illness. *Arch Gen Psychiat*, 1977, *34*, 1223–1225.

Tepper SJ and Haas JF. Prevalence of tardive dyskinesia. *J Clin Psychiat*, 1979, *40*, 508–516.

Thach BT, Chase TN, and Bosma JF. Oral facial dyskinesia associated with prolonged use of antihistaminic decongestants. *New Engl J Med*, 1975, *293*, 486–487.

Thompson GN. Cerebral lesions simulating schizophrenia: three case reports. *Biol Psychiat*, 1970, *2*, 59–64.

Thornton JE and Stahl SM. Case report of tardive dyskinesia and parkinsonism associated with amoxapine therapy. *Am J Psychiat*, 1984, *141*, 704–705.

Todd R, Lippmann S, Manshadi M, and Chang A. Recognition and treatment of rabbit syndrome, an uncommon complication of neuroleptic therapies. *Am J Psychiat*, 1983, *140*, 1519–1520.

Tolosa ES. Modification of tardive dyskinesia and spasmodic torticollis by apomorphine. *Arch Neurol*, 1978, *35*, 459–462.

Tolosa ES. Clinical features of Meige's disease (idiopathic orofacial dystonia). *Arch Neurol*, 1981, *38*, 147–151.

Tolosa ES and Klawans HL. Meige's disease. A clinical form of facial convulsion, bilateral and medial. *Arch Neurol*, 1979, *36*, 635–637.

Tyrer P, Alexander MS, Regan A, and Lee I. An extrapyramidal syndrome after lithium therapy. *Br J Psychiat*, 1980, *136*, 191–194.

Uhrbrand L and Faurbye A. Reversible and irreversible dyskinesia after treatment with perphenazine, chlorpromazine, reserpine and electroconvulsive therapy. *Psychopharmacologia*, 1960, *1*, 408–418.

Van Putten T. Lithium-induced disabling tremor. *Psychosomatics*, 1978, *19*, 27–31.

Varga E, Sugerman AA, Varga V, Zomorodi A, Zomorodi W, and Menken M. Prevalence of spontaneous oral dyskinesias in the elderly. *Am J Psychiat*, 1982, *139*, 329–331.

Vestergaard P, Amdisen A, and Schou M. Clinically significant side effects of lithium treatment. *Acta Psychiat Scand*, 1980, *62*, 193–200.

Villeneuve A. The rabbit syndrome. A peculiar extrapyramidal reaction. *Can Psychiat Assoc J*, 1972, *17*, SS69–SS72.

Wald D and Lerner J. Lithium in the treatment of periodic catatonia: a case report. *Am J Psychiat*, 1978, *135*, 751–752.

Warburton JW. Depressive symptoms in parkinson patients referred for thalamotomy. *J Neurol Neurosurg Psychiat*, 1967, *30*, 368–370.

Wasserman S and Yahr MD. Choreic movements induced by the use of methadone. *Arch Neurol*, 1980, *37*, 727–728.

Wegner JT and Kane JM. Follow-up study on the reversibility of tardive dyskinesia. *Am J Psychiat*, 1982, *139*, 368–369.

Wegner JT, Struve FA, Kantor JS, and Kane JM. Relationship between the β-mitten EEG pattern and tardive dyskinesia. *Arch Gen Psychiat*, 1979, *36*, 599–603.

Weinberger DR and Kelly MJ. Catatonia and malignant syndrome: a possible complication of neuroleptic administration. *J Nerv Ment Dis*, 1977, *165*, 263–268.

Weinberger DR and Wyatt RJ. Catatonic stupor and neuroleptic drugs. *JAMA*, 1978, *239*, 1846.

Weiner WJ, Goetz CG, Nausieda PA, and Klawans HL. Respiratory dyskinesias: extrapyramidal dysfunction and dyspnea. *Ann Int Med*, 1978a, *88*, 327–331.

Weiner WJ and Luby ED. Persistent akathisia following neuroleptic withdrawal. *Ann Neurol*, 1983, *13*, 466–467.

Weiner WJ, Nausieda PA, and Glantz RH. Meige syndrome (blepharospasm–oromandibular dystonia) after long-term neuroleptic therapy. *Neurology*, 1981, *31*, 1555–1556.

Weiner WJ, Nausieda PA, and Klawans HL. Methylphenidate-induced chorea: case report and pharmacologic implications. *Neurology*, 1978b, *28*, 1041–1044.

Weiner WJ and Werner TR. Mania-induced remission of tardive dyskinesia in manic–depressive illness. *Ann Neurol*, 1982, *12*, 229–230.

Weiss BL, Foster G, Reynolds CF III, and Kupfer DJ. Psychomotor activity in mania. *Arch Gen Psychiat*, 1974, *31*, 379–383.

Wilson LG. Viral encephalopathy mimicking functional psychosis. *Am J Psychiat*, 1976, *133*, 165–170.

Wilson RL, Waziri R, Nasrallah HA, and McCalley-Whitters M. The lateralization of tardive dyskinesia. *Biol Psychiat*, 1984, *19*, 629–635.

Yarden PE and Discipio WJ. Abnormal movements and prognosis in schizophrenia. *Am J Psychiat*, 1971, *125*, 317–323.

Yassa R, Nair V, and Schwartz G. Tardive dyskinesia and the primary psychiatric diagnosis. *Psychosomatics*, 1984, *25*, 135–138.

Young RR. Essential–familial tremor and other action tremors. *Semin Neurol*, 1982, *2*, 386–391.

Zorumski CF and Bakris GL. Choreoathetosis associated with lithium: case report and literature review. *Am J Psychiat*, 1983, *140*, 1621–1622.

Chapter 13

Secondary Psychoses, Delusions, and Schizophrenia

Psychosis is defined as a loss of reality testing such that affected individuals cannot evaluate the accuracy of their perceptions or thoughts and make incorrect inferences about external reality (*Diagnostic and statistical manual of mental disorders,* 1980). Delusions are specific false beliefs that are firmly held despite evidence to the contrary and that are not endorsed by members of patients' cultures or subcultures (*Diagnostic and statistical manual of mental disorders,* 1980; Jaspers, 1963). Delusions must be distinguished from hallucinations and from confabulation. Hallucinations are false perceptions and have a delusional aspect only if patients endorse them as reality. Confabulations are spontaneous untruths occurring in patients with amnesia and frequently changing with each interview.

This chapter reviews secondary psychoses and symptomatic delusions, describes the neurologic aspects of schizophrenia, and briefly reviews the pharmacological treatment of nonaffective psychotic disorders. Affective disturbances are presented in Chapter 14.

SECONDARY PSYCHOSES

A wide variety of neurological, toxic, and metabolic disorders can have secondary psychosis as their presenting manifestation or as one aspect that emerges during the course of the disease. The principal etiologies of secondary psychoses are presented in Tables 13-1, 13-2, and 13-3.

Neurological Diseases with Secondary Psychoses

Table 13-1 lists the neurological diseases that can produce secondary psychoses. Psychoses are particularly common among the extrapyramidal diseases and among traumatic, infectious, neoplastic, and vascular disorders affecting the limbic system and subcortical structures (Cummings, 1985; Davison and Bagley, 1969).

Extrapyramidal Disorders

Psychoses are not uncommon in postencephalitic Parkinson's disease. Delusions were the principal neuropsychiatric manifestation of the disease in 25 percent of Fairweather's large sample (Fairweather, 1947), and similar high frequencies of schizophrenialike disorders and paranoia were noted by others (Bromberg, 1930; Kirby and Davis, 1921; Menninger, 1926; Sands, 1928). Among patients with idiopathic Parkinson's disease (paralysis agitans), nonaffective psychosis is much less common. Individuals with paralysis agitans and schizophrenialike disorders have rarely been reported, and most psychoses unrelated to depression are induced by the drugs required to treat the Parkinson's disease (Celesia and Barr, 1970; Celesia and Wanamaker, 1972; Crow et al., 1976; Hollister and Glazener, 1961; Mindham, 1970; Moskovitz et al., 1978; Postma and van Tilburg, 1975).

Psychosis is common in the course of Huntington's disease and may be the presenting feature (Caine and Shoulson, 1983; Garron, 1973; James et al., 1969; Rosenbaum, 1941). Of 102 patients studied by Dewhurst et al. (1969), psychosis was present in 50 percent at the time of admission and was the principal reason for admission in 10 percent. Among patients with Sydenham's chorea—chorea associated with rheumatic fever in childhood—as many as 20 percent had psychosis concomitantly with the movement disorder (Hammes, 1922).

Psychoses also occur among patients with Wilson's disease, idiopathic basal ganglia calcification, and the spinocerebellar degenerations. Wilson's disease patients may manifest schizophrenialike illnesses with paranoid delusions and auditory hallucinations indistinguishable from those occurring in idiopathic schizophrenia (Beard 1959; Gysin and Cooke, 1950; Jackson and Zimmerman, 1919; Scheinberg, 1981; Scheinberg and Sternlieb, 1984). Idiopathic basal ganglia calcification commonly presents in the third or fourth decade of life with a schiz-

TABLE 13-1.   Neurological Causes of Secondary Psychoses

Extrapyramidal disturbances	Diseases affecting myelin
Postencephalitic Parkinson's disease	Multiple sclerosis
Idiopathic Parkinson's disease	Metachromatic leukodystrophy
Huntington's disease	Adrenoleukodystrophy
Syndenham's chorea	Marchiafava-Bignami disease
Wilson's disease	
Idiopathic basal ganglia calcification	Primary cortical dementias
Spinocerebellar degeneration	Alzheimer's disease
	Pick's disease
CNS infections	
	Other acquired CNS disturbances
Viral encephalitis	
Herpes	Epilepsy
Nonherpetic	Primary generalized seizures
	Complex partial seizures
Rabies	
Mumps	Cerebrovascular disease
Asian influenza	Posttraumatic encephalopathy
Mononucleosis	Postanoxic encephalopathy
Unidentified	Neoplasms
	Hydrocephalus
Slow virus diseases	
	Miscellaneous disorders
Jakob-Creutzfeldt disease	
Subacute sclerosing panencephalitis	Leber's hereditary aptic atrophy
	Cerebral lipidoses
Cerebral malaria	Niemann-Pick disease
Syphilis	Narcolepsy
Trypanosomiasis	
Schistosomiasis	

ophrenialike illness (Bennett et al., 1959; Bruyn et al., 1964; Cummings et al., 1983; Francis, 1979; Kalamboukis and Molling, 1962; Kasanin and Crank, 1935). Psychosis is less common in patients with spinocerebellar degenerations but has been observed in association with Friedreich's ataxia and olivopontocerebellar degeneration (Chandler and Bebin, 1956; Davies, 1949; Hamilton et al., 1983; Keddie, 1969; Richards et al., 1974; Shepherd, 1955).

CNS Infections

A variety of central nervous system (CNS) infections produce psychosis as a prominent clinical manifestation. Herpes simplex encephalitis preferentially involves the medial temporal lobes and inferior frontal lobes—cerebral cortical areas included in the limbic system—and frequently presents with psychosis, delusions, and/or auditory hallucinations as the earliest expressions of the infection (Drachman and Adams, 1962; Johnson et al., 1972; Rennick et al., 1973; Williams and Lerner, 1978). Nonherpetic viral encephalitides producing psychosis have included rabies, mumps encephalitis, infectious mononucleosis, and encephalitis associated with Asian influenza as well as a number of cases of encephalitis in which the causal organism was

not identified (Greenbaum and Lurie, 1948; Keddie, 1965; Misra and Hay, 1971; Nash, 1983; Raymond and Williams, 1948; Still, 1958).

Two slow virus diseases—Jakob-Creutzfeldt disease and subacute sclerosing panencephalitis—may have psychosis as a premonitory manifestation prior to the emergence of the progressive dementia (Goldhammer et al., 1972; Lorand et al., 1962; Risk and Haddad, 1979).

Nonviral causes of infectious psychoses have included cerebral malaria, CNS syphilis, trypanosomiasis, and schistosomiasis (Arieti, 1946; Blankfein and Chirico, 1965; Blocker et al., 1968; Nash, 1983; Rothschild, 1940; Schube, 1934).

Diseases Affecting Myelin

Multiple sclerosis is more likely to be associated with depression than with psychosis, but in some cases progressive demyelination has resulted in a psychotic disorder (Geocaris, 1957; Langworthy et al., 1941). Marchiafava-Bignami disease, an acquired demyelinating disorder affecting the corpus callosum and white matter of the frontal lobes, is a rare condition occurring primarily in chronic alcoholics. It has occasionally

TABLE 13-2. Metabolic Disorders Associated with Secondary Psychoses

Systemic illnesses	Deficiency state
Uremia and dialysis dementia	Thiamine (Wernicke-Korsakoff syndrome)
Hepatic encephalopathy	Vitamin B_{12}
Pancreatic encephalopathy	Folate
Anoxia (cardiopulmonary insufficiency)	Niacin
Subacute bacterial endocarditis	
Hyponatremia	Inflammatory disorders
Hypercalcemia	
Hypoglycemia	Systemic lupus erythematosus
Porphyria	Temporal arteritis
Postoperative and intensive care unit psychoses	Sarcoidosis
Endocrine disturbances	
Addison's disease (adrenal insufficiency)	
Cushing's disease (hyperadrenalism)	
Hypothyroidism	
Hyperthyroidism	
Hypoparathyroidism	
Hyperparathyroidism	
Panhypopituitarism	
Recurrent menstrual psychosis	
Postpartum psychosis	

been associated with a symptomatic psychosis (Freeman, 1980).

Inherited diseases of myelin producing psychoses include metachromatic leukodystrophy and adrenoleukodystrophy (Betts et al., 1968; Muller et al., 1969; Powell et al., 1975; Rumani, 1981).

Primary Cortical Dementias

Primary degenerative diseases of the cerebral cortex such as Alzheimer's disease and Pick's disease exhibit psychoses much less frequently than do diseases whose major impact is on limbic system or subcortical structures. Larson et al. (1963) found psychoses in 15 percent of their large series of Alzheimer patients. Cummings (1985) noted that the delusions in Alzheimer's disease are simple, loosely held, and often transient. Typically, Alzheimer patients with delusions believe that family members or others are trying to steal their money or home or that uninvited and unwelcome strangers are coming into the house.

Pick's disease patients with delusions have been reported, but, like Alzheimer's disease, Pick's disease is not frequently associated with symptomatic psychoses (Bouton, 1940; Malamud and Boyd, 1940).

Other Acquired CNS Disturbances

Psychosis is associated with both primary generalized epilepsy and with epilepsy manifest by complex partial seizures (Chapter 9). Psychosis has its highest association with temporal lobe epilepsy and is more common with seizures originating from left-sided epileptic foci (Slater et al., 1963; Toone, 1981; Trimble, 1981).

Cerebrovascular disorders such as infarctions, aneurysms, and arteriovenous malformations have produced psychoses. Psychotic manifestations are particularly common with lesions affecting limbic structures in the subcortical regions, temporal lobes, or temporoparietal areas (Cummings, 1985; Trimble and Cummings, 1981; Vaillant, 1965). Left hemispheric lesions manifest themselves primarily as ideas of reference and persecution (Benson, 1973), whereas right-sided lesions tend to produce delusions with visual hallucinations (Levine and Finklestein, 1982; Peroutka et al., 1982).

Traumatic brain injuries are also followed by an increased incidence of schizophrenialike psychoses (Hillbom, 1951, 1960; Nasrallah et al., 1981; Shapiro, 1939; Thompson, 1970). The traumatic lesions are concentrated in the temporal and inferior frontal regions, and in most series the psychoses have been more commonly associated with left-sided damage.

Cerebral neoplasms manifesting psychosis share the anatomic characteristics noted for epileptic, traumatic, and vascular lesions. Tumor-related psychoses occur with masses affecting the brainstem, temporal lobes, or frontal lobes (Gal, 1958; Leeks, 1967; Scott, 1970; White and Cobb, 1955; Wilson and Rupp, 1946).

Other acquired conditions associated with symptomatic psychoses include hydrocephalus and postan-

TABLE 13-3. Toxic Encephalopathies Associated with
            Secondary Psychoses

Drugs

  Anticholinergic agents
  Dopaminergic agents

    Amantadine hydrochloride
    Levodopa
    Bromocriptine

  Endocrine agents
  Appetite suppressants
  Antituberculous agents
  Anticonvulsants
  Antimalarials
  Antidepressants
  Antihypertensive agents
  Hallucinogens
    (LSD, cannabis, mescaline, psilocybin, PCP, etc.)
  Miscellaneous drugs

    Amphetamines
    Cimetidine
    Disulfiram
    Corticosteroids
    Benzodiazepines
    Digitalis
    Bromide

    Diethylpropion
    Podophyllin
    Actifed
    Isosafrol
    Cocaine
    Methylphenidate
    Ibuprofin
    Baclofen

    Lidocaine
    Procainamide
    Phenylephrine
    Ephedrine
    Procaine penicillin
    Metrizamide

  Withdrawal syndromes

    Alcohol
    Sedative–hypnotics
    Stimulants

Metals

  Mercury
  Arsenic
  Manganese
  Thallium
  Bismuth

---

oxic encephalopathy (Brierley and Cooper, 1962;
Davison and Bagley, 1969; Price and Tucker, 1964; Rice
and Gendelman, 1973).

Miscellaneous Secondary Psychoses

In addition to the disorders described in the preceding sections, a number of other neurological conditions with secondary psychoses have been described, including Leber's hereditary optic atrophy, Niemann-Pick disease, and inherited cerebral lipidoses (Bates, 1964; Davison and Bagley, 1969; Fox and Kane, 1967). A few cases of narcolepsy with psychosis have been reported. Most often, psychosis in a narcoleptic patient will be a product of treatment with psychostimulants, but in a few instances psychosis not attributable to medications have been described (Coren and Strain, 1965; Eilenberg and Woods, 1962; Pfefferbaum and Berger, 1977).

Metabolic Disorders with Secondary Psychoses

A large number of endogenous metabolic disturbances and systemic illnesses have produced secondary psychoses as part of their clinical presentation. In most cases, the psychosis is accompanied by evidence of an acute metabolic encephalopathy (fluctuating arousal, impaired attention, etc.), but the psychosis is occasionally the sole behavioral expression of the disorder. Table 13-2 outlines the metabolic causes of secondary psychoses.

Kidney diseases leading to uremia may produce psychotic states, and psychosis is also common among patients with dialysis dementia (Burks et al., 1976; Chokroverty et al., 1976; Schreiner, 1959). Similarly, hepatic encephalopathy and pancreatic failure may each produce secondary psychosis as one manifestation of their clinical symptomatology (Read et al., 1967; Rothermich and von Haam, 1941). Cerebral anoxia associated with pulmonary or cardiac insufficiency can cause psychosis or exacerbate an existing idiopathic psychosis. In a study of patients with subacute bacterial endocarditis, 60 percent had behavioral abnormalities, including some with paranoid psychoses (Nash, 1983). Serum abnormalities, including hyponatremia, hypoglycemia, and hypercalcemia, can also cause symptomatic cerebral dysfunction with psychosis (Burnell and Foster, 1972; Nash, 1983; Weizman et al., 1979). Acute intermittent porphyria produces encephalopathy with psychosis along with abdominal pain and peripheral neuropathy (Roth, 1945). Postoperative and intensive care unit psychoses appear to be determined by multiple factors, including sensory deprivation, sleep deprivation, electrolyte imbalance, drug administration, and organ failure (Gotze and Dahme, 1980; Kornfeld et al., 1965).

Endocrine disturbances are commonly associated with secondary psychoses. Adrenal insufficiency and excess, hypo- and hyperthyroidism, hypo- and hyperparathyroidism, and panhypopituitarism have all produced secondary psychoses in some patients (Asher, 1949; Bursten, 1981; Cleghorn, 1951; Fitz and Hallman, 1952; Gorman and Wortis, 1947; Green and Swanson, 1941; Hanna, 1970; Sanders, 1962; Spillane, 1951; Wijsenbeek et al., 1964). Recurrent psychoses have also been associated with the menstrual disorders, and endocrinologic factors are suspected to contribute to postpartum psychoses (Nash, 1983).

Deficiency states associated with psychosis include thiamine deficiency producing Korsakoff's psychosis, vitamin B_{12} deficiency, folate deficiency, and niacin deficiency (Bowman, 1935; Cutting, 1978a; Smith, 1960; Strachan and Henderson, 1967; Sydenstricker 1943).

Inflammatory diseases causing secondary psychoses include systemic lupus erythematosus, temporal arteritis, and sarcoidosis (Cares et al., 1957; Grant and McMenemey 1966; MacNeill et al., 1976; Stern and Robbins, 1960).

Toxic Encephalopathies

Toxic encephalopathies induced by drugs and metals, like those caused by endogenous metabolic disturbances, are also associated with secondary psychoses (Table 13-3). Drugs that may produce psychoses include anticholinergic agents, dopaminergic drugs (amantadine hydrochloride, levodopa, bromocriptine), antituberculous agents, anticonvulsants, endocrine agents, antimalarials, appetite suppressants, antidepressants, antihypertensive agents, hallucinogens, and a variety of miscellaneous drugs, including diethylpropion, podophyllin, actifed, isosafrol, cocaine, methylphenidate, ibuprofen, baclofen, lidocaine, procainamide, phenylephrine, ephedrine, procaine, penicillin, metrizamide, amphetamines, cimetidine, disulfiram, corticosteroids, benzodiazepines, digitalis, bromides, etc. (Adler et al., 1980; Ames, 1958; Askevold, 1959; Barnhart and Bowden, 1979; Beamish and Kiloh, 1960; Cohen, 1977; Cohen and Ditman, 1963; Goodwin, 1971; Hausner, 1980; Jefferson and Marshall, 1981; Lewis and Smith, 1983; Medical Letter, 1984; Moser et al., 1953; Moskovitz et al., 1978; Nash, 1983; Paykel et al., 1982; Remick et al., 1981).

Abrupt withdrawal of drugs can also precipitate a toxic psychosis with delusions. The principal agents capable of producing withdrawal syndromes when abruptly discontinued include alcohol, sedative-hypnotics, and psychostimulants such as amphetamines, cocaine, and even sympathomimetics (Devaugh-Geiss and Pandurangi, 1982).

Metal intoxications associated with secondary psychosis include the encephalopathies associated with excess mercury, arsenic, manganese, thallium, and bismuth (Abd ed Naby and Hassanein, 1965; Grunfeld and Hinostroza, 1964; Jefferson and Marshall, 1981; Schenk and Stolk, 1967; Vroom and Greer, 1972).

Generalizations Concerning Secondary Psychoses

The lists presented in the preceding section demonstrate that delusions have been associated with most neurological illnesses and with a wide variety of metabolic and toxic disorders. Within this diversity, however, certain patterns are apparent, and these may help in distinguishing the secondary psychoses from idiopathic psychiatric disorders and contribute to an understanding of the pathophysiology of secondary psychoses. The diseases that produce secondary psychoses are more common in the middle and late life, whereas the idiopathic psychoses commonly begin in the second or third decade. Onset of a psychosis in the fifth decade or later should thus stimulate consideration of a secondary psychosis and initiation of a search for an underlying neurological or toxic–metabolic disturbance. Likewise, many idiopathic psychiatric disorders have a genetic contribution, and the appearance of a psychosis in a patient with no family history of psychiatric disorder should increase the clinician's index of suspicion that the psychosis may be secondary to a structural or metabolic CNS disturbance.

There is a correlation between the integrity of the patient's intellect and the form and content of the delusions of an accompanying secondary psychosis. Patients with diseases such as Alzheimer's disease, Pick's disease, and multi-infarct dementia where intellectual function is significantly impaired tend to manifest delusions that are loosely held and poorly structured. On the other hand, disorders such as the extrapyramidal syndromes and many neoplastic, traumatic, and demyelinating disturbances that have less profound effects on neuropsychological abilities are often accompanied by complex, intricately structured, and rigidly held delusions (Cummings, 1985).

Anatomic correlates with the form and content of delusions are also evident. Delusions are less common, and when they occur, are more simply structured in diseases that involve the cerebral cortex and have relatively less impact on subcortical structures. On the other hand, delusions are much more common and may be more complex and richly structured in diseases that have direct involvement of the limbic system or its projections to rostral brainstem, basal ganglia, or thalamus (Cummings, 1985; Davison and Bagley, 1969). Schizophrenialike disorders appear to be more common with epileptic or traumatic lesions located in the left hemisphere (Chapter 9) (Hillbom, 1960; Trimble, 1981). Right hemisphere lesions produce delusions accompanied by visual hallucinations (Levine and Finkelstein,

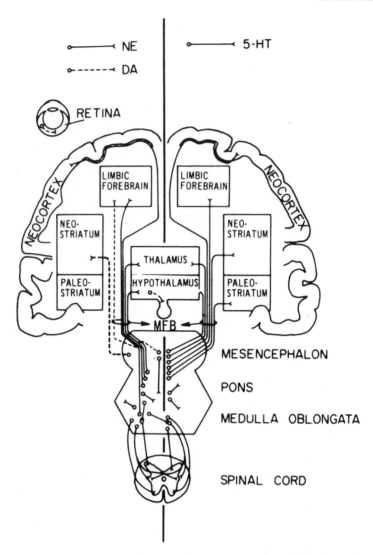

Figure 13-1. Diagram showing the distribution of the major neurotransmitter systems of the brain and demonstrating the vulnerability of these systems to disruption by appropriately placed limbic and subcortical lesions. Reproduced from Anden N-E, Dahlstrom A, Fuxe K, Larsson K, Olson L, Ungerstedt U. Ascending monoamine neurons to the diencephalon. *Acta Physiol Scand*, 1966, *67*, Fig. 10. With permission from the publisher.

1982; Peroutka et al., 1982), and brainstem lesions often have associated eye movement abnormalities (Trimble and Cummings, 1981). Cummings and colleagues (Cummings, 1985; Cummings et al., 1983; Trimble and Cummings, 1981) have suggested that the striking similarity between psychoses associated with limbic–subcortical disorders and idiopathic schizophrenia reflect the fact that limbic and subcortical lesions are anatomically located so as to disrupt ascending monoaminergic pathways and affect transmitter systems implicated in idiopathic schizophrenia (Fig. 13-1).

DELUSIONS

Most of the secondary psychoses are manifested by paranoid delusions, ideas of reference, and persecutory thoughts. In some cases, however, delusions have a specific theme or are confined to a single topic. Table 13-4 presents the principal content-specific delusions and lists the neurological and metabolic disorders that have been associated with them. These specific types of delusion have been associated with both idiopathic psychoses (mania, depression, schizophrenia, delusional disorder) and with neurological and toxic–metabolic conditions.

Schneiderian first-rank symptoms are specific psychotic symptoms that occur primarily in schizophrenia but have also been noted in a small number of patients with manic, depressive, and neurological psychoses (Carpenter et al., 1973; Ianzito et al., 1974). First-rank symptoms include aberrations of thought such as thought insertion, thought withdrawal, and thought broadcasting as well as certain types of auditory hallucination, delusional perception, and passivity experiences involving the feeling that bodily sensations, or one's emotions, impulses, or actions are imposed from outside (Table 13-5). Neurological and metabolic diseases producing first-rank symptoms include idiopathic basal ganglia calcification, posttraumatic encephalopathy, temporal lobe neoplasms, postencephalitic parkinsonism, temporal lobe epilepsy, viral encephalitis, cerebrovascular disease, hydrocephalus, hypothyroidism, Addison's disease, isosafrol, LSD, amphetamines, diethylpropion, clonazepam, podophyllin, actifed, inderal, and metrizamide encephalopathy (Bowers, 1972; Bromberg, 1930; Cummings et al., 1983; De Fine Olivarius and Roder, 1970; Gal, 1958; Gershon et al., 1979; Keitner et al., 1984; Leighton, 1982; Menninger, 1926; Mirsa and Hay, 1971; Nasrallah et al., 1982; Petursson, 1979; Reveley and Reveley, 1983; Slater et al., 1963; Stoudemire et al., 1981; Trimble and Cummings, 1981; White et al., 1982).

The Capgras syndrome is a specific delusional belief in which the patient is convinced that some important person (usually the spouse) has been replaced by an identical-appearing impostor. This syndrome occurs most commonly in schizophrenia but has also been described in manic–depressive psychosis, paraphrenia, and postpartum psychosis (Cohn et al., 1977; Enoch, 1963; Merrin and Silberfarb, 1976). Neurological disorders producing the Capgras syndrome include intracerebral hemorrhage, posttraumatic encephalopathy, temporal lobe epilepsy, postencephalitic parkinsonism, varicella encephalitis, and migraine (Alexander et al., 1979; Chawla and Virmani, 1977; Christodoulou, 1977; Hayman and Abrams, 1977; MacCallum, 1973; Rudnick, 1982; Weston and Whitlock, 1971). Among reported cases with structural lesions, there is a preponderance of right hemispheric lesions, suggesting that right-sided dysfunction may predispose to this particular delusional misinterpretation (Alexander et al., 1979; Hayman and Abrams, 1977; Quinn, 1981; Wilcox and Waziri, 1983). Metabolic disorders reported to produce the Capgras syndrome include vitamin B_{12} deficiency, hepatic encephalopathy, pneumonia, malnutrition, diabetic encephalopathy, hypothyroidism, and pseudohypoparathyroidism (Hay et al., 1974; MacCallum, 1973; Medakusira and Hall, 1981; Pies, 1982; Zucker et al., 1981).

Two syndromes that resemble the Capgras syndrome are the Fregoli syndrome and the intermetamorphosis syndrome. The *Fregoli syndrome* refers to a delusion wherein the patient believes that a persecutor is able to take on the appearance of others in the patient's environment, changing faces like an actor (Enoch and Trethowan, 1979). In the intermetamorphosis syndrome one believes that those in one's environment begin to look like a persecutor or other object of the delusion. Both of these syndromes have been noted in schizophrenia and in behavioral syndromes associated with epilepsy (Christodoulou, 1976; Malliaras et al., 1978).

Delusional jealousy is one of the most common monosymptomatic delusions. Also known as the *Othello syndrome,* delusional jealousy is manifested by an unjustified conviction of the spouse's infidelity. Delusional jealousy occurs in idiopathic psychoses as well as in Huntington's disease, encephalitis, CNS neoplasms, Alzheimer's disease, multiple sclerosis, epilepsy, Parkinson's disease, general paresis, and drug intoxication (Keddie, 1965; Mooney, 1965; Shepherd, 1961).

Delusions of infestation (acrophobia, parasitophobia) or the delusional belief that one's body is inhabited by worms or insects has been observed in vitamin B_{12} deficiency, iron deficiency, and toxic psychoses (Pope, 1970; Wilson, 1952). In lycanthropy or werewolfism one believes that one has been turned into a wolf. The syndrome has been produced by LSD use and an undiagnosed primary dementing illness (Surawicz and Banta, 1975).

Heutoscopy (the syndrome of doubles, the doppelgänger) is the delusion that one has an exact double. The double may or may not be visible. It occurs primarily in schizophrenia but is also observed in migraine, toxic psychoses, encephalitis, posttraumatic encephalopathy, epilepsy, and intracranial hemorrhage (Christodoulou, 1978; Damas Mora et al., 1980). The syndrome of doubles must be distinguished from autoscopy, where one has an hallucination of oneself but recognizes that the experience is hallucinatory.

De Clerambault syndrome or erotomania is a delusional belief, most common in women, that an older, more influential male is in love with her despite outward evidence to the contrary. The patient may pursue her victim relentlessly, trying to establish contact and allow him to demonstrate his love. The syndrome has occurred in schizophrenia, with toxic psychoses, with epilepsy, and with CNS tumors (Lovett Doust and Christie, 1978).

A few delusions that have more closely determined associations with specific CNS lesions have been mentioned in previous chapters. Denial of illness must be regarded as a delusional belief in one's well-being; thus anosognosia syndromes, such as denial of hemiparesis

TABLE 13-4.   Specific Delusions and Their Neurological and Metabolic Etiologies

Schneiderian first-rank symptoms	CNS disorders
	    Idiopathic basal ganglia calcification
	    Posttraumatic encephalopathy
	    Temporal lobe neoplasm
	    Postencephalitic parkinsonism
	    Temporal lobe epilepsy
	    Viral encephalitis
	    Cerebrovascular disease
	    Hydrocephalus
	
	Metabolic disorders
	    Hypothyroidism
	    Metrizamide encephalopathy
	    Addison's disease
	    Isosafrol
	    LSD
	    Amphetamines
	    Diethylpropion
	    Clonazepam
	    Podophyllin
	    Actifed
	    Inderal

Capgras syndrome	CNS disorders
	    Intracerebral hemorrhage
	    Posttraumatic encephalopathy
	    Temporal lobe epilepsy
	    Postencephalitic parkinsonism
	    Viral encephalitis
	    Migraine
	
	Metabolic disorders
	    Vitamin B_{12} deficiency
	    Hepatic encephalopathy
	    Pneumonia
	    Malnutrition
	    Diabetic encephalopathy
	    Hypothyroidism
	    Pseudohypoparathyroidism

Fregoli syndrome	Temporal lobe epilepsy
Intermetamorphosis syndrome	Cerebral dysrhythmia

Delusional jealousy (Othello syndrome)	CNS disorders
	    Huntington's disease
	    Encephalitis
	    CNS neoplasm
	    Alzheimer's disease
	    Multiple sclerosis
	    Epilepsy
	    Parkinson's disease
	    General paresis
	
	Metabolic disorders
	    Drug intoxication

Delusions of infestation (acraphobia, parasitophobia)	Metabolic disorders
	    Vitamin B_{12} deficiency
	    Iron deficiency
	    Toxic psychoses

(continued)

TABLE 13-4. *(continued)*

Lycanthropy (werewolfism)	CNS disorders
	    Degenerative dementia
	
	Metabolic disorders
	    LSD intoxication

Heutoscopy (the double, doppelgänger)	CNS disorders
	    Encephalitis
	    Posttraumatic encephalopathy
	    Intracranial hemorrhage
	    Migraine
	    Epilepsy
	
	Metabolic disorders
	    Toxic psychoses

De Clerambault syndrome (erotomania)	CNS disorders
	    Epilepsy
	    Meningioma
	
	Metabolic disorders
	    Toxic psychosis

Modified from Cummings JL. Organic delusions: phenomenology, anatomic correlations, and review. *Br J Psychiatr,* 1985, Table IV. With permission from the publisher.

and denial of blindness (Anton's syndrome) are delusional syndromes (Bergman, 1957; Cutting, 1978b; Reddlich and Dorsey, 1945; Symonds and Mackenzie, 1957). Occasional patients with anosognosia develop a delusional conviction that a third limb exists on the paretic side (Weinstein et al., 1954). Anosognosic syndromes are commonly associated with unilateral neglect and occur with posterior hemispheric lesions (Chapter 5). Reduplicative paramnesia is another delusion closely correlated with specific CNS lesions. This is the belief that one has been relocated, usually to a position closer to one's home. It occurs in patients with right hemispheric lesions in conjunction with frontal lesions or during recovery from acute confusional states (Chapter 4) (Benson et al., 1976; Fisher, 1982).

NEUROLOGICAL ASPECTS OF SCHIZOPHRENIA

Schizophrenia is an idiopathic neuropsychiatric disorder characterized by bizarre, persecutory, or religious delusions; auditory hallucinations; illogical thinking with losening of associations and poverty of information content; and deterioration from a previous level of functioning. The disease develops in adolescence or early adulthood, and the active phase is often preceded by a prodrome of deteriorating abilities and social withdrawal. The course of the disease is life-long, although periods of active illness are followed by remissions or a residual phase similar to the prodromal period (*Diagnostic and statistical manual of mental disorders,* 1980). The abnormalities of verbal output characterizing the speech of some schizophrenics are described in Chapter 3.

Attempts to subdivide schizophrenia into clinical types that have clinical or prognostic significance have generally met with failure, but one classification scheme that identifies two groups with differing prognoses in-

TABLE 13-5. Schneiderian First-Rank Symptoms

Thought aberrations

  Thought insertion
  Thought withdrawal
  Thought broadcasting

Auditory hallucinations

  Thoughts spoken aloud
  Voices arguing about or discussing the patient
  Voices commenting on the patient's actions

Delusional Perception

  Delusional interpretation of a normal perception

Passivity experience

  Bodily sensations imposed from outside
  Affect imposed or controlled from outside
  Impulses imposed and controlled from outside
  Motor actions imposed or controlled from outside

TABLE 13-6.   Characteristics of Two Subgroups of Schizophrenia

Type I	Type II
Positive symptoms: hallucinations; delusions, thought disorder	Negative symptoms: flattening of affect, poverty of speech, loss of drive, social withdrawal
Neuropsychological deficits absent	Neuropsychologic deficits common
Normal CT scan	CT scan reveals ventricular dilation and sulcal widening
Few "soft signs" on examination	More neurologic "soft signs" on examination
Better premorbid adjustment	Poor premorbid adjustment
Good response to neuroleptics	Poor response to neuroleptics
Good prognosis	Poor prognosis
Family history of psychosis more common	Family history of psychosis less common
Postulated pathology: increased dopamine receptors	Postulated pathology: cell loss
Postulated etiology: inherited disorder of dopamine metabolism or dopamine receptors	Postulated etiology: acquired CNS insult with injury to limbic or limbic-related areas

Data from Crow (1980) and Cummings and Benson (1983).

volves separating those with predominantly negative symptoms from those whose clinical picture is dominated by positive symptoms (Table 13-6). The negative symptom group is characterized by a predominance of flattened affect, social withdrawal, retardation, poverty of speech, and the presence of neuropsychological impairment. Patients with negative symptoms are more likely to have abnormal computerized tomograms, "soft signs" on neurological examination, a history of an abnormal personality and poor premorbid adjustment, poor response to neuroleptics, poor prognosis, and less evidence of genetic or inherited contributions to their illness. The etiology of this form of schizophrenia appears to be an acquired CNS insult with cell loss in the limbic system and related areas. The clinical picture contrasts with positive symptom schizophrenia, which appears to be an inherited disorder of dopamine receptors or dopamine metabolism and is characterized by absence of or less pronounced neuropsychological or CT abnormalities, few abnormalities on neurological examination, better premorbid functioning, better prognosis, and better response to neuroleptics (Andreason, 1982; Andreason and Olsen, 1982; Andreason et al., 1982a,b; Crow, 1980; Cummings and Benson, 1983; Donnelly et al., 1980; Golden et al., 1980a; Johnstone et al., 1978; Quitkin et al., 1976). Positive symptoms include marked delusions and prominent hallucinations. There are a number of schizophrenic patients whose symptoms and history are sufficiently mixed to make assignment to one of these subgroups difficult, but this classification appears to correlate well with several neurobiologic parameters within the schizophrenic syndrome and provides guidelines for determining prognosis and predicting treatment response.

Neurological examination of schizophrenic patients may reveal catatonic-type motor signs (Chapter 12) or neurological "soft signs" such as minor movements of the resting limb when testing the contralateral limb, posturing of the hands and arms when walking on toes or heels, pseudoathetosis of the outstretched fingers, and slowed fine finger movements. Testing of oculomotor pursuit movements in schizophrenics reveals that the usually smooth following movements are broken into a number of small saccadic steps (Cegalis and Sweeney, 1979; Holzman et al., 1973, 1974, 1977). These pursuit alterations occur in a majority of schizophrenics but have also been observed in a variety of neurological disorders and in a few normal control subjects (Brezinova and Kendell, 1977; Levin et al., 1982). In addition to abnormalities of smooth pursuit movements, schizophrenics have occasional bursts of horizontal eye movements and alterations of blink rates (decreased blinking in chronic schizophrenia, increased in acute schizophrenic exacerbations) (Karson, 1983; Stevens, 1978).

Computerized tomography reveals abnormalities in 20–50 percent of schizophrenic patients. The characteristic abnormalities include dilation of the lateral and third ventricles and sulcal enlargement, particularly of the Sylvian fissure. The presence of these radiological abnormalities correlates with the existence of neuropsychological deficits. The CT abnormalities are present in young as well as older patients and are independent of disease duration or type and amount of treatment (Andreasen et al., 1982a,b; Donnelly et al., 1980; Golden et al., 1980a,b; Johnstone et al., 1976; Nasrallah et al., 1982; Pandurangi et al., 1984; Reveley et al., 1984; Schulz et al., 1983; Weinberger et al., 1979a,b, 1982; Woods and Wolf, 1983). A few studies have suggested that there is an increased frequency of reversal or absence of the normal cerebral asymmetries (larger and longer left posterior hemisphere and right anterior hemisphere in normals) and alterations in brain density (Golden et al., 1981; Luchins et al., 1979; Tsai et al., 1983).

Electroencephalographic studies in schizophrenics reveal an increased incidence of nonspecific abnormalities (Abenson, 1970; Small, 1983). Power spectral analyses and depth electrode studies of freely moving schizophrenics reveal alterations that temporally coincide with bizarre behavior. The alterations originate in deep limbic and temporal lobe structures (Hanley et al., 1972; Petersen, 1953; Sem-Jacobsen et al., 1955; Stevens and Livermore, 1982). Evoked potential studies have suggested abnormalities in both frontal and posterior hemispheric function (Morihisa et al., 1983; Morstyn et al., 1983). Regional cerebral blood flow studies show diminished frontal lobe activation during psychological testing and suggest that the left hemisphere is more abnormal than the right (Franzen and Ingvar, 1975; Gur et al., 1983; Mathew et al., 1982; Ariel et al., 1983). Positron emission tomography demonstrates that the frontal lobes of schizophrenics are relatively hypometabolic compared to posterior hemispheric regions (Brodie et al., 1984; Farkas et al., 1984).

Postmortem studies of the brains of schizophrenic patients have revealed three main types of alteration: (1) neuronal loss and gliosis, (2) changes in concentrations of monoamines in various brain regions, and (3) changes in monoamine receptor density or sensitivity. Histological studies have revealed loss of neurons and gliosis in the brainstem, including the areas involved in the manufacture and transport of monoaminergic neurotransmitters. Structural alterations in the cerebral cortex have been observed with less consistency (Bogerts et al., 1983; Colon, 1972; Fisman, 1975; Stevens, 1982; Weinberger et al., 1983). Preliminary neurochemical investigations have shown increased concentrations of dopamine in the nucleus accumbens and the anterior perforated substance and increased noradrenalin in the septal and striatal regions (Bird et al., 1979; Crow et al., 1979; Farley et al., 1978). Monoaminergic receptor studies have demonstrated increased dopamine-receptor activity in these same subcorticolimbic structures (Lee et al., 1978; Owen et al., 1978). Alterations in dopamine concentrations and receptor sensitivity might be expected in patients treated with dopamine-blocking agents, but similar changes were found in the small number of untreated schizophrenics and in those that had remained drug-free for at least 1 year.

The pathogenesis of schizophrenia is not understood, but the success of dopamine-blocking drugs in treating many of the most florid manifestations of schizophrenia and the production of schizophrenialike psychoses by drugs such as levodopa and amphetamines that act on dopaminergic systems suggest that dopaminergic overactivity is an important aspect of the pathophysiology (Baldessarini, 1977; Crow et al., 1977, 1978; Snyder et al., 1974). This hypothesis is supported by the neurochemical and neuropathological data cited earlier and by the presence of schizophreniclike symptoms in secondary psychoses associated with subcorticolimbic pathology. Relatively few postmortem studies have been accomplished thus far, however, and not all have revealed dopamine system abnormalities. In addition, neuroleptic agents control some psychotic symptoms but have little impact on the negative symptoms of schizophrenia. Although dopaminergic hyperactivity may be an important element in the production of schizophrenia, therefore, it is likely that additional changes are also involved.

TREATMENT OF PSYCHOSIS

Treatment of psychosis is necessary not only because the thought disorganization, delusions, and hallucinations make it impossible for psychotic patients to work effectively and have successful social interactions, but also because action on delusional beliefs may lead these patients to harm themselves or others. The major thrust of treatment of the secondary psychoses is directed at correcting the underlying condition. Psychoses associated with metabolic and toxic disorders usually abate when metabolic balance is restored or toxic exposure eliminated. Psychoses associated with structural diseases of the CNS and the idiopathic psychoses must be treated with neuroleptic medications.

Table 13-7 presents a list of the commonly used neuroleptic agents. Their relative potency compared to chlorpromazine, the usual and extreme dosage ranges, and their most common side effects are also shown. Choice of an antipsychotic agent is based on the side-effect profile, the response of the patient to previous treatment regimens, and the experience of the clinician with each drug or class of drugs. Highest dosages are required during the acute psychotic episodes and should be reduced to the lowest possible levels between psychotic exacerbations, but the rate of relapse is high if neuroleptics are completely discontinued (Baldessarini, 1980; Hollister, 1972; Kessler and Waletzky, 1981).

Absorption of neuroleptic medications from the gastrointestinal tract is erratic and unpredictable and is poorer for those agents with prominent anticholinergic properties or when anticholinergic agents are coadministered. Peak serum concentrations are usually found 2–4 hours after oral administration. The elimination

TABLE 13-7. Dosages and Side-Effects of Commonly Used Neuroleptic Drugs

Drug Class	Generic Name	Common Proprietary Brand Name	Relative Potency[a]	Usual Dosage Range (Oral mg)
Phenothiazines	Chlorpromazine	Thorazine	100	300–800
	Thioridazine	Mellaril	100	200–600
	Perphenazine	Trilafon	10	8–34
	Trifluoperazine	Stelazine	5	6–20
	Fluphenazine	Prolixin	2	2.5–20
Thioxanthene	Thiothixene	Navane	5	6–30
Butyrophenones	Haloperidol	Haldol	2	6–20
Dibenzoxazepines	Loxapine	Loxitane	10	60–100
Indolics	Molindone	Moban	10	50–225

[a]Dosage equivalent to 100 mg of chlorpromazine.
Data from Baldesserini (1980) and Hollister (1977).

half-life for most agents is 10–20 hours; steady plasma levels are reached in 5–10 days when patients are maintained on fixed dosages; and biologic effects persist for at least 24 hours after a single oral dose. Antipsychotic agents are metabolized by hepatic microsomal enzymes and are excreted in the urine and bile. Plasma levels are poor predictors of clinical response and play a useful role in management primarily when there is concern over erratic absorption, when drug interactions that influence absorption or metabolism are suspected, or when there is a lack of clinical improvement despite administration of standard or larger than usual dosages (Baldessarini, 1980; Meltzer et al., 1983). Fluphenazine is available in enanthate and decanoate oil-suspension preparations that can be administered intramuscularly (IM) every other week for patients whose compliance is poor or whose absorption of orally administered forms is inadequate (Bassuk and Schoonover, 1977).

Neuroleptics interact with relatively few other drugs, but they do enhance the effects of sedative–hypnotics, analgesics, and alcohol. Thioridazine may partially negate the inotropic effect of digitalis (Baldessarini, 1980). Phenothiazines form a precipate when combined with caffeine, and caffeine-containing beverages may lower serum levels and diminish clinical effectiveness (Kulhanek et al., 1979; Lever and Hague, 1964; Mikkelsen, 1978). Barbiturates stimulate hepatic microenzymes and lower neuroleptic plasma levels through rapid metabolism. (Other interactions between neuroleptics and anticonvulsants are reviewed in Chapter 9.)

Neuroleptic agents have a wide range of possible side effects. The three principal effects are sedation, extrapyramidal effects, and postural hypotension. In general, the low-potency agents such as chlorpromazine and thioridazine have the greatest sedative and hypotensive effects and are least likely to induce parkinsonism and acute dystonic reactions; high-potency agents such as trifluoperazine, fluphenazine, and haloperidol have the opposite response profile (Table 13-7) (Baldessarini, 1980; Hollister, 1977). Table 13-8 lists the major side effects and idiosyncratic reactions reported with neuroleptic agents. (Not all the reactions listed in the table have been described with each neuroleptic agent.) Adequate management of a patient treated with antipsychotic drugs should include surveillance of possible effects on the central and autonomic nervous systems, as well as on the gastrointestinal, hematologic, dermatologic, ophthalmologic, endrocrine, and cardiovascular systems (Ayd 1972, 1974; Baldessarini, 1980; DePaulo and Ayd, 1982; Hollister, 1977).

Neuroleptic malignant syndrome refers to a rare complication of neuroleptic therapy characterized by muscular rigidity, hyperthermia, autonomic instability, and stupor. If unrecognized or untreated, the syndrome may cause death, but the lethal course of the syndrome has been aborted by administration of dantrolene, amantadine, and bromocriptine (Goulon et al., 1983; Granato et al., 1983; Henderson and Wooten, 1981; Morris et al., 1980; Zubenko and Pope, 1983).

The interactions between seizures and neuroleptic drugs are described in Chapter 9, the extrapyramidal effects of antipsychotic agents are presented in Chapter 12, and their effects on sexual function are included in Chapter 17.

Extreme Dosage Range (Oral mg)	Sedative Effects	Extra pyramidal Effects	Hypotensive Effects
25–2000	+ + +	+ +	+ +
50–800	+ + +	+	+ +
4–64	+ +	+ + +	+
2–60	+	+ + +	+
1–30	+	+ + +	+
6–60	+ + +	+ +	+ +
1–100	+	+ + +	+
20–250	+	+ +	+
15–400	+ +	+	0

TABLE 13-8.   Side Effects of Neuroleptic Medications

Central nervous system

  Akathisia
  Acute dystonic reactions
  Parkinsonism
  Tardive dyskinesia
  Seizures
  Neuroleptic malignant syndrome

Autonomic nervous system

  Orthostatic hypotension
  Dry mouth
  Blurred vision
  Urinary retention
  Inhibition of ejaculation
  Constipation
  Tachycardia
  Paralytic ileus
  Nasal congestion

Gastrointenstinal

  Jaundice (cholestatic)

Hematologic

  Leukocytosis
  Leukopenia
  Eosinophilia
  Agranulocytosis
  Hemolytic anemia, thrombocytopenic purpura, pancytopenia
  Aplastic anemia

Dermatologic

  Urticaria
  Photosensitivity
  Abnormal skin pigmentation

Ophthalmologic

  Corneal opacities
  Lens opacities
  Pigmentary retinopathy

Metabolic

  Weight gain

Endocrinologic

  Increased prolactin (may lead to glactorrhea), serum glucose
  Decreased adrenocorticotrophin, somatotrophin, luteinizing
  hormone, follicle-stimulating hormone, vasopressin,
  testosterone, oxytocin, corticosteroids, insulin, estrogens,
  progestins
  Amenorrhea
  Gynecomastia
  Decreased libido

Cardiovascular

  Orthostatic hypotension
  EKG changes—prolongation of Q-T and P-R intervals, blunted
  T waves, S-T segment depression

REFERENCES

Abd el Naby S and Hassanein M. Neuropsychiatric manifestations of chronic manganese poisoning. *J Neurol Neurosurg Psychiat*, 1965, *28*, 282–288.

Abenson MH. EEGs in chronic schizophrenia. *Br J Psychiat*, 1970, *116*, 421–425.

Adler AE, Sndja L, and Wilets G. Cimetidine toxicity manifested as paranoia and hallucinations. *Am J Psychiat*, 1980, *137*, 1112–1113.

Alexander MP, Stuss DT, and Benson DF. Capgras syndrome: a reduplicative phenomenon. *Neurology*, 1979, *29*, 334–339.

Ames F. A clinical and metabolic study of acute intoxication with *cannabis sativa* and its role in the model psychoses. *J Ment Sci*, 1958, *104*, 972–999.

Andreasen NC. Negative symptoms in schizophrenia. *Arch Gen Psychiat*, 1982, *39*, 784–788.

Andreasen NC and Olsen S. Negative *V* positive schizophrenia. *Arch Gen Psychiat*, 1982, *39*, 789–794.

Andreasen NC, Olsen SA, Dennert JW, and Smith MR. Ventricular enlargement in schizophrenia: relationship to positive and negative symptoms. *Am J Psychiat*, 1982a, *139*, 297–302.

Andreasen NC, Smith MK, Jacoby CG, Dennert JW, and Olsen SA. Ventricular enlargement in schizophrenia: definition and prevalence. *Am J Psychiat*, 1982b, *139*, 292–296.

Ariel RN, Golden CJ, Berg RA, Quaife MA, Dirksen JW, Forsell T, Wilson J, and Graber B. Regional cerebral blood flow in schizophrenics. *Arch Gen Psychiat*,1983, *40*, 258–263.

Arieti S. Histopathologic changes in cerebral malaria and their relation to psychotic sequels. *Arch Neurol Psychiat*, 1946, *56*, 79–104.

Asher R. Myxoedematous madness.*Br Med J*, 1949, *2*, 555–562.

Askevold F. The occurrence of paranoid incidents and abstinence delirium in abusers of amphetamine. *Acta Psychiat Neurol Scand*, 1959, *34*, 145–164.

Ayd FJ Jr. Haloperidol: fifteen years of clinical experience. *Dis Nerv Syst*, 1972, *33*, 459–469.

Ayd FJ Jr. A critical evaluation of molindone (Moban): a new indole derivative neuroleptic. *Dis Nerv Syst*, 1974, *35*, 447–452.

Baldessarini RJ. Schizophrenia. *New Engl J Med*, 1977, *297*, 988–995.

Baldessarini RJ. Drugs and the treatment of psychiatric disorders. In Gilman AG, Goodman LS, and Gilman A (Eds.): *Goodman and Gilman's the pharmacologic basis of therapeutics*, 6th ed. New York, Macmillan Publishing Company, 1980, pp. 391–447.

Barnhart CC and Bowden CL. Toxic psychosis with cimetidine. *Am J Psychiat*, 1979, *136*, 725–726.

Bassuk EL and Schoonover SC. *The practitioner's guide to psychoactive drugs*. New York, Plenum Medical Book Company, 1977.

Bates GM Jr. Leber's disease and schizophrenia. *Am J Psychiat*, 1964, *120*, 1017–1019.

Beamish P and Kiloh LG. Psychoses due to amphetamine consumption. *J Ment Sci*, 1960, *106*, 337–343.

Beard AW. The association of hepatolenticular degeneration with schizophrenia. *Acta Psychiat Neurol*, 1959, *34*, 411–428.

Bennett JC, Maffley RH, and Steinbach HL. The significance of bilateral basal ganglia calcification. *Radiology*, 1959, *72*, 368–377.

Benson DF. Psychiatric aspects of aphasia. *Br J Psychiat*, 1973, *123*,555–566.

Benson DF, Gardner H, and Meadows JC. Reduplicative paramnesia. *Neurology*, 1976, *26*, 147–151.

Bergman PS. Cerebral blindness. *Arch Neurol Psychiat*, 1957, *78*, 568–584.

Betts TA, Smith WT, and Kelly RE. Adult metachromatic leukodystrophy (sulphatide lipidosis) simulating schizophrenia. *Neurology*, 1968, *18*, 1140–1142.

Bird ED, Spokes EGS, and Iversen LL. Increased dopamine concentration in limbic areas and brain from patients dying with schizophrenia. *Brain*, 1979, *102*, 347–360.

Blankfein RJ and Chirico A-M. Cerebral schistosomiasis. *Neurology*, 1965, *15*, 957–967.

Blocker WW Jr, Kastl AJ Jr, and Daroff RB. The psychiatric manifestations of cerebral malaria. *Am J Psychiat*, 1968, *125*, 192–196.

Bogerts B, Hantsch T, and Herzer M. A morphometric study of the dopamine-containing cell groups in the mesencephalon of normals, Parkinson patients, and schizophrenics. *Biol Psychiat*, 1983, *18*, 951–969.

Bouton SM Jr. Pick's disease: clinicopathologic case reports. *J Nerv Ment Dis*, 1940, *91*, 9–30.

Bowers MB Jr. Acute psychosis induced by psychotomimetic drug abuse. I. Clinical findings. *Arch Gen Psychiat*, 1972, *27*, 437–440.

Bowman KM. Psychoses with pernicious anaemia. *Am J Psychiat*, 1935, *92*, 371–392.

Brezinova V and Kendell RE. Smooth pursuit eye movements of schizophrenia and normal people under stress. *Br J Psychiat*, 1977, *130*, 59–63.

Brierley JB and Cooper JE. Cerebral complications of hypotensive anesthesia in a healthy adult. *J Neurol Neurosurg Psychiat*, 1962, *25*, 24–30.

Brodie JD, Christman DR, Corona JF, Fowler JS, Gomez-Mont F, Jaeger J, Micheels PA, Rotrosen J, Russell JA, Volkow ND, Wikler A, Wolf AP, and Wolkin A. Patterns of metabolic activity in the treatment of schizophrenia. *Ann Neurol*, 1984, *15* (Suppl.), S166–S169.

Bromberg W. Mental states in chronic encephalitis. *Psychiat Quart*, 1930, *4*, 537–566.

Bruyn GW, Bots GThAM, and Staal A. Familial bilateral vascular calcification in the central nervous system. *Psychiat Neurol Neurochir*, 1964, *67*, 342–376.

Burks JS, Huddlestone J, Alfrey AC, Norenberg MD, and Lewin E. A fatal encephalopathy in chronic haemodialysis patients. *Lancet*, 1976, *1*, 764–768.

Burnell GM and Foster TA. Psychosis with low sodium syndrome. *Am J Psychiat*, 1972, *128*, 133–134.

Bursten N. Psychoses associated with thyrotoxicosis. *Arch Gen Psychiat*, 1981, *4*, 262–273.

Caine ED and Shoulson I. Psychiatric syndromes in Huntington's disease. *Am J Psychiat*, 1983, *140*, 728–733.

Cares RM, Gordon BS, and Kreuger E. Boeck's sarcoid in chronic meningo-encephalitis. *J Neuropathol Exp Neurol*, 1957, *16*, 544–554.

Carpenter WT Jr, Strauss JS, and Muleh S. Are there pathognomonic symptoms in schizophrenia? *Arch Gen Psychiat*, 1973, *28*, 847–852.

Cegalis JA and Sweeney JA. Eye movements in schizophrenia: a quantitative analysis. *Biol Psychiat*, 1979, *14*, 13–26

Celesia GG and Barr AN. Psychosis and other psychiatric manifestations of levodopa therapy. *Arch Neurol*, 1970, *23*, 193–200.

Celesia GG and Wanamaker WM. Psychiatric disturbances in Parkinson's disease. *Dis Nerv Syst*, 1972, *33*, 577–583.

Chandler JH and Bebin J. Hereditary cerebellar ataxia. *Neurology*, 1956, *6*, 187–195.

Chawla HM and Virmani V. Capgras phenomenon in a case of temporal lobe epilepsy. *Folia Psychiat Neurol Jap*, 1977, *31*, 615–617.

Chokroverty S, Breutman ME, Berger V, and Reyes MG. Progressive dialytic encephalopathy. *J Neurol Neurosurg Psychiat*, 1976, *39*, 411–419.

Christodoulou GN. Delusional hyper-identification of the Frigoli type. *Acta Psychiat Scand*, 1976, *54*, 305–314.

Christodoulou GN. The syndrome of Capgras. *Br J Psychiat*, 1977, *130*, 556–564.

Christodoulou GN. Syndrome of subjective double. *Am J Psychiat*, 1978, *135*, 249–251.

Cleghorn RA. Adrenal cortical insufficiency: psychological and neurological observations. *Can Med Assoc*, 1951, *65*, 449–454.

Cohen S. Angel dust. *JAMA*, 1977, *238*, 515–516.

Cohen S and Ditman KS. Prolonged adverse reactions to lysergic acid diethylamide. *Arch Gen Psychiat*, 1963, *8*, 475–480.

Cohn CK, Rosenblatt S, and Faillace LA. Capgras' syndrome presenting as postpartum psychosis. *South Med J*, 1977, *70*, 942.

Colon EJ. Quantitative cytoarchitectonics of the human cerebral cortex in schizophrenic dementia. *Acta Neuropathol*, 1972, *20*, 1–10.

Coren HA and Strain JJ. A case of narcolepsy with psychosis. *Comp Psychiat*, 1965, *6*, 191–199.

Crow TJ. Molecular pathology of schizophrenia: more than one disease process? *Br Med J*, 1980, *280*, 66–68.

Crow TJ, Baker HF, Cross AJ, Joseph MH, Lofthouse R, Langden A, Owen F, Riley GJ, Glover V, and Killpack WS. Monoamine mechanisms in chronic schizophrenia: postmortem neurochemical findings. *Br J Psychiat*, 1979, *134*, 249–256.

Crow TJ, Deakin JFW, and Longden A. The nucleus accumbens—possible site of antipsychotic action of neuroleptic drugs? *Psychol Med*, 1977, *7*, 213–221.

Crow TJ, Johnstone EC, Longden A, and Owen F. Dopamine and schizophrenia. *Adv Biochem Psychopharm*, 1978, *19*, 301–309.

Crow TJ, Johnstone EG, and McClelland HA. The coincidence of schizophrenia and parkinsonism: some neurochemical implications. *Psychol Med*, 1976, *6*, 227–233.

Cummings JL. Organic delusions: phenomenology anatomic correlations, and review. *Br J Psychiat*, 1985, *146*, 184–197.

Cummings JL and Benson DF. *Dementia: a clinical approach.* Boston, Butterworths, 1983.

Cummings J, Gosenfeld LF, Houlihan JP, and McCaffrey T. Neuropsychiatric disturbances associated with idiopathic

calcification of the basal ganglia. *Biol Psychiat*, 1983, *18*, 591–601.

Cutting J. The relationship between Korsakov's syndrome and "alcoholic dementia." *Br J Psychiat*, 1978a, *132*, 240–251.

Cutting J. Study of anosognosia. *J Neurol Neurosurg Psychiat*, 1978b, *41*, 548–555.

Damas Mora JMR, Jenner FA, and Eacoh SE. On heutoscopy or the phenomenon of the double: case presentation and review of the literature. *Br J Med Psychol*, 1980, *53*, 75–83.

Davies DL. Psychiatric changes associated with Friedreich's ataxia. *J Neurol Neurosurg Psychiat*, 1949, *12*, 246–250.

Davison K and Bagley OR. Schizophrenia-like psychoses associated with organic disorders of the central nervous system: a review of the literature. *Br J Psychiat*, 1969, (Special Issue No. 4), 113–184.

De Fine Olivarius B and Roder E. Reversible psychosis and dementia in myxedema. *Acta Psychiat Scand*, 1970, *46*, 1–12.

DePaulo JR Jr and Ayd FT Jr. Loxapine: fifteen years' clinical experience. *Psychosomatics*, 1982, *23*, 261–271.

Deveaugh-Geiss J and Pandurangi A. Confusional paranoid psychosis after withdrawal from sympathomimetic amines: two case reports. *Am J Psychiat*, 1982, *139*, 1190–1191.

Dewhurst K, Oliver J, Trick KLK, and McKnight AL. Neuropsychiatric aspects of Huntington's disease. *Confin Neurol*, 1969, *31*, 258–268.

Diagnostic and statistical manual of mental disorders, 3rd ed. Washington, D.C., American Psychiatric Association, 1980.

Donnelly EF, Weinberger DR, Waldman IN, and Wyatt RJ. Cognitive impairment associated with morphological brain abnormalities on computed tomography in chronic schizophrenic patients. *J Nerv Ment Dis*, 1980, *168*, 305–308.

Drachman DA and Adams RD. Herpes simplex and acute inclusion-body encephalitis. *Arch Neurol*, 1962, *7*, 45–63.

Eilenberg D and Woods LW. Narcolepsy with psychosis: report of two cases. *Mayo Clin Proc*, 1962, *37*, 561–566.

Enoch MD. The Capgras syndrome. *Acta Psychiat Scand*, 1963, *39*, 437–462.

Enoch MD and Trethowan WH. *Uncommon psychiatric syndromes,* 2nd ed. Bristol, England, John Wright and Sons Ltd., 1979.

Fairweather DS. Psychiatric aspects of the postencephalitic syndrome. *J Ment Sci*, 1947, *93*, 201–254.

Farkas T, Wolf AP, Jaeger J, Brodie JD, Christman DR, and Fowler JS. Regional brain glucose metabolism in chronic schizophrenia. *Arch Gen Psychiat*, 1984, *41*, 293–300.

Farley IJ, Price KS, McCullough E, Deck JHN, Hordynski W, and Hornykiewicz O. Norepinephrine in chronic paranoid schizophrenia: above-normal levels in limbic forebrain. *Science*, 1978, *200*, 456–457.

Fisher CM. Disorientation for place. *Arch Neurol*, 1982, *39*, 33–36.

Fisman M. The brain stem in psychosis. *Br J Psychiat*, 1975, *126*, 414–422.

Fitz TE and Hallman BL. Mental changes associated with hyperparathyroidism. *Arch Int Med*, 1952, *89*, 547–551.

Fox JT Jr and Kane FT Jr. Niemann-Pick's disease manifesting as schizophrenia. *Dis Nerv Syst*, 1967, *28*, 194.

Francis AF. Familial basal ganglia calcification and schizophreniform psychosis. *Br J Psychiat*, 1979, *135*, 360–362.

Franzen G and Ingvar DH. Absence of activation in frontal structures during psychological testing of chronic schizophrenics. *J Neurol Neurosurg Psychiat*, 1975, *38*, 1027–1032.

Freeman AM III. Delusions, depersonalization and unusual psychopathological symptoms. In Hall RCW (Ed.): *Psychiatric presentations of medical illness*. New York, SP Medical and Scientific Books, 1980, pp. 75–89.

Gal P. Mental symptoms in cases of tumor of temporal lobe. *Am J Psychiat*, 1958, *115*, 157–160.

Garron DC. Huntington's chorea and schizophrenia. *Adv Neurol*, 1973, *1*, 729–734.

Geocaris K. Psychotic episodes heralding the diagnosis of multiple sclerosis. *Menninger Clin Bull*, 1957, *21*, 107–116.

Gershan ES, Goldstein RE, Moss AJ, and Van Kammen DP. Psychosis with ordinary doses of propranolol. *Ann Int Med*, 1979, *90*, 938–939.

Golden CJ, Graber B, Coffman J, Berg RA, Newlin DB, and Bloch S. Structural brain deficits in schizophrenia. *Arch Gen Psychiat*, 1981, *38*, 1014–1017.

Golden CJ, Graber B, Moses TA, and Zatz LM. Differentiation of chronic schizophrenics with and without ventricular enlargement by the Luria-Nebraska neuropsychological battery. *Internat J Neurosci*, 1980a, *11*, 131–138.

Golden CJ, Moses JA Jr, Zelazowski R, Graber B, Zatz LM, Horvath TB, and Berger PA. Cerebral ventricular size and neuropsychological impairment in young chronic schizophrenics. *Arch Gen Psychiat*, 1980b, *37*, 619–623.

Goldhammer Y, Bubis JJ, Sarova-Pinhas I, and Braham J. Subacute spongiform encephalopathy and its relation to Jakob-Creutzfeldt disease: report of six cases. *J Neurol Neurosurg Psychiat*, 1972, *35*, 1–10.

Goodwin FK. Behavioral effects of dopa in man. *Semin Psychiat*, 1971, *3*, 477–492.

Gorman WF and Wortis SB. Psychosis in Addison's disease. *Dis Nerv Syst*, 1947, *8*, 267–271.

Gotze P and Dahme B. Psychopathological syndromes and neurological disturbances before and after open-heart surgery. In Speidel H and Rodewald G (Eds.): *Psychic and neurological dysfunctions after open-heart surgery*. New York, Thieme Stratton, Inc., 1980, pp. 48–67.

Goulon M, de Rohan-Chabot P, Elkharrat D, Gajdos P, Bismuth C, and Conso F. Beneficial effects of dentrolene in the treatment of neuroleptic malignant syndrome: a report of two cases. *Neurology*, 1983, *33*, 516–518.

Granato JE, Stern BJ, Ringel A, Karim AH, Krumholz A, Coyle J, and Adler S. Neuroleptic malignant syndrome: successful treatment with dantrolene and bromocriptine. *Ann Neurol*, 1983, *14*, 89–90.

Grant HC and McMenemey WH. Giant cell encephalitis in a dement. *Neuropath Pol*, 1960, Suppl. 4, 735–740.

Greenbaum JV and Lurie LA. Encephalitis as a causative factor in behavior disorders of children. *JAMA*, 1948, *136*, 923–931.

Green JA and Swanson LW. Psychosis in hypoparathyroidism with a report of five cases. *Ann Int Med*, 1941, *14*, 1233–1236.

Grunfeld O and Hinostroza G. Thallium poisoning. *Arch Int Med*, 1964, *114*, 132–138.

Gur RE, Skolnick BE, Gur RC, Caroff S, Riegar W, Obrist WD, Younkin D, and Reivich M. Brain function in psychiatric disorders. *Arch Gen Psychiat*, 1983, *40*, 1250–1254.

Gysin WM and Cooke ET. Unusual mental symptoms in a case of hepatolenticular degeneration. *Dis Nerv Syst*, 1950, *28*, 305–309.

Hamilton NG, Frick RB, Takahashi T, and Hopping MW. Psychiatric symptoms and cerebellar pathology. *Am J Psychiat*, 1983, *140*, 1322–1326.

Hammes EM. Psychoses associated with Sydenham's chorea. *JAMA*, 1922, *79*, 804–807.

Hanley J, Rickles WR, Crandall PH, and Walter RD. Automatic recognition of EEG correlates of behavior in a chronic schizophrenic patient. *Am J Psychiat*, 1972, *128*, 1524–1528.

Hanna SM. Hypopituitarism (Sheehan's syndrome) presenting with organic psychosis. *J Neurol Neurosurg Psychiat*, 1970, *33*, 192–193.

Hausner RS. Amantadine-associated recurrence of psychosis. *Am J Psychiat* 1980, *137*, 240–242.

Hay GG, Jolley DJ, and Jones RG. A case of the Capgras syndrome in association with pseudo-hypoparathyroidism. *Acta Psychiat Scand*, 1974, *50*, 73–77.

Hayman MA and Abrams R. Capgras' syndrome and cerebral dysfunction. *Br J Psychiat*, 1977, *130*, 68–71.

Henderson VW and Wooten GF. Neuroleptic malignant syndrome: a pathogenetic role for dopamine receptor blockade? *Neurology*, 1981, *31*, 132–137.

Hillbom E. Schizophrenia-like psychoses after brain trauma. *Acta Psychiat Neurol Scand*, 1951, Suppl. 60, 36–47.

Hillbom E. After-effects of brain injuries. *Acta Psychiat Neurol Scand*, 1960, *35* (Suppl. 142), 1–135.

Hollister LE. Mental disorders—antipsychotic and antimanic drugs. *New Engl J Med*, 1972, *286*, 984–987.

Hollister LE. Antipsychotic medications and the treatment of schizophrenia. In Barchas JD, Berger PA, Ciarnaello RD, and Elliot GR (Eds.): *Psychopharmacology from theory to practice*. New York, Oxford University Press, 1977, pp. 121–150.

Hollister LE and Glazener FS. Concurrent paralysis agitans and schizophrenia. *Dis Nerv Syst*, 1961, *22*, 187–189.

Holzman PS, Kringlen E, Levy DL, Proctor LR, Haberman SJ, and Yasillo NJ. Abnormal pursuit eye movement in schizophrenia. *Arch Gen Psychiat*, 1977, *34*, 802–805.

Holzman PS, Proctor LR, and Hughes DW. Eye-tracking patterns in schizophrenia. *Science*, 1973, *181*, 179–181.

Holzman PS, Proctor LR, Levy DL, Yasillo NJ, Meltzer HY, and Hurt SW. Eye-tracking dysfunctions in schizophrenic patients and their relatives. *Arch Gen Psychiat*, 1974, *31*, 143–151.

Ianzito BM, Cadoret RJ, and Pugh DP. Thought disorder in depression. *Am J Psychiat*, 1974, *131*, 703–707.

Jackson JA and Immerman SL. A case of pseudosclerosis associated with a psychosis. *J Nerv Ment Dis*, 1919, *49*, 5–13.

James WE, Mefferd RB Jr, and Kimbell I Jr. Early signs of Huntington's chorea. *Dis Nerv Syst* 1969, *30*, 550–559.

Jaspers K. *General psychopathology* (translated by Hoenig J and Hamilton MW). Chicago, University of Chicago Press, 1963.

Jefferson JW and Marshall JR. *Neuropsychiatric features of medical disorders*. New York, Plenum Medical Book Company, 1981.

Johnson KP, Rosenthal MS and Lerner PI. Herpes simplex encephalitis. *Arch Neurol*, 1972, *27*, 103–108.

Johnstone EC, Crow TJ, Frith CD, Husband J, and Kreel L. Cerebral ventricular size and cognitive impairment in chronic schizophrenia. *Lancet*, 1976, *2*, 924–926.

Johnstone EC, Crow TJ, Frith CD, Stevens M, Kreel L, and Husband J. The dementia of dementia praecox. *Acta Psychiat Scand*, 1978, *57*, 305–324.

Kalamboukis Z and Molling P. Symmetrical calcification of the brain in the predominance of the basal ganglia and cerebellum. *J Neuropathol Exp Neurol*, 1962, *21*, 364–371.

Karson CN. Spontaneous eye-blink rates and dopaminergic systems. *Brain*, 1983, *106*, 643–653.

Kasanin J and Crank RP. A case of extensive calcification in the brain. *Arch Neurol Psychiat*, 1935, *34*, 164–178.

Keddie KMG. Toxic psychosis following mumps. *Br J Psychiat*, 1965, *111*, 691–696.

Keddie KMG. Hereditary ataxia, presumed to be of the Menzel type, complicated by paranoid psychosis in a mother and two sons. *J Neurol Neurosurg Psychiat*, 1969, *32*, 82–87.

Keitner GI, Sabaawi M, and Haier RJ. Isosafrole and schizophrenia-like psychosis. *Am J Psychiat*, 1984, *141*, 997–998.

Kessler KA and Waletzky JP. Clinical use of antipsychotics. *Am J Psychiat*, 1981, *138*, 202–208.

Kirby GH and Davis TK. Psychiatric aspects of epidemic encephalitis. *Arch Neurol Psychiat*, 1921, *5*, 491–551.

Kornfeld DS, Zimberg S, and Malm JR. Psychiatric complications of open-heart surgery. *New Engl J Med*, 1965, *273*, 287–292.

Kulhanek F, Linde OK, and Meisenberg G. Precipitation of antipsychotic drugs in interaction with coffee and tea. *Lancet*, 1979, *2*, 1130.

Langworthy OR, Kolb LC, and Androp S. Disturbances of behavior in patients with disseminated sclerosis. *Am J Psychiat*, 1941, *98*, 243–249.

Larson T, Sjogren T, and Jacobson G. Senile dementia. *Acta Psychiat Scand*, 1963, Suppl. 167, 1–259.

Lee T, Seeman P, Tourtellotte WW, Farley IJ, and Hornykeiwicz O. Binding of ^{3}H-neuroleptics and ^{3}H-apomorphine in schizophrenic brains. *Nature*, 1978, *274*, 897–900.

Leeks SR. A mid-brain lesion presenting as schizophrenia. *New Zeal Med J*, 1967, *66*, 311–314.

Leighton KM. Paranoid psychosis after abuse of actifed. *Br Med J*, 1982, *284*, 789–790.

Lever PG and Hague JR. Observations on phenothiazine con-centrates and diluting agents. *Am J Psychiat*, 1964, *120*, 1000–1002.

Levin S, Jones A, Stark L, Mervin EL, and Holzman PS. Identification of abnormal patterns in eye movements of schizophrenic patients. *Arch Gen Psychiat*, 1982, *39*, 1125–1130.

Levine DN and Finkelstein S. Delayed psychosis after right temporoparietal stroke or trauma: relation to epilepsy. *Neurology*, 1982, *32*, 267–273.

Lewis DA and Smith RE. Steroid-induced psychiatric syndromes. *J Affect Dis*, 1983, *5*, 319–322.

Lorand B, Nagy T and Tariska S. Subacute progressive panencephalitis. *World Neurol*, 1962, *3*, 376–394.

Lovett Doust JW and Christie H. The pathology of love: some clinical variants of de Clerambault's syndrome. *Soc Sci Med*, 1978, *12*, 99–106.

Luchins DJ, Weinberger DR, and Wyatt RT. Schizophrenia. Evidence of a subgroup with reversed cerebral asymmetry. *Arch Gen Psychiat*, 1979, *36*, 1309–1311.

MacCallum WAG. Capgras symptoms with an organic basis. *Br J Psychiat*, 1973, *123*, 639–652.

MacNeill A, Grennan DM, Werd D, and Dick WC. Psychiatric problems in systemic lupus erythematosus. *Br J Psychiat*, 1976, *128*, 442–445.

Medakusira S and Hall TB III. Capgras syndrome in a patient with myxedema. *Am J Psychiat*, 1981, *138*, 1506–1508.

Malamud N and Boyd DA Jr. Pick's disease with atrophy of the temporal lobes. *Arch Neurol Psychiat*, 1940, *43*, 210–222.

Malliaras DE, Kossouvitsa YT, and Christodoulou GN. Organic contributors to the intermetamorphosis syndrome. *Am J Psychiat*, 1978, *135*, 985–987.

Mathew RJ, Duncan GC, Weinman ML, and Barr DL. Regional cerebral blood flow in schizophrenia. *Arch Gen Psychiat*, 1982, *39*, 1121–1124.

Medical letter. Drugs that cause psychiatric symptoms. *Med Let*, 1984, *26*, 75–78.

Meltzer HY, Kane JM, and Kolakowska T. Plasma levels of neuroleptics, prolactin levels and clinical response. In Coyle TJ and Enna ST (Eds.): *Neuroleptics: neurochemical, behavioral, and clinical perspectives*. New York, Raven Press, 1983, pp. 255–279.

Menninger KA. Influenza and schizophrenia. *Am J Psychiat*, 1926, *82*, 469–529.

Merrin EL and Silverfarb PM. The Capgras phenomenon. *Arch Gen Psychiat*, 1976, *33*, 965–968.

Mikkelsen EJ. Caffeine and schizophrenia. *J Clin Psychiat*, 1978, *39*, 732–736.

Mindham RHS. Psychiatric symptoms in parkinsonism. *J Neurol Neurosurg Psychiat*, 1970, *33*, 188–191.

Misra PC and Hay GG. Encephalitis presenting as acute schizophrenia. *Br Med J*, 1971, *1*, 532–533.

Mooney HB. Pathologic jealousy and psychochemotherapy. *Br J Psychiat*, 1965, *111*, 1023–1042.

Morihisa JM, Duffy FH, and Wyatt RJ. Brain electrical activity mapping (BEAM) in schizophrenic patients. *Arch Gen Psychiat*, 1983, *40*, 719–728.

Morris HH III, McCormick WF, and Reinarz JA. Neuroleptic malignant syndrome. *Arch Neurol*, 1980, *37*, 462–463.

Morstyn R, Duffy FH, and McCorkley RW. Altered P300 topography in schizophrenia. *Arch Gen Psychiat*, 1983, *40*, 729–734.

Moser M, Syner J, Malitz S, and Mattingly JW. Acute psychosis as a complication of hydralazine therapy in essential hypertension. *JAMA*, 1953, *152*, 1329–1331.

Moskovitz C, Moses H III, and Klawans HL. Levodopa-induced psychosis: a kindling phenomenon. *Am J Psychiat*, 1978, *135*, 669–675.

Muller D, Pilz H, and Ter Meulen V. Studies on adult metachromatic leukodystrophy. Part I. Clinical, morphological and histochemical observations in two cases. *J Neurol Sci*, 1969, *9*, 567–584.

Nash DL. Delusions. In Cavenar JO Jr and Brodie HKH (Eds.): *Signs and symptoms in psychiatry*. Philadelphia, JB Lippincott, 1983, pp. 455–481.

Nasrallah HA, Fowler RC, and Jud LL. Schizophrenia-like illness following head injury. *Psychosomatics*, 1981, *22*, 359–361.

Nasrallah HA, Jacoby CG, McCalley-Whitters M, and Kuperman S. Cerebral ventricular enlargement in subtypes of chornic schizophrenia. *Arch Gen Psychiat*, 1982, *39*, 774–777.

Owen F, Crow TJ, Poulter M, Gross AJ, Longden A, and Riley GJ. Increased dopamine-receptor sensitivity in schizophrenia. *Lancet*, 1978, *1*, 223–226.

Pandurangi AK, Dewan MJ, Lee SH, Ramachandran T, Levy BF, Boucher M, Yozawitz A, and Major L. The ventricular system in chronic schizophrenic patients in a controlled computed tomography study. *Br J Psychiat*, 1984, *144*, 172–176.

Paykel ES, Fleminger R, and Watson JP. Psychiatric side effects of antihypertensive drugs other than reserpine. *J Clin Psychopharm*, 1982, *2*, 14–39.

Peroutka SJ, Sohmer BH, Kumer AJ, Folstein M, and Robinson RG. Hallucinations and delusions following a right temporoparieto-occipital infarction. *Johns Hopkins Med J*, 1982, *151*, 181–185.

Petersen MC, Bickford G, Sem-Jacobsen CW, and Dodge HW Jr. The depth electrogram in schizophrenic patients. *Proc Mayo Clin*, 1953, *28*, 170–175.

Petursson H. Diethylpropion and paranoid psychosis. *Aust New Zeal J Psychiat*, 1979, *13*, 67–68.

Pfefferbaum A and Berger PA. Narcolepsy, paranoid psychosis, and tardive dyskinesia: a pharmacological dilemma. *J Nerv Ment Dis*, 1977, *164*, 293–297.

Pies R. Capgras phenomenon, delirium, and transient hepatic dysfunction. *Hosp Comm Psychiat*, 1982, *33*, 382–383.

Pope FM. Parasitophobia as the presenting symptom in vitamin B_{12} deficiency. *Practitioner*, 1970, *204*, 421–422.

Postma JU and van Tilburg W. Visual hallucinations and delirium during treatment with amantadine (symmetrel). *J Am Geriat Soc*, 1975, *23*, 212–215.

Powell H, Tindall R, Schultz P, Paa D, O'Brien J, and Lampert P. Adrenoleukodystrophy. *Arch Neurol*, 1975, *32*, 250–260.

Price TRP and Tucker GJ. Psychiatric and behavioral manifestations of normal pressure hydrocephalus. *J Nerv Ment Dis*, 1964, *164*, 51–55.

Quinn D. The capgras syndrome: two case reports and a review. *Can J Psychiat*, 1981, *26*, 126–129.

Quitkin F, Rifkin A, and Klein DF. Neurologic soft signs in schizophrenia and character disorders. *Arch Gen Psychiat*, 1976, *33*, 845–853.

Ramani SV. Psychosis associated with frontal lobe lesions in Schilder's cerebral sclerosis: a case report with CT scan evidence. *J Clin Psychiat*, 1981, *42*, 250–252.

Raymond RW and Williams RL. Infectious mononucleosis with psychosis. *New Engl J Med*, 1948, *239*, 542–544.

Read AE, Sherlock S, Laidlaw J, and Walker JG. The neuropsychiatric syndromes associated with chronic liver disease and extensive portal-systemic collateral circulation. *Quart J Med*, 1967, *36*, 135–150.

Redlich FC and Dorsey JF. Denial of blindness by patients with cerebral disease. *Arch Neurol Psychiat*, 1945, *53*, 407–417.

Remick RA, O'Kane J, and Sparling TG. A case report of toxic psychosis with low-dose propranolol therapy. *Am J Psychiat*, 1981, *138*, 850–851.

Rennick PM, Nolan DC, Bauer RB, and Lerner AM. Neuropsychologic and neurologic follow-up after herpes hominis encephalitis. *Neurology*, 1973, *23*, 42–47.

Reveley AM and Reveley MA. Aqueduct stenosis and schizophrenia. *J Neurol Neurosurg Psychiat*, 1983, *46*, 18–22.

Reveley AM, Reveley MA, and Murray RM. Cerebral ventricular enlargement in non-genetic schizophrenia: a controlled twin study. *Br J Psychiat*, 1984, *144*, 89–93.

Rice E and Gendelman S. Psychiatric aspects of normal pressure hydrocephalus. *JAMA*, 1973, *223*, 409–412.

Richards F II, Cooper MR, Pearce LA, Cowan RJ, and Spurr CL. Familial spinocerebellar degeneration, hemolytic anemia, and glutathione deficiency. *Arch Int Med*, 1974, *134*, 534–537.

Risk WS and Hadded FS. The variable natural history of subacute sclerosing panencephalitis. *Arch Neurol*, 1979, *86*, 610–614.

Rosenbaum D. Psychosis with Huntington's disease. *Psychiat Quart*, 1941, *15*, 93–99.

Roth N. The neuropsychiatric aspects of porphyria. *Psychosom Med*, 1945, *7*, 291–301.

Rothermich NO and von Haam E. Pancreatic encephalopathy. *J Clin Endocrinol*, 1941, *1*, 872–881.

Rothschild D. Dementia paralytica accompanied by manic-depressive and schizophrenic psychoses. *Am J Psychiat*, 1940, *96*, 1043–1060.

Rudnick DF. The paranoid-erotic syndromes. In Friedmann CTH and Fagnet RA (Eds.): *Extraordinary disorders of human behavior*. New York, Plenum Press, 1982, pp. 99–119.

Sanders V. Neurologic manifestations of myxedema. *New Engl J Med*, 1962, *266*, 547–552, 599–603.

Sands IJ. The acute psychiatric type of epidemic encephalitis. *Am J Psychiat*, 1928, *84*, 975–987.

Scheinberg IH. Neurological and behavioral aspects of Wilson's disease. In Alexander PE (Ed.): *Electrolytes and neuropsychiatric disorders.* New York, SP Medical and Scientific Books, 1981, pp. 113–120.

Schienberg IH and Steinlieb I. *Wilson's disease.* Philadelphia, WB Saunders Company, 1984.

Schenk VWD and Stolk PJ. Psychosis following arsenic (possibly thallium) poisoning. *Psychiat Neurol Neurochir,* 1967, *70,* 31–37.

Schreiner GE. Mental and personality changes in the uremic syndrome. *Med Ann DC,* 1959, *28,* 316–323.

Schube PG. Emotional states of general paresis. *Am J Psychiat,* 1934, *91,* 625–638.

Schulz SC, Koller MM, Kishore PR, Hamer RM, Gehl JJ, and Friedel RO. Ventricular enlargement in teenage patients with schizophrenic spectrum disorder. *Am J Psychiat,* 1983, *140,* 1592–1595.

Scott M. Transitory psychotic behavior following operation for tumors of the cerebello-pontine angle. *Psychiat Neurol Neurochir,* 1970, *73,* 37–48.

Sem-Jacobson CW, Petersen MC, Lazarte JA, Dodge HW Jr, and Holman CB. Intracerebral electrographic recordings from psychotic patients during hallucinations and agitation. *Am J Psychiat,* 1955, *112,* 278–288.

Shapiro LB. Schizophrenia-like psychosis following head injuries. *Ill Med J,* 1939, *76,* 250–253.

Shepherd M. Report of a family suffering from Friedreich's disease peroneal muscular atrophy, and schizophrenia. *J Neurol Neurosurg Psychiat,* 955, *18,* 297–304.

Shepherd M. Morbid jealousy: some clinical and social aspects of a psychiatric symptom. *J Ment Sci,* 1961, *107,* 687–753.

Slater E, Beard AW and Glithero E. The schizophrenia-like psychoses of epilepsy. *Br J Psychiat,* 1963, *109,* 95–150.

Small JG. EEG in schizophrenia. In Hughes JR and Wilson WP (Eds.): *EEG and evoked potentials in psychiatry and behavioral neurology.* Boston, Butterworths, 1983, pp. 25–40.

Smith ADM. Megaloblastic madness. *Br Med J,* 1960, *2,* 1840–1845.

Synder SH, Banerjee SP, Yamamura HI, and Greenberg D. Drugs, neurotransmitters, and schizophrenia. *Science,* 1974, *184,* 1243–1253.

Spillane JD. Nervous and mental disorders in Cushing's syndrome. *Brain,* 1951, *74,* 72–94.

Stern M and Robbins ES. Psychoses in systemic lupus erythematosis. *Arch Gen Psychiat,* 1960, *3,* 205–212.

Stevens JR. Disturbances of ocular movements and blinking in schizophrenia. *J Neurol Neurosurg Psychiat,* 1978, *41,* 1024–1030.

Stevens JR. Neuropathology of schizophrenia. *Arch Gen Psychiat,* 1982, *39,* 1131–1139.

Stevens JR and Livermore A. Telemetered EEG in schizophrenia: spectral analysis during abnormal behavior episodes. *J Neurol Neurosurg Psychiat,* 1982, *45,* 385–395.

Still RML. Psychosis following Asian influenza in Barbados. *Lancet,* 1958, *3,* 20–21.

Stoudemire A, Baker N, and Thompson TL II. Delirium induced by topical application of podophyllin: a case report. *Am J Psychiat,* 1981, *138,* 1505–1506.

Strachan RW and Henderson JG. Dementia and folate deficiency. *Quart J Med,* 1967, *36,* 189–204.

Surawicz FG and Banta R. Lycanthropy revisited. *Can Psychiat Assoc J,* 1975, *20,* 537–542.

Sydenstricker VP. Psychic manifestations of nicotinic acid deficiency. *Proc Roy Soc Med,* 1943, *36,* 169–171.

Symonds C and Mackenzie I. Bilateral loss of vision from cerebral infarction. *Brain,* 1957, *80,* 415–455.

Thompson GN. Cerebral lesions simulating schizophrenia: three case reports. *Biol Psychiat,* 1970, *2,* 59–64.

Toone B. Psychoses in epilepsy. In Reynolds EH and Trimble MR (Eds.): *Epilepsy and psychiatry.* New York, Churchill Livingston, 1981, pp. 113–137.

Trimble MR. *Neuropsychiatry.* New York, John Wiley & Sons, 1981.

Trimble MR and Cummings JL. Neuropsychiatric disturbances following brainstem lesions. *Br J Psychiat,* 1981, *138,* 56–59.

Tsai LY, Nasrallah HA, and Jacoby CG. Hemispheric asymmetries on computed tomographic scans in schizophrenia and mania. *Arch Gen Psychiat,* 1983, *40,* 1286–1289.

Vaillant G. Schizophrenia in a woman with temporal lobe arterio-venous malformation. *Br J Psychiat,* 1965, *111,* 307–308.

Vroom FQ and Greer M. Mercury vapor intoxication. *Brain,* 1972, *95,* 305–318.

Weinberger DR, Delisi LE, Perman GP, Targum S, and Wyatt RJ. Computed tomography in schizophreniform disorder and other acute psychiatric disorders. *Arch Gen Psychiat,* 1982, *39,* 778–783.

Weinberger DR, Torrey EF, Neophytides AN, and Wyatt RJ. Lateral cerebral ventricular enlargement in chronic schizophrenia. *Arch Gen Psychiat,* 1979a, *36,* 735–739.

Weinberger DR, Torrey EF, Neophytides AN, and Wyatt RJ. Structural abnormalities in the cerebral cortex of chronic schizophrenic patients. *Arch Gen Psychiat,* 1979b, *36,* 935–939.

Weinberger DR, Wagner RL and Wyatt RJ. Neuropathological studies of schizophrenia: a selective review. *Schiz Bull,* 1983, *9,* 193–212.

Weinstein EN, Kahn RL, Malitz S, and Rozanski J. Delusional reduplication of parts of the body. *Brain,* 1954, *77,* 45–60.

Weizman A, Eldar M, Shoenfeld Y, Hirschorn M, Wijsenbeck H, and Pinkhas J. Hypercalcemia-induced psychopathology in malignant diseases. *Br J Psychiat,* 1979, *135,* 363–366.

Weston MJ and Whitlock FA. The capgras syndrome following head injury. *Br J Psychiat,* 1971, *119,* 25–31.

White JC and Cobb S. Psychological changes associated with giant pituitary neoplasms. *Arch Neurol Psychiat,* 1955, *74,* 383–396.

White MC, Silverman JJ, and Harbison JW. Psychosis associated with clonazepam therapy for bleparospasm. *J Nerv Ment Dis,* 1982, *170,* 117–119.

Wijsenbeek H, Kriegel Y and Landau B. A paranoid state in a

patient suffering from Sheehan syndrome. *Am J Psychiat*, 1964, *120*, 1120–1122.

Wilcox J, and Waziri R. The Capgras symptom and nondominant cerebral dysfunction. *J Clin Psychiat*, 1983, *44*, 70–72.

Williams BB and Lerner AM. Some previously unrecognized features of herpes simplex virus encephalitis. *Neurology*, 1978, *28*, 1193–1196.

Wilson G and Rupp C. Mental symptoms associated with extramedullary posterior fossa tumors. *Trans Am Neurol Assoc*, 1946, *71*, 104–106.

Wilson JW. Delusions of parasitosis (acraphobia). *Arch Dermatol*, 1952, *66*, 577–585.

Woods BT and Wolf J. A reconsideration of the relation of ventricular enlargement to duration of illness in schizophrenia. *Am J Psychiat*, 1983, *140*, 1564–1570.

Zubenko G and Pope HG Jr. Management of a case of neuroleptic malignant syndrome with bromocriptine. *Am J Psychiat*, 1983, *140*, 1619–1620.

Zucker DK, Livingston RL, Nakra R, and Clayton PJ. B_1 deficiency and psychiatric disorders: case report and literature review. *Biol Psychiat*, 1981, *16*, 197–205.

Chapter 14

Disturbances of Mood and Affect

Mood refers to the internal emotional experience of an individual (happiness, sadness, anger, etc.), whereas *affect* is the external expression of emotion. In most cases mood and affect are congruent, with the external affect accurately reflecting the individual's internal mood, and this has given rise to the common practice of referring to pathological disturbances of mood as affective disorders. In some cases, however, mood and affect may be dissociated. In disorders such as pseudobulbar palsy and certain types of epileptic seizure, the patient may cry or laugh when the corresponding mood is lacking. This chapter presents the neurological aspects of disturbances of mood and affect.

MOOD DISORDERS

Depression

Depression refers to a mood alteration with prominent sadness, hopelessness, irritability, and anhedonia. To be considered indicative of a major depressive disorder, the symptoms must persist for at least 2 weeks and be complicated by at least four of the following: alterations in appetite, sleep disturbance, psychomotor agitation or retardation, loss of libido, fatigue, cognitive impairment, and suicidal ideation (*Diagnostic and statistical manual of mental disorders,* 1980). The etiologies of depression, the clinical elements of the depression syndrome, and the neurological aspects of idiopathic depression are discussed in this chapter. In this discussion *idiopathic depression* refers to the depression syndromes accompanying the primary affective disorders (major depression or depressed phase of a bipolar disorder), and *secondary depression* refers to mood alterations produced by identifiable neurological, toxic, or metabolic conditions.

Etiologies of Depression

The relative frequency of idiopathic and secondary depressions has not been fully determined, but it is estimated that approximately 30 percent of patients with

significant depressions have physical conditions contributing to or wholly accounting for the psychiatric illness (Whitlock, 1982). Table 14-1 presents the neurological and systemic–metabolic disorders that may produce depression syndromes.

Neurological disorders producing depression. A variety of neurological disorders produce depression in excess of what would be expected for the degree of disability resulting from any associated physical abnormalities. Depression is one of the cardinal features of subcortical dementia and is a common manifestation of the mental status alterations of extrapyramidal syndromes (Chapter 8). Depression is particularly common in Parkinson's disease, occurring in 47–71 percent of cases. It occurs with approximately equal frequency in idiopathic paralysis agitans and postencephalitic parkinsonism (Brown and Wilson, 1972; Celesia and Wanamaker, 1972; Horn 1974; Jackson et al., 1923, Mayeux et al., 1981; Mettler and Crandell, 1959; Mindham, 1970; Robins, 1976; Warburton, 1967). Depression accounts for 90 percent of all psychiatric dysfunction in patients with idiopathic Parkinson disease. In postencephalitic parkinsonism, depression occurs in conjunction with a variety of conduct disorders, schizophrenialike psychoses, and obsessive–compulsive disorders (Bromberg, 1930; Fairweather, 1947; Kirby and Davis, 1921; Mindham, 1970). The depression of parkinsonism correlates poorly with the degree of physical disability, the age of the patient, or the duration of the disease (Celesia and Wanamaker, 1972; Mayeux et al., 1981; Mindham, 1970; Robins, 1976; Warburton, 1967). Depression is more common among those with neuropsychological impairment, and depressed parkinsonians have lower levels of 5-hydroxyindoleacetic acid in their cerebrospinal fluid (CSF) than do nondepressed parkinsonians (Mayeux et al., 1981, 1983, 1984). The depression in parkinsonism must be distinguished from superficially depressed appearance produced by bradykinesia and masked face.

Treatment of Parkinson's disease with levodopa improves the motor disturbance but does not improve or forestall the occurrence of depression (Cherington, 1970; Marsh and Markham, 1973). The depression frequently

TABLE 14-1   Principal Neurological and Systemic Disorders Producing Depression

Neurological disorders

Extrapyramidal diseases

Parkinson's disease
Huntington's disease
Progressive supranuclear palsy
Cerebrovascular disease (especially anterior hemispheric lesions)
Cerebral neoplasms
Cerebral trauma
CNS infections
Multiple sclerosis
Epilepsy
Narcolepsy
Hydrocephalus

Systemic disorders

Infections

Viral
Bacterial

Endocrine disorders

Hyperthyroidism
Hypothyroidism
Hyperparathyroidism
Hypoparathyroidism
Cushing's syndrome (steroid excess)
Addison's disease (steroid insufficiency)
Hyperaldosteronism
Premenstrual depression

Inflammatory disorders

Systemic lupus erythematosus
Rheumatoid arthritis
Temporal arteritis
Sjögren's syndrome

Vitamin deficiencies

Folate
Vitamin B_{12}
Niacin
Vitamin C

Miscellaneous systemic disorders

Cardiopulmonary disease
Renal disease and uremia
Systemic neoplasms
Porphyria
Klinefelter's syndrome
Acquired immune deficiency syndrome
Postpartum affective disorders
Postoperative affective disorders

responds to treatment with tricyclic antidepressants and with electroconvulsive therapy (Anderson et al., 1980; Asnis, 1977; Denmark et al., 1961; Gillhespy and Mustard, 1963; Laitinen, 1969; Lebensohn and Jenkins, 1975; Mandell et al., 1961; Strauss, 1959; Strang, 1965; Yudofsky, 1979).

Depression is also particularly common in Huntington's disease. It occurs in approximately half the patients suffering from the disorder and may have either recurrent unipolar or bipolar manifestations (Caine and Shoulson, 1983; Dewhurst et al., 1969; Folstein et al., 1983; Goodman et al., 1966; McHugh and Folstein,

1975). Suicide accounts for 7 percent of the deaths of Huntington's disease patients, and suicide attempts occur in many more (Reed et al., 1958). Treatment of the depression associated with Huntington's disease with tricyclic antidepressants and electroconvulsive therapy has met with variable success (Caine and Shoulson, 1983; McHugh and Folstein, 1975; Whittier et al., 1961).

Depression is not unusual in progressive supranuclear palsy, occurring in conjunction in axial rigidity, supranuclear gaze palsy, pseudobulbar palsy, and dementia (Albert et al., 1974; Janati and Appel, 1984; Jackson et al., 1983). The depression may respond to treatment with tricyclic antidepressants (Kvale, 1982).

Depression is a common consequence of cerebrovascular disease (Folstein et al., 1977; Robinson et al., 1984; Trimble and Cummings, 1981). Depression is more common with frontal lobe lesions than with posterior hemispheric lesions and is more common and more severe with left-sided infarctions than with right-sided insults (Finklestein et al., 1982; Robinson and Price, 1982; Robinson and Szetela, 1981; Robinson et al., 1984). The increased incidence of depression with left anterior hemispheric lesions correlates with its increased incidence in patients with Broca's aphasia compared with Wernicke's aphasia (Robinson and Benson, 1981). The period of maximal vulnerability to depression occurs within the first 2 years after the infarct (Robinson and Price, 1982), and often improves when treated with tricyclic antidepressants (Lipsey et al., 1984). Depression has occured with arteriovenous malformations as well as with cerebral infarctions and hemorrhages (Lin et al., 1952; Remington and Jeffries, 1984).

Cerebral neoplasms and infections produce depression in some patients. Depression occurs in a minority of patients with frontal lobe tumors (euphoria is more common), occurs in approximately 20 percent of patients with temporal lobe tumors, and appears to be more common with left temporal than right temporal neoplasms (Avery, 1971; Brock and Wiesel, 1948; Hécaen, 1964; Keschner et al., 1936; Kolodny, 1929; Malamud, 1967; Strauss and Keschner, 1935). Central nervous system (CNS) infections may produce depression as one manifestation of cerebral dysfunction. Depression occurs as the presenting manifestation in some cases of viral encephalitis and of bacterial infections such as syphilis (Han et al., 1959; Sobin and Ozer, 1966).

Cerebral trauma may produce either euphoria or depression (Miller, 1966). Lishman (1968) found depression in 58 of 670 penetrating head injuries and euphoria in 10 of 670. Depression was correlated with depth of penetration of the injury, total amount of brain tissue destroyed, and duration of posttraumatic amnesia. Lishman (1968) also found that depression was associated predominantly with frontal lobe injury and was more common with right than left-sided damage. Robinson and coworkers confirmed the relationship between anterior location and depression but found depression to be more frequent and severe with left-sided lesions (Lipsey et al., 1983; Robinson and Szetela, 1981). Depression is also a feature of less severe injuries, occurring in up to 70 percent of patients with postconcussion syndromes (Merskey and Woodforde, 1972).

The most common mood changes associated with multiple sclerosis are euphoria (elevated mood) or eutonia (exaggerated sense of well-being), but in some cases depression may be the presenting or the dominant manifestation (Baretz and Stephenson, 1981; Borberg and Zahle, 1946; Brown and Davis, 1922; Goodstein and Ferrell, 1977; Matthews, 1979; Surridge, 1969; Whitlock and Siskind, 1980; Young et al., 1976). The mood changes remit and relapse like other manifestations of the disease, and occasional patients experience cyclical mood changes alternating between depression and euphoria (Kellner et al., 1984). Depression is more common among multiple sclerosis victims manifesting predominantly cerebral involvement and is less common among those with primary involvement of spinal cord and cerebellum, an observation suggesting that the depression is not a reaction to disability (Schiffer et al., 1983).

The relationship between epilepsy and depression is particularly complex (Chapter 9). Depression is second only to fear as an ictal affect and differs from other ictal experiences in that it may persist for several days following termination of the seizure (Daly, 1958; Weil, 1955, 1956; Williams, 1956). Depression is also the most common interictal psychiatric disorder and is associated with a high rate of suicide and suicide attempts (Betts, 1981; Gunn, 1973; Hancock and Bevilacqua, 1971; Hawton et al., 1980; Mackay, 1979). In addition, depression in epileptics may be a product of anticonvulsant therapy or reactive psychological changes or may occur as an independent affective illness.

Narcoleptic patients have a high rate of depression, although separation of a primary neurobiologic association from the effects of chronic stimulant medication or reactive psychologic changes is difficult (Kales et al., 1982; Krishnan et al., 1984; Roy, 1976).

Obstructive hydrocephalus may manifest depression along with dementia, incontinence, and gait disturbance. The mood disorder usually resolves when the hydrocephalus is relieved by shunting (Price and Tucker, 1977; Rice and Gendelman, 1973).

Systemic disorders producing depression. In addition to neurological disorders, a wide variety of systemic disturbances also produce depression (Table 14-1). In viral and bacterial infections depression may occur as a prodrome or as a persisting consequence, and elevated herpes virus titers have been identified in an ex-

TABLE 14-2   Drugs Implicated in Producing Depression Syndromes

Cardiac and antihypertensive drugs

Bethanidine	Digitalis
Clonidine	Prazosin
Guanethidine	Procainamide
Hydralazine	Veratrum
Methyldopa	Lidocaine
Propranolol	Oxprenolol
Reserpine	Methoserpidine

Sedatives and hypnotics

Barbiturates	Benzodiazepines
Chloral hydrate	Chlormethiazole
Ethanol	Chlorazepate

Steroids and hormones

Corticosteroids	Triamcinalone
Oral contraceptives	Norethisterone
Prednisone	Danazol

Stimulants and appetite suppressants

Amphetamine	Diethylpropion
Fenfluramine	Phenmetrazine

Psychotropic Drugs

Butyrophenones	Phenothiazines

Neurological agents

Amantadine	Carbamazepine
Bromocriptine	Methosuximide
Levodopa	Phenytoin
Tetrabenazine	Phenidione
Baclofen	

Analgesics and anti-inflammatory drugs

Fenoprofen	Phenacetin
Ibuprofen	Phenylbutazone
Indomethacin	Pentazocine
Opiates	Benzydamine

Antibacterial and antifungal drugs

Ampicillin	Griseofulvin
Sulfamethoxazole	Metronidazole
Clotrimazole	Nitrofurantoin
Cycloserine	Nalidixic acid
Dapsone	Sulfonamides
Ethionamide	Streptomycin
Tetracycline	Thiocarbanilide

Antineoplastic drugs

Azathioprine	6-Azauridine
C-Asparaginase	Bleomycin
Mithramycin	Trimethoprim
Vincristine	

Miscellaneous drugs

Acetazolamide	Anticholinesterases
Choline	Cimetidine

(continued)

186

TABLE 14-2.   *(continued)*

Cyproheptadine	Diphenoxylate
Disulfiram	Lysergide
Methysergide	Mebeverine
Meclizine	Metaclopramide
Pizotifen	Salbutamol

Data from Whitlock (1982) and Whitlock and Evans (1978).

cessive number of psychotically depressed patients (Halonen et al., 1974; Whitlock, 1982).

Depression is a major manifestation of endocrine dysfunction. It occurs in a majority of patients with Cushing's syndrome and hypothyroidism and is common in hyperthyroidism, hyper- and hypoparathyroidism, Addison's disease, and hyperaldosteronism (Cohen, 1980; Kelly et al., 1983; Lishman, 1978; Whitlock, 1982; Whybrow et al., 1969). Depression is also common during the premenstrual period, occurring in up to 40 percent of patients with premenstrual behavioral alterations (Halbreich et al., 1983; Rubinow et al., 1984).

Inflammatory disorders often produce depression. In most cases the depression is a consequence of inflammatory involvement of intracerebral vessels, and CNS immunologic activity probably contributes in some. Depression is frequent in systemic lupus erythematosus and may have a waxing and waning course along with other manifestations of the disease (Bennett et al., 1972; Bresnihan et al., 1979; Guze, 1967; MacNeill et al., 1976; Stern and Robbins, 1960). Depression is the most common prodrome of temporal arteritis and may dominate the clinical picture (Hamilton et al., 1971; Pauley and Hughes, 1960; Vereker, 1957). Depression has also been reported in rhematoid arthritis and the Sjögren syndrome (Whitlock, 1982).

Depression has been described, albeit less commonly, in a variety of other conditions, including vitamin deficiency states (folate, B_{12}, C), cardiopulmonary insufficiency, uremia, systemic neoplasms, prophyria, the Klinefelter syndrome, and acquired immune deficiency (AIDS) (Lishman, 1978; Rinieris et al., 1979; Sorensen and Nielsen, 1977; Whitlock, 1982). Postpartum psychoses and postoperative psychoses may also have major affective manifestations (Whitlock, 1982).

Drug-induced depressions.   As shown in Table 14-2, depression has been produced by cardiac and antihypertensive agents, sedatives and hypnotics, steroids and other hormonal agents, stimulants and appetite suppressants, psychotropic agents, drugs used in the treatment of neurological disorders (antiparkinsonian agents, antispastic drugs, anticonvulsants), analgesics and antiinflammatory drugs, antibacterial and antifungal agents, antineoplastic drugs, and a variety of miscellaneous drugs (Whitlock, 1982; Whitlock and Evans, 1978).

As a class of drugs, antihypertensives are most frequently implicated in the genesis of depression. Sedation occurs with many antihypertensive agents, and depression has been produced by reserpine, methyldopa, and propranolol hydrochloride (DeMuth and Ackerman, 1983; Paykel et al., 1982; Petrie et al., 1982; Quetsch et al., 1959). Depression occurred in approximately 25 percent of patients treated with reserpine, and in many cases the agent appeared to act by precipitating depression in predisposed individuals (Goodwin and Bunney, 1971; Jensen, 1959; Quetsch et al., 1959). When depression occurs in a patient receiving one of the implicated antihypertensive agents, the patient may be better managed by shifting to the use of diuretic or vasodilating agents.

Idiopathic psychiatric disorders with depression. Depression occurs in a variety of idiopathic psychiatric disorders (Table 14-3). It is the definitive manifestation of the major depressive episodes occurring in recurrent unipolar depression and in single episodes of depression such as late-onset depression or involutional melancholia, and it alternates with periods of mania in bipolar affective disorders. In cyclothymic disorders there are alternating periods of euphoria and depression that are not sufficiently severe to justify a diagnosis of bipolar affective disorder. Dysthymic disorder is characterized by a chronic depressed mood and anhedonia persisting for at least 2 years, and adjustment disorder with depressed features is a transient disorder occurring in reaction to a psychosocial stressor (*Diagnostic and statistical manual of mental disorders,* 1980). Depression may also occur in the course of schizophrenia, either during the psychotic episode or as the acute psychotic symptoms remit (McGlashan and Carpenter, 1976; Planansky and Johnston, 1978). Depression must be distinguished from grief reactions following a significant loss and from psychomotor retardation without mood alteration.

CLINICAL AND ANATOMIC CORRELATES OF THE DEPRESSION SYNDROME

Depression is a complex multifaceted syndrome comprised of several elements (Table 14-4). Each of these elements has neurological correlates, and neuro-

TABLE 14-3   Idiopathic Psychiatric Disorders with Depressed Mood

Major depressive episode

   Recurrent unipolar depression
   Single depressive episode
   Bipolar (manic–depressive) disorder

Cyclothymic disorder

Dysthymic disorder

Adjustment disorder with depressed mood

Schizophrenia with depression

logical disturbances can modify or imitate each specific manifestation of the depression syndrome. The mood associated with depression is characterized by feelings of sadness, hopelessness, worthlessness, anhedonia, guilt, and irritability. Papez's (1937) original proposal that the inner experience of emotion is mediated by a group of anatomically related structures located in the medial regions of the hemispheres—the limbic system—has been amply confirmed, and the anatomic boundaries of the limbic system have been extended to include the inferior frontal cortex and its connections, medial temporal lobe structures including hippocampus and amygdala, hypothalamus, anterior nuclei of the thalamus, cingulate gyrus, and rostral brainstem regions (Livingston and Escobar, 1971; MacLean, 1949, 1958; Powell and Hines, 1974; White, 1965; Williams, 1968; Yakovlev, 1948). The limbic system has important interfaces with the basal ganglia, suggesting that the limbic and extrapyramidal systems function together as a single unit mediating mood, motivation, and motion (Nauta, 1982; Nauta and Domesick, 1978). Biochemical theories relating affective disorders to disturbances of neurotransmitter function correlate well with the concept of limbic system mediation of mood. Norepinephrine, the principal neurotransmitter implicated in the pathogenesis of depression, originates in brainstem nuclei and is transported through ascending tracts to targets in the limbic system and the cerebral cortex (Fig. 13-1) (Anden et al., 1966; Bunney and Davis, 1965; Green and Costain, 1981; Schildkraut et al., 1967; Ungerstedt, 1971). Serotonergic and dopaminergic dysfunction have been suggested as the basis for biochemical subtypes of depression, and these transmitters likewise originate in brainstem nuclei and project to limbic system structures (Anden et al., 1966; Asberg et al., 1976; Green and Costain, 1981; Maas, 1975; Ungerstedt, 1971). The subcortical and limbic location of the structures and ascending projections mediating depression

TABLE 14-4   Major Clinical Elements of the Depression Syndrome

Mood change

Verbal expression

Affective expression (prosody)

Motoric manifestations

   Retardation–agitation
   Catatonia

Cognitive impairment

Neurovegetative disturbances

   Appetite alterations
   Sleep disturbances

      Early morning awakening, difficulty falling asleep, multiple awakenings
      Decreased REM latency

   Loss of libido

Neuroendocrinologic changes

   Abnormal dexamethasone suppression test (DST)
   Abnormal thyrotropin-releasing hormone test (TRH test)

provides an explanation for the tendency for subcortical, frontal, and limbic lesions to produce depression, whereas posterior hemispheric damage has no similar correlation. Norepinephrine is asymmetrically distributed to the hemispheres (Oke et al., 1978), and this asymmetry may underlie the tendency for depressions to occur more frequently and to be more severe with left-sided lesions (Finkelstein et al., 1982; Keschner et al., 1936; Robinson and Benson, 1981; Robinson and Price, 1982; Robinson and Szetela, 1981).

Clinicians have focused on the content of the verbal exchange with the patient for the diagnosis of depression. Identification often depends on the patient's self-report of feelings of sadness, worthlessness, and hopelessness. In their descriptions, depressed patients tend to use vague and qualified expression with considerable self-preoccupation, ideas of deprivation, exaggeration of problems and difficulties, and lack of words concerning action and achievement (Andreasen and Pfohl, 1976; Beck, 1963). Unfortunately, overdependence on this limited aspect of the depression syndrome may lead to under recognition of depression. Patients with right hemispheric lesions may deny the presence of existing symptoms of depression (Ross and Rush, 1981), and aphasic patients may be unable to communicate their moods. The latter consideration is particularly important in view of the high incidence of depression among patients with left-frontal lobe damage and nonfluent aphasia (Chapter 3) (Robinson and Benson, 1981).

As important as what is said is the way in which the message is communicated. The speech of the depressed patient is hypophonic and slowed, has increased speech pause time (the silent interval between phonations during automatic speech, e.g., counting), and has a tendency for volume decresendo at the end of sentences (Greden and Carroll, 1980; Greden et al., 1981). These speech characteristics may be modified by coexisting brain injuries. Right-sided anterior lesions and subcortical injuries disrupt speech prosody and inflection and make it impossible for the patient to generate an affective expression consistent with the inner distress (Ross and Rush, 1981). Pseudobulbar palsy (discussed later) may lead to the expression of an affect completely contrary to the mood of the patient or may release a mood-congruent emotional display out of proportion to the intensity of the experienced emotion.

The motoric manifestations are also an important aspect of the clinical phenomenology of depression. Although a few patients become agitated and hyperkinetic, most manifest varying degrees of psychomotor retardation. There is a facial masking with little or no response to emotional stimuli (Schwartz et al., 1976). The posture is bowed, steps shortened, and there is a paucity of spontaneous activity (Kupfer et al., 1974).

Overall, the appearance resembles parkinsonism without tremor and with little rigidity but with prominent bradykinesia. Patients with extrapyramidal syndromes and bradykinesia must be carefully evaluated for depression since depression may be overdiagnosed by attributing the movement disturbance to depression or underdiagnosed by assuming that the bradykinesia is entirely a product of the extrapyramidal disease. The identity between the bradykinesia of depression and that of the basal ganglia disorders suggests that the motor manifestations of depression are also mediated by dysfunction in subcortical structures (de Ajuriaguera, 1975; Mandell et al., 1962). This relationship is further supported by the high rate of depression among patients with extrapyramidal diseases (discussed earlier) and by the ability to improve the movements of depressed patients with levodopa and the movement of parkinsonian patients with electroconvulsive therapy (Asnis, 1977; Bunney et al., 1969, 1971; Lebensohn and Jenkins, 1975; Yudofsky, 1979).

Cognitive impairment is ubiquitous in depression. Memory, particularly recent recall and learning new information, is impaired (Glass et al., 1981; Henry et al., 1973; Miller, 1975; Sternberg and Jarvik, 1976; Weingartner et al., 1981), and the coordination of cognitive activities to solve complex problems is also disturbed (Silberman et al., 1983a). In the elderly, the cognitive consequences of depression may be sufficiently severe to produce a dementia syndrome (Chapter 8), and in children depression may be associated with learning disabilities (Brumback and Staton, 1983; Staton et al., 1981; Weintraub and Mesulam, 1983). Attempts to ascribe the major cognitive deficits of depression to one or the other hemisphere have produced conflicting results, and it appears that the cognitive disturbances of depression involve functions mediated by both hemispheres (Hommes and Panhuysen, 1971; Kronfol et al., 1978; Sackeim et al., 1983; Silberman et al., 1983b; Tucker et al., 1981). The intellectual abnormalities accompanying depression most closely resemble those occurring in the subcortical dementias of the extrapyramidal syndromes (Chapter 8), and the intellectual impairment correlates with other evidence suggesting subcortical dysfunction in depression.

Neurovegetative functions are also routinely altered in depression. Appetite is usually diminished, often leading to substantial weight loss. Sex drive is decreased, and constipation and disturbances of thirst and water homeostasis may occur (Zubenko et al., 1984). Sleep disturbances are also common. Occasionally, patients report increased sleep, but in most cases sleep is interrupted by early morning awakening, multiple nocturnal awakenings, or difficulty falling asleep. Studies of sleep architecture in depressed patients confirm these subjective reports and demonstrate a decreased latency to the onset of the first period of rapid-eye-movment (REM) sleep, diminished total REM sleep time, decreased Stage IV sleep, decreased total sleep time, and an increased number of awakenings (Coble et al., 1976; Kupfer et al., 1982; McCarley, 1982; Mendels and Hawkins, 1967). The number of phasic eye movements occurring in REM periods is decreased in depressions associated with systemic illnesses compared with primary idiopathic depressions (Foster et al., 1976). Sleep, libido, and appetite are mediated by brainstem and hypothalamic structures, and alterations in neurovegetative functions suggest involvement and alterations of these CNS areas by the processes producing the depression syndrome.

Neuroendocrinologic disturbances in depression confirm the presence of limbic-hypothalamic dysfunction. In primary endogenous depression, baseline cortisol secretion is elevated, and approximately 50 percent of patients have early escape of cortisol secretion from suppression by exogenously administered dexamethasone (Carroll et al., 1981; Gwirtsman et al, 1982b; Hirschfeld et al., 1983; Sachar et al., 1973; Stokes et al., 1984). These abnormalities indicate a release of hypothalamic–pituitary–adrenocortical function from normal corticolimbic inhibitory influences. Abnormalities in the dexamethasone suppression test are not specific to primary endogenous depression and have also been noted in mania, degenerative dementias, Cushing's syndrome, and a variety of other neuromedical disorders. Abnormalities of the hypothalamopituitary axis are also evident in the control of thyroid function. Response of thyrotrophin (thyroid-stimulating hormone) to administration of thyrotrophin-releasing hormone (TRH) is diminished in affective disorders (Kirkegaard et al., 1978; Loosen and Prange, 1982; Sternbach et al., 1982, 1983). Endogenously depressed patients also have attenuated prolactin responses to intramuscular methadone (Judd et al., 1982).

Computerized tomographic studies of depressed patients reveal an increased incidence of ventricular enlargement compared with age-matched controls (Jacoby and Levy, 1980; Pearlson et al., 1984; Rieder et al., 1983). No specific EEG abnormalities have been described in idiopathic depression, but EEG studies may reveal abnormalities in secondary depressions associated with metabolic or neurological disturbances (Shagrass, 1965; Small, 1983). Abnormalities of auditory and visual evoked responses are present but are not diagnostically specific (Buchsbaum et al., 1971; Shagrass, 1983), and cerebral blood flow is reduced in severe depression (Mathew et al., 1980). Studies of cerebral glucose metabolism by use of positron emission tomography show relative hypometabolism in the frontal regions, and in some cases the alterations are more severe on the left than on the right (Buchsbaum et al., 1984; Phelps et al., 1984). This distribution of metabolic change in spontaneous idiopathic depression correlates well with the production of depression by focal left anterior lesions produced by cerebrovascular disease (Robinson et al., 1984).

Taken together, the elements of the depression syndrome suggest that the major focus of dysfunction involves primarily the limbic–subcortical structures. These abnormalities are expressed in the mood, motoric, cognitive, neurovegetative, and neuroendocrine manifestations of the depression syndrome. The communication of the mood state is further elaborated by linguistic activities of the left hemisphere and the prosodic function of the right hemisphere. The major neurotransmitter abnormality implicated in depression involves norepinephrine, but roles for other neurotransmitters, neuroregulators, and neuromodulators appear likely. The distribution of these transmitters is consistent with a limbic–subcortical focus of dysfunction in depression. Autopsy confirmation of this hypothesis is not yet available, but the few pathologic studies accomplished demonstrate a depletion of striatal dopamine, diminished concentration of norepinephrine in the region of the red nucleus and adjacent structures, and generalized lowering of serotonin concentrations (Birkmayer and Riederer, 1975).

Mania

Mania is an affective syndrome featuring an elevated or expansive mood along with increased physical activity, pressured speech, flight of ideas or racing thoughts, grandiosity, decreased need for sleep, distractibility, and excessive involvement with high-risk activities. Mania occurs in the course of idiopathic manic–depressive illness or may be secondary to a variety of neurological, metabolic, and toxic disorders (*Diagnostic and statistical manual of mental disorders*, 1980).

Secondary Mania

Secondary mania is defined as a syndrome lasting for at least 1 week and characterized by elated and/or irritable mood and by at least two of the following: hyperactivity, pressured speech, flight of ideas, grandiosity, decreased sleep, distractibility, and lack of judgment. In addition, there must be no previous history of mania or depression, no evidence of delirium or dementia, and an identifiable association with neurological or medical illness or drug intoxication (Krauthammer and Klerman, 1978).

Etiologies of secondary mania. Table 14-5 lists the principal etiologies of secondary mania. Among neurologic disorders, extrapyramidal diseases have an important association with secondary mania. Huntington's disease is associated with mania in some patients, and the mood change may precede the appearance of a movement disorder or dementia (Folstein et al., 1983; McHugh and Folstein, 1975). Dewhurst et al. (1969) found hypomania in two of 102 patients and euphoria in 14. Manic symptoms have also been reported in postencephalitic Parkinson's disease and in Wilson's disease (Bromberg, 1930; Fairweather, 1947; Pandey et al., 1981).

General paresis of the insane caused by syphilis produces mania in approximately 10 percent of cases (Binder and Dickman, 1980; Bockner and Coltart, 1961; Dewhurst, 1969; Mapelli and Bellelli, 1982). Spirochetal invasion of the brain in general paresis preferentially involves the frontal lobes. Pick's disease, a degenerative disorder also involving anterior hemispheric structures, has likewise been associated with manic symptoms in some patients (Neumann, 1949). Viral encephalitis may produce mania as part of the acute encephalitic disorder or as a postencephalitic disturbance following recovery from the acute stage of the illness (Goldney and Temme, 1980; Steinberg et al., 1972; Weisert and Hendrie, 1977).

A variety of focal CNS lesions have produced mania, including several varieties of cerebral neoplasms, cerebral trauma, surgical procedures, cerebrovascular insults, multiple sclerosis, and temporal lobe epilepsy (Alpers, 1937; Bourgeois and Campagne, 1967; Cohen and Niska, 1980; Cohn et al., 1977; Cummings and Mendez, 1984; Flor-Henry, 1969; Forrest, 1982; Jamieson and Wells, 1979; and Jampala and Abrams, 1983; Kellner et al., 1984; Kemp et al., 1977; Malamud, 1967; Oppler, 1950; Oyewumi and Lapierre, 1981; Rosenbaum and Barry, 1975; Stern and Dancey, 1942; Van der Lugt and de Visser, 1967, 1967; Whitlock, 1982). Most focal lesions producing mania are located in the vicinity of the hypothalamus, and a majority have involved the right cerebral hemisphere.

Mania has also been associated with Klinefelter syndrome and the Kleine-Levin syndrome (Cameron and Landon, 1980; Jeffries and Lefebvre, 1973).

Systemic conditions associated with mania include uremia and hemodialysis, dialysis dementia, hyperthyroidism, pellagra, carcinoid syndrome, vitamin B_{12} deficiency, and postpartum psychosis (Cooper, 1967; Corn and Checkley, 1983; Goggans, 1983; Jack et al., 1983; Jefferson and Marshall, 1981; Josephson and Mackenzie, 1980; Kadrmas et al., 1979; Lehmann, 1966; Spivak and Jackson 1977; Villani and Weitzel, 1979).

A variety of drugs have, likewise, produced secondary manic syndromes. Levodopa and bromocriptine may produce mania in parkinsonian patients, and up to 12 percent of treated patients develop mania (Brook and Cookson, 1978; Lin and Ziegler, 1976; Ryback and

TABLE 14-5   Etiologies of Secondary Mania

Neurological disorders

  Extrapyramidal diseases

    Huntington's disease
    Postencephalitic Parkinson's disease
    Wilson's disease

  CNS infections

    General paresis
    Viral encephalitis

  Miscellaneous conditions

    Cerebral neoplasms
    Cerebral trauma
    Thalamotomy
    Cerebrovascular accidents
    Multiple sclerosis
    Temporal lobe epilepsy
    Pick's disease
    Kleine-Levin syndrome
    Klinefelter's syndrome

Systemic disorders

  Uremia and hemodialysis
  Dialysis dementia
  Hyperthyroidism
  Pellagra
  Carcinoid syndrome
  Vitamin B_{12} deficiency
  Postpartum mania

Drugs

  Levodopa
  Bromocriptine
  Sympathomimetics
  Isonaizid
  Procarbazine
  Bromide
  Cocaine
  Amphetamines
  Procyclidine
  Hydralazine
  Cylcobenzaprine
  Phencyclidine (PCP)
  Cimetidine
  Yohimbine
  Baclofen
  Metrizamide (following myelography)

Data from Cummings (1985), Cummings and Mendez (1984), and Krauthammer and Klerman (1978).

Schwab, 1971; Vlissides et al., 1978). Psychostimulants including sympathomimetics, isoniazid, cocaine, and amphetamines also produce manic behavior (Jefferson and Marhsall, 1981; Krauthammer and Klerman, 1978; McEvoy, 1981; Waters and Lapierre, 1981). Mania is the second most common neuropsychiatric disturbance induced by steroids, occurring in 30–35 percent of patients who develop behavioral disorders. High dosages of prednisone, female gender, and systemic lupus erythematosus as the underlying disorder appear to be factors that predispose to steroid-induced behavioral changes (Lewis and Smith, 1983; Ling et al., 1981). Additional agents capable of producing mania include procarbazine, procyclidine, hydralazine, cyclobenzaprine, phencyclidine, cimetidine, bromide, yohimbine and baclofen (Arnold et al., 1980; Coid and Strang, 1982; Harsch, 1984; Hubain et al., 1982; Krauthammer and Klerman, 1978; Price et al., 1984; Paykel et al., 1982; Rosen, 1979; Sayed, 1976; Titus, 1983). Mania has also been described as a toxic reaction following metrizamide myelography (Kwentus et al., 1984). The common property exhibited by many of these mania-inducing drugs is that their mechanism of action involves facilitation of monoaminergic neurotransmission.

Mania may also be induced by the administration of tricyclic antidepressants and monoamine oxidase (MAO) inhibitors (Cohen et al., 1980; Nasrallah et al., 1982; Pickar et al., 1982). Patients receiving these agents are depressed and thus fall outside the definition of secondary mania, but in some cases the patients have had no previous manic episodes.

Secondary mania should be considered in the differential diagnosis of any patient who develops manic behavior for the first time after the age of 50, has no history of psychiatric illness and no family history of emotional disturbances, or who suffers from a predisposing neurological or medical illness (Cummings and Mendez, 1984).

Pathogenesis of secondary mania. The mechanisms responsible for secondary mania have not been determined, but the clinical circumstances in which this disorder occurs suggests a tentative formulation. A majority of focal lesions associated with secondary mania are located in the region abutting on the third ventricle and impinging on midline and hypothalamic structures (Cummings and Mendez, 1984). Hypothalamic dysfunction may account for the alterations in sleep, appetite, and libido noted in manic episodes. The elevated and expansive mood is more difficult to explain and may have contributions from both midline and lateralized structures. The deep medial regions of the brain contain a series of reward-oriented nuclei whose activation is sufficiently agreeable to produce vigorous self-stimulation through appropriately placed electrodes in the brains of experimental animals (Olds, 1958), and pleasurable experiences have also been produced in humans by similarly placed local stimulations accomplished during the course of surgical procedures (Delgado, 1969). The same areas are also rich in euphoriant enkephalins capable of mood elevation (Whitlock, 1982).

Hemisphere-specific factors may also play a role in secondary mania. A majority of focal lesions producing manic behavior have been located in the right cerebral hemisphere (Cummings and Mendez, 1984). Experimentally, infarction of the right cerebral hemisphere produces significantly more locomotor hyperactivity when compared with left hemispheric infarction (Robinson, 1979). In humans, destructive lesions of the right hemisphere have tended to produce mood elevation, whereas left hemispheric dysfunction is more likely to produce depression and catastrophic reactions (Gainotti, 1972; Perria et al., 1961; Sackeim et al., 1982). Thus a right hemispheric location may facilitate the occurrence of mania with an appropriately placed perihypothalamic lesion.

Idiopathic Manic–Depressive Illness

Idiopathic manic–depressive illness is a cyclic bipolar mood disorder in which periods of mania alternate with episodes of depression. During the manic period, the patient's mood is one of expansive elation often combined with and sometimes overshadowed by irritability and hostility. Physical hyperactivity is accompanied by pressured speech and flight of ideas. In some cases, rhyming and punning may be evident in the spontaneous verbal output. Paranoid ideation and delusions, usually of a grandiose type, are present in the advanced stages. Appetite and libido are increased, and the need for sleep is diminished. Insight and judgment are impaired, and reckless monetary investments, risk-taking behavior, and encounters with the police are common. The first manic episode usually occurs between the ages of 20 and 25 and persists for 3–6 months. Between one-quarter and one-third of patients will have more than one episode, and the interval between episodes is typically 3–4 years but may be considerably shorter (Angst, 1980; Carlson and Goodwin, 1973; Durbin and Martin, 1977; Kolb, 1973; Lorenz and Cobb, 1952; Weiss et al., 1974). The intellect is unimpaired between episodes, but the patients, particularly if elderly, may be in acute confusional states during the manic period (Lipowski, 1983).

Most laboratory studies of manic patients are normal, but many patients have elevated concentrations of erythrocyte choline and increased levels of 3-methoxy-4-hydroxyphenylglycol (the chief metabolite of norepinephrine) in CSF (Jope et al., 1980; Swann et al., 1983).

Manic–depressive illness appears to be largely a genetically determined disorder. The risk of the disorder is increased 25 times in the families of affected patients, and the concordance rate for the disorder in monozygotic twins is 75 percent (Allen, 1976; Kolb, 1973). Patients with no predisposing family history have a higher frequency of EEG abnormalities and more evidence of perinatal insults (Dalen, 1965; Hays, 1976). Such patients may represent examples of secondary mania resulting from early cerebral injury.

The differential diagnosis of idiopathic manic–depressive illness includes two groups of disorders: 1) the secondary manias, and 2) other episodic psychoses. The secondary manias were presented earlier. Recurrent psychoses are presented in Table 14-6. These include neurological disorders such as migraine, epilepsy, and the Kleine-Levin syndrome; metabolic disorders such as hepatic encephalopathy, uremia, prophyria, hypoglycemia, cardiopulmonary failure, and diabetes; toxic disturbances, including recurrent drug ingestion or withdrawal and drug-induced flashbacks; and idiopathic psychiatric disorders such as periodic psychosis of puberty and menstrual-related periodic psychosis, recurrent unipolar depression, periodic catatonia, borderline states, and schizophenia (Berlin et al., 1982; Endo et al., 1978; Gjessing, 1983; Goldstein and Halbreich, 1984; Lisanksy et al., 1984; Nomura et al., 1983; Teja, 1976; Tupin, 1984). Recurrent cycloid psychoses differing from classic affective and schizophrenic disorders have been described by some clinicians (Leonard, 1961).

Rage, Eutonia, and Other Mood Disturbances

Although depression and mania are the best studied mood disturbances, they are not the only possible deviations in mood state. Rage, eutonia, and indifference or placidity are other mood alterations occurring in neurological disorders. Rage has been described in postictal confusional states following complex partial seizures and in patients with hypothalamic neoplasms (Malamud, 1957; Reeves and Plum, 1969).

Multiple sclerosis produces a number of affective alterations. Depression (discussed earlier) occurs in some patients, whereas others develop euphoria or eutonia. *Euphoria* refers to the feeling of mental well-being and *eutonia* to a feeling of physical well-being. Eutonia is rare in disorders other than multiple sclerosis (Trimble and Grant, 1982).

Indifference or placidity may be viewed as the pathological loss of affective investment. Disorders manifesting such indifference include anosognosia (Chapter 5), frontal lobe disturbances (Chapter 6), Alzheimer's disease and other dementias (Chapter 8), and bilateral temporal lobe lesions such as the Klüver-Bucy syndrome (Lilly et al., 1983).

TABLE 14-6   Principal Disorders with Recurrent Psychoses

Neurological disorders

  Migraine
  Epilepsy
  Kleine-Levin syndrome

Metabolic disturbances

  Hepatic encephalopathy
  Porphyria
  Hypoglycemia
  Cardiopulmonary failure
  Diabetes
  Uremia

Toxic encephalopathies

  Recurrent drug or alcohol ingestion
  Drug-induced flashbacks
  Drug or alcohol withdrawal

Psychiatric disorders

  Periodic psychosis of puberty
  Menstrual-related periodic psychosis
  Manic–depressive illness
  Recurrent unipolar depression
  Schizophrenia
  Cycloid psychosis
  Periodic catatonia
  Borderline personality

Treatment of Mood Disorders

Antidepressant Agents

Table 14-7 presents the comparative pharmacology of the principal antidepressant agents. Tricyclic agents remain the most commonly used group of antidepressant drugs and act primarily by inhibiting the reuptake of monoamines into the presynaptic neuron terminal. Amitriptyline acts primarily on serotonin reuptake, desipramine on norepinephrine uptake, and nortriptyline and imipramine on both monoamine transmitters (Rosenbaum et al., 1979a). The average half-life for most tricyclics is 10–30 hours (Richardson and Richelson, 1984).

The main side effects of the tricyclic antidepressants relate to their anticholinergic activity. Anticholinergic effects include urinary retention, constipation and delayed gastric emptying time, blurred vision, confusion, and sedation. The principal cardiovascular affect is cardiac intraventricular conduction delay. Miscellaneous adverse side effects include postural hypotension, skin reactions, liver toxicity, and agranulocytosis. Central nervous system side effects involve postural tremor, myoclonus, seizures, and psychosis (Baldessarini, 1980;

TABLE 14-7   Comparative Pharmacology of the Principal Antidepressant Agents

Class and Agent	Common Proprietary Preparation (Manufacturer)	Daily Dosage Range (mg)[a]	Relative Anticholinergic Potency[b]
Tricyclic			
Amitriptyline	Elavil (Merck, Sharp & Dohme), Endep (Roche)	150–300	5.5
Trimipramine	Surmontil (Ives)	100–300	1.7
Doxepin	Sinequan (Roerig), Adapin (Pennwalt)	150–300	1.3
Imipramine	Tofranil (Geigy), Janimine (Abbott)	150–300	1.1
Protriptyline	Vivactil (Merck Sharp & Dohme)	15–60	4.0
Nortriptyline	Aventyl (Lilly), Pamelor (Sandoz)	75–150	0.7
Desipramine	Norpramin (Merrell Dow) Pertofrane (USV Pharmaceutical)	150–250	0.5
Amoxapine	Ascendin (Lederle)	150–300	0.1
Tetracyclic			
Maprotiline	Ludiomil (CIBA)	50–300	0.2
Trazodone	Desyrel (Mead Johnson Pharmaceutical)	100–400	0.003
Benzodiazepine			
Alprazolam	Xanax (Upjohn)	0.75–4.0	—
MAO inhibitors			
Phenelzine	Nardil (Parke-Davis)	15–75	—
Isocarboxazid	Marplan (Roche)	10–50	—
Tranylcypromine	Parnate (Smith Kline & French)	20–40	—

Data from Baldessarini (1980); Berger (1977); Feighner (1981); Feighner et al. (1983); Richardson and Richelson (1984); and Richelson (1983).
[a]Dosages in elderly patients should be adjusted to approximately half those shown (Thompson et al; 1983).
[b]Based on data from muscarinic receptors of human caudate nucleus (Richelson, 1983).

Lippman et al., 1977; Rosenbaum et al., 1979a; Spector and Schnapper, 1981). The use of antidepressants in patients with seizures is presented in Chapter 9, and tricyclic-induced movement disorders are discussed in Chapter 12.

Interactions between tricyclic antidepressants and other drugs are important in specific clinical circumstances. Reduced serum binding with potential toxicity can be produced by phenytoin, phenylbutazone, aspirin, aminopyrine, scopolamine, and phenothiazines. Drugs that interfere with the metabolism of tricyclic antidepressants and raise serum levels include neuroleptic agents, methylphenidate, and some steroids such as oral contraceptives. Drugs accelerating metabolism and lowering antidepressant levels include barbiturates and alcohol. The antidepressant activity of tricyclic agents

is antagonized by α-methyldopa, clonidine, and propranolol. Tricyclic drugs increase the sedation induced by alcohol, may produce hypertensive crises in combination with epinephrine, increase the anticoagulant effect of dicumarol, and increase the hypotensive effect of chlorothiazide (Baldessarini, 1980; Hollister, 1978; Rosenbaum et al., 1979a).

In addition to standard tricyclic antidepressant agents, a number of other antidepressant drugs are available for use in specific circumstances. Amoxapine differs from other tricyclic antidepressants in that it has both neuroleptic dopamine-blocking effects as well as antidepressant effects (Donlon, 1981; Smith and Ayd, 1981). Nontricyclic antidepressants in clinical use include maprotiline, trazodone, and alprazolam. Maprotiline is a tetracyclic antidepressant with weak anticholinergic and cardiovascular effects but relatively prominent seizure-inducing effects (Chapter 9) (Feighner, 1981; Gwirtsman et al., 1983b). Trazodone is a noncyclic antidepressant that selectively inhibits the reuptake of serotonin (Riblet and Taylor, 1981). It has few anticholinergic or cardiovascular side effects (Gershon and Newton, 1980; Himmelhoch, 1981). Priapism has been reported as an unusual side effect (Scher et al., 1983), and sedation is common. Alprazolam is a benzodiazepine with both anxiolytic and antidepressant properties. Sedation and gastrointestinal distress are the most common adverse effects (Feighner et al., 1983).

Monoamine oxidase inhibitors exert their antidepressant action by blocking the deamination of neurotransmitter monoamines and thus increasing their availability at the synapse. Side effects of MAO inhibitors include hepatotoxicity, tremors, insomnia, hyperhydrosis, and orthostatic hypotension. Monoamine oxidase inhibitors intensify the effects of monoaminergic compounds, including levodopa and amphetamines and prolong the effects of anesthetics, sedatives, antihistamines, alcohol, anticholinergic agents, and tricyclic antidepressants (Baldessarini, 1980). The most serious reaction observed in patients receiving MAO inhibitors is hypertensive crisis when tyramine-containing foods are ingested. Tyramine is most abundant in cheeses, wine, beer, sherry, pickled herring, lox, snails, chicken liver, yeast, figs, raisins, sauerkraut, coffee, citrus fruits, broad beans, chocolate, soy sauce, and cream (Baldessarini, 1980; Bassuk and Schoonover, 1977).

Electroconvulsive Therapy

Patients who cannot tolerate pharmacotherapy for depression because of toxic side effects or unacceptable drug interactions, who fail to respond to antidepressant drug regimens, or who require more rapid relief from depressive symptoms may be candidates for electroconvulsive therapy (ECT). Electroconvulsive therapy is contraindicated in patients with increased intracranial pressure and should be used with caution in those with cardiac disease or profound medical illnesses but can be safely used in those with other neurological disorders complicated by depression. Electroconvulsive therapy effectively treats depression in 60–90 percent of patients with major depressive episodes (with psychotic and/or neurovegetative disturbances) and provides relief from depression in up to 50 percent of those failing to respond to pharmacotherapy (Frankel et al., 1978; Kendell, 1981; Taylor, 1982).

Side effects of ECT include an amnesia that has both anterograde and retrograde components. The retrograde amnesia shrinks to within a short period of initiating the treatment, but the patient may remain amnesic for the time surrounding the shock administration. Memory function recovers completely within 6 months of terminating the usual course of 6–14 treatments (Squire, 1982; Squire and Chace, 1975). Left unilateral ECT has more impact on verbal memory, whereas right unilateral ECT produces more disturbances of nonverbal memory. Unilateral treatments also produce a brief contralateral hemiparesis, reflex asymmetry, and contralateral neglect (Kriss et al., 1981). Patients predisposed to epilepsy may experience an increased frequency of seizures following ECT (Devinsky and Duchowny, 1983). Permanent cognitive deficits are not produced by ECT unless the patient receives an excessive number of treatments, and most patients experience an improvement in cognition as their depression resolves (Malloy et al., 1982; Weeks et al., 1981).

Antimanic Agents

Two pharmacologic agents have antimanic properties: lithium and carbamazepine (Table 14-8). Lithium effectively treats mania–hypomania and also provides prophylactic protection against the recurrence of mania in bipolar affective disorders. It also has antidepressant qualities and is useful in ameliorating recurring unipolar and bipolar depression (Baldessarini, 1980; Rosenbaum et al., 1979b). Lithium is effective in secondary mania produced by CNS damage (Herlihy and Herlihy, 1979; Kemp et al., 1977; Mehta, 1976; Oyewumi and Lapierre, 1981; Rosenbaum and Barry, 1975; Young et al., 1977). Lithium has a short half-life (6–12 hours) and usually is administered three times daily in dosages of 900–1800 mg/day. The desired therapeutic serum level is 0.8–1.5 mEq/l; acutely manic patients should have serum levels in the upper therapeutic range, and euthymic patients receiving lithium for prophylactic purposes should be maintained with levels in the lower range. A wide variety of adverse side effects have been described with lithium, and patients receiving lithium must be carefully monitored for evidence of toxicity. The typical signs of toxicity include edema, gastrointestinal distress with diarrhea, nausea and vomiting, an action tremor, polyuria and polydypsia, and confusion (Bach et al., 1979; Bone et al., 1980; Lyskowski et al., 1982; Schou et al., 1970; Vestergaard et al., 1980). Some patients may develop toxic symptoms despite "normal" therapeutic levels (Speirs and Hirsch, 1978). Lithium may induce nephrogenic diabetes insipidus, and a few patients have developed interstitial nephritis and renal insufficiency (Ramsey and Cox, 1982). Endocrinologic effects of lithium include hypothyroidism and hyperparathyroidism (Fieve and Platman, 1968; Franks et al., 1982; Rosenbaum et al., 1979b). An action tremor is the most common neurological side effect of lithium

TABLE 14-8 Pharmacologic Properties of Antimanic Agents

	Lithium	Carbamazepine
Dosage range	900–1800 mg/d	600–1800 mg/d
Half-life	6–12 hours	8–15 hours
Days to reach steady state level	5–6 days	2–5 days
Therapeutic serum level	0.8–1.5 mEq/l	4–12 µg/ml
Side effects	Edema; thyroid dysfunction; polyuria, polydypsia; hyperparathyroidism; leukocytosis; diarrhea; nephropathy; ataxia, tremor; myoclonus; EEG changes and seizures; acute confusional state; neuropathy; choreoathetosis; parkinsonism	Nystagmus, ataxia, lethargy; oral-lingual dyskinesia; leukopenia, thrombocytopenia; hepatotoxicity; rash; systemic lupus erythematosus; diplopia; ophthalmoplegia
Drug interactions	Serum levels increased by diuretics (thiazides, furosemide, ethacrynic acid)	Decreased serum phenytoin and warfarin levels; serum levels decreased by phenobarbital

therapy, but a profusion of other neurological effects have been reported including peripheral neuropathy, ataxia, myoclonus, EEG changes, seizures, cogwheel rigidity, parkinsonism, and choreoathetosis (Brust et al., 1979; Reches et al., 1981; Rosen and Stevens, 1983; Shopsin and Gerson, 1975; Tyrer et al., 1980; Van Putten, 1978; Zorumski and Bakris, 1983). In some cases the neurological deficits are permanent, persisting after discontinuation of lithium therapy (Apte and Langston, 1983; Donaldson and Cunningham, 1983). Lithium may also aggravate a preexisting tardive dyskinesia (Beitman, 1978; Crews and Carpenter, 1977). The most important drug interaction concerning lithium involves the coadministration of diuretics. Sodium depleting diuretics (thiazides, furosemide, ethacrynic acid) may increase lithium retention and lead to toxicity (Baldessarini, 1980).

Carbamazepine is an iminostilbene compound useful in the management of paroxysmal pain syndromes and epilepsy (Chapter 9) and also exhibiting significant antimanic properties (Ballenger and Post, 1980; Okuma et al., 1973, 1979, 1981; Post et al., 1983). The pharmacology, side effects, and drug interactions of carbamazepine are presented in Chapter 9.

DISTURBANCES OF AFFECT

Disturbances of mood—the emotion experienced by the patient—must be distinguished from affect—the emotion expressed by the patient. In normal circumstances, mood and affect are congruent but in many neurological disturbances the two may become dissociated. There are three principal conditions in which CNS lesions result in alterations of affect: 1) pseudobulbar palsy, 2) ictal affective alterations, and 3) dysprosody.

Pseudobulbar Palsy

Exaggerated emotional expression with unintended laughing or unmotivated weeping occur in pseudobulbar palsy. The emotion expressed may be completely unrelated to the mood of the patient or may reflect the appropriate feeling but is out of proportion to the intensity of the emotion experienced (Ironside, 1956; Langworthy and Hesser, 1940). In most cases the patients have episodes of either laughing or crying; however, they may have both, or one may turn into the other, making it difficult to judge from the facial contortion which emotion is present. Once initiated, the emotional expression is very difficult or impossible to arrest, and the hyperbolic emotional exhibition may lead to great embarrassment for the patient. Martin (1950) reported a 25-year-old man who had an attack of uncontrollable laughter while attending his mother's funeral. He also described a 23-year-old woman who began laughing uncontrollably when a boxer was knocked from the ring and fell almost at her feet. In both cases the pseudobulbar palsy was associated with acute subarachnoid hemorrhage. A few patients have literally died laughing when acute pseudobulbar palsy with sustained laughter was initiated by a fatal neurological event. Martin (1950) commented that "this is the greatest mockery of all, that the patient should be forced to laugh as a portent of his own doom."*

In addition to unintended laughing and crying, pseudobulbar palsies have several other clinical features (Table 14-9). The three cardinal features are disturbed emotional expression (pseudobulbar affect), dysarthria, and dysphagia (Langworthy and Hesser, 1940). The dysarthria is usually severe and is characterized by imprecise articulation, slow rate, low pitch, and a strained–strangled sound of effortful phonation (Darley et al., 1975). Occasionally the dysarthria is so profound that the patient is completely unintelligible or even anarthric (Cummings et al., 1983; Lloyd, 1980). Lieberman and Benson (1977) observed a patient with amyotrophic lateral sclerosis and severe pseudobulbar palsy who could not speak and eventually communicated only through eye-movement Morse code. Loss of coordination of mastication and swallowing leads to dysphagia and may be life-threatening. Wilson (1924) described a patient who was unable even to voluntarily open his mouth. To allow the patient to eat, a house physician sat at the foot of the patient's bed and yawned until the patient reflexly yawned in response and the food was inserted into his mouth by a nurse! Drooling is common as the dysphagia progresses and swallowing of saliva is impaired.

Examination of the face of pseudobulbar patients reveals a variety of signs of upper motor neuron dysfunction (Haymaker, 1969; Langworthy and Hesser, 1940; Tilney and Morrison, 1912). The face is masked, showing little spontaneous emotional expression in the resting state. Paralysis of the facial muscles is common. Weakness of forced lip and eye closure is present, the patient has difficulty grimacing or voluntarily contracting the platysma, and tongue protrusion is weak. The jaw jerk is exaggerated, and muscle stretch reflexes of the orbicularis oris and orbicularis oculi are increased. Palatal movement is diminished when the patient is asked to phonate (say "ah"), but the reflex response to posterior pharyngeal stimulation is hyperactive. Disorders of respiration, particularly Cheyne-Stokes breathing, may be present. Not all these findings are present in every case, but a careful search will usually reveal some confirmatory signs in the patient whose emotional lability is on the basis of pseudobulbar palsy.

In addition to the disturbances of faciolinguorespiratory function, the diseases producing pseudobulbar palsy cause a variety of other neurological abnormalities (Table 14-9) (Langworthy and Hesser, 1940; Til-

TABLE 14-9.   Clinical Characteristics of the Pseudobulbar Syndrome

Unmotivated laughing or crying
Dysarthria
Dysphagia (often with drooling)
Weakness of volitional facial movements
Brisk jaw jerk
Exaggerated facial muscle stretch reflexes
Increased gag reflex
Cheyne-Stokes respiration
Associated neurological findings
Supranuclear ophthalmoplegia
Extrapyramidal disturbances
Limb weakness
Increased muscle stretch reflexes
Limb rigidity
Extensor plantar responses

ney and Morrison 1912). There may be supranuclear gaze palsies, particularly paralysis of upward gaze. Combined pyramidal and extrapyramidal disturbances also occur and are manifested by limb weakness and rigidity, shuffling gait, loss of associated movements, increased muscle stretch reflexes, and extensor plantar responses.

Anatomically, pseudobulbar palsy is produced by bilateral lesions located anywhere between the origin of the corticobulbar tracts in the cerebral cortex and their termination in the brainstem nuclei. Fibers innervating the jaw and facial muscles, the pharynx and larynx, and the tongue are involved.

The differential diagnosis of pseudobulbar palsy includes all diseases producing bilateral disturbances of upper motor neurons or their descending axons (Davison and Kelman, 1939; Langworthy and Hesser, 1940; Tilney and Morrison, 1912). Most cases are secondary to bilateral vascular infarctions of the cortex or the internal capsule. Multiple small infarctions involving the fibers of the internal capsule and resulting from hypertensive cerebrovascular disease (lacunar state) are a particularly common cause of pseudobulbar palsy, but atherosclerotic and embolic vascular occlusions, cerebral hemorrhage, basilar artery aneurysms, syphilitic cerebrovascular disease, and inflammatory vascular disorders must also be considered. Multiple sclerosis, traumatic cerebral insults, and amyotrophic lateral sclerosis account for many of the remaining cases. Several cases of extrinsic neoplasms pressing against the brainstem and causing a pseudobulbar state have been reported, including cerebellopontine angle tumors (Achari and Colover, 1976; Wood et al., 1958), clivus meningiomas,

---

*From Martin JP. Fits of laughter (sham mirth) in organic cerebral disease. Brain, 1950, 73, p. 464.

and chordomas (Cantu and Drew, 1966; Ironside, 1956). Intrinsic brainstem tumors have also produced the syndrome (Stern and Brown, 1957). Brainstem encephalitis, tuberculous meningitis, syringobulbia, and degenerative conditions such as Friedreich's ataxia are rare causes of pseudobulbar palsy. Pathological laughter and pseudobulbar states have also been reported in extrapyramidal disorders, including Wilson's disease, dystonia musculorum deformans (Ironside, 1956; Davison and Kelman, 1939) and progressive supranuclear palsy (Behraman et al., 1969). Rarely an apparently unilateral lesion of the limbic system will result in the acute onset of sustained laughter, which gradually subsides over a period of days or weeks (Swash, 1972). Such lesions may produce bilateral dysfunction by indirect effects such as edema or impaired circulation, or an acute unilateral lesion may be sufficient to disinhibit laughter mechanisms.

The unifying pathophysiological principle of pseudobulbar palsy is that bilateral interruption of descending cortical fibers disinhibits responses integrated at lower CNS levels. There is bilateral volitional facial weakness, but the facial muscles overreact in emotional expression; the patient may be unable to produce any propositional speech but cannot control involuntary laughing and weeping; the palate fails to move with attempted phonation but is reflexly hyperactive; or there may be a supranuclear ophthalmoplegia, but reflex oculocephalic eye movements in all planes are intact. The supranuclear lesions disturb volitional control of the faciorespiratory synkinesis, but leave subcortical and brainstem mechanisms intact. The pseudobulbar affect results from release of intrinsic motor programs of the limbic system and related subcortical structures (Cummings et al., 1983).

Ictal Affect

Alterations of emotional expression in epilepsy may be secondary to mood changes induced by focal seizure activity or may be sham emotional responses induced by the seizure. Because patients are frequently amnesic for the period of the seizure, distinction between the two causes of altered expression may be impossible in some cases. The two principal affective alterations described in epilepsy involve laughing and crying. Ictal affective expressions may occur in the course of complex partial seizures, infantile spasms, or seizures associated with hypothalamic lesions.

In adults, ictal affect is usually a manifestation of limbic epilepsy, with the inciting lesion located in the temporal or frontal lobes (Louiseau et al., 1971). The term "gelastic epilepsy" is applied to seizures manifesting laughter as an ictal automatism (Daly and Mulder, 1957). Ictal crying has been called *quiritarian* (Sethi

and Rao, 1976) meaning to cry or scream or *dacrystic* (Offen et al., 1976) meaning to tear. Laughter as an ictal manifestion is much more common than crying, and both may occasionally occur in the same patient (Offen et al., 1976; Sethi and Rao, 1976). The laughter is inappropriate and stereotyped, and occurs without a precipitating stimulus. There is frequently an associated alteration in consciousness, and other seizure manifestations may be evident. Postictal confusion may occur and the patient is usually amnesic for the event. Psychomotor phenomena accompanying the laughter may include running in cursive epilepsy (Chen and Forster, 1973), macropsia and metamorphopsia (Lehtinen and Kivalo, 1965), déjà vu feelings (Chen and Forster, 1973; Ironside, 1956), olfactory hallucinations (Roubicek, 1946), feelings of sexual orgasm (Jacome et al., 1980; Roubicek, 1946), or limb and verbal automatisms (Ames and Enderstein, 1975; Daly and Mulder, 1957). When consciousness persists during the attacks, the laughter is usually recalled as being disagreeable and incongruous, not a pleasurable experience as the affect would suggest (Lehtinen and Kivalo, 1965; Roger et al., 1967; Roubicek, 1946; Sethi and Rao, 1976). An EEG obtained during an attack will show paroxysmal abnormalities, and interictal EEGs are often abnormal. The ictal episodes diminish in frequency with appropriate treatment.

In infantile spasms, a form of primary generalized seizure disorder occurring in infants and young children and resulting from a wide variety of CNS disturbances, laughter may be one manifestation of the seizure activity. The laughter varies from prolonged violent attacks lasting for as long as several minutes to short periods of giggling or grinning (Druckman and Chao, 1957). The epileptic nature of the laughter is indicated by the lack of external precipitants, the odd nature of the laughter (mothers recognize it as not in character for their children), the accompanying manifestations of epilepsy (motor seizure activity), and the response to anticonvulsants.

The third clinical syndrome in which ictal laughter occurs is in association with deep midline lesions involving the hypothalamus (Gumpert et al., 1970; Louiseau et al., 1971; Money and Hosta, 1967; Sher and Brown, 1976). Neoplasms are a frequent cause of this syndrome, but a variety of lesions have been reported, including astrocytomas of the mamillary bodies, colloid cysts of the third ventricle, dysraphic states, pituitary adenomas, hypothalamic hamartomas, papillomas of the third ventricular choroid plexus, and hypothalamic gliomas (Sher and Brown, 1976). In addition to ictal laughter, the hypothalamic lesions may produce precocious puberty (Money and Hosta, 1967), chiasmal blindness (Ironside, 1956), central fever (Gumpert et al., 1970), or other evidence of hypothalamic dysfunction. The associated seizure manifestations include brief lapses of consciousness, eye deviation, and flushing.

Dysprosody

Prosody refers to the affective and inflectional coloring of speech based on syllable and word stress, speech rhythm and cadence, and syllable and word pitch shifts (Monrad-Krohn, 1947). These aspects of language expression along with gesture and mimicry are most responsible for investing speech with its emotional content, and any modification of prosodic ability distorts the patients' abilities to communicate their emotional states. Prosody is altered by lesions in a variety of locations in the brain. Basal ganglionic, cerebellar, and brainstem disorders produce dysarthria as well as alterations of pitch, volume, and stress that disturb prosody. Patients with Broca's aphasia are also dysprosodic. They express themselves in single-word replies or short phrases, and the melody of speech is abnormal. Inflection, however, is maintained in Broca's aphasia, and patients can often communicate considerable emotional information by the way they inflect their remaining verbal output. Right hemisphere lesions affecting the frontal lobe (right hemisphere equivalent of Broca area) impair the patients' use of prosody to express their internal emotional states (Ross, 1981; Ross and Mesulum, 1979; Ross et al., 1981; Weintraub et al., 1981). The dysprosody reduces the patients' abilities to elaborate their feelings and makes it difficult for the patients' families and clinicians to appreciate their emotions.

REFERENCES

Achari AN and Colover J. Posterior fossa tumors with pathological laughter. *JAMA*, 1976, *235*, 1469–1471.

Albert ML, Feldman RG, and WIllis AL. The "subcortical dementia" of progressive supranuclear palsy. *J Neurol Neurosurg Psychiat*, 1974, *37*, 121–130.

Allen MG. Twin studies in affective illness. *Arch Gen Psychiat*, 1976, *33*, 1476–1478.

Alpers BJ. Relation of the hypothalamus to disorders of personality. *Arch Neurol Psychiat*, 1937, *38*, 291–303.

Ames FR and Enderstein O. Ictal laughter: a case report with clinical cinefilm, and EEG observation. *J Neurol Neurosurg Psychiat*, 1975, *38*, 11–17.

Anden N-E, Dahlstrom A, Fuxe K, Larsson K, Olson L, and Ungerstedt U. Ascending monoamine neurons to the telencephalon and diencephalon. *Acta Physiol Scand*, 1966, *67*, 313–326.

Anderson J, Aabro E, Gulmann N, Hjelmsted A, and Pedersen HE. Anti-depressive treatment in Parkinson's disease. *Acta Neurol Scand*, 1980, *62*, 210–219.

Andreasen NJC and Pfohl B. Linguistic analysis of speech in affective disorders. *Arch Gen Psychiat*, 1976, *33*, 1361–1367.

Angst J. Clinical typology of bipolar illness. In Belmaker RH and van Praag HM (Eds.): *Mania. An evolving concept.* Lancaster, England, MTP Press, 1980, pp. 61–76.

Apte SN and Langston JW. Permanent neurological deficits due to lithium toxicity. *Ann Neurol*, 1983, *13*, 453–455.

Arnold ES, Rudd SM, and Kirshner H. Manic psychosis following withdrawal from baclofen. *Am J Psychiat*, 1980, *137*, 1466–1467.

Ashberg M, Thoren P, Traskman L, Bertilsson L, and Ringberger V. "Serotonin depression"—a biochemical subgroup within the affective disorders? *Science*, 1976, *191*, 478–480.

Asnis G. Parkinson's disease, depression, and ECT: a review and case report. *Am J Psychiat*, 1977, *134*, 191–195.

Avery TL. Seven cases of frontal tumour with psychiatric presentation. *Br J Psychiat*, 1971, *119*, 19–23.

Baldessarini R. Drugs and the treatment of psychiatric disorders. In Gilman AG, Goodman LS, and Gilman P (Eds.): *Goodman and Gillman's pharmacological basis of therapeutics*, 6th ed. New York, Macmillan Publishing Company, 1980, pp. 391–447.

Ballenger JC and Post RM. Carbamazepine in manic–depressive illness: a new treatment. *Am J Psychiat*, 1980, *137*, 782–790.

Baretz RM and Stephenson GR. Emotional responses to multiple sclerosis. *Psychosomatics*, 1981, *22*, 117–127.

Bassuk EL and Schoonover SC. *The practitioner's guide to psychactive drugs.* New York, Plenum Medical Book Company, 1977.

Bech P, Thomsen J, Prytz S, Vendsborg PB, Zilstorff K, and Rafaelson OJ. The profile and severity of lithium-induced side effects in mentally healthy subjects *Neuropsychobiology*, 1979, *5*, 160–166.

Beck AT. Thinking and depression. I. Idiosyncratic content and cognitive distortions. *Arch Gen Psychiat*, 1963, *9*, 324–333.

Behraman S, Carroll JD, Janota I, Matthews WB. Progressive supranuclear palsy. *Brain*, 1969, *92*, 663–678.

Beitman BD. Tardive dyskinesia reinduced by lithium carbonate. *Am J Psychiat*, 1978, *135*, 1229–1230.

Bennett R, Hughes GRV, Bywaters EGL, and Holt PJL. Neuropsychiatric problems in systemic lupus erythematosus. *Br Med J*, 1972, *4*, 342–345.

Berger PA. Antidepressant medications in the treatment of depression. In Barchas JD, Berger PA, Ciaranello RD, and Elliot GR (Eds.): *Psychopharmacology from theory to practice*. New York, Oxford University Press, 1977, pp. 174–207.

Berlin FS, Bergey GK, and Money T. Periodic psychosis of puberty: a case report. *Am J Psychiat*, 1982, *139*, 119–120.

Betts TA. Depression, anxiety, and epilepsy. In Reynolds EH and Trimble MR (Eds.): *Epilepsy and psychiatry*. New York, Churchill Livingston, 1981, pp. 60–71.

Binder RL and Dickman WA. Psychiatric manifestations of neurosyphilis in middle-aged patients. *Am J Psychiat*, 1980, *137*, 741–742.

Birkmayer W and Riederer P. Biochemical post-mortem findings in depressed patients. *J Neurol Trans*, 1975, *37*, 95–109.

Bockner S and Coltart N. New cases of GPI. *Br Med J*, 1961, *1*, 18–20.

Bone S, Roose SP, Dunner DL, and Fieve RR. Incidence of side effects in patients on long-term lithium therapy. *Am J Psychiat*, 1980, *137*, 103–104.

Borberg NC and Zahle U. On the psychopathology of disseminated sclerosis. *Acta Psychiat Neurol Scand*, 1946, *21*, 75–89.

Bourgeois M and Campagne A. Maniaco-depressive et syndrome de Garcin. *Ann Med Psychol*, 1967, *125* (Suppl. 2), 451–460.

Bresnihan B, Hohmeister R, Cutting J, Travers RL, Waldburger M, Black C, Jones T, and Hughes GRV. The neuropsychiatric disorder in systemic lupus erythematosus: evidence for both vascular and immune mechanisms. *Ann Rheum Dis*, 1979, *38*, 301–306.

Brock S and Wiesel B. Psychotic symptoms masking the onset in cases of brain tumor. *Med Clin N Am*, 1948, *32*, 759–767.

Bromberg W. Mental states in chronic encephalitis. *Psychiat Quart*, 1930, *4*, 537–566.

Brook NM and Cookson IB. Bromocriptine-induced mania? *Br Med J*, 1978, *1*, 790.

Brown GL and Wilson WP. Parkinsonism and depression. *South Med J*, 1972, *65*, 540–545.

Brown SII and Davis TK. The mental symptoms of multiple sclerosis. *Arch Neurol Psychiat*, 1922, *7*, 629–634.

Brumback RA and Staton RD. Learning disability and childhood depression. *Am J Orthopsychiat*, 1983, *53*, 269–281.

Brust JMC, Hammer JS, Challenor Y, Healton EB, and Lesser RP. Acute generalized polyneuropathy accompanying lithium poisoning. *Ann Neurol*, 1979, *6*, 360–362.

Buchsbaum MS, Cappelletti J, Ball R, Hazlett E, King AC, Johnson J, Wu J, and De Lisi LE. Positron emission tomographic image, measurement in schizophrenia and affective disorders. *Ann Neurol*, 1984, *15* (Suppl.), S157–S165.

Buchsbaum M, Goodwin F, Murphy D, and Borge G. AER in affective disorders. *Am J Psychiat*, 1971, *128*, 19–25.

Bunney WF Jr, Brodie HKH, Murphy DL, and Goodwin FK. Studies of alphamethyl-para-tyrosine, dopa, and tryptophan in depression and mania. *Am J Psychiat*, 1971, *127*, 872–881.

Bunney WE Jr and Davis JM. Norepinephrine in depressive reactions. *Arch Gen Psychiat*, 1965, *13*, 483–494.

Bunney WE, Janowsky DS, Goodwin FK, Davis JM, Brodie HKH, Murphy DL, and Chase TN. Effects of dopa on depression. *Lancet*, 1969, *1*, 885–886.

Caine ED and Shoulson I. Psychiatric syndromes in Huntington's disease. *Am J Psychiat*, 1983, *140*, 728–733.

Cantu RC and Drew JH. Pathological laughing and crying associated with a tumor ventral to the pons. *J Neurosurg*, 1966, *24*, 1024–1026.

Cammeron OG and Landon SG. Lithium carbonate treatment of mania associated with Klinefelter's syndrome. *JAMA*, 1980, *243*, 1712.

Carlson GA and Goodwin FK. The stages of mania. *Arch Gen Psychiat*, 1973, *28*, 221–228.

Carroll BJ, Feinberg M, Greden JF, Tarika J, Albalo AA, Haskett RF, James N McI, Kronfol Z, Luhr N, Steinr M, de Vigne JP, and Young E. A specific laboratory test for the diagnosis of melancholia. *Arch Gen Psychiat*, 1981, *38*, 15–22.

Celesia GG and Wanamaker WM. Psychiatric disturbances in Parkinson's disease. *Dis Nerv Sys*, 1972, *33*, 577–583.

Chen R-C and Forster FM. Cursive epilepsy and gelastic epilepsy. *Neurology*, 1973, *23*, 1019–1029.

Cherington M. Parkinsonism, L-dopa, and mental depression. *J Am Geriat Soc*, 1970, *18*, 513–516.

Coble P, Foser G, and Kupfer DJ. Electroencephalographic sleep diagnosis of primary depression. *Arch Gen Psychiat*, 1976, *33*, 1124–1127.

Cohen MR and Niska RW. Localized right cerebral hemisphere dysfunction and recurrent mania. *Am J Psychiat*, 1980, *137*, 847–848.

Cohen RM, Pickar D, and Murphy DL. Myoclonus-associated hypomania during MAO-inhibitor treatment. *Am J Psychiat*, 1980, *137*, 105–106.

Cohen SI. Cushing's syndrome: a psychiatric study of 29 patients. *Br J Psychiat*, 1980, *136*, 120–124.

Cohn CK, Wright JR III, and De Vaul RA. Post head trauma syndrome in an adolescent treated with lithium carbonate—case report. *Dis Nerv Syst*, 1977, *38*, 630–631.

Coid J and Strang J. Mania secondary to procylidine ("kemadrin") abuse. *Br J Psychiat*, 1982, *141*, 81–84.

Cooper AT. Hypomanic psychosis precipitated by hemodialysis. *Comp Psychiat*, 1967, *8*, 168–172.

Corn TH and Checkley SA. A case of recurrent mania with recurrent hyperthyroidism. *Br J Psychiat*, 1983, *143*, 74–76.

Crews EL and Carpenter AE. Lithium-induced aggravation of tardive dyskinesia. *Am J Psychiat*, 1977, *134*, 933.

Cummings JL. Organic delusions: phenomenology, anatomical correlations and review. *Br J Psychiat*, 1985, *146*, 184–197.

Cummings JL, Benson DF, Houlihan JP, and Gosenfeld LF. Mutism: loss of neocortical and limbic vocalization. *J Nerv Ment Dis*, 1983, *171*, 255–259.

Cummings JL and Mendez MF. Secondary mania with focal cerebrovascular lesions. *Am J Psychiat*, 1984, *141*, 1084–1087.

Dalen P. Family history, the electroencephalogram and perinatal factors in manic conditions. *Acta Psychiat Scand*, 1965, *41*, 527–563.

Daly D. Ictal affect. *Am J Psychiat*, 1958, *115*, 97–108.

Daly DD and Mulder DW. Gelastic epilepsy. *Neurology*, 1957, *7*, 189–192.

Darley FL, Bronson ME, and Brown JR. *Motor speech disorders*. Philadelphia, WB Saunders Company, 1975.

Davison C and Kelman H. Pathologic laughing and crying. *Arch Neurol Psychiat*, 1939, *42*, 595–643.

De Ajuriaguerra J. The concept of akinesia. *Psychol Med*, 1975, *5*, 129–137.

Delgado JMR. *Physical control of the mind*. New York, Harper and Row, 1969.

DeMuth GW and Ackerman SH, α-methyldopa and depression: a clinical study and review of the literature. *Am J Psychiat*, 1983, *140*, 534–538.

Denmark JC, David JDP, and McComb SG. Imipramine hydrochloride (Tofranil) in parkinsonism. *Br J Clin Pract*, 1961, *15*, 523–524.

Devinski O and Duchowny MS. Seizures after convulsive therapy: a retrospective case survey. *Neurology*, 1983, *33*, 921–925.

Dewhurst K. The neurosyphilitic psychoses today. *Br J Psychiat*, 1969, *115*, 31–38.

Dewhurst K, Oliver J, Trick KLK, and McKnight ML. Neuropsychiatric aspects of Huntington's disease. *Confin Neurol*, 1969, *31*, 258–268.

Diagnostic and statistical manual of mental disorders, 3rd ed. Washington, D.C., American Psychiatric Association, 1980.

Donaldson I MacG and Cunningham J. Persisting neurologic sequelae of lithium carbonate therapy. *Arch Neurol*, 1983, *40*, 747–751.

Donlon PT. Amoxapine: a newly marketed tricyclic antidepressant. *Psychiat Ann*, 1981, *11*, 379–383.

Druckman R and Chao D. Laughter in epilepsy. *Neurology*, 1957, *7*, 26–36.

Durbin M and Martin RL. Speech in mania: syntactic aspects. *Brain Lang*, 1977, *4*, 208–218.

Endo M, Daiguji M, Asano Y, Yamashita I, and Talcahashi S. Periodic psychosis recurring in association with menstrual cycle. *J Clin Psychiat*, 1978, *37*, 456–466.

Fairweather DS. Psychiatric aspects of the post-encephalitic syndrome. *J Ment Sci*, 1947, *93*, 201–254.

Feighner JP. Clinical efficacy of the newer antidepressants. *J Clin Psychopharm*, 1981, Suppl. No. 6, 23S–26S.

Feighner JP, Aden GC, Fabre LF, Rickels K, and Smith WT. Comparison of alprazolam, imipramine, and placebo in the treatment of depression. *JAMA*, 1983, *249*, 3057–3064.

Fieve RR and Platman S. Lithium and thyroid function in manic–depressive psychosis. *Am J Psychiat*, 1968, *125*, 527–530.

Finklestein S, Benowitz LI, Baldessarini RJ, Arana GW, Levine D, Woo E, Bear D, Moya K, and Stoll AL. Mood, vegetative disturbance, and dexamethasone suppression test after stroke. *Ann Neurol*, 1982, *12*, 463–468.

Flor-Henry P. Psychosis and temporal lobe epilepsy. *Epilepsia*, 1969, *10*, 363–395.

Folstein SE, Franz ML, Jensen BA, Chase GA, and Folstein MF. Conduct disorder and affective disorder among the offspring of patients with Huntington's disease. *Psychol Med*, 1983, *13*, 45–52.

Folstein MF, Maiberger R, and McHugh PR. Mood disorder as a specific complication of stroke. *J Neurol Neurosurg Psychiat*, 1977, *40*, 1018–1020.

Forrest DV. Bipolar illness after right hemispherectomy. *Arch Gen Psychiat*, 1982, *39*, 817–819.

Foster FG, Kupfer DJ, Coble P, and McPartland RJ. Rapid eye movement sleep density. *Arch Gen Psychiat*, 1976, *33*, 1119–1123.

Frankel FH, Bidder TG, Fink M, Mandel MR, Small IF, Wayne GJ, Squire LR, Dutton EN, and Gurel L. *Electroconvulsive therapy. Task Force Report 14*. Washington, D.C., American Psychiatric Association, 1978.

Franks RD, Dubovsky SL, Lifshitz M, Cohen P, Subryan V, and Walker SH. Long-term lithium carbonate therapy causes hyperparathyroidism. *Arch Gen Psychiat*, 1982, *39*, 1074–1077.

Gainotti G. Emotional behavior and hemispheric side of the lesion. *Cortex*, 1972, *8*, 41–55.

Gershon S and Newton R. Lack of anticholinergic side effects with a new antidepressant—Trazodone. *J Clin Psychiat*, 1980, *41*, 100–104.

Gillhespy RO and Mustard DM. The evaluation of imipramine in the treatment of Parkinson's disease. *Br J Clin Pract*, 1963, *17*, 205–208.

Gjessing LR. An essay on the syndrome of catatonia periodica. In Hatotani N and Nomura T (Eds.): *Neurobiology of periodic psychoses*. New York, Igaku-Shoin, 1983, pp. 15–45.

Glass RM, Uhlenhuth EH, Hartel FW, Matuzas W, and Fischman M. Cognitive dysfunction and imipramine in outpatient depressives. *Arch Gen Psychiat*, 1981, *38*, 1048–1051.

Goggans FC. A case of mania secondary to vitamin B12 deficiency. *Am J Psychiat*, 1983, *141*, 300–301.

Goldney RD and Temme PB. Case report: manic depressive psychosis following infectious mononucleosis. *J Clin Psychiat*, 1980, *41*, 322–323.

Goldstein S and Halbreich U. Hormone-related transient psychoses. In Tupin JP, Halbreich U, and Pena JJ (Eds.): *Transient psychosis: diagnosis, management and evaluation*. New York, Brunner-Mazel, 1984, pp. 61–79.

Goodman RM, Hall CL Jr, Terango L, Perrine GA Jr, and Roberts PL. Huntington's chorea. *Arch Neurol*, 1966, *15*, 345–355.

Goodstein RK and Ferrell RB. Multiple sclerosis—presenting as depressive illness. *Dis Nerv Syst*, 1977, *38*, 127–131.

Goodwin FK and Bunney WE Jr. Depression following reserpine: a reevaluation. *Semin Psychiat*, 1971, *3*, 435–448.

Greden JF, Albala AA, Smokler IA, Gardner R, and Carroll BJ. Speech pause time: a marker of psychomotor retardation among endogenous depressives. *Biol Psychiat*, 1981 *16*, 851–859.

Greden JF and Carroll BJ. Decrease in speech pause time with treatment of endogenous depression. *Biol Psychiat*, 1980 *15*, 575–587.

Green AR and Costain DW. *Pharmacology and biochemistry of psychiatric disorders*. New York, John Wiley & Sons, 1981.

Gumpert J, Hansotia P, and Upton A. Gelastic epilepsy. *J Neurol Neurosurg Psychiat*, 1970, *33*, 479–483.

Gunn J. Affective and suicidal symptoms in epileptic prisoners. *Psychol Med*, 1973, *3*, 108–114.

Guze SB. The occurrence of psychiatric illness in systemic lupus erythmatosus. *Am J Psychiat*, 1967, *123*, 1562–1570.

Gwirtsman HE, Ahles S, Halaris A, DeMet E, and Hill MA. Therapeutic superiority of maprotiline versus doxepin in geriatric depression. *J Clin Psychiat*, 1983a, *44*, 449–453.

Gwirtsman H, Gerner RH, and Sternbach H. The overnight dexamethasone suppression test: clinical and theoretical review. *J Clin Psychiat*, 1983b, *43*, 321–327.

Hahn RD, Webster B, Weickhardt G, Thomas E, Timberlake W, Solomon H, Stokes JH, Moore TE, Heyman A, Gammon G, Gleeson GA, Curtis AC, and Cutler JC. Penicillin treatment of general paresis (dementia paralytica). *Arch Neurol Psychiat*, 1959, *81*, 557–590.

Halbreich U, Endicott J, and Nee J. Premenstrual depressive changes. *Arch Gen Psychiat*, 1983, *40*, 535–542.

Halonen PE, Rimon R, Arohonka K, and Jantti V. Antibody levels to herpes simplex type I, measles and rubella virus in psychiatric patients. *Br J Psychiat*, 1974, *125*, 461–465.

Hamilton CR Jr, Shelley WM, and Tumulty DA. Giant cell arteritis and polymyalgia rheumatica. *Medicine*, 1971, *50*, 1–27.

Hancock JC and Bevilacqua AR. Temporal lobe dysrhythmia and impulsive or suicidal behavior. *South Med J*, 1971, *64*, 1189–1193.

Harsch HH. Mania in two patients following cyclobenzoprine. *Psychosomatics*, 1984, *25*, 791–793.

Hawton K, Fagg J, and Marsack P. Association between epilepsy and attempted suicide. *J Neurol Neurosurg Psychiat*, 1980, *43*, 168–170.

Haymaker W. *Bing's local diagnosis in neurological diseases*. St. Louis, CV Mosby Company, 1969.

Hays P. Etiological factors in manic-depressive psychoses. *Arch Gen Psychiat*, 1976, *33*, 1187–1188.

Hécaen H. Mental symptoms associated with tumors of the frontal lobe. In Warren JM and Akerk K (Eds.): *The frontal granular cortex and behavior*. New York, McGraw-Hill Book Company, 1964, pp. 335–352.

Henry GM, Weingartner H, and Murphy DL. Influence of affective states and psychoactive drugs on verbal learning and memory. *Am J Psychiat*, 1973, *130*, 966–971.

Herlihy CE Jr and Herlihy CE. Lithium and organic brain syndrome. *J Clin Psychiat*, 1979, *40*, 455.

Himmelhoch JM. Cardiovascular effects of trazodone in humans. *J Clin Psychopharm*, 1981, *1* (Suppl. No. 6), 76S–81S.

Hirschfeld RMA, Koslow SH, and Kupfer DJ. The clinical utility of the dexamethasone suppression test in psychiatry. *JAMA*, 1983, *250*, 2172–2174.

Hollister LE. Tricyclic antidepressants. *New Engl J Med*, 1978, *299*, 1106–1109, 1168–1172.

Hommes OR and Panhuysen LHHM. Depression and cerebral dominance. *Psychiat Neurol Neurochir*, 1971, *74*, 259–270.

Horn S. Some psychological factors in parkinsonism. *J Neurol Neurosurg Psychiat*, 1974, *37*, 27–31.

Hubain PP, Soboski J, and Menlewicz J. Cimetidine-induced mania. *Neuropsychobiology*, 1982, *8*, 223–224.

Ironside R. Disorders of laughter due to brain lesions. *Brain*, 1956, *79*, 589–609.

Jack RA, Rivers-Bulkeley NT, and Robin PL. Secondary mania as a presentation of progressive dialysis encephalopathy. *J Nerv Ment Dis*, 1983, *171*, 193–195.

Jackson JA, Free GBM, and Pike HV. The psychic manifestations in paralysis agitans. *Arch Neurol Psychiat*, 1923, *10*, 680–684.

Jackson JA, Jankovic J, and Ford J. Progressive supranuclear palsy: clinical features and response to treatment in 16 patients. *Ann Neurol*, 1983, *13*, 273–278.

Jacoby RT and Levy R. Computed tomography in the elderly. 3. Affective disorder. *Br J Psychiat*, 1980, *136*, 270–275.

Jacome DE, McLain LW Jr, and Fitzgerald R. Postictal reflex gelastic seizures. *Arch Neurol*, 1980, *37*, 249–251.

Jamieson RC and Wells CE. Manic psychosis in a patient with multiple metastatic brain tumors. *J Clin Psychiat*, 1979, *40*, 280–282.

Jampala VC and Abrams R. Mania secondary to left and right hemisphere damage. *Am J Psychiat*, 1983, *140*, 1197–1199.

Janati A and Appel AR. Psychiatric aspects of progressive supranuclear palsy. *J Nerv Ment Dis*, 1984, *172*, 85–89.

Jefferson JW and Marshall Jr. *Neuropsychiatric features of medical disorders*. New York, Plenum Medical Book Company, 1981.

Jeffries JJ and Lefebvre A. Depression and mania associated with Kleine-Levin-Critchley syndrome. *Can Psychiat Assoc J*, 1973, *18*, 439–444.

Jensen K. Depressions in patients treated with reserpine for arterial hypertension. *Acta Psychiat Neurol Scand*, 1959, *34*, 195–204.

Jope RS, Jenden DJ, Ehrlich BE, Diamond JM, and Gosenfeld LF. Erythrocyte choline concentrations are elevated in manic patients. *Proc Natl Acad Sci (USA)*, 1980, *77*, 6144–6146.

Josephson AM and Mackenzie TB. Thyroid-induced mania in hypothyroid patients. *Br J Psychiat*, 1980, *137*, 222–228.

Judd LL, Risch SC, Parker DC, Janowsky DS, Segal DS, and Huey LY. Blunted prolactin response. A neuroendocrine abnormality manifested by depressed patients. *Arch Gen Psychiat*, 1982, *39*, 1413–1416.

Kadrmas A, Winokur G, and Crowe R. Postpartum mania. *Br J Psychiat*, 1979, *135*, 551–554.

Kales A, Soldatos CR, Bixler EO, Caldwell A, Cadieux RJ, Verrechio JM, and Kales JD. Narcolepsy–cataplexy. II.

Psychosocial consequences and associated psychopathology. *Arch Neurol*, 1982, *39*, 169–171.

Kellner CH, Davenport Y, Post RM, and Ross RJ. Rapidly cycling bipolar disorder in multiple sclerosis. *Am J Psychiat*, 1984, *141*, 112–113.

Kelly WF, Checkley SM, Bender DA, and Mashiter K. Cushing's syndrome and depression—a prospective study of 26 patients. *Br J Psychiat*, 1983, *142*, 16–19.

Kemp K, Lion JR, and Magram G. Lithium in the treatment of a manic patient with multiple sclerosis: a case report. *Dis Nerv Syst*, 1977, *38*, 210–211.

Kendell RE. The contribution of ECT to the treatment of affective disorders. In Palmer RL (Ed.): *Electroconvulsive therapy: an appraisal*. New York, Oxford University Press, 1981, pp. 28–36.

Keschner M, Bender MB, and Strauss I. Mental symptoms in cases of tumor of the temporal lobe. *Arch Neurol Psychiat*, 1936, *35*, 572–596.

Kirby GH and Davis TK. Psychiatric aspects of epidemic encephalitis. *Arch Neurol Psychiat*, 1921, *5*, 491–551.

Kirkegaard C, Bjrum N, Cohn D, Lauridsen B. Thyrotrophin-releasing hormone (TRH) stimulation test in manic–depressive illness. *Arch Gen Psychiat*, 1978, *35*, 1017–1021.

Kolb LC. *Modern clinical psychiatry*, 8th ed. Philadelphia, WB Saunders Company, 1973.

Kolodny A. Symptomatology of tumor of the frontal lobe. *Arch Neurol Psychiat* 1929, *21*, 1107–1127.

Krauthammer C and Klerman GL. Secondary mania. *Arch Gen Psychiat*, 1978, *35*, 1333–1339.

Krishnan RR, Volow MR, Miller PP, and Carwile ST. Narcolepsy: preliminary retrospective study of psychiatric and psychosocial aspects. *Am J Psychiat*, 1984, *141*, 428–431.

Kriss A, Halliday AM, and Pratt RTC. Transitory electrophysiological and neurological asymmetries following unilateral ECT. In Palmer RL (Ed.): *Electroconvulsive therapy: an appraisal*. New York, Oxford University Press, 1981, pp. 236–252.

Kronfol Z, Hamsher K deS, Digre K, and Waziri R. Depression and hemispheric functions: changes associated with unilateral ECT. *Br J Psychiat*, 1978, *132*, 560–567.

Kupfer DJ, Shaw DH, Ulrich R, Coble PA, and Spiker DG. Application of automated REM analysis in depression. *Arch Gen Psychiat*, 1982, *39*, 569–573.

Kupfer DJ, Weiss BL, Foster FG, Detre TP, Delgado J, and McPortland R. Psychomotor activity in affective states. *Arch Gen Psychiat*, 1974, *30*, 765–768.

Kvale JN. Amitriptyline in the management of progressive supranuclear palsy. *Arch Neurol*, 1982, *39*, 387–388.

Kwentus JA, Silverman JJ, and Sprague M. Manic syndrome after metrizamide myelography. *Am J Psychiat*, 1984, *141*, 700–702.

Laitinen L. Desipramine in treatment of Parkinson's disease. *Acta Neurol Scand*, 1969, *45*, 109–113.

Langworthy OR and Hesser FH. Syndrome of pseudobulbar palsy. *Arch Int Med*, 1940, *65*, 106–121.

Lebensohn ZM and Jenkins RB. Improvement of parkinson-

ism in depressed patients treated with ECT. *Am J Psychiat*, 1975, *132*, 283–285.

Lehmann J. Mental disturbances followed by stupor in a patient with carcinoidosis. *Acta Psychiat Scand*, 1966, *42*, 153–161.

Lehtinen L and Kivalo A. Laughter epilepsy. *Acta Neurol Scand*, 1965, *41*, 255–261.

Leonard K. Cycloid psychoses-endogenous psychoses which are neither schizophrenic nor manic–depressive. *J Ment Sci*, 1961, *107*, 633–648.

Lewis DA and Smith RE. Steroid-induced psychiatric syndromes. *J Affect Disord*, 1983, *5*, 319–332.

Lieberman A and Benson DF. Control of emotional expression in pseudobulbar palsy. *Arch Neurol*, 1977, *34*, 717–719.

Lilly R, Cummings JL, Benson DF, and Frankel M. The human Klüver-Bucy syndrome. *Neurology*, 1983, *33*, 1141–1145.

Lin T-Y and Ziegler D. Psychiatric symptoms with initiation of carbidopa-levodopa treatment. *Neurology*, 1976, *26*, 679–700.

Lin T-Y, Greenblatt M, and Solomon HC. Agitated depression associated with arteriovenous aneurysm of left frontal lobe. *New Engl J Med*, 1952, *247*, 631–633.

Ling MHM, Perry PJ, and Tsuang MT. Side effects of corticosteroid therapy. *Arch Gen Psychiat*, 1981, *38*, 471–477.

Lipowski ZT. Transient cognitive disorders (delirium, acute confusional states) in the elderly. *Am J Psychiat*, 1983, *140*, 1426–1436.

Lippmann S, Moskovitz R, and O'Tuama L. Tricyclic-induced myoclonus. *Am J Psychiat*, 1977, *134*, 90–91.

Lipsey JR, Robinson RG, Pearlson GD, Rao K, and Price TR. Nortriptyline treatment of post-stroke depression: a double-blind study. *Lancet*, 1984, *1*, 297–300.

Lipsy JR, Robinson RG, Pearlson GD, Rao K, and Price TR. Mood change following bilateral hemisphere brain injury. *Br J Psychiat*, 1983, *14*, 266–273.

Lisansky J, Strassman RT, Janowsky D, and Risch SC. Drug-induced psychoses. In Tupin JP, Halbreich U, and Pena JJ (Eds.): *Transient psychosis: diagnosis, management and evaluation*. New York, Brunner-Mazel, 1984, pp. 80–110.

Lishman WA. Brain damage in relation to psychiatric disability after head injury. *Br J Psychiat*, 1968, *114*, 373–410.

Lishman WA. *Organic psychiatry*. London, Blackwell Scientific Publications, 1978.

Livingston KE and Escobar A. Anatomical bias of the limbic system concept. *Arch Neurol*, 1971, *24*, 17–21.

Lloyd JH. Pseudobulbar palsy. *Internat Clin*, 1908, *4*, 210–220.

Loosen PT and Prange AJ Jr. Serum thyrotropin response to thyrotropin-releasing hormone in psychiatric patients: a review. *Am J Psychiat*, 1982, *139*, 405–416.

Lorenz M and Cobb S. Language behavior in manic patients. *Arch Neurol Psychiat*, 1952, *67*, 763–770.

Louiseau P, Cahadon F, and Cahadon S. Gelastic epilepsy. *Epilepsia*, 1971, *12*, 313–323.

Lyskowski J, Nasrallah HA, Dunner FJ, and Bucher K. A longitudinal survey of side effects in a lithium clinic. *J Clin Psychiat*, 1982, *43*, 284–286.

Maas JW. Biogenic amines and depression. *Arch Gen Psychiat*, 1975, *32*, 1357–1361.

Mackay A. Self-poisoning—a complication of epilepsy. *Br J Psychiat*, 1979, *134*, 277–282.

MacLean PD. Psychosomatic disease and the "visceral brain." *Psychosom Med*, 1949, *11*, 338–353.

MacLean PD. Contrasting functions of limbic neocortical systems of the brain and their relevance to psychophysiological aspects of medicine. *Am J Med*, 1958, *25*, 611–626.

MacNeill A, Grennan DM, Ward D, and Dick WC. Psychiatric problems in systemic lupus erythematosus. *Br J Psychiat*, 1976, *128*, 442–445.

Malamud N. Psychiatric symptoms and the limbic lobe. *Bull LA Neurol Soc*, 1957, *22*, 131–139.

Malamud N. Psychiatric disorder with intracranial tumors of limbic system. *Arch Neurol*, 1967, *17*, 113–123.

Malloy FW, Small IF, Miller MJ, Milstein U, and Stout JR. Changes in neuropsychological test performance after electroconvulsive therapy. *Biol Psychiat*, 1982, *17*, 61–67.

Mandell AJ, Markham C, and Fowler W. Parkinson's syndrome, depression and imipramine. *Calif Med*, 1961, *95*, 12–14.

Mandell AJ, Markham CH, Tallman FF, and Mandell MP. Motivation and ability to move. *Am J Psychiat*, 1962, *119*, 544–549.

Mapelli G and Bellelli T. Secondary mania. *Arch Gen Psychiat*, 1982, *39*, 743.

Marsh GG and Markham CH. Does levodopa alter depression and psychopathology in parkinsonism patients? *J Neurol Neurosurg Psychiat*, 1973, *36*, 925–935.

Martin JP. Fits of laughter (sham mirth) in organic cerebral disease. *Brain*, 1950, *73*, 453–464.

Mathew RJ, Meyer JS, Francis DJ, Semchuk KM, Mortel K, and Claghorn JL. Cerebral blood flow in depression. *Am J Psychiat*, 1980, *137*, 1449–1450.

Matthews WB. Multiple sclerosis presenting with acute remitting psychiatric symptoms. *J Neurol Neurosurg Psychiat*, 1979, *42*, 859–863.

Mayeux R, Stern Y, Rosen J, and Leventhal J. Depression, intellectual impairment, and Parkinson disease. *Neurology*, 1981, *31*, 645–650.

Mayeux R, Stern Y, Cote L, and Williams JBW. Clinical and biochemical features of depression in Parkinson's disease. *Ann Neurol*, 1983, *14*, 135–136.

Mayeux R, Stern Y, Cote L, and Williams JBW. Altered serotonin metabolism in depressed patients with Parkinson's disease. *Neurology*, 1984, *34*, 642–646.

McCarley RW. REM sleep and depression: common neurobiological control mechanisms. *Am J Psychiat*, 1982, *139*, 565–570.

McEvoy JP. Organic brain syndromes. *Ann Int Med*, 1981, *95*, 213–220.

McGlashan TH and Carpenter WT Jr. Post-psychotic depression in schizophrenia. *Arch Gen Psychiat*, 1976, *33*, 231–239.

McHugh PR and Folstein MF. Psychiatric syndromes in Huntington's chorea: a clinical and phenomenologic study. In Benson DF and Blumer D (Eds.): *Psychiatric aspects of neurologic disease*. New York, Grune & Stratton, 1975, pp. 267–285.

Mehta DB. Lithium and affective disorders associated with organic brain impairment. *Am J Psychiat*, 1976, *133*, 236.

Mendels J and Hawkins DR. Sleep and depression. *Arch Gen Psychiat*, 1967, *16*, 344–354.

Merskey H and Woodforde JM. Psychiatric sequelae of minor head injury. *Brain*, 1972, *95*, 521–528.

Mettler FA and Crandell A. Relation between parkinsonism and psychiatric disorder. *J Nerv Ment Dis*, 1959, *129*, 551–563.

Miller H. Mental sequelae of head injury. *Proc Roy Soc Med*, 1966, *59*, 257–261.

Miller WR. Psychological deficit in depression. *Psychol Bull*, 1975, *82*, 238–260.

Mindham RHS. Psychiatric symptoms in parkinsonism. *J Neurol Neurosurg Psychiat*, 1970, *33*, 188–191.

Money J and Hosta G. Laughing seizures with sexual precocity: report of two cases. *Johns Hopkins Med J*, 1967, *120*, 326–336.

Monrad-Krohn GH. Dysprosody or altered "melody of language." *Brain*, 1947, *70*, 405–415.

Nasrallah HA, Lyskowski J, and Schroeder D. TCA-induced mania: differences between switchers and nonswitchers. *Biol Psychiat*, 1982, *17*, 271–274.

Nauta WJH. Limbic innervation of the striatum. In Friedhoff AJ and Chase TN (Eds.): *Gilles de la Tourette syndrome*. New York, Raven Press, 1982, pp. 41–47.

Nauta WJH and Domesick VB. Crossroads of limbic and striatal circuitry: hypothalamo-nigral connections. In Livingston KE and Hornykiewicz O (Eds.): *Limbic mechanisms*. New York, Plenum Press, 1978, pp. 75–93.

Neumann MA. Pick's disease *J Neuropath Exp Neurol*, 1949, *8*, 255–282.

Nomura J, Hisamatsu K, Hatotani N, Higashimura T, and Kamiya S. Studies on the cerebrohepatic relationship with reference to the pathogenesis of acute psychoses. In Hatotani N and Nomura J (Eds.): *Neurobiology of periodic psychoses*. New York, Igaku-Shoin, 1983, pp. 201–214.

Nurnberg HG, Prudic J, Fiori M, and Freedman EP. Psychopathology complicating acquired immune deficiency syndrome (AID's). *Am J Psychiat*, 1984, *141*, 95–96.

Offen ML, Davidoff DW, Troost BT, and Richey ET. Dacrystic epilepsy. *J Neurol Neurosurg Psychiat*, 1976, *39*, 829–834.

Oke A, Keller R, Mefford I, and Adams RN. Lateralization of norepinephrine in human thalamus. *Science*, 1978, *200*, 1411–1413.

Okuma T, Inanaga K, Otsuki S, Sarai K, Takahashi R, Hazama H, Mori A, and Watanabe M. Comparison of the antimanic efficacy of carbamazepine and chlorpromazine: a double-blind controlled study. *Psychopharmacology*, 1979, *66*, 211–217.

Okuma T, Inanaga K, Otsuki S, Sarai K, Takahashi R, Hazama H, Mori A, and Watanabe S. A preliminary double-blind study on the efficacy of carbamazepine in prophylaxis of manic–depressive illness. *Psychopharmacology*, 1981, *73*, 95–96.

Okuma T, Kishimoto A, Inoue K, Matsumoto H, Ogura A, Matsushita T, Nakao T, and Ogura C. Antimanic prophylactic effects of carbamazepine (Tegretol) on manic depressive psychosis. *Folia Psychiat Neurol Japon*, 1973, *27*, 283–297.

Olds J. Self stimulation of the brain. *Science*, 1958, *127*, 315–324.

Oppler W. Manic psychosis in a case of parasagittal meningioma. *Arch Neurol Psychiat*, 1950, *64*, 417–430.

Oyewumi KL and Lapierve YA. Efficacy of lithium in treating mood disorders occurring after brainstem injury. *Am J Psychiat*, 1981, *138*, 110–112.

Pandey RS, Sreenivas KN, Patih NM, and Swamy HS. Dopamine β-hydroxylase in a patient with Wilson's disease and mania. *Am J Psychiat*, 1981, *138*, 1628–1629.

Papez JW. A proposed mechanism of emotion. *Arch Neurol Psychiat*, 1937, *38*, 725–743.

Paulley JW and Hughes JP. Giant-cell arteritis, or arteritis of the aged. *Br Med J*, 1960, *2*, 1562–1567.

Paykel ES, Fleminger R, and Watson JP. Psychiatric side effects of antihypertensive drugs other than reserpine. *J Clin Psychopharmacol*, 1982, *2*, 14–39.

Pearlson GP, Garbacz DJ, Tompkins RH, Ahn HS, Gutterman DF, Veoff AE, and DePaulo JR. Clinical correlates of lateral ventricular enlargement in bipolar affective disorder. *Am J Psychiat*, 1984, *141*, 253–256.

Perria L, Rosadini G, and Rossi GF. Determination of side of cerebral dominance with amobarbital. *Arch Neurol*, 1961, *4*, 173–181.

Petrie WM, Maffucci RJ, and Woosley RL. Propranolol and depression. *Am J Psychiat*, 1982, *139*, 92–94.

Phelps ME, Mazziota JC, Baxter C, and Gerner R. Positron emission tomographic study of affective disorders: problems and strategies. *Ann Neurol*, 1984, *15* (Suppl.), S149–S156.

Pickar D, Murphy DL, Cohen RM, Campbell IC, and Lipper S. Selective and nonselective monoamine oxidase inhibitors. *Arch Gen Psychiat*, 1982, *39*, 535–540.

Planansky K and Johnston R. Depressive syndrome in schizophrenia. *Acta Psychiat Scand*, 1978, *57*, 207–218.

Post RM, Uhde TW, Ballenger JC, and Squillace KM. Prophylactic efficacy of carbamazepine in manic–depressive illness. *Am J Psychiat*, 1983, *140*, 1602–1604.

Powell EW and Hines G. The limbic system: an interface. *Behav Biol*, 1974, *12*, 149–164.

Price LH, Charney DS, and Heninger GR. Three cases of manic symptoms following yohimbine administration. *Am J Psychiat*, 1984, *141*, 1267–1268.

Price TRP and Tucker GJ. Psychiatric and behavioral manifestations of normal pressure hydrocephalus. *J Nerv Ment Dis*, 1977, *164*, 51–55.

Quetsch RM, Achor RWP, Litin EM, and Faucett RL. Depressive reactions in hypertensive patients. *Circulation*, 1959, *19*, 366–375.

Ramsey TA and Cox M. Lithium and the kidney: a review. *Am J Psychiat* 1982, *139*, 443–449.

Reches A, Tietler J, and Lavy S. Parkinsonism due to lithium carbonate poisoning. *Arch Neurol*, 1981, *38*, 471.

Reed TE, Chandler JH, Hughes EM, and Davidson RT. Huntington's chorea in Michigan. I. Demography and genetics. *Am J Hum Genet*, 1958, *10*, 201–225.

Reeves AG and Plum F. Hyperphagia, rage, and dementia accompanying a ventromedial hypothalamic neoplasm. *Arch Neurol*, 1969, *20*, 616–624.

Remington G and Jeffries JJ. The role of cerebral arteriovenous malformations in psychiatric disturbances: case report. *J Clin Psychiat*, 1984, *45*, 226–229.

Riblet LA and Taylor DP. Pharmacology and neurochemistry of trazodone. *J Clin Psychopharm*, 1981, *1* (Suppl. No. 6), 17S–22S.

Rice E and Gendelman S. Psychiatric aspects of normal pressure hydrocephalus. *JAMA*, 1973, *223*, 409–412.

Richardson JW III and Richelson E. Antidepressants: a clinical update for medical practitioners. *Mayo Clin Proc*, 1984, *59*, 330–337.

Richelson E. Antimuscarinic and other receptor-blocking properties of antidepressants. *Mayo Clin Proc*, 1983, *58*, 40–46.

Rieder RO, Mann LS, Weinberger DR, van Kammen DP, and Post RM. Computed tomographic scans in patients with schizophrenia, schizoaffective and bipolar affective disorders. *Arch Gen Psychiat*, 1983, *40*, 735–739.

Rinieris PM, Malliaras DE, Batrinos ML, and Stefanis CN. Testosterone treatment of depression in two patients with Klinefelter's syndrome. *Am J Psychiat*, 1979, *136*, 986–988.

Robins AH. Depression in patients with parkinsonism. *Br J Psychiat*, 1976, *128*, 141–145.

Robinson RG. Differential behavioral and biochemical effects of right and left hemispheric infarction in the rat. *Science*, 1979, *205*, 707–710.

Robinson RG and Benson DF. Depression in aphasic patients: frequency, severity, and clinical–pathological correlations. *Brain Lang*, 1981, *14*, 282–291.

Robinson RG, Kubos KL, Starr LB, Rao K, and Price TR. Mood disorders in stroke patients. *Brain*, 1984, *107*, 81–93.

Robinson RG and Price TR. Post-stroke depressive disorders: a follow-up study of 103 patients. *Stroke*, 1982, *13*, 635–641.

Robinson RG and Szetela B. Mood change following left hemisphere brain injury. *Ann Neurol*, 1981, *9*, 447–453.

Roger J, Lob H, Waltregny A, and Gastaut H. Attacks of epileptic laughter; on 5 cases. *Electroenceph Clin Neurophysiol*, 1967, *22*, 279.

Rosen A. Case report: symptomatic mania and phencyclidine abuse. *Am J Psychiat*, 1979, *136*, 118–119.

Rosen PB and Stevens R. Action myoclonus in lithium toxicity. *Ann Neurol*, 1983, *13*, 221–222.

Rosenbaum AH and Barry MJ Jr. Positive therapeutic response to lithium in hypomania secondary to organic brain syndrome. *Am J Psychiat*, 1975, *132*, 1072–1073.

Rosenbaum AH, Maruta T, and Richelson E. Drugs that alter mood. I. Tricyclic agents and monoamine oxidase inhibitors. *Mayo Clin Proc*, 1979a, *54*, 335–344.

Rosenbaum AH, Maruta T, and Richelson E. Drugs that alter mood. II. Lithium. *Mayo Clin Proc*, 1979b, *54*, 401–407.

Ross ED. The aprosodias. *Arch Neurol*, 1981, *38*, 561–569.

Ross ED, Horney JH, deLacoste-Utamsing C, and Purdy PD. How the brain integrates affective and propositional language into a unified behavioral function. *Arch Neurol*, 1981, *38*, 745–748.

Ross ED and Mesulam M-M. Dominant language functions of the right hemisphere? *Arch Neurol*, 1979, *36*, 144–148.

Ross ED and Rush AJ. Diagnosis and neuroanatomical correlates of depression in brain-damaged patients. *Arch Gen Psychiat*, 1981, *38*, 1344–1354.

Roubicek J. Laughter in epilepsy, with some general introductory notes. *J Ment Sci*, 1946, *92*, 734–755.

Roy A. Psychiatric aspects of narcolepsy. *Br J Psychiat*, 1976, *128*, 562–565.

Rubinow DR, Roy-Byrne P, Hoban C, Gold PW, and Post RM. Prospective assessment of menstrually related mood disorders. *Am J Psychiat*, 1984, *141*, 684–686.

Ryback RS and Schwab RS. Manic response to levodopa therapy. *New Engl J Med*, 1971, *285*, 788–789.

Sachar EJ, Hellman L, Roffwarg HP, Halpern FS, Fukushima DK, and Gallagher TF. Disrupted 24-hour patterns of cortisol secretion in psychotic depression. *Arch Gen Psychiat*, 1973, *28*, 19–24.

Sackeim HA, Decina P, Epstein P, Bruder GE, and Malitz S. Possible reversed affective lateralization in a case of bipolar disorder. *Am J Psychiat*, 1983, *140*, 1191–1193.

Sackeim HA, Greenberg MS, Weiman AL, Gur RC, Hungerbuhler JP, and Geschwind N. Hemispheric asymmetry in the expression of positive and negative emotions. *Arch Neurol*, 1982, *39*, 210–218.

Sayed AJ. Mania and bromism: a case report and a look to the future. *Am J Psychiat*, 1976, *133*, 228–229.

Scher M, Krieger JN, and Juergens S. Trazodone and priapism. *Am J Psychiat*, 1983, *140*, 1362–1363.

Schiffer RB, Caine ED, Bamford KA, and Levy S. Depressive episodes in patients with multiple sclerosis. *Am J Psychiat*, 1983, *140*, 1498–1500.

Schildkraut JJ, Schanberg SM, Breese GR, and Kopin IJ. Norepinephrine metabolism and drugs used in the affective disorders: a possible mechanism of action. *Am J Psychiat*, 1967, *124*, 600–608.

Schou M, Boastrup PC, Grof P, Weis P, and Angst J. Pharmacological and clinical problems of lithium prophylaxis. *Br J Psychiat*, 1970, *100*, 615–619.

Schwartz GE, Fair PL, Salt P, Mandel MR, and Klerman GL. Facial muscle patterning to affective imagery in depressed and nondepressed subjects. *Science*, 1976, *192*, 489–491.

Sethi PK and Rao S. Gelastic, quiritarian, and cursive epilepsy. *J Neurol Neurosurg Psychiat*, 1976, *39*, 823–828.

Shagrass C. The EEG in affective disorders. In Wilson WP (Ed.): *Applications of electroencephalography in psychiatry*. Durham, North Carolina, Duke University Press, 1965, pp. 146–167.

Shagrass C. Evoked potentials in adult psychiatry. In Hughes JR and Wilson WP (Eds.): *EEG and evoked potentials in psychiatry and behavioral neurology*. Boston, Butterworths, 1983, pp. 169–210.

Sher PK and Brown SB. Gelastic epilepsy. *Am J Dis Childh*, 1976, *130*, 1126–1131.

Shopsin B and Gerson S. Cogwheel rigidity related to lithium maintenance. *Am J Psychiat*, 1975, *132*, 536–538.

Silberman EK, Weingartner H, and Post RM. Thinking disorder in depression. *Arch Gen Psychiat*, 1983a, *40*, 775–780.

Silberman EK, Weingartner H, Stillman R, Chen H-J, and Post RM. Altered lateralization of cognitive processes in depressed women. *Am J Psychiat*, 1983b, *140*, 1340–1341.

Small JG. EEG in affective disorders. In Hughes JR and Wilson WP (Eds.): *EEG and evoked potentials in psychiatry and behavioral neurology*. Boston, Butterworths, 1983, pp. 41–54.

Smith RS Jr and Ayd FT Jr. A critical appraisal of amoxapine. *J Clin Psychiat*, 1981, *42*, 238–242.

Sobin A and Ozer MN. Mental disorders in acute encephalitis. *J Mt Sinai Hosp*, 1966, *33*, 73–82.

Sorensen K and Nielsen J. Twenty psychotic males with Klinefelter's syndrome. *Acta Psychiat Scand*, 1977, *56*, 249–255.

Spector RH and Schnapper R. Amitriptyline-induced ophthalmoplegia. *Neurology*, 1981, *31*, 1188–1190.

Speirs J and Hirsch SR. Severe lithium toxicity with "normal" serum concentrations. *Br Med J*, 1978, *1*, 815–816.

Spivak JL and Jackson DL. Pellagra: an analysis of 18 patients and a review of the literature. *Johns Hopkins Med*, 1977, *140*, 295–309.

Squire LR. Neuropsychological effects of ECT. In Abrams R and Essman WB (Eds.): *Electroconvulsive therapy. Biological foundations and clinical applications*. New York, SP Medical and Scientific Books, 1982, pp. 169–186.

Squire LR and Chace PM. Memory functions six to nine months after electroconvulsive therapy. *Arch Gen Psychiat*, 1975, *32*, 1157–1564.

Staton RD, Wilson H, and Brumback RA. Cognitive improvement associated with tricyclic antidepressant treatment of childhood major depressive illness. *Percept Motor Skills*, 1981, *53*, 219–234.

Steinberg D, Hirsch SR, Marston SD, Reynolds K, and Sutton RNP. Influenza infection causing manic psychosis. *Br J Psychiat*, 1972, *120*, 531–535.

Stern K and Dancey TE. Glioma of the diencephalon in a manic patient. *Am J Psychiat*, 1942, *98*, 716–719.

Stern M and Robbins ES. Psychoses in systemic lupus erythmatosus. *Arch Gen Psychiat*, 1960, *3*, 205–212.

Stern WE and Brown WJ. Pathological laughter. *J Neurosurg*, 1957, *14*, 129–139.

Sternbach H, Garner RH, and Gwirtsman HE. The thyrotropin releasing hormone stimulation test: a review. *J Clin Psychiat*, 1982, *43*, 4–6.

Sternbach HA, Gold MS, Pottash AC, and Extein I. Thyroid failure and protirelin (thyrotropin-releasing hormone) test abnormalities in depressed outpatients. *JAMA*, 1983, *249*, 1618–1620.

Sternberg DE and Jarvik ME. Memory functions in depression. *Arch Gen Psychiat*, 1976, *33*, 219–224.

Stokes PE, Stoll PM, Koslow SH, Maas JW, Davis JM, Swann AC, and Robins E. Pretreatment DST and hypothalamic-pituitary-adrenocortical function in depressed patients and comparison groups. *Arch Gen Psychiat*, 1984, *41*, 257–267.

Strang RR. Imipramine in treatment of parkinsonism: a double-blind placebo study. *Br Med J*, 1965, *2*, 33–34.

Strauss H. Office treatment of depressive states with a new drug (imipramine). *NY State J Med*, 1959, *59*, 2906–2910.

Strauss I and Keschner M. Mental symptoms in cases of tumor of the frontal lobe. *Arch Neurol Psychiat*, 1935, *33*, 986–1005.

Surridge D. An investigation into some psychiatric aspects of multiple sclerosis. *Br J Psychiat*, 1969, *115*, 749–764.

Swann AC, Secunda S, Davis JM, Robins E, Hanin I, Koslow SH, and Maas JW. CSF monoamine metabolities in mania. *Am J Psychiat*, 1983, *140*, 396–400.

Swash M. Released involuntary laughter after temporal lobe infarction. *J Neurol Neurosurg Psychiat*, 1972, *35*, 108–113.

Taylor MA. Indications for electroconvulsive treatment. In Abrams R and Essmar WB (Eds.): *Electroconvulsive therapy. Biologic foundations and clinical applications*. New York, SP Medical and Scientific Books, 1982, pp. 7–39.

Teja JS. Periodic psychosis of puberty. *J Nerv Ment Dis*, 1976, *162*, 52–57.

Thompson TL II, Moran MG, and Nies AS. Psychotropic drug use in the elderly. *New Engl J Med*, 1983, *308*, 134–138, 194–199.

Tilney F and Morrison JF. Pseudobulbar palsy clinically and pathologically considered with the clinical report of five cases. *J Nerv Ment Dis*, 1912, *39*, 505–535.

Titus JP. Cimetidine-induced mania in depressed patients. *J Clin Psychiat*, 1983, *44*, 267–268.

Trimble MR and Cummings JL. Neuropsychiatric disturbances following brainstem lesions. *Br J Psychiat*, 1981, *138*, 56–59.

Trimble MR and Grant I. Psychiatric aspects of multiple sclerosis. In Benson DF and Blumer D (Eds.): *Psychiatric aspects of neurologic disease*, Vol. 2. New York, Grune & Stratton, 1982, pp. 279–298.

Tucker DM, Stenslie CE, Roth RS, and Shearer SL. Right frontal lobe activation and right hemisphere performance. Decrement during a depressed mood. *Arch Gen Psychiat*, 1981, *38*, 169–174.

Tupin JP. Borderline states and psychosis. In Tupin JP, Halbreich U, and Pena JJ (Eds.): *Transient psychosis: diagnosis, management and evaluation*. New York, Brunner-Mazel, 1984, pp. 15–27.

Tyrer P, Alexander MS, Regan A, and Lee I. An extrapyramidal syndrome after lithium therapy. *Br J Psychiat*, 1980, *136*, 191–194.

Ungerstedt U. Stereotaxic mapping of the monoamine pathways of the rat brain. *Acta Physiol Scand*, 1971, Suppl. *367*, 1–48.

Van de Lught PJM and de Visser AP. Two patients with a vital expansive syndrome following a cerebrovascular accident. *Psychiat Neurol Neurochir*, 1967, *70*, 349–359.

Van Putten T. Lithium-induced disabling tremor. *Psychosomatics*, 1978, *19*, 27–31.

Vereker R. The psychiatric aspects of temporal arteritis. *J Ment Sci*, 1957, *98*, 280–286.

Vestergaard P, Amdisen A, and Schou M. Clinically significant side effects of lithium treatment. *Acta Psychiat Scand*, 1980, *62*, 193–200.

Villani S and Weitzel WD. Secondary mania. *Arch Gen Psychiat*, 1979, *36*, 1031.

Vlissides D, Gill D, and Castelow J. Bromocriptine-induced mania? *Br Med J*, 1978, *1*, 510.

Warburton JW. Depressive symptoms in Parkinson patients referred for thalamotomy. *J Neurol Neurosurg Psychiat*, 1967, *30*, 368–370.

Waters BGH and Lapierre YD. Secondary mania associated with sympathomimetic drug use. *Am J Psychiat*, 1981, *138*, 837–838.

Weeks D, Freeman CPL, and Kendell R. Does ECT produce enduring cognitive deficits? In Palmer RL (Ed.): *Electroconvulsive therapy: an appraisal*. New York, Oxford University Press, 1981, pp. 159–181.

Weil AA. Depressive reactions associated with temporal lobe uncinate seizures. *J Nerv Ment Dis*, 1955, *121*, 505–510. 505–510.

Weil AA. Ictal depression and anxiety in temporal lobe epilepsy. *Am J Psychiat*, 1956, *113*, 149–157.

Weingartner H, Cohen RM, Murphy DL, Martello J, and Gerdt C. Cognitive processes in depression. *Arch Gen Psychiat*, 1981, *38*, 42–47.

Weintraub S, Mesulam M-M, and Kramer L. Disturbances in prosody. *Arch Neurol*, 1981, *38*, 742–744.

Weintraub S and Mesulam M-M. Developmental learning disabilities of the right hemisphere. *Arch Neurol*, 1983, *40*, 463–468.

Weisert KN and Hendrie HC. Secondary mania? A case report. *Am J Psychiat*, 1977, *134*, 929–930.

Weiss BL, Foster G, Reynolds CF III, and Kupfer DJ. Psychomotor activity in mania. *Arch Gen Psychiat*, 1974, *31*, 379–383.

White LE Jr. A morphologic concept of the limbic lobe. *Int Rev Neurobiol*, 1965, *8*, 1–34.

Whitlock FA. *Symptomatic affective disorders*. New York, Academic Press, 1982.

Whitlock FA and Evans LEJ. Drugs and depression. *Drugs*, 1978, *18*, 53–71.

Whitlock FA and Siskind MM. Depression as a major symptom of multiple sclerosis. *J Neurol Neurosurg Psychiat*, 1980, *43*, 861–865.

Whittier J, Haydu G, and Crawford J. Effect of imipramine (Tofranil) on depression and hyperkinesia in Huntington's disease. *Am J Psychiat*, 1961, *118*, 79.

Whybrow PC, Prange AJ Jr, and Treadway CR. Mental changes accompanying thyroid gland dysfunction. *Arch Gen Psychiat*, 1969, *20*, 48–63.

Williams D. The structure of emotions reflected in epileptic experiences. *Brain*, 1956, *79*, 29–67.

Williams D. Man's temporal lobe. *Brain*, 1968, *91*, 639–654.

Wilson SAK. Pathological laughing and crying. *J Neurol Psychopathol*, 1924, *4*, 299–333.

Wood MW, Svien HJ, and Daly D. Involuntary laughter. *Mayo Clin Proc*, 1958, *33*, 267–275.

Yakovlev PI. Brain, motility, and behavior. *J Nerv Ment Dis*, 1948, *107*, 313–335.

Young AC, Saunders J, and Ponsford JR. Mental change as an early feature of multiple sclerosis. *J Neurol Neurosurg Psychiat*, 1976, *39*, 1008–1013.

Young LD, Taylor I, and Holmstrom V. Lithium treatment of patients with affective illness associated with organic brain symptoms. *Am J Psychiat*, 1977, *134*, 1405–1407.

Yudofsky SC. Parkinson's disease, depression and electroconvulsive therapy: a clinical and neurobiologic synthesis. *Comp Psychiat*, 1979, *20*, 579–581.

Zorumski CF and Bakris GL. Choreoathetosis associated with lithium: case report and literature review. *Am J Psychiat*, 1983, *140*, 1621–1622.

Zubenko GS, Altesman RI, Cassidy JW, and Barreira PT. Disturbances of thirst and water homeostatis in patients with affective illness. *Am J Psychiat*, 1984, *141*, 436–437.

Personality Alterations, Hysteria, Anxiety, and Obsessive–Compulsive Disorder

The disturbances grouped in this chapter share the common feature of being long-term behavioral patterns characterizing the individual's typical feelings, moods, and adaptive functions. In some cases the behaviors are lifelong and are a product of hereditary or congenital factors: in others the behaviors follow an acquired CNS disorder and are related to the location and extent of brain dysfunction. This chapter presents the neurobiology of personality alterations, hysteria, anxiety, and obsessive–compulsive disorder.

PERSONALITY ALTERATIONS

The term "personality" refers to one's habitual feelings, moods, attitudes, and patterns of behavior, including the way one responds to, perceives, and thinks about the environment and oneself (*Diagnostic and statistical manual of mental disorders,* 1980; McHugh and Folstein, 1975). A diagnosis of personality disorder is warranted when the behavioral patterns are sufficiently inflexible and maladaptive to cause impaired adaptive functioning or significant subjective distress.

The identification of personality disorders is difficult and controversial, and combinations of different personality characteristics are common (Millon, 1981). Table 15-1 presents one approach to the classification of personality disorders and lists the neurological factors that may contribute to their occurrence. Most types of personality disorder (dependent, histrionic, narcissistic, compulsive, passive–aggressive, schizoid, avoidant, schizotypal) have not been associated with specific neurological conditions, although all personality styles are influenced by genetic factors that guide the development of brain structure and function and ultimately contribute to personality function (Millon, 1981).

Several of the personality disorders listed in Table 15-1 have been associated with neurological conditions.

Of patients with antisocial personalities, 40–60 percent exhibit EEG abnormalities. The EEG changes are particularly likely to include temporal lobe dysrhythmia or slowing of posterior background rhythms (Chapter 11) (Arthurs and Cahoon, 1964; Gibbens et al., 1959; Harper et al., 1972; Hill, 1952; Knott, 1965; Levy and Kennard, 1953; Small, 1966; Williams, 1969). Minor abnormalities on neurological examination, the occurrence of epilepsylike experiences, and deficits on neuropsychological tests are also common among individuals with antisocial personalities (Bach-y-Rita and Veno, 1974; Krynicki, 1978; Lewis, 1976; Lewis et al., 1979; Pontius and Yudowitz, 1980; Yeudall et al., 1982). Children with hyperactivity and learning disorders are predisposed to develop antisocial personalities in adulthood, an observation that further supports a relationship between brain dysfunction and antisocial behavior (Hogenson, 1974; Mendelson et al., 1971; Morrison and Minkoff, 1975; Virkkunen and Nuutila, 1976).

Borderline personality disorders have also been associated with childhood hyperactivity and with a variety of other neurological disorders, including epilepsy, cerebral trauma, and encephalitis. Patients with borderline personality associated with brain dysfunction are more likely to be male and develop aberrant personality patterns at an earlier age of onset than do patients with idiopathic borderline syndromes (Andrulonis et al., 1980).

Paranoid personality has followed brain damage and has been reported with injury lateralized to either hemisphere (Benson, 1973; Gaspirini et al., 1978; Leftoff, 1983).

The "organic" personality syndrome described in the *Diagnostic and statistical manual of mental disorders* (1980) is characterized by emotional lability and impaired impulse control. It most closely resembles the personality alteration that follows damage to the orbitofrontal aspects of the brain as discussed in the following paragraphs and in Chapter 6.

TABLE 15-1.   Personality Disorders *(Diagnostic and Statistical Manual of Mental Disorders,* 1980) and Their Neurological
Correlates

Personality Disorder	Associated Neurological Condition
Dependent personality	Genetic neurobiologic contributions
Histrionic personality	Genetic neurobiologic contributions
Narcissistic personality	Genetic neurobiologic contributions
Compulsive personality	Genetic neurobiologic contributions
Passive–aggressive personality	Genetic neurobiologic contributions
Schizoid personality	Genetic neurobiologic contributions
Avoidant personality	Genetic neurobiologic contributions
Schizotypal personality	Genetic neurobiologic contributions
Antisocial personality	EEG abnormalities common; hyperactivity in childhood
Borderline personality	Brain damage; hyperactivity in childhood; epilepsy
Paranoid personality	Brain damage
Organic personality	Orbitofrontal lobe damage

The principal clue that an acquired neurological disorder is responsible for a particular personality pattern is the occurrence of the sudden *change* in the patient's behavioral style. Regardless of the type of change manifested, the patient who suddenly exhibits an altered personality is often harboring a neurological illness. The types of personality changes induced by neurological disease may be quite variable, and most current personality nosologies are inadequate to account for the diversity of personality changes that have been noted in patients with neurological disturbances. Table 15-2 lists some of the personality changes reported in patients with specific neurological conditions.

Damage to the frontal lobe may produce different behavioral alterations depending on the site of the lesion (Chapter 6). Patients with orbitofrontal injuries lack tact and restraint. They are often irritable, facetious, and euphoric and tend to be uncritical, disinhibited, and impulsive. Patients with lesions of the frontal lobe convexities, on the other hand, are apathetic, are indifferent, and lack initiative. Combinations of convexity and orbitofrontal symptoms are common (Arseni et al., 1966; Blumer and Benson, 1975; Faust, 1966; Hunter et al., 1968). Frontal lobe syndromes occur with frontal neoplasms, demyelinating disorders, degenerative diseases, and infectious and inflammatory illnesses and are particularly common following closed head injury (Brooks and McKinley, 1983; Hunter et al., 1968; Lishman, 1968, 1973).

Correlation of personality alterations with the lateralization of brain injuries has received little study, but a few observations are available. Patients with left hemisphere lesions may become depressed or paranoid (Ben-

son, 1973; Gaspirini et al., 1978; Leftoff, 1983). Patients who sustain right hemisphere damage as adults manifest denial of illness and tend to be abnormally euthymic (Gainotti, 1972; Gasparini et al., 1978). Injury to the right hemisphere occurring early in life has been reported to lead to a personality pattern characterized by shyness, depression, isolation, and schizoid behavior (Weintraub and Mesulam, 1983).

The existence of a personality pattern specifically associated with epilepsy is controversial, but considerable evidence suggests that patients with seizure disorders, particularly those with complex partial seizures, are subject to several types of personality alteration (Trimble, 1983). One characteristic personality change consists of interpersonal viscosity, circumstantial speech, religiosity and increased attention to nascent philosophical concerns, hyposexuality, and hypergraphia (Chapter 9) (Bear and Fedio, 1977; Bear et al., 1982; Hermann and Riel, 1981; Roberts et al., 1982; Waxman and Geschwind, 1974). The personality syndrome is not pathognomonic of epilepsy and occurs in other psychiatric disorders (Mungas, 1982), but its emergence after the onset of a limbic system injury implies the existence of a relationship between the lesion site and the development of the behavioral characteristics. Pond and Bidwell (1959–1960) found this type of personality alteration in approximately 5 percent of all epileptics followed in general medical practices in Great Britain. Another peronality pattern found in epileptics is the borderline personality disorder (Andrulonis et al., 1980). The borderline syndrome is characterizied by impulsivity, unstable and intense interpersonal relationships, intense anger and poor control of temper, identity dis-

TABLE 15-2.   Neurological Disorders with Associated Personality Alterations

Neurological Condition	Personality Alteration
Frontal lobe damage	
Orbitofrontal	Lack of tact and restraint; facetious; euphoric; impulsive and disinhibited
Frontal convexity	Apathetic, indifferent; lack initiative
Lateralized hemispheric injury	
Left	Paranoia, depression
Right	Adult onset: denial, neglect, paranoia
	Childhood onset: shyness, depression, social isolation
Epilepsy	Epileptic personality: viscosity, circumstantiality, religiosity, hyposexuality, hypergraphia
	Borderline personality, paranoia
Bilateral limbic system lesions	Placidity
Hyperactivity, learning disability	Antisocial personality
	Borderline personality

turbances, affective instability, physically self-damaging activities, and chronic feelings of emptiness or boredom (*Diagnostic and statistical manual of mental disorders,* 1980).

Children with attention-deficit syndromes, hyperactivity, and learning disabilities are at increased risk for the development of antisocial and borderline personality disorders in their adult years (Andrulonis et al., 1980; Hogenson, 1974; Mendelson et al., 1971; Morrison and Minkoff, 1975; Virkkunen and Nuutila, 1976).

Placidity is a personality alteration that has frequently been observed in association with bilateral limbic system lesions. It has been reported in patients with the Klüver-syndrome, the Wernicke-Korsakoff syndrome, and following frontal lobotomy (Lilly et al., 1983; Parkin, 1984).

Personality alterations occur with many neurological disorders in addition to those described here, but this aspect of neuropsychiatry has received little systematic study. Alterations in personality also overlap with the chronic changes in mood described in Chapter 14.

HYSTERIA

The term "hysteria" has been used in a variety of ways to describe a plethora of clinical disorders (Chodoff and Lyons, 1958; Weintraub, 1983). It may describe a particular personality disorder (hysterical or *histrionic personality*) characterized by self-dramatization; excessive attention seeking; overreaction to minor events; irrational emotional outbursts; vain and demanding behavior; dependence; and a tendency toward manipulative suicide threats, gestures, or attempts (*Diagnostic and*

statistical manual of mental disorders, 1980). Hysteria has also been applied to a disorder characterizied by phobias and anxiety, called *anxiety hysteria. Hysterical conversion reaction* refers to the occurrence of neurological symptoms in the absence of confirmatory signs of neurological disease or in excess of any disability attributable to an existing neurological condition. Hysteria has also been used synonymously with the *Briquet syndrome,* somatization disorder characterizied by the presence of at least 15 symptoms involving at least nine somatic areas and occurring predominantly in young women with complicated medical histories but without identifiable medical disease (Guze, 1975; Murphy, 1982; Perley and Guze, 1962). *Epidemic* or *mass hysteria* refers to the occurrence of similar physical symptoms or unusual behaviors that affect a group of individuals and have no identifiable neurological or medical cause (Small and Nicholi, 1982). Hysteria has also been applied to the excessive emotional displays that may occur in individuals who receive unexpected favorable or unfavorable news, and it has been used as a term of approbrium. With all these different usages, it might justifiably be asked whether the term has any real meaning at all and whether it might appropriately be discarded. The concept of hysteria, however, is one of the oldest in medicine and is likely—whatever its value—to persist (Ey, 1982; Merskey, 1979).

The form of hysteria of greatest concern in neuropsychiatry is the hysterical conversion reaction. Conversion symptoms are usually defined as neurological abnormalities that cannot be explained on the basis of the patient's clinical findings. Table 15-3 presents conversion symptoms observed in four studies in which the relative proportion of complaints was reported. Mutism,

TABLE 15-3. Relative Frequency of Symptoms in Four Studies of Hysterical Conversion Reactions

Symptom	Carter (1949) (Percent of Cases)	Farley et al. (1968) (Percent of Cases)	Guze et al. (1971) (Percent of Cases)	Folks et al. (1984) (Percent of Cases)
Paralysis	23	8	10	26
Ataxia	—	—	13	—
Aphonia	29	—	13	—
Anesthesia	—	14	14	16
Blindness	3	26	9	5
Deafness	—	4	4	—
Amnesia	23	0	8	—
Unconsciousness	—	10	8	3
Convulsions	6	8	4	13
Miscellaneous	16	30	17	37
Total	100 (N = 100)	100 (N = 50)	100 (N = 209)	100 (N = 62)

paralysis, anesthesia, blindness, and amnesia are among the most commonly described symptoms (Carter, 1949; Farley et al., 1968; Folks et al., 1984; Guze et al., 1971). Hysterical convulsions are discussed in Chapter 9.

The significance of conversion symptoms is controversial. The psychoanalytic school of thought conceives of the symptoms as symbolically significant physical symptoms substituted for repressed instinctual and unacceptable impulses. An alternative psychodynamic explanation suggests that the symptoms represent a form of nonverbal communication between patient and physician by which the patient can covertly transmit personal needs or distress (Chodoff, 1974). Some believe that the patient simply exaggerates existing symptoms to focus the physician's attention, whereas others suggest that the symptoms arise directly from existing physical disturbances too subtle to be detected by the clinician. Whatever the explanation of the symptoms, they rarely occur in the absence of significant neurological, phsychiatric, or medical disturbances. A majority of patients presenting with a chief complaint of having a lump in the throat (globus hystericus), for example, will be found on examination to have an esophageal lesion (Malcomson, 1968). Follow-up studies of patients presenting to general medical or neurologic hospitals with conversion symptoms reveal that 50–70 percent will develop diagnoseable neurologic conditions within the next few years (Merskey and Buhrich, 1975; Merskey and Trimble, 1979; Slater, 1965; Whitlock, 1967), whereas patients with conversion reactions assessed in psychiatric institutions are found to be suffering from personality disorders, alcoholism, depression, and/or schizophrenia (Guze et al., 1971; Stefansson et al., 1976; Ziegler et al., 1960). The personality disorders most

likely to be associated with conversion reactions are the passive–aggressive, dependent, antisocial, and histrionic types (Chodoff and Lyons, 1958; Guze et al., 1971; Merskey and Trimble, 1979). The death rate from suicide and from fatal neuromedical illnesses is significantly increased in follow-up studies of patients presenting with conversion symptoms, an observation that emphasizes the seriousness with which this clinical syndrome must be regarded by the clinician (Slater, 1965; Stefansson et al., 1976).

Given the difficulties of defining, understanding, and diagnosing conversion symptoms as well as the high rate of medical, neurological, and psychiatric disturbances among patients presenting with them, the most defensible clinical course is to regard the conversion reaction as an important harbinger of an underlying condition that must be identified and treated.

ANXIETY

Anxiety disorders are characterizied by feelings of dread, fear, or foreboding in the absence of an appropriate threatening situation. The anxiety may be persistent (generalized anxiety disorder), episodic (panic disorder), present only in specific circumstances (phobic disorder), or reexperienced periodically after a particularly threatening experience (posttraumatic stress disorder) (Brown et al., 1984; *Diagnostic and statistical manual of mental disorders*, 1980). Some nosologies include obsessive–compulsive disorder among the anxiety states, but phenomenological and neurobiological information (presented later) suggest that it may represent a separate category of neuropsychiatric disturbance.

In addition to the subjective elements of anxiety such as dread, foreboding, and the fear of dying or losing control, there are also perceptual, cognitive, autonomic, and motoric manifestations of anxiety (Table 15-4) (Cohen and Ross, 1983; *Diagnostic and statistical manual of mental disorders*, 1980; Hall, 1980). Perceptual changes involve feelings of derealization and depersonalization and may include hallucinations. Cognitive alterations are manifest by poor attention and concentration and an impaired ability to organize and pursue a coherent line of thought. The autonomic aspects of anxiety are manifold and involve the cardiovascular system (tachycardia, palpitation, hypertension, syncope), respiratory system (dyspnea, hyperventilation), gastrointestinal system (anorexia, diarrhea), and genitourinary system (urinary frequency, urgency, hesitancy), as well as increased perspiration and pupillary dilatation. Motorically, anxious individuals are restless and hypervigilant, and have an action tremor and brisk muscle stretch reflexes.

Anxiety is triggered when anticipation of punishing, novel, or innately fear-inducing stimuli produces the perceptual, cognitive, autonomic, and motoric phenomenon disussed in the preceding paragraph. Anxiety may be learned—as in classical conditioning—or may result from direct end organ activation by autonomic stimulants such as amphetamines, vasopressors, and sympathomimetics. Anxiety proneness, particularly for phobias and panic disorder, also has an important hereditary contribution (Crowe et al., 1983; Harris et al., 1983; Leckman et al., 1983; Torgelsen, 1983). Anxiety is a product of the interaction of genetic, neuromedical, and experiential–dynamic factors, therefore, with each playing more or less of a role in individual cases. Table 15-5 presents the differential diagnosis of conditions associated with anxiety. The neuromedical conditions and agents most likely to be associated with anxiety symptoms include posttraumatic and postconcussive syndromes, hypoxia, hyperthyroidism, hypoglycemia, pheochromocytoma, alcohol and drug withdrawal and administration of caffeine, amphetamines, vasopressor agents, lactic acid, and sympathomimetic drugs (Hall, 1980; Jefferson and Marshall, 1981; Mackenzie and Popkin, 1983; Pitts, 1969). Anxiety may also be prominent in the course of mania, depression, and schizophrenia as well as in the primary idiopathic anxiety disorders.

Gray (1982) has constructed a neurophysiological model of anxiety, proposing that excessive activity in the limbic system overstimulates the behavioral system responsible for surveillance, vigilance, and stimulus evaluation. The excessive activation results secondarily in the perceptual, cognitive, motoric, and autonomic phenomena comprising the anxious state. γ-Aminobutyric acid, norepinephrine, and serotonin all play a role in

TABLE 15-4.   Components of the Anxiety Syndrome

Emotional aspects
Feelings of terror, apprehension, tension, dread, panic
Perceptual aspects
Derealization, depersonalization, hallucination
Cognitive aspects
Poor attention span and concentration
Disruption of organized thinking
Autonomic and visceral manifestations
Palpitations
Light-headedness
Tachycardia and hypertension
Hyperventilation and dyspnea
Increased perspiration
Tingling of extremities (occasional carpopedal spasm)
Anorexia
Diarrhea
Pupillary dilatation
Syncope
Urinary frequency, urgency, hesitancy
Motoric manifestations
Action tremor
Vigilant, fearful facial expression
Pacing, restlessness
Exaggerated muscle stretch reflexes

Data from Cohen and Ross (1983), *Diagnostic and statistical manual of mental disorders* (1980), and Hall (1980).

the arousal and limbic system activity. Anxiolytic agents modify the excessive activation, and behavior therapy permits habituation of the limbic response to anxiogenic stimuli (Gray, 1982; Hoehn-Saric, 1982; Kandel,1983).

Anxiety disorders can be significantly modified by psychotherapy and pharmacotherapy. Behavioral conditioning techniques have been the most successful form of psychotherapy, and the benzodiazepines are currently the most useful pharmacological agents (Table 15-6). The most important side effects of benzodiazepines are sedation, depression, and irritability, and some agents (e.g., lorazepam) have an adverse effect on memory function (Baldessarini, 1980; Healy et al., 1983). Decreased levels of consciousness and respiratory depression are reported with toxic doses. Physical dependence may occur with chronic administration leading to withdrawal symptoms when the drug is rapidly discontinued. The long half-life of several of the agents may lead to gradual accumulation to toxic levels, particularly in elderly patients (Greenblatt and Shader, 1974, 1978).

Propanediols (meprobamate), antihistamines (hydroxyzine, diphenhydramine), and barbiturates have been used in the treatment of anxiety but have more side ef-

TABLE 15-5.   Disorders Associated with Anxiety

Neurological Disorders	Miscellaneous conditions
	Hypoglycemia
Cerebral neoplasms	Carcinoid syndrome
Cerebral trauma and postconcussive syndromes	Systemic malignancies
Cerebrovascular disease	Premenstrual syndrome
Subarachnoid hemorrhage	Febrile illnesses and chronic infections
Migraine	Porphyria
Encephalitis	Infectious mononucleosis
Cerebral syphilis	Posthepatitis syndrome
Multiple sclerosis	Uremia
Wilson's disease	
Huntington's disease	
Epilepsy	Toxic Conditions
	Alcohol and drug withdrawal
Systemic Conditions	Amphetamines
	Sympathomimetic agents
Hypoxia	Vasopressor agents
Cardiovascular Disease	Caffeine and caffeine withdrawal
Cardiac arrhythmias	Penicillin
Pulmonary insufficiency	Sulfonamides
Anemia	Cannabis
	Mercury
Endocrine disturbances	Arsenic
Pituitary dysfunction	Phosphorus
Thyroid dysfunction	Organophosphates
Parathyroid dysfunction	Carbon disulfide
Adrenal dysfunction	Benzene
Pheochromocytoma	
Virilization disorders of females	Idiopathic Psychiatric Disorders
Inflammatory disorders	Depression
Lupus erythematosus	Mania
Rheumatoid arthritis	Schizophrenia
Polyarteritis nodosa	Anxiety disorders
Temporal arteritis	
	Generalized anxiety
Deficiency states	Panic attacks
Vitamin B_{12} deficiency	Phobic disorders
Pellagra	Posttraumatic stress disorder

Data from Hall (1980) and Jefferson and Marshall (1981).

fects than do benzodiazepines and are now rarely used in anxiety disorders (Baldessarini, 1980; Tinklenberg, 1977). Beta-adrenergic blocking agents (e.g., propranolol, atenolol) may be useful in the management of anxiety, particularly when the manifestations are primarily somatic (Csernansky and Hollister, 1983).

OBSESSIVE–COMPULSIVE DISORDER

Obsessive–compulsive disorder is characterized by involuntary recurrent ego-dystonic thoughts, images, or impulses (obsessions) and the performance of repetitive, stereotyped, involuntary acts or rituals (compulsions)

TABLE 15-6. Benzodiazepine Agents Used in Management of Anxiety

Agent	Common Proprietary Preparation (Manufacturer)	Dosage (mg) (range)	Serum Half-Life (hours)
Chlordiazepoxide	Librium (Roche)	15–60 (10–100)	5–30
Clorazepate dipotassium	Tranxene (Abbott)	30 (7.5–90)	36–200
Diazepam	Valium (Roche)	4–40 (2–40)	20–50
Lorazepam	Ativan (Wyeth)	2–6 (1–10)	10–20
Oxazepam	Serax (Wyeth)	30–60 (30–120)	3–21
Alprazolam	Xanax (Upjohn)	0.75–1 (0.75–4)	11–14

Data from Baldessarini (1980); Greenblatt and Shader (1978); and Owen (1983).

(*Diagnostic and statistical manual of mental disorders,* 1980). Obsessional thoughts include ideas of dirt, disease, and sexual activities or aggressive acts. Compulsions typically involve cleaning, checking, counting, avoiding, and repeating specific activities (Akhtar et al., 1975; Goodwin et al., 1969; Stern and Cobb, 1978). Obsessive–compulsive neurosis or disorder must be distinguished from compulsivity as a behavioral trait and from the obsessive–compulsive personality disorder where the compulsive behavior is not experienced as ego-alien and is manifest as a rigid perfectionistic behavioral style.

Table 15-7 lists the conditions associated with obsessive–compulsive disorder and with compulsive behaviors. There is a prominent association between obsessive–compulsive disorder and specific extrapyramidal syndromes. It occurs with increased frequency in postencephalitic parkinsonism, idiopathic parkinsonism, Gilles de la Tourette syndrome, and manganese-induced parkinsonism and may be increased in the Meige's syndrome. The most dramatic examples of an association between obsessive–compulsive disorder and a neurological illness occurred in cases of postencephalitic parkinsonism following the 1919–1926 epidemic of von Economo encephalitis lethargica (Fairweather, 1947; Grimshaw, 1964; Holt, 1937; Schilder, 1938; Schwab et al., 1951). Jelliffe (1929a,b) and Wexberg (1937) described patients with postencephalitic parkinsonism who had simultaneous attacks of obsessions or compulsions and oculogyric crises. During the period of forced gaze deviation, patients had intrusive thoughts of murder or rape, forced counting, paranoid feelings, or repetitive irrelevant thoughts. Forced shouting or grunting resembling Tourette syndrome also occurred in some patients (Onuaguluchi, 1961; Van Bogaert, 1934; Wohlfart et al., 1961). Among other causes of parkinsonian syndromes, obsessive–compulsive disorders have occasionally been observed in patients with idiopathic Parkinson

disease and parkinsonism associated with cerebrovascular disease and occurs frequently in patients with parkinsonism due to manganese toxicity (Mena et al., 1967; Mindham, 1970; Penalver, 1955; Schuler et al., 1957). An excess of obsessions and compulsions has also been noted among patients with Meige's syndrome, the id-

TABLE 15-7. Disorders Associated with Obsessive–Compulsive Behavior

Obsessive–compulsive disorder

  Neurological disturbances

    Postencephalitic parkinsonism
    Manganese-induced parkinsonism
    Idiopathic Parkinson's disease
    Cerebrovascular disease (with parkinsonism)
    Meige's syndrome
    Gilles de la Tourette syndrome
    Levodopa therapy in parkinsonism
    Amphetamine toxicity
    Cerebral trauma
    Cerebral neoplasms

  Psychiatric disturbances

    Obsessive–compulsive disorder
    Depression
    Schizoprenia

Differential diagnosis of obsessional or compulsive behaviors

  Neurological conditions

    Personality alterations associated with complex partial seizures
    Ictal obsessions (''forced thinking'')
    Autism
    Perseveration
    Echolalia
    Hypermetamorphosis in Klüver-Bucy syndrome

  Psychiatric disorders

    Compulsive personality

iopathic blepharospasm–oromandibular dystonia syndromes (Jankovic and Ford, 1983). Possibly related to the occurrence of obsessive–compulsive disorder among patients with extrapyramidal syndromes is its emergence as a manifestation of levodopa or amphetamine toxicity (Ellinwood, 1967; Jenike, 1983). Levodopa and amphetamine both act through monoaminergic transmitters present in subcortical structures and may produce obsessions and compulsions by mechanisms similar to those involved in the production of obsessive compulsive disorders in extrapyramidal diseases.

Obsessive–compulsive disorder is present in between 30 and 90 percent of patients with Gilles de la Tourette syndrome (Cohen et al., 1980; Eldridge et al., 1977; Eriksson and Persson, 1969; Fernando, 1967; Montgomery et al., 1982; Morphew and Sim, 1969; Nee et al., 1980, 1982; Walsh, 1962). The compulsions take the form of touching, skipping, counting, echolalia, coprolalia, echopraxia, or ritualization of daily activities. Obsessions include involuntary internalized cursing; intrusive violent and sexual images; and ego-alien concerns about death, self-harm and harm to others, dirt, feces, and contamination.

Obsessive–compulsive disorders also occur in a few patients with posttraumatic and neoplastic CNS injuries (Achte, 1955; Andy et al., 1981; Jenike, 1983; McKeon et al, 1984). In most cases the damage has been frontotemporal in location.

Idiopathic obsessive–compulsive disorder begins in late adolescence or early adulthood, exhibits a fluctuating course with exacerbations and remissions, and has a tendency to improve gradually over time (Grimshaw, 1965; Jenike, 1983; Kringlen, 1965; Pollitt, 1957). There is an increased incidence of neuropsychological abnormalities, enlarged ventricles, and abnormal birth histories in patients with obsessive–compulsive disorder, suggesting a role for an early CNS insult in its pathogenesis (Behar et al., 1984; Capstick and Seldrup, 1977; Insel et al., 1983). The occurrence of obsessions and compulsions in Gilles de la Tourette syndrome, the many similarities between the course and manifestations of obsessive–compulsive disorder and Gilles de la Tourette syndrome, and the increased incidence of obsessive–compulsive disorder among family members of Gilles de la Tourette syndrome patients suggest that obsessive–compulsive disorder and Gilles de la Tourette syndrome may share common neurobiologic mechanisms.

Patients with obsessions and compulsions show no special vulnerability to psychosis, but schizophrenia may occasionally present with obsessions and compulsions, and such phenomena are also common in late-life agitated depressions (Gittleson, 1966; Lewis, 1967; Rosen, 1957; Welner et al., 1976).

Compulsive or obsessional behaviors in the absence of obsessive–compulsive disorder occur in a number of neuropsychiatric conditions. In epilepsy, obsessions may occur as ictal "forced thinking," or they may be one manifestation of the altered personality that occurs in some patients with complex partial seizures (Chapter 9) (Brickner et al., 1940; Hill and Mitchel, 1953). Preservation occurs in many CNS disorders and is compulsive in that the patients are unable to control the purposeless repetition of the perseverated performance (Allison, 1966). Likewise, echolalia is the compulsive repetition of what is heard and occurs in transcortical aphasias, dementia syndromes, and mental retardation (Chapter 3) (Stengel, 1947). Both perseveration and echolalia are evident in autistic syndromes (Damasio and Maurer, 1978; Hauser et al., 1975; Rutter, 1974; Sorosky et al., 1968). The hypermetamorphosis—involuntary attraction to and manipulation of environmental objects—that occurs in the Klüver-Bucy syndrome also has a compulsive aspect (Lilly et al., 1983). Finally, compulsivity may be a behavioral trait in normal personalities or may be a dominant, rigid, and unyielding (but ego-syntonic) behavioral pattern in patients with compulsive personality disorders (*Diagnostic and statistical manual of mental disorders*, 1980).

Obsessive–compulsive disorder has proved to be remarkably resistant to therapy. Pharmacological agents that have been at least partially successful in relieving the symptoms include neuroleptics, antidepressants, benzodiazepines, and clonidine hydrochloride (Altschuler, 1962; Ananth, 1976; Burrell et al., 1974; de Silva and Wijewickrama, 1976; Knesevich, 1982; O'Regan, 1970; Tesar and Jenike, 1984; Trethowan and Scott, 1955). Nonpharmacological treatment strategies have included electroconvulsive therapy (ECT) and behavior modification techniques (Mellman and Gorman, 1984; Steketee et al., 1982), and severe cases frequently improve following medial limbic leukotomy (Bridges et al., 1973; Mitchell-Heggs et al., 1976; Tan et al., 1971).

REFERENCES

Achte KA. On compulsive neuroses of brain-injured. *Acta Psychiat Neurol Scand*, 1955, Suppl. 137, 88–89.

Akhtar S, Wig NN, Varma KK, Pershad D and Verma SK. A phenomenological analysis of symptoms in obsessive–compulsive neurosis. *Br J Psychiat*, 1975, *127*, 342–348.

Allison RS. Perseveration as a sign of diffuse and focal brain damage. *Br Med J*, 1966, *2*, 1027–1032, 1095–1101.

Altschuler M. Massive doses of trifluoperazine in the treatment of compulsive rituals. *Am J Psychiat*, 1962, *119*, 367–368.

Ananth J. Treatment of obsessive–compulsive neurosis: pharmacological approach. *Psychosomatics*, 1976, *17*, 180–184.

Andrulonis DA, Glueck BC, Stroebel CF, Vogel NG, Shapiro AL, and Aldridge DMA. Organic brain dysfunction and the borderline syndrome. *Psychiat Clin N Am*, 1980, *4*, 47–66.

Andy OJ, Webster JS, and Carranza J. Frontal lobe lesions and behavior. *South Med J*, 1981, *74*, 968–972.

Arseni C, Boetz MI, Alexandru S, and Simionescu MD. Bilateral defect of frontal and orbital lobes. *Internat J Neurol*, 1966, *5*, 430–441.

Arthurs RGS and Cahoon EB. A clinical and electroencephalographic survey of psychopathic personality. *Am J Psychiat*, 1964, *120*, 875–877.

Bach-y-Rita G and Veno A. Habitual violence: a profile of 62 men. *Am J Psychiat*, 1974, *131*, 1015–1017.

Baldessarini RJ. Drugs and the treatment of psychiatric disorders. In Gilman RG, Goodman LS, and Gilman A (Eds.): *Goodman and Gilman's pharmacological basis of therapeutics*, 6th ed. New York, Macmillan Publishing Company, 1980, pp. 391–447.

Bear DM and Fedio P. Quantitative analysis of interictal behavior in temporal lobe epilepsy. *Arch Neurol*, 1977, *34*, 454–467.

Bear DM, Levin K, Blumer D, Chetham D, and Ryder J. Interictal behavior in hospitalized temporal lobe epileptics: relationship to idiopathic psychiatric syndromes. *J Neurol Neurosurg Psychiat*, 1982, *45*, 481–488.

Behar D, Rapaport JL, Berg CJ, Denckla MB, Mann L, Cox C, Fedio P, Zahn T, and Wolfman MG. Computerized tomography and neuropsychological test measures in adolescents with obsessive–compulsive disorder. *Am J Psychiat*, 1984, *141*, 363–369.

Benson DF. Psychiatric aspects of aphasia. *Br J Psychiat*, 1973, *123*, 555–566.

Blumer D and Benson DF. Personality changes with frontal and temporal lobe lesions. In Benson DF and Blumer D (Eds.): *Psychiatric aspects of neurologic disease*. New York, Grune & Stratton, 1975, pp. 151–169.

Brickner RM, Rosner AA, and Munro R. Physiological aspects of the obsessive state. *Psychosom Med*, 1940, *2*, 369–383.

Bridges PK, Goktepe EV, Maratos J, Brown A, and Young L. A comparative review of patients with obsessional neurosis and with depression treated by neurosurgery. *Br J Psychiat*, 1973, *123*, 663–674.

Brooks DN and McKinlay W. Personality and behavioral change after severe blunt head injury—a relative's view. *J Neurol Neurosurg Psychiat*, 1983, *46*, 336–344.

Brown JJ, Murlow CD, and Stoudemire GA. The anxiety disorders. *Ann Int Med*, 1984, *100*, 558–564.

Burrell RH, Culpan RH, Newton KJ, Ogg GJ, and Short JHW. Use of bromazepam in obsessional, phobic, and related states. *Curr Med Res Opin*, 1974, *2*, 430–436.

Capstick N and Seldrup J. Obsessional states. A study in the relationship between abnormalities at the time of birth and the subsequent development of obsessional symptoms. *Acta Psychiat Scand*, 1977, *56*, 427–431.

Carter AB. The prognosis of certain hysterical symptoms. *Br Med J*, 1949, *1*, 1076–1079.

Chodoff P. The diagnosis of hysteria: an overview. *Am J Psychiat*, 1974, *131*, 1073–1078.

Chodoff P and Lyons H. Hysteria, the hysterical personality, and "hysterical" conversion. *Am J Psychiat*, 1958, *114*, 734–740.

Cohen DJ, Detlor J, Young JG, and Shaywitz BA. Clonidine ameliorates Gilles de la Tourette syndrome. *Arch Gen Psychiat*, 1980, *37*, 1350–1357.

Cohen SI and Ross RN. *Handbook of clinical psychobiology and pathology*, Vol 2. New York, Hemisphere Publishing Company, 1983.

Crowe RR, Noyes R, Pauls DL, and Slymen D. A family study of panic disorder. *Arch Gen Psychiat*, 1983, *40*, 1065–1069.

Csernansky J and Hollister L. Beta blockers and benzodiazepines in the treatment of anxiety. *Hosp Form*, 1983, *18*, 67–72.

Damasio AR and Maurer RG. A neurological model for childhood autism. *Arch Neurol*, 1978, *35*, 777–786.

de Silva FRP and Wijewickrama HS deS. Clomipramine in phobic and obsessional states: preliminary report. *New Zeal Med J*, 1976, *84*, 4–6.

Diagnostic and statistical manual of mental disorders, 3rd ed. Washington, D.C., American Psychiatric Association, 1980.

Eldridge R, Sweet R, Lake CR, Ziegler M, and Shapiro AK. Gilles de la Tourette syndrome: clinical, genetic, psychologic, and biochemical aspects of 21 selected families. *Neurology*, 1977, *27*, 115–124.

Ellinwood EH. Amphetamine psychoses: I. Description of the individuals and the process. *J Nerv Ment Dis*, 1967, *144*, 273–283.

Eriksson B and Persson T. Gilles de la Tourette's syndrome. Two cases with organic brain injury. *Br J Psychiat*, 1969, *115*, 351–353.

Ey H. History and analysis of the concept. In Roy A (Ed.): *Hysteria*. New York, John Wiley & Sons, 1982, pp. 3–19.

Fairweather DS. Psychiatric aspects of the post-encephalitic syndrome. *J Ment Sci*, 1947, *93*, 201–254.

Farley J, Woodruff RA Jr, and Guze SB. The prevalence of hysteria and conversion symptoms. *Br J Psychiat*, 1968, *114*, 1121–1125.

Faust CI. Different psychological consequences due to superior frontal and orbito-basal lesions. *Internat J Neurol*, 1966, *5*, 410–421.

Fernando SJM. Gilles de la Tourette syndrome. *Br J Psychiat*, 1967, *113*, 607–617.

Folks DG, Ford CV, and Regan WM. Conversion symptoms in a general hospital. *Psychosomatics*, 1984, *25*, 285–295.

Gainotti G. Emotional behavior and hemispheric side of the lesion. *Cortex*, 1977, *8*, 41–55.

Gaspirini WG, Satz P, Heilman KM, and Coolidge FL. Hemispheric asymmetries of affective processing as determined by the Minnesota Multiphasic Personality Inventory. *J Neurol Neurosurg Psychiat*, 1978, *41*, 470–473.

Gibbens TCN, Pond DA, and Stafford-Clark D. A follow-up study of criminal psychopaths. *J Ment Sci*, 1959, *105*, 108–115.

Gittleson NL. The phenomenology of obsessions in depressive psychosis. *Br J Psychiat*, 1966, *112*, 261–264.

Goodwin DW, Guze SB, and Robins E. Follow-up studies in obsessional neurosis. *Arch Gen Psychiat*, 1969, *20*, 182–187.

Gray JB. *The neuropsychology of anxiety*. New York, Oxford University Press, 1982.

Greenblatt DJ and Shader RI. Benzodiazepines. *New Engl J Med*, 1974, *291*, 1011–1015, 1239–1243.

Greenblatt DJ and Shader RI. Pharmacokinetic understanding of antianxiety drug therapy. *South Med J*, 1978, *71* (Suppl. 1), 2–9.

Grimshaw L. Obsessional disorder and neurological illness. *J Neurol Neurosurg Psychiat*, 1964, *27*, 229–231.

Grimshaw L. The outcome of obsessional disorder. A follow-up study of 100 cases. *Br J Psychiat*, 1965, *111*, 1051–1056.

Guze SB. The validity and significance of the clinical diagnosis of hysteria (Briquet's syndrome). *Am J Psychiat*, 1975, *132*, 138–141.

Guze SB, Woodruff RA, and Clayton PJ. A study of conversion symptoms in psychiatric out-patients. *Am J Psychiat*, 1971, *128*, 643–646.

Hall RC. Anxiety. In Hall RC (Ed.): *Psychiatric presentations of medical illness*. New York, SP Medical and Scientific Books, 1980, pp. 13–35.

Harper MA, Morris M, and Bleyerveld J. The significance of an abnormal EEG in psychopathic personalities. *Aust New Zeal J Psychiat*, 1972, *6*, 215–224.

Harris EL, Noyes R Jr, Crowe RR, and Chaudhry DR. Family study of agoraphobia. *Arch Gen Psychiat*, 1983, *40*, 1061–1064.

Hauser SL, DeLong GR, and Rosman NP. Pneumographic findings in the infantile autism syndrome. *Brain*, 1975, *98*, 667–688.

Healey M, Pickens R, Meisch R, and McKenna T. Effects of clorazepate, diazepam, lorazepam, and placebo on human memory. *J Clin Psychiat*, 1983, *44*, 436–439.

Hermann BP and Riel P. Interictal personality and behavioral traits in temporal lobe and generalized epilepsy. *Cortex*, 1981, *17*, 125–128.

Hill D. EEG in episodic psychotic and psychopathic behavior. *Electroenceph Clin Neurophysiol*, 1952, *4*, 419–442.

Hill D and Mitchell W. Epileptic anamesis. *Folia Psychiat*, 1953, *56*, 718–725.

Hoehn-Saric R. Neurotransmitters in anxiety. *Arch Gen Psychiat*, 1982, *39*, 735–742.

Hogenson DI. Reading failure and juvenile delinquency. *Bull Orton Soc*, 1974, *24*, 164–169.

Holt WL Jr. Epidemic encephalitis. *Arch Neurol Psychiat*, 1937, *38*, 1135–1144.

Hunter R, Blackwood W, and Bull J. Three cases of frontal meningiomas presenting psychiatrically. *Br Med J*, 1968, *3*, 9–16.

Insel TR, Donnelly EF, Lalakea ML, Alterman IS, and Murphy DL. Neurological and neuropsychological studies of patients with obsessive–compulsive disorder. *Biol Psychiat*, 1983, *18*, 741–751.

Jankovic J and Ford J. Blepharospasm and orofacial-cervical dystonia: clinical and pharmacological findings in 100 patients. *Ann Neurol*, 1983, *13*, 402–411.

Jefferson JW and Marshall JR. *Neuropsychiatric features of medical disorders*. New York, Plenum Medical Book Company, 1981.

Jelliffe SE. Oculogyric crises as compulsion phenomena in postencephalitis: their occurrence, phenomenology and meaning. *J Nerv Ment Dis*, 1929a, *69*, 59–68, 165–184, 278–297, 415–426, 531–551, 666–679.

Jelliffe SE. Psychologic components in postencephalitic oculogyric crises. *Arch Neurol Psychiat*, 1929b, *21*, 491–532.

Jenike MA. Obsessive compulsive disorder. *Comp Psychiat*, 1983, *24*, 99–115.

Kandel ER. From metapsychology to molecular biology: explorations into the nature of anxiety. *Am J Psychiat*, 1983, *140*, 1277–1293.

Knesevich JW. Successful treatment of obsessive–compulsive disorder with clonidine hydrochloride. *Am J Psychiat*, 1982, *139*, 364–365.

Knott JR. Electroencephalograms in psychopathic personality and in murderers. In Wilson WP (Ed.): *Applications of electroencephalography in psychiatry*. Durham, North Carolina, Duke University Press, 1965, pp. 19–29.

Kringlen E. Obsessional neurotics. A long-term follow-up. *Br J Psychiat*, 1965, *111*, 709–722.

Krynicki VE. Cerebral dysfunction in repetitively assaultive adolescents. *J Nerv Ment Dis*, 1978, *166*, 59–67.

Leckman JF, Weissman MM, Merikangas KR, Pauls DL, and Prusoff BA. Panic disorder and major depression. *Arch Gen Psychiat*, 1983, *40*, 1055–1060.

Leftoff S. Psychopathology in the light of brain injury: a case study. *J Clin Neuropsychol*, 1983, *5*, 51–63.

Levy S and Kennard M. A study of the electroencephalogram as related to personality structure in a group of inmates of a state penitentiary. *Am J Psychiat*, 1953, *109*, 832–839.

Lewis A. *Inquiries in psychiatry*. New York, Science House, 1967.

Lewis DO. Delinquency, psychomotor epileptic symptoms, and paranoid ideation: a triad. *Am J Psychiat*, 1976, *133*, 1395–1398.

Lewis DO, Shanock SS, Pincus JH, and Glazer GH. Violent juvenile delinquents. *J Am Acad Child Psychiat*, 1979, *18*, 307–319.

Lilly R, Cummings JL, Benson DF, and Frankel M. The human Klüver-Bucy syndrome. *Neurology*, 1983, *33*, 1141–1145.

Lishman WA. Brain Damage in relation to psychiatric disability after head injury. *Br J Psychiat*, 1968, *114*, 373–410.

Lishman WA. The psychiatric sequelae of head injury: a review. *Psychol Med*, 1973, *3*, 304–318.

Mackenzie TB and Popkin MK. Organic anxiety syndrome. *Am J Psychiat*, 1983, *140*, 342–344.

Malcomson KG. Globus hystericus vel pharyngis. *J Laryngol Otol*, 1968, *82*, 219–230.

McHugh PR and Folstein MF. Psychiatric syndromes of Huntington's chorea: a clinical and phenomenologic study. In Benson DF and Blumer D (Eds.): *Psychiatric aspects of neurologic disease*. New York, Grune & Stratton, 1975, pp. 267–285.

McKeon J, McGuffin P, and Robinson P. Obsessive–compulsive neurosis following head-injury. A report of four cases. *Br J Psychiat*, 1984, *144*, 190–192.

Mellman LA and Gorman JM. Successful treatment of obsessive–compulsive disorder with ECT. *Am J Psychiat*, 1984, *141*, 596–597.

Mena I, Marin O, Fuenzalida S, and Cotzias GC. Chronic manganese poisoning. *Neurology*, 1967, *17*, 128–136.

Mendelson W, Johnson N, and Stewart MA. Hyperactive children as teenagers: a follow-up study. *J Nerv Ment Dis*, 1971, *153*, 273–279.

Merskey H. *The analysis of hysteria*. London, Bailliere Tindall, 1979.

Merskey H and Buhrich NA. Hysteria and organic brain disease. *Br J Psychiat*, 1975, *48*, 359–366.

Merskey H and Trimble M. Personality, sexual adjustment, and brain lesions in patients with conversion symptoms. *Am J Psychiat*, 1979, *136*, 179–182.

Millon T. *Disorders of personality. DSM III: Axis II*. New York, John Wiley & Sons, 1981.

Mindham RHS. Psychiatric symptoms in parkinsonism. *J Neurol Neurosurg Psychiat*, 1970, *33*, 188–191.

Mitchell-Heggs N, Kelly D, and Richardson A. Stereotactic limbic leucotomy: a follow-up at 16 months. *Br J Psychiat*, 1976, *128*, 226–240.

Montgomery MA, Clayton PJ, and Friedhoff AJ. Psychiatric illness in Tourette syndrome patients and first degree relatives. In Friedhoff AJ and Chase TN (Eds.): *Gilles de la Tourette syndrome*. New York, Raven Press, 1982, pp. 335–339.

Morphew JA and Sim M. Gilles de la Tourette syndrome: a clinical and psychopathological study. *Br J Med Psychol*, 1969, *42*, 293–301.

Morrison JR and Minkoff K. Explosive personality as a sequel to the hyperactive child syndrome. *Comp Psychiat*, 1975, *16*, 343–348.

Mungas D. Interictal behavior abnormality in temporal lobe epilepsy. *Arch Gen Psychiat*, 1982, *39*, 108–111.

Murphy GE. The clinical management of hysteria. *JAMA*, 1982, *247*, 2559–2564.

Nee LE, Caine ED, Polinsky RJ, Eldridge R, and Ebert MH. Gilles de la Tourette syndrome: clinical and family study of 50 cases. *Ann Neurol*, 1980, *7*, 41–49.

Nee LE, Polinsky RJ and Ebert MH. Tourette syndrome: clinical and family studies. In Friedhoff AJ and Chase TN (Eds.): *Gilles de la Tourette syndrome*. New York, Raven Press, 1982, pp. 291–295.

Onuaguluchi G. Crises in post-encephalitic parkinsonism. *Brain*, 1961, *84*, 395–414.

O'Regan JB. Treatment of obsessive–compulsive neurosis with haloperidol. *Can Med Assoc J*, 1970, *103*, 167–168.

Owen JA. Alprazolam: a new benzodiazepine approved for anxiety disorders. *Hosp Form*, 1983, *18*, 950–954.

Parkin AJ. Amnesic syndrome: a lesion-specific disorder? *Cortex*, 1984, *20*, 475–508.

Penalver R. Manganese Poisoning. *Indust Med Surg*, 1955, *24*, 1–7.

Perley MJ and Guze SB. Hysteria—the stability and usefulness of clinical criteria. *New Engl J Med*, 1962, *266*, 421–426.

Pitts FN Jr. The biochemistry of anxiety. *Sci Am*, 1969, *220*(2), 69–74.

Pollitt J. Natural history of obsessional states. *Br Med J*, 1957, *1*, 194–198.

Pond DA and Bidwell BH. A survey of epilepsy in fourteen general practices. II. Social and psychological aspects. *Epilepsia*, 1959–1960, *1*, 285–299.

Pontius AA and Yudowitz BS. Frontal lobe system dysfunction in some criminal actions as shown in the narratives test. *J Nerv Ment Dis*, 1980, *168*, 111–117.

Roberts JKA, Robertson MM, and Trimble MR. The lateralizing significance of hypergraphia in temporal lobe epilepsy. *J Neurol Neurosurg Psychiat*, 1982, *45*, 131–138.

Rosen I. The clinical significance of obsessions in schizophrenia. *J Ment Sci*, 1957, *103*, 773–786.

Rutter M. The development of infantile autism. *Psychol Med*, 1974, *4*, 147–163.

Schilder P. The organic background of obsessions and compulsions. *Am J Psychiat*, 1938, *94*, 1397–1416.

Schuler P, Oyanguren H, Maturana V, Valenzuela A, Cruz E, Plaza V, Schmidt E, and Haddad R. Manganese poisoning. *Indust Med Surg*, 1957, *26*, 167–173.

Schwab RS, Fabing HD, and Prichard JS. Psychiatric symptoms and syndromes in Parkinson's disease. *Am J Psychiat*, 1951, *107*, 901–907.

Slater E. Diagnosis of "hysteria." *Br Med J*, 1965, *1*, 1395–1399.

Small GW and Nicholi AM Jr. Mass hysteria among school children. *Arch Gen Psychiat*, 1982, *39*, 721–724.

Small JG. The organic dimension of crime. *Arch Gen Psychiat*, 1966, *15*, 82–89.

Sorosky AD, Ornitz EM, Brown MB, and Ritvo ER. Systematic observations of autistic behavior. *Arch Gen Psychiat*, 1968, *18*, 439–449.

Stefansson JG, Messina JA, and Meyerowitz S. Hysterical neurosis, conversion type: clinical and epidemiological considerations. *Acta Psychiat Scand*, 1976, *53*, 119–138.

Steketee G, Foa EB, and Grayson JB. Recent advances in the behavioral treatment of obsessive–compulsives. *Arch Gen Psychiat*, 1982, *39*, 1365–1371.

Stengel E. Clinical and psychological study of echo-reactions. *J Ment Sci*, 1947, *93*, 598–612.

Stern RS and Cobb JP. Phenomenology of obsessive–compulsive neurosis. *Br J Psychiat*, 1978, *132*, 233–239.

Tan E, Marks IM, and Marset P. Bimedial leukotomy in obsessive–compulsive neurosis. *Br J Psychiat*, 1971, *118*, 155–164.

Tesar GE and Jenike MA. Alprazolam as treatment for a case of obsessive–compulsive disorder. *Am J Psychiat,* 1984, *141,* 689–690.

Tinklenberg JR. Antianxiety medications and the treatment of anxiety. In Barchas JD, Berger PA, Ciaranello RD, and Elliot GR (Eds.): *Psychopharmacology.* New York, Oxford University Press, 1977, pp. 226–242.

Torgersen S. Genetic factors in anxiety disorders. *Arch Gen Psychiat,* 1983, *40,* 1085–1089.

Trethowan WH and Scott PAL. Chlorpromazine in obsessive-compulsive and allied disorders. *Lancet,* 1955, *1,* 781–785.

Trimble MR. Personality disturbances in epilepsy. *Neurology,* 1983, *33,* 1332–1334.

Van Bogaert L. Ocular paroxysms and palilalia. *J Nerv Ment Dis,* 1934, *80,* 48–61.

Virkkunen M and Nuutila A. Specific reading retardation, hyperactive child syndrome, and juvenile delinquency. *Acta Psychiat Scand,* 1976, *54,* 25–28.

Walsh PJF. Compulsive shouting and Gilles de la Tourette syndrome. *Br J Clin Practs,* 1962, *16,* 651–655.

Waxman SG and Geschwind N. Hypergraphia in temporal lobe epilepsy. *Neurology,* 1974, *24,* 629–636.

Weintraub MI. *Hysterical conversion reactions.* New York, SP Medical and Scientific Books, 1983.

Weintraub S and Mesulam M-M. Developmental learning disabilities of the right hemisphere. *Arch Neurol,* 1983, *40,* 463–468.

Welner A, Reich T, Robins E, Fishman R, and Van Doran T. Obsessive–compulsive neurosis: record follow-up, and family studies. I. Inpatient record study. *Comp Psychiat,* 1976, *17,* 527–539.

Wexberg E. Remarks on the psychopathology of oculogyric crises in epidemic encephalitis. *J Nerv Ment Dis,* 1937, *85,* 56–69.

Whitlock FA. The etiology of hysteria. *Acta Psychiat Neurol Scand,* 1967, *43,* 144–162.

Williams D. Neural factors related to habitual aggression. *Brain,* 1969, *92,* 503–520.

Wohlfart G, Ingvar DH, and Hellberg A-M. Compulsory shouting (Benedek's "Klazomania") associated with oculogyric spasms in chronic epidemic encephalitis. *Acta Psychiat Neurol Scand,* 1961, *36,* 369–377.

Yeudall LT, Fromm-Auch D, and Davies P. Neuropsychological impairment of persistent delinquency. *J Nerv Ment Dis,* 1982, *170,* 257–265.

Ziegler FJ, Imboden JB, and Meyer E. Contemporary conversion reactions: a clinical study. *Am J Psychiat,* 1960, *116,* 901–910.

Chapter 16

Hallucinations

Hallucinations are sensory experiences that occur without external stimulation of the relevant sensory organ (*Diagnostic and statistical manual of mental disorders,* 1980). They may occur in any sensory modality—visual, auditory, tactile, olfactory, or gustatory. The hallucinations may be appreciated as such or may be misinterpreted as real sensory perceptions in the case of psychosis. Hallucinations occur in the course of a large number of pathological processes and may occasionally occur in normal individuals in the absence of any disease. The neuropsychiatric differential diagnosis and pathophysiology of hallucinations in each sensory modality are presented in this chapter.

VISUAL HALLUCINATIONS

A visual hallucination has been defined operationally as a symptom in which the patient claims to see something or behaves as though having seen something that the observer cannot see (Lessell, 1975.) Some classifications distinguish between hallucinations and pseudohallucinations according to whether the image is considered real (true hallucinations) or is recognized to be a false sensory experience (pseudohallucinations) (Hare, 1973; Sedman, 1966a). In this discussion, all images are considered hallucinations, and patients who endorse them as real are discussed as suffering from psychosis in addition to hallucinations. Visual hallucinations occur in a wide variety of ophthalmologic, neurological, toxic–metabolic, and idiopathic psychiatric disorders.

Differential Diagnosis

Table 16-1 presents a systematic approach to the differential diagnosis of visual hallucinations. Ophthalmologic disorders that reduce or eliminate the patient's vision frequently produce hallucinations. They have been described by patients suffering acute blindness from traumatic enucleation and in patients with poor vision secondary to cataract formation or diseases of the macula,

choroid, or retina (Bartlet, 1951; Berrios and Brook, 1984; Cohn, 1971; Levine, 1980; Opie, 1968; White, 1980). Hallucinations commonly occur following ocular surgery, particularly if both eyes are patched in the post-operative period. Such post-surgical hallucinations are more likely to occur if a toxic psychosis is also present (Linn et al., 1953; Ziskind et al., 1960). The hallucinations associated with reduced vision are usually fully formed, brightly colored images of people, animals, flowers, or scenery. Brief, unformed flashes of light may also occur with ocular pathology and are noted with vitreous detachment (Moore's lightning streaks), with sudden ocular motion in individuals with no ocular pathology (flick phosphenes), or may be induced by sound in patients with a variety of ocular disorders (auditory-visual synesthesia) (Jacobs et al., 1981; Lessell and Cohen, 1979; Nebel, 1957). Hallucinations must be distinguished from entoptic phenomena such as particles floating in the vitreous humor, Haidingers brushes (nerve bundles made visible by macular edema) and Scheerer's phenomenon (red blood cells circulating in the paramacular region) (Priestly and Foree, 1955).

The Charles Bonnet syndrome, although formerly considered a condition with spontaneous visual hallucinations in the elderly, now appears to be associated with ocular pathology in most cases, and the onset of hallucinations in aged individuals should lead to a search for eye disease (Berrios and Brook, 1982; Damas-Mora et al., 1982).

Optic nerve disease, particularly optic neuritis, is also associated with brief unformed visual hallucinations. The phosphenes occur with movement of the eyes or may be induced by sounds (Davis et al., 1976; Jacobs et al., 1981; Lessell and Cohen, 1979).

Focal lesions in a number of locations in the brain are associated with visual hallucinations. Lesions in the midbrain region produce the syndrome of peduncular hallucinosis. In this condition there are complex visual hallucinations that typically occur in the evenings; are associated with disturbances of the sleep–wake cycle; and are usually viewed as benign, entertaining phenom-

TABLE 16-1. Differential Diagnosis of Visual
Hallucinations

Ophthalmologic disorders

Enucleation
Cataract formation
Macular, choroidal, retinal disease
Vitreous traction

Central nervous system disorders

Optic nerve disease
Brainstem lesions (peduncular hallucinosis)
Hemisphere lesions
Epilepsy
Migraine
Narcolepsy

Medical illnesses

Acute confusional states

Toxic disturbances

Acute confusional states
Alcohol and drug withdrawal
Hallucinogenic agents

Idiopathic psychiatric disorders

Schizophrenia
Depression
Mania
Conversion reaction

"Normal" individuals

Dreams
Hypnagogic hallucinations
Hypnosis
Childhood (imaginary companions)
Sensory deprivation
Sleep deprivation
Intense emotional experience

ena. Other evidence of brainstem dysfunction is usually present (Dunn et al., 1983; Garrel et al., 1967;
Rozanski, 1952; Smith et al., 1971). Auditory–visual
synesthesia has also occasionally been described by patients with lesions involving the upper brainstem (Vike
et al., 1984).

Hemispheric lesions can produce visual hallucinations in two clinical circumstances: as part of focal seizure activity or as release phenomena associated with
visual field defects (Cogan, 1973). Release hallucinations are generally formed images, lasting from minutes to hours. They are variable in content, may be
modified by altering the visual input such as opening
or closing the eyes, and tend to occur within the field
defect (Brust and Behrens, 1977; Critchley, 1939;
Hoppe, 1921; Horrax, 1923; Lance, 1976; Lance et al.,

1974; Pick, 1904; Weinberger and Grant, 1940). The
underlying pathological lesion is usually an infarction
or neoplasm, but any focal lesion within the visual pathways in the temporal, parietal, or occipital lobes may
produce release hallucinations. Hallucinations have occasionally been reported with frontal lobe lesions, but
this is rare and when described they have usually been
associated with mass lesions capable of exerting distant effects on the temporal lobes or brainstem (Schneider et al., 1961). Release hallucinations are more
frequently associated with right- than left-sided lesions
(Lessell, 1975).

Ictal hallucinations occurring as expressions of seizure activity can usually be distinguished from release
hallucinations on the basis of their clinical features (Table 16-2) (Cogan, 1973). Ictal hallucinations are brief,
stereotyped visual experiences (Bender and Kanzer,
1941; Fischer-Williams et al., 1964; Guinena and Taher,
1955; Jackson and Beevor, 1889; Kennedy, 1911; King
and Marsan, 1977; Mooney et al., 1965; Russell and
Whitty, 1955). There may or may not be an associated
visual field defect; they rarely are lateralized to one portion of the visual field; and when they are formed, they
often consist of visual recollections of past experiences
(Gloor et al., 1982; Mundy-Castle, 1951; Robinson and
Watt, 1947). Epileptic lesions in primary and associative cortex give rise to unformed hallucinations (flashes,
lights, colors, etc.), whereas more anterior foci situated
in the temporal lobe produce formed hallucinations and
remembered scenes (Cogan, 1973; Cushing, 1922; Parkinson et al., 1952; Sanford and Bair, 1939.) Consciousness may be altered during or after an ictal hallucination,
and there may be ictal motor phenomena such as head
or eye deviation. A variety of visual distortions, including macropsia, micropsia, and metamorphopsia,
also occur as ictal visual phenomena, either without
hallucinations or concomitantly with them (Willanger
and Klee, 1966). Like release hallucinations, ictal hallucinations are more often associated with right- than
left-sided lesions (Hécaen and Albert, 1978). These observations regarding ictal hallucinations have largely
been reproduced and confirmed by stimulation of the
occipitotemporal cortex during surgical procedures (Brindley and Lewin, 1968; Foerster, 1931; Horowitz et al.,
1968; Penfield and Perot, 1963; Weingarten et al., 1977).

Two syndromes causing visual hallucinations and
unassociated with focal CNS lesions are migraine and
narcolepsy. Visual hallucinations occur in about half of
all patients with migraine (Selby and Lance, 1960). The
most common hallucination is a fortification-type zig-
zag spectrum often associated with a scotoma, but fully
formed complex hallucinations may also occur (Gowers,
1895; Hachinski et al., 1973; Haas, 1982; Peatfield and
Rose, 1981). The migrainous aura may also include

TABLE 16-2. Distinction Between Ictal and Release Hallucinations Associated with Hemispheric Lesions

Ictal Hallucinations	Release Hallucinations
Brief (seconds to minutes)	Longer duration (minutes to hours)
Stereotyped	Variable content
Unformed with posterior lesions; formed with temporal lesions	Usually formed regardless of lesion location
Visual field defect not necessarily present	Visual field defect usually present
Seldom lateralized	Typically lateralized to side of visual field defect
Hallucination content (if formed) often a visual memory	Content usually novel
Unaltered by environmental activities	May be modified by environmental alterations (e.g., opening or closing the eyes)
Consciousness altered during or after ictal event	No associated alteration of consciousness

macropsia and micropsia, a clinical complex call the "Alice in Wonderland syndrome" after Lewis Carroll, whose personal experiences with migraine were utilized in that famous tale (Klee and Willanger, 1966; Todd, 1955.)

Narcolepsy, in its fully expressed form, consists of a tetrad of sleep attacks, cataplexy, sleep paralysis, and hallucinations (Chapter 17) (Dement et al., 1966; Sours, 1963; Zarcone, 1973). The hallucinations occur in 20–50 percent of narcoleptics and are noted most often in the drowsy period as the patient is falling asleep (hypnagogic hallucinations). Hypnopompic hallucinations occurring just as the patient is awakening occur in a smaller number of cases. Hypnagogic visions occur most commonly in association with nocturnal sleep and rarely occur with daytime narcoleptic attacks. The hallucinations are primarily visual, but auditory and somesthetic hallucinations have been reported as well as macropsia and micropsia (Roth, 1980). The hallucinations are accompanied by EEG changes characteristic of rapid-eye-movement (REM) or dreaming sleep and represent the intrusion of dreams into the drowsy state (Dement et al., 1966; Hishikawa and Kaneko, 1965; Zarcone, 1973). Hypnagogic hallucinations unaccompanied by other evidence of narcolepsy can occur in normal individuals and have been described in a variety of psychiatric disorders, including schizophrenia, depression, paranoid state, and puerperal psychosis (McDonald, 1971).

Hallucinations frequently occur in the course of acute confusional states induced my medical illnesses (Chapter 7). They have been noted in 40–75 percent of delirious patients. In delirium, the hallucinations are relatively brief, are often nocturnal, and may be regarded as real (Lipowski, 1980). The patients are often fearful and respond to the hallucinations with self-protective measures. The visions are typically formed, moving,

silent images but in some cases may be accompanied by auditory or tactile hallucinations.

Among toxin-related disturbances, hallucinations occur in three major circumstances: nonspecific acute confusional states, alcohol and sedative withdrawal, and hallucinogen-induced conditions (Table 16-3). Any drug when taken in excess may produce an acute confusional state with concomitant hallucinations. In some cases hallucinations may occur as the primary manifestation of toxicity with little evidence of delirium or confusion. Among agents that have been reported to produce hallucinations and may be particularly prone to cause this symptom are cimetidine, antidepressants, digoxin, sympathomimetics, quinidine, anticholinergics, antibiotics, hormonal agents, bromocriptine, levodopa, amantadine hydrochloride, narcotics, antimalarials, phenacetin, disulfiram, propranolol, heavy metals, metrizamide, and bromide (Adler et al., 1980; Albala et al., 1983; Brawley and Duffield, 1972; Closson, 1983; Escobar and Karno, 1982; Fisher, 1981, Goetz et al., 1982; Jarvik, 1970; Kane and Keeler, 1964; Klein, 1964; Levin, 1960; Parkes et al., 1976; Postma and van Tilburg, 1975; Sholomskas, 1980; Shopsin et al., 1975).

Hallucinations are also common during withdrawal states, occurring in up to 75 percent of those manifesting an acute abstinence syndrome (Lipowski, 1980). Withdrawal syndromes develop following abrupt cessation of intake of a variety of agents, including alcohol, barbiturates, benzodiazepines, chloral hydrate, paraldehyde, meprobamate, methaqualone, opioid compounds, and cocaine (Berger and Tinklenberg, 1977; Deiker and Chambers, 1978; Heiman, 1942; Lipowski, 1980). The type of hallucination is very similar to that described earlier for medical illnesses. Zoopsia, or hallucinations of animals, is particularly common in— although not limited to—withdrawal syndromes (Critchley, 1939). Alcohol and sedative–hypnotics produce chronic

TABLE 16-3. Pharmacologic Agents Associated with Visual Hallucinations

Hallucinogens	Hormonal agents	
Indole hallucinogens	Steroids	
LSD	Thyroxin	
Dimethyltryptamine	Antibiotics	
Psilocybin		
Psilocin	Sulfonamides	
Harmine	Penicillin	
Mescaline	Tetracycline	
Amphetamines	Bromide	
Cocaine	Digoxin	
Cannabinols	Sympathomimetics	
	Cimetidine	
Tetrahydrocannabinol	Propranolol	
Other hallucinogens	Phenacetin	
	Disulfiram	
Phencyclidine (PCP)	Narcotics	
Ketamine	Antimalarials	
Nitrous oxide	Heavy metals	
Miscellaneous agents that may cause hallucinations	Metrizamide	
Antidepressants	Drugs associated with withdrawal syndromes	
Imipramine	Ethyl alcohol	
Maprotiline	Barbiturates	
Antiparkinsonian agents	Benzodiazepines	
	Chloral hydrate	
Anticholinergic drugs	Paraldehyde	
Amantadine hydrochloride	Meprobamate	
Levodopa	Methaqualone	
Bromocriptine	Opiates and Cocaine	

suppression of REM sleep, and withdrawal is associated with REM rebound. At the time that visual hallucinations emerge during alcohol withdrawal, REM sleep accounts for a majority of sleep time and begins almost immediately when the patient falls asleep. This suggests that visual hallucinations associated with alcohol withdrawal, like those occurring in narcolepsy, are a product of dream phenomena intruding into the waking state (Greenberg and Pearlman, 1967; Gròss et al., 1966).

Hallucinogens (psychotomimetics, utopiates) are pharmacological agents that produce perceptual distortions and hallucinations. The latter are usually associated with concomitant alterations in affect and cognition resembling those occurring in the psychoses, as well as with physiological alterations such as mydriasis, elevated heart rate and blood pressure, increased muscle tone, tachypnea, and nausea (Brawley and Duffield, 1972). In general, hallucinogens do not produce an acute confusional state, and hallucinations are disproportionately prominent compared to other drug-induced changes. Several classes of agent are included among the hallucinogens including compounds with an indole structure such as lysergic acid diethylamide (LSD), dimethyltryptamine, psilocybin pscilocin, har-

mine, mescaline, amphetamines, and cocaine; cannabinols such as tetrahydrocannabinol; and a variety of other agents such as phencyclidine, ketamine, and nitrous oxide (Table 16-3) (Brawley and Duffield, 1972; Grinspoon and Bakalar, 1979; Jarvik, 1970; Watson, 1977). Self-reports and studies of subjects who have ingested LSD and mescaline reveal that in the preliminary stages one sees nonpatterned or geometric shapes; this progresses to more structured geometric images such as lattices, chessboards, cobwebs, funnels, and spirals; finally, fully formed images of landscapes, people, and animals may appear. Visual distortions, movement of patterns, and alterations in color intensity are common (Critchley, 1939; Grinspoon and Bakalar, 1979; Klüver, 1966; Malitz et al., 1962; Siegel, 1977). Brief recurrences of the visual experiences (''flashbacks'') may occur for several years following exposure to LSD (Abraham, 1983; Horowitz, 1969; Rosenthal, 1964).

Auditory hallucinations are far more characteristic of the idiopathic psychiatric illnesses than visual hallucinations, but the latter are not uncommon. Between 24 and 46 percent of acute schizophrenics and up to 72 percent of chronic schizophrenics report having had visual hallucinations at some time during the course of their illnesses (Goodwin et al., 1971; Mott et al., 1965).

The visual hallucinations of schizophrenia may occur with auditory hallucinations, or they may be visual memories, bizarre, fragmented images, or even unformed flashes of light. Visual hallucinations have been reported in 10–70 percent of patients with affective disorders (Bowman and Raymond, 1931; Goodwin et al., 1971), and in up to 75 percent of patients with hysteria (Fitzgerald and Wells, 1977; Goodwin et al., 1971). Hallucinations occurring in the context of major affective disorders usually are mood congruent.

Finally, visual hallucinations occur in normal individuals in specific circumstances (Table 16-1). The best examples of unbidden spontaneous visual images are dreams. These unique visual hallucinations are common to the experience of all intact individuals, meet most definitions of visual hallucinations, and are pathological only when not confined to the sleep state (Lessell, 1975). Children may have imaginary companions and play objects that they "see" with realitylike clarity (Bender and Vogel, 1941; Weiner 1961), and they also appear to be more likely to respond to emotional stress with hallucinatory syndromes (Egdell and Kolvin, 1972; Esman, 1967). In adults, visual hallucinations occur during periods of sleep deprivation, as a product of suggestion during hypnosis, and as hypnagogic phenomena (McDonald, 1971; Ribstein, 1976; West et al., 1962). In addition, hallucinations occur during sensory deprivation, a state that may share essential features with hallucinations that are reported with blindness of all types (Flynn, 1962; Heron, 1957). Hallucinations occur during intense emotional experiences such as in the course of grief reactions and appear to be influenced by the cultural experiences of the involved individuals (MacDonald and Oden, 1977; Matchett, 1972). Hallucinations have also been described by many "visionaries" who found them to be sources of guidance and inspiration; thus, hallucinations played a role in the lives of Socrates, St. Paul, Joan of Arc, Mohammed, Luther, Moses, Pascal, Swedenborg, George Fox, Shelley, William Blake, Bunyan, Napoleon, Raphael, Schumann, Goethe, Byron, and Walter Scott (McGowan, 1939; Medlicott, 1958).

Phenomenology

Specific features of visual hallucinations may facilitate identification of the clinical disorders from which they originate. The characteristics that distinguish ictal and release hallucinations are described in Table 16-2. The form of epileptic hallucinations has localizing significance: posterior occipital lesions produce unformed, simple flashes; the patterns become more complex if the focus is located in visual association cortex; and more anteriorly placed lesions in the medial temporal lobe produce complex, formed images and visual memories (Editoral, *Br Med J*, 1977). Release hallucinations, on the other hand, have little localizing value. They occur with lesions of the eye, optic nerve and chiasm, and cerebral hemispheres.

Lilliputian hallucinations— visions of tiny human and animal figures named for the diminutive inhabitants of the Isle of Lilliput described by Swift in *Gulliver's Travels* (Swift, 1960)—are distinctive but appear to have little etiologic significance. They have been described in toxic and metabolic disorders, hypnagogic states, structural CNS disturbances, epilepsy, ocular diseases, affective disturbances and schizophrenia (Alexander, 1926; Goldin, 1955; Leroy, 1922, 1926; Lewis, 1961; Savitsky and Tarachow, 1941). Hallucinations of giants— Brobdingnagian hallucinations—have been recorded in a small number of confusional states (Fleming, 1923; Thomas and Fleming, 1934). Lilliputian and Brobdingnagian hallucinations involve seeing small and large individuals, respectively, and must be distinguished from micropsia and macropsia, where the entire scene, along with an included figure, appears altered in size.

Autoscopy (heutoscopy) is another striking hallucinatory experience in which one sees one's own image. Such hallucinations have occurred in epilepsy, brain tumors, cerebral trauma, subarachnoid hemorrhage, cerebral syphilis, migraine, postencephalitic parkinsonism, typhus and other infectious diseases, drug intoxications, schizophrenia, and depression (Dewhurst and Pearson, 1955; Lhermitte, 1951; Lippman, 1953; Lukianowicz, 1958). If the patient endorses the vision as a true double or believes that a double exists even though invisible, the syndrome merges into the delusion of the double or the doppelgänger (Chapter 13) (Christodoulou, 1978; Damas-Mora et al., 1980). The syndrome is put to literary use in Dostoyevsky's *The Double*, Edgar Allen Poe's *William Wilson*, Steinbeck's *Great Valley*, and Oscar Wilde's *The Portrait of Dorian Gray* (Lhermitte, 1951.)

"Psychedelic" hallucinations consisting of geometric forms, spirals, funnels and chessboards are most characteristic of the hallucinogenic drugs (Grinspoon and Bakalar, 1979; Klüver, 1966; Mitchell, 1896; Siegel, 1977) but also occur with sensory deprivation (Heron, 1957) and have been described in CNS disorders such as during recovery from acute viral encephalitis and with acute occipital lobe insults (Mize, 1980).

Illusions are misperceptions or perceptual distortions of an existing external stimulus (McGowan, 1939). They differ from hallucinations in that the perceptual activity has its original stimulus in the external environment. Although illusions and hallucinations can be differentiated clinically, the distinction has little etiologic significance since both phenomena are found in the same disorders. Illusions occur in epilepsy, migraine, and narcolepsy, and with hallucinogens (Roth, 1980; Siegel, 1977; Willanger and Klee, 1966).

Palinopsia is a unique form of visual hallucination that involves the persistence or recurrence of visual images after the exciting stimulus has been removed (Bender et al., 1968; Critchley, 1951). The image remains when the patient changes direction of gaze and may spontaneously recur for up to several hours. The phenomenon usually begins abruptly with a cerebral infarction, neoplasm, or trauma and persists only a few days, but in some cases it has endured for years (Cummings et al., 1982). Palinopsia can occur with lesions of either hemisphere but is most common with acute damage to the posterior aspect of the right hemisphere (Kinsbourne and Warrington, 1963; Meadows and Munro, 1977; Michel and Troost, 1980). Originally considered as an ictal manifestation, palinopsia shares many features with hallucinations originating from hemispheric lesions involving the visual radiations, suggesting that it is a unique type of release hallucination (Cummings et al., 1982).

Pathophysiology

The remarkable similarity of many aspects of visual hallucinations suggests that a few basic CNS mechanisms are responsible for generation of most of the images. The most common situation in which hallucinations emerge involves the reduction of visual input. This occurs in sensory isolation; enucleation; cataract formation; retinal, choroidal, or macular disease; optic nerve and tract disease; and with hemispheric lesions involving the geniculocalcarine pathways. The blindness may be partial or total or monocular or hemianoptic and in all cases may be associated with hallucinations of similar character. West (1962) proposed a "perceptual release theory" that suggests that decreased sensory input results in release of spontaneous activity of CNS structures normally mediating perceptual experience. This basic mechanism might also account for hallucinations associated with diminished arousal in narcolepsy, hypnotic and trance states, confusional states, and some idiopathic psychiatric disorders. Physiologically, profound and permanent defects in visual pathways produces occipital slowing and spontaneous occipital spiking on the EEG (Chatta and Lombroso, 1972). This observation supports the perceptual-release concept and creates a link between hallucinations produced by decreased visual input and ictal hallucinations.

Another basic mechanism associated with several types of visual hallucination involves the appearance of dreams in the waking state. Dreams themselves are a unique variety of visual hallucinations occurring in normal individuals. The emancipation of dreams from the sleep state appears to account for hypnagogic hallucinations occurring in normal individuals and in narcoleptics and for hallucinations occurring during alcohol withdrawal and may play a role in the hallucinations of peduncular hallucinosis where a consistent diurnal pattern has been observed.

The ability of the hallucinogens to induce vivid hallucinatory experiences is not understood. An effect on retinal function has been demonstrated but is insufficient to account for the diversity of their actions or the similarity between hallucinogen-induced visions and those of certain CNS lesions (Horowitz, 1964; Jacobsen, 1963; Krill et al., 1960). Lysergic acid diethylamide is also capable of inducing hallucinations in patients who have been enucleated demonstrating the independence of the LSD effects of ocular function. Hallucinogens antagonize the functions of serotonin in the brainstem and may exert effects on brainstem arousal, sleep and dream mechanisms or have secondary effects on cerebral cortical activity (Brawley and Duffield, 1972; Jacobs, 1978). An effect on memory function with generation of spontaneous images from memory stores may also play a role in the production of the hallucinations (Jarvik, 1970). Any or all of these effects or some as yet undiscovered action of these drugs may account for their hallucinogenic capacity.

Anatomically, a majority of hallucinations associated with structural hemispheric lesions or epileptic foci arise from the right cerebral hemisphere. This hemisphere mediates nonverbal visuospatial and visuoperceptual activity, and the tendency for hallucinations to arise from lesions of this hemisphere reflects this specialization. Removal of the temporal lobes diminishes the hallucinogenic effects of LSD, suggesting that, within the hemispheres, temporal lobe structures play a major role in mediating the effects of hallucinogenic agents. (Serafetinides, 1965).

Hallucinations can thus be correlated with a few basic mechanisms—perceptual release, ictal discharges, dream intrusions, neurochemical effects. These few mechanisms, along with a few CNS principles (i.e., specialization of right cerebral hemisphere for visuoperceptual processing), provide the foundations for understanding many aspects of these unique experiential phenomena.

AUDITORY HALLUCINATIONS

Auditory hallucinations, unlike visual hallucinations, are much more characteristic of idiopathic psychiatric disorders than of neuromedical or toxic disorders. An important exception to this observation is the common occurrence of auditory hallucinations in schizo-phrenialike psychoses that may be associated with a variety of neurological and toxic–metabolic disorders (Chapter 13). Table 16-4 presents the disorders to be considered in the differential diagnosis of auditory hallucinations. Deafness produced by disease of the middle ear (e.g., otosclerosis) or of the inner ear and auditory nerve can produce both unformed and formed hallucinations. The unformed hallucinations are referred to as *tinnitus* and consist of buzzing or tones of varying pitch and timbre. The formed hallucinations are comprised of melodies, organ music, hymns, songs, and—occasionally—voices. In some cases the content can be influenced by imagining or vocalizing a song or melody (Hammeke et al., 1983; Miller and Crosby, 1979; Ross et al., 1975; Rozanski and Rosen, 1952). Deafness and auditory hallucinations appear to predispose to the development of a paranoid syndrome, particularly in the elderly (Cooper and Curry, 1976; Rhein, 1913). The association between auditory hallucinations and deafness resembles the similar correlation of visual hallucinations with blindness and of phantom limbs with amputation.

Among central nervous system (CNS) disorders, partial seizures may give rise to auditory hallucinations. Currie and colleagues (1971) studied 514 patients with temporal lobe epilepsy and found that 17 percent had auditory hallucinations as one component of their seizures. Crude sensations were five times more common than elaborate, formed sounds or voices. The hallucinations are brief, stereotyped sensory impressions and, if formed, may be trivial sentences, previously heard phrases, or commands (Karagulla and Robertson, 1955).

Central nervous system neoplasms also give rise to auditory hallucinations in 3–10 percent of cases (Courville, 1928; Critchley, 1939; Tarachow, 1941). The hallucinations may be either formed or unformed and are associated predominantly with frontal and temporal lobe tumors. Vascular lesions have also rarely been associated with auditory hallucinations (Anastasopoulos, 1967).

Auditory hallucinations may occur as part of delirious psychoses in the course of toxic and metabolic encephalopathies or during withdrawal states. Alcoholic hallucinosis is a unique auditory hallucinatory syndrome related to chronic alcoholism and alcohol withdrawal. The hallucinations are usually vocal in nature and typically consist of accusatory, threatening, and critical voices directed at the patient. The voices begin in the withdrawal period in a majority of cases and usually cease within a few days. In a few cases, however, the auditory hallucinations become chronic, persisting for years. The patient may have no insight into the unreality of the experiences and may act on directions received from the voices or may seek protec-

TABLE 16-4. Etiologies of Auditory Hallucinations

Peripheral lesions

Middle ear disease
Inner ear disease
Auditory nerve disease

Central nervous system disorders

Epilepsy
Neoplasms
Vascular lesions

Toxic–metabolic disturbances

Chronic alcoholic hallucinosis

Idiopathic psychiatric disorders

Schizophrenia
Mania
Depression
Conversion symptoms
Multiple personality

tion from them with relatives or police (Surawicz, 1980; Victor and Hope, 1958).

Auditory hallucinations are most characteristic of the idiopathic psychoses. They occur in 60–90 percent of schizophrenic patients and up to 80 percent of patients with affective psychoses (Bowman and Raymond, 1931; Goodwin et al., 1971; Lowe, 1973; Mott et al., 1965; Small et al., 1966). The hallucinations vary from ''inner voices'' sensed by the patient to vivid hallucinations heard as if coming from the outside (Sedman, 1966b). Some patients may hear their own thoughts spoken aloud (''gadenkenlautwerden''). Schizophrenic patients experience the voices as objective, involuntarily present and having unique and immediate relevance to them, but a minority expect that other members of the public should be able to hear them (Aggernaes, 1972; Aggernaes and Nyeborg, 1972; Larkin, 1979). There is a tendency for some patients with affective disorders to lateralize their hallucinations to the right side of space (Alpert and Silvers, 1970; Gruber et al., 1984). Auditory hallucinations, like visual hallucinations, reflect the predominant mood state of the individual when they occur in the affective disorders.

In addition to their occurrence in the psychoses, auditory hallucinations also occur as manifestations of hysterical conversion reactions and in the syndrome of multiple personality (Bliss et al., 1983; Levinson, 1966; Mckegney, 1967; Siomopoulos, 1971). The presence of auditory hallucinations in these syndromes contributes to their frequent misdiagnosis as schizophrenia.

Auditory hallucinations must be distinguished from palinacousis. In the latter, there is a persistence or late recurrence of existing auditory stimuli. Palinacousis has been associated with a variety of cerebral lesions (particularly neoplasms and infarctions), and the lesions usually involve the temporal lobe (Jacobs et al., 1973; Malone and Leiman, 1983).

TACTILE, SOMATIC AND PHANTOM LIMB HALLUCINATIONS

Phantom limb, or the sensation that an amputated extremity still exists, is a very common postsurgical somatic hallucination. Of 73 soldiers who had traumatic amputations and were seen within 6 months following injury, Carlen and colleagues (1978) found that all had had phantom limb sensations and 67 percent had had phantom limb pains. Typically, the phantom is described as tingling or as being numb (as opposed to the absence of sensation that characterizes a normal limb). The phantom is usually of normal size and shape and is correctly aligned with the stump. Occasionally, phantoms may seem to be of distorted size or configuration or to occupy an odd position or may feel as if they are moving. The peripheral portions of the limb, particularly the digits, are the most prominent and enduring parts of the phantom. With time, the phantom begins to recede and fade. Frequently, the hand or foot feels as though it is gradually approaching, and is then absorbed into, the stump. This process takes from a few months to several years and may never be complete (Henderson and Smyth, 1948; Russell, 1949). Phantom limbs may also occur in acute hemiplegia, where the abrupt onset of unilateral paralysis is accompanied by the impression that a third upper or lower limb has come into existence (Weinstein et al., 1954). In addition to phantom limbs, phantom organs may appear after loss of virtually any body part. Phantom breasts, for example, are not uncommon in women who have had mastectomies (Jarvis, 1970).

The impression of distortion in body shape or appearance (somatic hallucinations) occur in a number of clinical circumstances. Alterations in the size, shape, or position of the entire body or parts of the body may constitute the aura preceding an attack of migraine (Lippman, 1952). Such alterations may also occasionally occur in toxic–metabolic enecphalopathies and under the influence of hallucinogenic drugs (Lunn, 1965). Fantastic bodily transformation with delusional endorsement of their occurrence may also emerge in the course of psychoses. Schizophrenic patients and, less frequently, patients with psychotic depression may feel as though transformed into animals, members of the opposite sex, or historical personages, or they may experience sensa-

tions of changes in body shape, size, or mass, as well as splitting, loss, or addition of body parts (Angyal, 1935; Bychowski, 1943; Connolly and Gittleson, 1971; Lukianowicz, 1976).

More elementary tactile hallucinations such as feeling insects crawling on the skin or feeling electricity pass through the body occur in a wide variety of neurological and psychiatric disorders and are particularly common in toxic and metabolic disturbances (Berrios, 1982). Tactile (haptic) hallucinations are reported by 15–50 percent of schizophrenics and approximately 25 percent of patients with affective disorders (Goodwin et al., 1971; Mott et al., 1965). Tactile hallucinations occur with about 1 percent of cerebral neoplasms (Tarachow, 1941). Formication hallucinations, the feeling that insects are crawling on the skin, are common in alcohol and drug withdrawal. Their occurrence in cocaine withdrawal is graphically described in Burrough's *Naked Lunch* (Burroughs, 1959).

OLFACTORY AND GUSTATORY HALLUCINATIONS

Olfactory and gustatory (taste) hallucinations are the least common hallucinations recorded in clinical investigations. Olfactory hallucinations are well known in epilepsy, where they are associated with medial temporal lobe lesions and complex partial seizures (uncinate seizures) (Daly, 1975). Such hallucinations may also occur in migraine and in both cases are usually described as unpleasant (Wolberg and Ziegler, 1982). Olfactory hallucinations have also been described in multi-infarct dementia, Alzheimer's disease, and alcoholic psychosyndromes (Bromberg and Schilder, 1934). Among psychiatric disorders, olfactory hallucinations occur in depression and in at least 20–25 percent of patients with Briquet's syndrome (Goodwin et al., 1971; Rupert et al., 1961). In depression, the hallucinations are commonly mood congruent smells of death, decay, and personal filth. Similar delusional beliefs that one is emitting a foul odor characterize the olfactory reference syndrome (Davidson and Mukherjee, 1982; Pryse-Phillips, 1971). In this disorder, one develops the monosymptomatic belief that one is the source of an offensive odor. The syndrome may be a stable monosymptomatic delusion or a form of hypochondriasis or may progress to an affective disorder (Bishop, 1980; Videbech, 1967).

Gustatory hallucinations occur in manic–depressive illness, schizophrenia, Briquet's syndrome, and partial seizures (Bowman and Raymond, 1931; Daly, 1975; Goodwin et al., 1971).

REFERENCES

Abraham HD. Visual phenomenology of the LSD flashback. *Arch Gen Psychiat*, 1983, *40*, 884–889.

Adler LE, Sadja L, and Wiletz G. Cimetidine toxicity manifested as paranoia and hallucinations. *Am J Psychiat*, 1980, *137*, 1112–1113.

Aggernaes A. The experienced reality of hallucinations and other psychological phenomena. *Acta Psychiat Scand*, 1972, *48*, 220–238.

Aggernaes A and Nyeborg O. The reliability of different aspects of the experienced reality of hallucinations in clear states of consciousness. *Acta Psychiat Scand*, 1972, *48*, 239–252.

Albala AA, Weinberg N, and Allen SM. Maprotiline-induced hypnopompic hallucinations. *J Clin Psychiat*, 1983, *44*, 149–150.

Alexander MC. Lilliputian hallucinations. *J Ment Sci*, 1926, *72*, 187–191.

Alpert M and Silvers KN. Perceptual characteristics distinguishing auditory hallucinations in schizophrenia and acute alcoholic psychoses. *Am J Psychiat*, 1970, *127*, 298–302.

Anastasopoulos GK. Aphasic disorders and verbal hallucinations. *J Neurol Sci*, 1967, *4*. 83–93.

Angyal A. The perceptual basis of somatic delusions in a case of schizophrenia. *Arch Neurol Psychiat*, 1935, *34*, 270–279.

Bartlet JEA. A case of organized visual hallucinations in an old man with cataract, and their relation to the phenomena of the phantom limb. *Brain*, 1951, *79*, 363–373.

Bender L and Vogel BF. Imaginary companions of children. *Am J Orthopsychiat*, 1941, *11*, 56–68.

Bender MB, Feldman M, and Sobin AJ. Palinopsia. *Brain*, 1968, *91*, 321–338.

Bender MB and Kanzer MG. Metamorphopsia and other psychovisual disturbances in a patient with tumor of the brain. *Arch Neurol Psychiat*, 1941, *45*, 481–485.

Berger PA and Tinklenberg JR. Treatment of abusers of alcohol and other addictive drugs. In Barchas JD, Berger PA, Ciaranello RD, and Elliot GR (Eds.): *Psychopharmacology*. New York, Oxford University Press, 1977, pp. 355–385.

Berrios GE. Tactile hallucinations: conceptual and historical aspects. *J Neurol Neurosurg Psychiat*, 1982, *45*, 285–293

Berrios GE and Brook P. The Charles Bonnet syndrome and the problem of visual perceptual disorders in the elderly. *Age Ageing*, 1982, *11*, 17–23.

Berrios GE and Brook P. Visual hallucinations and senory delusions in the elderly. *Br J Psychiat*, 1984, *144*, 662–684.

Bishop ER Jr. An olfactory reference syndrome— monosymptomatic hypochondriasis. *J Clin Psychiat*, 1980, *41*, 57–59.

Bliss EL, Larson EM, and Nakashima SR. Auditory hallucinations and schizophrenia. *J Nerv Ment Dis*, 1983, *171*, 30–33.

Bowman KM and Raymond AF. A statistical study of hallucinations in the manic-depressive psychoses. *Am J Psychiat*, 1931, *88*, 299–309.

Brawley P and Duffield JC. The pharmacology of hallucinogens. *Pharm Rev*, 1972, *24*, 31–66.

Brindley GS and Lewin WS. The sensations produced by electrical stimulation of the visual cortex. *J Physiol*, 1968, *196*, 479–493.

Bromberg W and Schilder P. Olfactory imagination and olfactory hallucinations. *Arch Neurol Psychiat*, 1934, *32*, 467–492.

Brust JCM and Behrens MM. ''Release hallucinations'' as the major symptom of posterior cerebral artery occlusion: a report of 2 cases. *Ann Neurol*, 1977, *2*, 432–436.

Burroughs WS. *Naked Lunch*. New York, Grove Press, 1959.

Bychowski G. Disorders in the body-image in the clinical pictures of psychoses. *J Nerv Ment Dis*, 1943, *97*, 310–335.

Carlen PL, Wall PD, Nadvorna H, and Steinbach T. Phantom limbs and related phenomena in recent traumatic amputations. *Neurology*, 1978, *28*, 211–217.

Chatta AS and Lombroso CT. Electroencephalographic changes in childhood optic neuritis. *Electroenceph Clin Neurophysiol*, 1972, *33*, 81–88.

Christodoulou GN. Syndrome of subjective doubles. *Am J Psychiat*, 1978, *135*, 249–251.

Closson RG. Visual hallucinations as the earliest symptom of digoxin intoxication. *Arch Neurol*, 1983, *40*, 386.

Cogan DG. Visual hallucinations as release phenomena. *Albrecht v. Graefes Arch Klin exp ophthalmol*, 1973, *188*, 139–150.

Cohn R. Phantom vision. *Arch Neurol*, 1971, *25*, 468–471.

Connolly FH and Gittleson NL. The relationship between delusions of sexual change and olfactory and gustatory hallucinations in schizophrenia. *Br J Psychiat*, 1971, *119*, 443–444.

Cooper AF and Curry AR. The pathology of deafness in the paranoid and affective psychoses of later life. *J Psychosomat Res*, 1976, *20*, 97–105.

Courville CB. Auditory hallucinations provoked by intracranial tumors. *J Nerv Ment Dis*, 1928, *67*, 265–274.

Critchley M. Neurological aspect of visual and auditory hallucinations. *Br Med J*, 1939, *2*, 634–639.

Critchley M. Types of visual perseveration: ''paliopsia'' and ''illusory visual spread.'' *Brain*, 1951, *74*, 267–299.

Cummings JL, Syndulko K, Goldberg Z, and Treiman DM. Palinopsia reconsidered. *Neurology*, 1982, *32*, 444–447.

Currie S, Heathfield KWG, Henson RA and Scott DF. Clinical course and prognosis of temporal lobe epilepsy. *Brain*, 1971, *94*, 173–190.

Cushing H. The field defects produced by temporal lobe lesions. *Brain*, 1922, *44*, 341–396.

Daly DD. Ictal clinical manifestations of complex partial seizures. *Adv Neurol*, 1975, *11*, 57–82.

Damas-Mora JMR, Jenner FA, and Eacott SE. On heutoscopy or the phenomenon of the double: case presentation and review of the literature. *Br J Med Psychol*, 1980, *53*, 75–83.

Damas-Mora J, Skelton-Robinson M, and Jenner FA. The

Charles Bonnet syndrome in perspective. *Psychol Med,* 1982, *12,* 251–261.

Davidson M and Mukherjee S. Progression of olfactory reference syndrome to mania: a case report. *Am J Psychiat,* 1982, *139,* 1623–1624.

Davis FA, Bergen D, Schauf C, McDonald I, and Deutsch W. Movement phosphenes in optic neuritis: a new clinical sign. *Neurology,* 1976, *26,* 1100–1104.

Deiker T and Chambers HE. Structure and content of hallucinations in alcohol withdrawal and functional psychosis. *J Stud Alc,* 1978, *39,* 1831–1840.

Dement W, Rechschaffen A, and Gulevich G. The nature of the narcoleptic sleep attack. *Neurology,* 1966, *16,* 18–33.

Dewhurst K and Pearson J. Visual hallucinations of the self in organic disease. *J Neurol Neurosurg Psychiat,* 1955, *18,* 53–57.

Diagnostic and statistical manual of mental disorders, 3rd ed., Washington D.C., American Psychiatric Association, 1980.

Dunn DW, Weisberg LA, and Nadell J. Peduncular hallucinations caused by brainstem compression. *Neurology,* 1983, *33,* 1360–1361.

Editorial. Localisation of visual hallucinations. *Br Med J,* 1977, *2,* 147–148.

Egdell HG and Kolvin I. Childhood hallucinations. *J Child Psychol Psychiat* 1972, *13,* 279–287.

Escobar JI and Karno M. Chronic hallucinosis from nasal drops. *JAMA,* 1982, *247,* 1859–1860.

Esman AH. Visual hallucinoses in young children. *Psychoanal Study Child,* 1967, *17,* 334–343.

Fischer-Williams M, Bickford RG, and Whisnant JP. Occipito-parieto-temporal seizure discharge with visual hallucinations and aphasia. *Epilepsia,* 1964, *5,* 279–292.

Fisher CM. Visual disturbances associated with quinidine and quinine. *Neurology,* 1981, *31,* 1569–1571.

Fitzgerald BA and Wells CE. Hallucinations as a conversion reaction. *Dis Nerv Syst,* 1977, *38,* 381–383.

Fleming GWTH. A case of Lilliputian hallucinations with a subsequent single macroscopic hallucination. *J Ment Sci,* 1923, *69,* 86–89.

Flynn WR. Visual hallucinations in sensory deprivation. *Psychiat Quart,* 1962, *36,* 55–59.

Foerster O. The cerebral cortex in man. *Lancet,* 1931, *2,* 309–312.

Garrel S, Fau R, Perret J, and Chatelain R. Disturbances of sleep in two brain-stem vascular syndromes, one with anatomo-clinical confirmation. *Electroenceph Clin Neurophysiol,* 1967, *23,* 290.

Gloor P, Olivier A, Quesney LF, Andermann F, and Horowitz S. The role of the limbic system in experiential phenomena of temporal lobe epilepsy. *Ann Neurol,* 1982, *12,* 129–144.

Goetz CG, Tanner CM, and Klawans HL. Pharmacology of hallucinations induced by long-term drug therapy. *Am J Psychiat,* 1982, *139,* 494–497.

Goldin S. Lilliputian hallucinations. *J Ment Sci,* 1955, *101,* 569–576.

Goodwin DW, Alderson P and Rosenthal R. Clincial signifi-

cance of hallucinations in psychiatric disorders. *Arch Gen Psychiat,* 1971, *24,* 76–80.

Gowers WR. Subjective visual sensation. *Trans Ophthalmol Soc,* 1895, *15,* 1–38.

Greenberg R and Pearlman C. Delirium tremens and dreaming. *Am J Psychiat,* 1967, *124,* 133–142.

Grinspoon L and Bakalar JB. *Psychedelic drugs reconsidered.* New York, Basic Books, 1979.

Gross MM, Goodenough D, Tobin M, Halpert E, Lepove A, Perlstein A, Sirota M, Dibianco J, Fuller R, and Kishner I. Sleep disturbances and hallucinations in the acute alcoholic psychoses. *J Nerv Ment Dis,* 1966, *142,* 493–514.

Gruber LN, Mangat BS, and Abou-Taleb H. Laterality of auditory hallucinations in psychiatric patients. *Am J Psychiat,* 1984, *141,* 586–588.

Guinena YH and Taher Y. Psychosensory seizures "visual and auditory" of primary subcortical origin. *Electoenceph Clin Neurophysiol,* 1955, *7,* 425–428.

Haas DC. Prolonged migraine aural status. *Ann Neurol,* 1982, *11,* 197–199.

Hachinski VC, Porchawka J, and Steele JC. Visual symptoms in the migraine syndrome. *Neurology,* 1973, *23,* 570–579.

Hammeke TA, McQuillen MP, and Cohen BA. Musical hallucinations associated with acquired deafness. *J Neurol Neurosurg Psychiat,* 1983, *46,* 570–572.

Hare EH. A short note on pseudo-hallucinations. *Br J Psychiat,* 1973, *122,* 469–476.

Hécaen H and Albert ML. *Human neuropsychology.* New York, John Wiley & Sons, 1978.

Heiman M. Visual hallucinations during paradehyde addiction. *J Nerv Ment Dis,* 1942, *96,* 251–260.

Henderson WR and Smyth GE. Phantom limbs. *J Neurol Neurosurg Psychiat,* 1948, *11,* 88–112.

Heron W. The pathology of boredom. *Sci Am,* 1957, *196,* 52–56.

Hishikawa Y and Kaneko Z. Electroencephalographic study on narcolepsy. *Electroenceph Clin Neurophysiol,* 1965, *18,* 249–259.

Hoppe H. A syndrome of the visuopathic cortical area—based on stabile hallucinations and defective visual association in a sane person. *Trans Am Neurol Assoc,* 1921, *47,* 247–253.

Horowitz MJ. The imagery of visual hallucinations. *J Nerv Ment Dis,* 1964, *138,* 513–522.

Horowitz MJ. Flashbacks: recurrent intrusive images after the use of LSD. *Am J Psychiat,* 1969, *126,* 565–569.

Horowitz MJ, Adams JE, and Rutkin BB. Visual imagery of brain stimulation. *Arch Gen Psychiat,* 1968, *19,* 469–486.

Horrax G. Visual hallucinations as a cerebral localizing phenomenon. *Arch Neurol Psychiat,* 1923, *10,* 532–547.

Jackson JH and Beevor CE. Case of tumour of the right temporo-sphenoidal lobe bearing on the localisation of the sense of smell and on the interpretation of a particular variety of epilepsy. *Brain,* 1889, *12,* 346–357.

Jacobs BL. Dreams and hallucinations: a common neurochemical mechanism mediating their phenomenological similarities. *Neurosci Biobehav Rev,* 1978, *2,* 59–69.

Jacobs L, Feldman M, Diamond SP, Bender MB. Palinacousis:

persistent or recurring auditory sensations. *Cortex*, 1973, 9, 275–287.

Jacobs L, Karpik A, Bozian D, and Gothgen S. Auditory-visual synesthesia. *Arch Neurol*, 1981, 38, 211–216.

Jacobsen E. The clinical pharmacology of the hallucinogens. *Clin Pharm Ther*, 1963, 4, 480–503.

Jarvik M. Drugs, hallucinations and memory. In Keup W. (Ed.): *Origin and mechanisms of hallucinations*. New York, Plenum Press, 1970, pp. 457–459.

Kane FT Jr and Keeler MH. Visual hallucinations while receiving imipramine. *Am J Psychiat*, 1964, 121, 611–612.

Karagulla S and Robertson EE. Psychical phenomena in temporal lobe epilepsy and in the psychoses. *Br Med J*, 1955, 1, 748–752.

Kennedy F. The symptomatology of temporosphenoidal tumors. *Arch Int Med*, 1911, 8, 317–350.

King DW and Marsan CA. Clinical features and ictal patterns in epileptic patients with EEG temporal lobe foci. *Ann Neurol*, 1977, 2, 138–147.

Kinsbourne M and Warrington EK. A study of visual perseveration. *J Neurol Neurosurg Psychiat*, 1963, 26, 468–475.

Klee A and Willanger R. Disturbances of visual perception in migraine. *Acta Neurol Scand*, 1966, 42, 400–414.

Klein DF. Visual hallucinations with imipramine. *Am J Psychiat*, 1964, 121, 911–914.

Klüver H. *Mescal and mechanisms of hallucinations*. Chicago, University of Chicago Press, 1966.

Krill AE, Wieland AM, and Ostfeld AM. The effect of two hallucinogenic agents on human retinal function. *Arch Ophthalmol*, 1960, 64, 724–733.

Lance JW. Simple formed hallucinations confined to the area of a specific visual field defect. *Brain*, 1976, 99, 719–734.

Lance JW, Cooper B and Misbach J. Visual hallucinations as a symptom of right parieto-occipital lesions. *Proc Aust Assoc Neurol*, 1974, 11, 209–217.

Larkin AR. The form and content of schizophrenic hallucinations. *Am J Psychiat*, 1979, 136, 940–942.

Leroy R. The syndrome of Lilliputian hallucinations. *J Nerv Ment Dis*, 1922, 56, 325–333.

Leroy R. The affective states in Lilliputian hallucinations. *J Ment Sci*, 1926, 72, 179–186.

Lessell S. Higher disorders of visual function: positive phenomena. In Glaser JS and Smith JL (Eds.): *Neuroophthalmology*, Vol. VIII. St. Louis, CV Mosby Company, 1975, pp. 27–44.

Lessell S and Cohen MM. Phosphenes induced by sound. *Neurology*, 1979, 29, 1524–1527.

Levin M. Bromide hallucinosis. *Arch Gen Psychiat*, 1960, 2, 429–433.

Levine AM. Visual hallucinations and cataracts. *Ophthalmol Surg*, 1980, 11, 95–98.

Levinson H. Auditory hallucinations in a case of hysteria. *Br J Psychiat*, 1966, 112, 19–26.

Lewis DJ. Lilliputian hallucinations in the functional psychoses. *Can Psychiat Assoc J*, 1961, 6, 177–201.

Lhermitte J. Visual hallucinations of the self. *Br Med J*, 1951, 1, 431–434.

Linn L, Kahn RL, Coles R, Cohen J, Marshall D, and Weinstein EA. Patterns of behavior disturbance following cataract extraction. *Am J Psychiat*, 1953, 110, 281–289.

Lipowski ZJ. *Delirium. Acute brain failure in man*. Springfield, Illinois, Charles C Thomas, Publisher, 1980.

Lippman CW. Certain hallucinations peculiar to migraine. *J Nerv Ment Dis*, 1952, 116, 346–351.

Lippman CW. Hallucinations of physical duality in migraine. *J Nerv Ment Dis*, 1952, 117, 345–350.

Lowe GR. The phenomenology of hallucinations as an aid to differential diagnosis. *Br J Psychiat*, 1973, 123, 621–623.

Lukianowicz N. Autoscopic phenomena. *Arch Neurol Psychiat*, 1958, 80, 199–220.

Lukianowicz N. ''Body image'' disturbances in psychiatric disorders. *Br J Psychiat*, 1967, 113, 31–47.

Lunn V. On body hallucinations. *Acta Psychiat Scand*, 1965, 41, 387–399.

MacDonald WS and Oden CW Jr. Aumakua: behavioral direction visions in Hawaiians. *J Abnorm Psychol*, 1977, 86, 189–194.

Malitz S, Wilkens B, and Esecover H. A comparison of drug-induced hallucinations with those seen in spontaneously occurring psychoses. In West LJ (Ed.): *Hallucinations*. New York, Grune & Stratton, 1962, pp. 50–63.

Malone GL and Leiman HI. Differential diagnosis of palinacousis in a psychiatric patient. *Am J Psychiat*, 1983, 140, 1067–1068.

Matchett WF. Repeated hallucinatory experiences as part of the mourning process among Hopi indian women. *Psychiatry*, 1972, 35, 185–194.

McDonald C. A clinical study of hypnagogic hallucinations. *Br J Psychiat*, 1971, 118, 543–547.

McGowan PK. The significance of auditory and visual hallucinations. *Br Med J*, 1939, 2, 631–634.

Mckegney FP. Auditory hallucination as a conversion symptom. *Comp Psychiat*, 1967, 8, 80–89.

Meadows JC and Munro SSF. Palinopsia. *J Neurol Neurosurg Psychiat*, 1977, 40, 5–8.

Medlicott RW. An inquiry into the significance of hallucinations with special reference to their occurrence in the sane. *Internat Rec Med*, 1958, 171, 664–677.

Michel EM and Troost BT. Palinopsia: cerebral localization with computed tomography. *Neurology*, 1980, 30, 887–889.

Miller TC and Crosby TW. Muscial hallucinations in a deaf elderly patient. *Ann Neurol*, 1979, 5, 301–302.

Mitchell SW. The effects of *Anhelonium Lewinii* (the mescal button). *Br Med J*, 1896, 2, 1625–1629.

Mize K. Visual hallucinations following viral encephalitis: a self report. *Neuropsychologia*, 1980, 18 193–202.

Mundy-Castle AC. A case in which visual hallucinations related to past experience were evoked by photic stimulation. *Electroenceph Clin Neurophysiol*, 1951, 3, 353–356.

Nebel BR. The phosphene of quick eye motion. *Arch Ophthalmol*, 1957, 58, 235–243

Opie EL. Relation of visual illusions to memory. *Dis Nerv Syst*, 1968, 29, 552–556.

Parkes JD, Debono AG, and Marsden CD. Bromocriptine in parkinsonism: long-term treatment, dose response, and comparison with levodopa. *J Neurol Neurosurg Psychiat*, 1976, *39*, 1101–1107.

Parkinson D, Rucker CW, Craig W Mck. Visual hallucinations associated with tumors of the occipital lobe. *Arch Neurol Psychiat*, 1952, *68*, 66–68.

Peatfield RC and Rose C. Migrainous visual symptoms in a woman without eyes. *Arch Neurol*, 1981, *38*, 466.

Penfield W and Perot P. The brain's record of auditory and visual experience. *Brain*, 1963, *86*, 595–696.

Pick A. The localizing diagnostic significance of so-called hemianopic hallucinations, with remarks on bitemporal scintillating scotomata. *Am J Med Sci*, 1904, *127*, 82–92.

Postma JU and van Tilburg W. Visual hallucinations and delirium during treatment with amantadine (symmetrel). *J Am Geriat Soc*, 1975, *23*, 212–215.

Priestly BS and Foree K. Clinical significance of some entoptic phenomena. *Arch Ophthalmol*, 1955, *53*, 390–397.

Pryse-Phillips W. An olfactory reference syndrome. *Acta Psychiat Scan*, 1971, *47*, 484–509.

Rhein JHW. Hallucinations of hearing and diseases of the ear. *NY Med J*, 1913, *97*, 1236–1238.

Ribstein M. Hypnagogic hallucinations. *Adv Sleep Res*, 1976, *3*, 145–160.

Robinson PK and Watt AC. Hallucinations of remembered scenes as an epileptic aura. *Brain*, 1947, *70*, 440–448.

Rosenthal SH. Persistent hallucinosis following repeated administration of hallucinogenic drugs. *Am J Pschyiat*, 1964, *121*, 238–244.

Ross ED, Jossman PB, Bell B, Sabin T, and Geschwind N. Musical hallucinations in deafness. *JAMA*, 1975, *231*, 620–621.

Roth B. *Narcolepsy and hypersomnia*. New York, S. Karger, 1980.

Roth B and Brůhová S. Dreams in narcolepsy, hypersomnia, and dissociated sleep disorders. *Exp Med Surg*, 1969, *27*, 187–209.

Rozanski J. Peduncular hallucinõsis following vertebral angiography. *Neurology*, 1952, *2*, 341–349.

Rozanski J and Rosen H. Musical hallucinosis in otosclerosis. *Confinia Neurol*, 1952, *12*, 49–54.

Rupert SL, Hollender MH, and Mehrhof EG. Olfactory hallucinations. *Arch Gen Psychiat*, 1961, *5*, 313–318.

Russell WR. Painful amputation stumps and phantom limbs. *Br Med J*, 1949, *1*, 1024–1026.

Russell WR and Whitty CWM. Studies in traumatic epilepsy. 3. Visual fits. *J Neurol Neurosurg Psychiat*, 1955, *18*, 79–96.

Sanford HS and Bair HL. Visual disturbances associated with tumors of the temporal lobe. *Arch Neurol Psychiat*, 1939, *42*, 21–43.

Savitsky N and Tarachow S. Lilliputian hallucinations during convalescence of scarlet fever. *J Nerv Ment Dis*, 1941, *93*, 310–312.

Schneider RC, Crosby EC, Bagchi BK, and Calhoun HD. Temporal or occipital lobe hallucinations triggered from frontal lobe lesions. *Neurology*, 1961, *11*, 172–179.

Sedman G. A phenomenological study of pseudohallucinations and related experiences. *Acta Psychiat Scand*, 1966a, *42*, 35–70.

Sedman G. "Inner voices." Phenomenological and clinical aspects. *Br J Psychiat*, 1966b, *112*, 485–490.

Selby G and Lance JW. Observations on 500 cases of migraine and allied vascular headache. *J Neurol Neurosurg Psychiat*, 1960, *23*, 23–32.

Serafetinides EA. The significance of the temporal lobes and of hemispheric dominance in the production of the LSD-25 symptomatology in man: a study of epileptic patients before and after temporal lobectomy. *Neuropsychologia*, 1965, *3*, 69–79.

Sholomskas AJ. An old side effect revisited: visual hallucinations. *Psychiat Ann*, 1980, *10*, 475–480.

Shopsin B, Hirsch J, and Gershon S. Visual hallucinations and propranolol. *Biol Psychiat*, 1975, *10*, 105–107.

Siegel RK. Hallucinations. *Sci Am*, 1977, *237*, (4), 132–140.

Siomopoulos V. Hysterical psychosis: psychopathological aspects. *Br J Med Psychol*, 1971, *44*, 95–100.

Small IF, Small JG, and Andersen JM. Clinical characteristics of hallucinations of schizophrenia. *Dis Nerv Syst*, 1966, *27*, 349–353.

Smith RA, Gelles DB, and Vanderhaeghen JJ. Subcortical visual hallucinations. *Cortex*, 1971, *7*, 162–168.

Sours JA. Narcolepsy and other disturbances in the sleep–waking rhythm: a study of 115 cases with review of the literature *J Nerv Ment Dis*, 1963, *137*, 525–542.

Surawicz FG. Alcoholic hallucinosis: a missed diagnosis. *Can J Psychiat*, 1980, *25*, 57–63.

Swift J. *Gulliver's travels*. New York, New American Library, 1960.

Tarachow S. The clinical value of hallucinations in localizing brain tumors. *Am J Psychiat*, 1941, *97*, 1434–1442.

Thomas CJ and Fleming GWTH. Lilliputian and Brobdingnagian hallucinations occurring simultaneously in a senile patient. *J Ment Sci*, 1934, *80*, 94–102.

Todd J. The syndrome of Alice in Wonderland. *Canad Med Assoc J*, 1955, *73*, 701–704.

Victor M and Hope JM. The phenomenon of auditory hallucinations in chronic alcoholism. *J Nerv Ment Dis*, 1958, *126*, 451–481.

Videbach Th. Chronic olfactory paranoid syndromes. *Acta Psychiat Scand*, 1967, *42*, 187–213.

Vike J, Jabbari B, and Maitland CG. Auditory-visual synesthesia. *Arch Neurol*, 1984, *41*, 680–681.

Watson SJ. Hallucinogens and other psychotomimetics: biological mechanisms. In Barchas JD, Berger PA, Ciaranello RD, and Elliot GR (Eds.): *Psychopharmacology*. New York, Oxford University Press, 1977, pp. 341–354.

Weinberger LM and Grant FC. Visual hallucinations and their neuro-optical correlates. *Arch Ophthalmol*, 1940, *23*, 166–199.

Weiner MF. Hallucinations in children. *Arch Gen Psychiat*, 1961, *5*, 544–553.

Weingarten SM, Cherlow DG, and Holmgren E. The relationship of hallucinations to the depth structures of the temporal lobe. *Acta Neurochir*, 1977, Suppl. 24, 199–216.

Weinstein EA, Kahn RL, Malitz S, and Rozanski J. Delusional reduplication of parts of the body. *Brain*, 1954, *77*, 45–60.

West LJ. A general theory of hallucinations and dreams. In

West LJ (Ed.): *Hallucinations*. New York, Grune & Stratton, 1962, pp. 275–291.

West LJ, Janszen HH, Lester BK, and Cornelisoon FS Jr. The psychosis of sleep deprivation. *Ann Acad Sci*, 1962, *96*, 66–70.

White NJ. Complex visual hallucinations in partial blindness due to eye disease. *Br J Psychiat*, 1980, *136*, 284–286.

Willanger R and Klee A. Metamorphopsia and other visual disturbances with latency occurring in patients with diffuse cerebral lesions. *Acta Neurol Scand*, 1966, *42*, 1–18.

Wolberg FL and Ziegler DK. Olfactory hallucinations in migraine. *Arch Neurol*, 1982, *39*, 382.

Yoss RE and Daly DD. Narcolepsy in children. *Pediatrics*, 1960, *25*, 1025–1033.

Zarcone V. Narcolepsy. *New Engl J Med*, 1973, *288*, 1156–1166.

Ziskind E, Jones H, Filante W, and Goldberg J. Observations on mental symptoms in eye patched patients: hypnagogic symptoms in sensory deprivation. *Am J Psychiat*, 1960, *116*, 893–900.

Chapter 17

Disturbances of Sleep, Appetite, and Sexual Behavior

Disorders of sleep, appetite, and sexual behavior are grouped together in this chapter because they involve alterations in basic life functions. Sometimes called "vegetative" functions for contrast with more volitional aspects of behavior, they are not passively automatic and may be modified by a wide variety of neurological, medical, and idiopathic psychiatric disturbances. The clinical characteristics and differential diagnosis of behavioral alterations in each of the three areas are presented.

SLEEP DISORDERS

Sleep disturbances can be divided into disorders of excessive sleepiness (hypersomnias), disorders in which the patient is unable to sleep adequately (insomnias), and a variety of sleep-related conditions that do not alter the total amount of sleep but are nocturnal in occurrence (parasomnias) (Table 17-1).

Hypersomnias

Narcolepsy

Narcolepsy is a disorder of excessive somnolence characterized by sudden irresistible attacks of sleep. The sleep attacks often occur in combination with other features of a clinical tetrad including cataplexy, sleep paralysis, or hypnagogic hallucinations (Kales et al., 1982; Roth, 1980; Sours, 1963; Zarcone, 1973). Narcoleptic sleep attacks most commonly begin between the ages of 15 and 25 and persist throughout life. Onset of this disorder rarely occurs before the age of 10 or after the age of 50. Most patients have between one and six attacks per day. The disorder has a prevalence in the population of 0.3–1 percent and is more common in men than women. A majority of cases appear to be sporadic, but familial occurrence of narcolepsy is not uncommon, and 10–30 percent demonstrate autosomal dominant in-

heritance of the disorder (Kales et al., 1982; Roth, 1980; Sours, 1963; Zarcone, 1973). Sleep attacks are the first manifestation of the disorder in 90 percent of cases, but a majority eventually develop other elements of the syndrome, with the narcolepsy–cataplexy combination being most common (Roth, 1980; Sours, 1963). *Cataplexy* refers to the sudden loss of muscular tone and occurs in 60 percent of narcoleptic patients; sleep paralysis is the inability to move during the transition period from sleep and wakefulness and occurs in 20–40 percent of patients; and hypnagogic and hypnopompic hallucinations are visual or auditory hallucinations occurring on falling asleep or awakening, respectively, and are experienced by 15–50 percent of narcolepsy patients (Roth, 1980).

Pathophysiologically, narcolepsy results from an aberrant intrusion of rapid-eye-movement (REM) sleep into the waking state. The sleep attack itself represents the sudden onset of REM sleep, the sleep paralysis and cataplexy result from the loss of muscle tone that accompanies REM sleep, and the hallucinations reflect the dreams that occur during REM periods (Zarcone, 1973). Electroencephalographic studies also reveal the abrupt onset of REM sleep coincident with the occurrence of the narcoleptic sleep attack (Dement et al., 1966; Hishikawa and Kaneko, 1965). In addition to the classic clinical and EEG characteristics, narcoleptic patients also have disturbed nocturnal sleep and episodes of unrecalled automatic behavior. Narcoleptic patients are at increased risk for personality disorders, depression, and, occasionally, psychoses (Eilenberg and Wood, 1962; Kirshnan et al., 1984; Roth, 1980; Roy, 1976).

In addition to idiopathic and hereditary narcolepsy, symptomatic forms of narcolepsy secondary to structural neurological insults have also been reported. The majority of CNS disorders associated with narcolepsy involve the brainstem, where they can influence neurological mechanisms mediating sleep processes. Narcolepsy has been noted to occur with von Economo encephalitis lethargica, with malarial brainstem infections, and with a variety of other forms of viral encephalitis

TABLE 17-1. Classification of Sleep Disorders

Hypersomnias	**Insomnias** *(continued)*
Narcolepsy	Other psychiatric disorders
Primary	Transient and situational disturbances
Secondary	Toxic–metabolic disorders with insomnia
Sleep apnea	Sleep apnea
Occlusive type	Miscellaneous insomnias
Central type	With nocturnal myoclonus
Mixed forms	With restless legs
Toxic–metabolic hypersomnias	With CNS disorders
Medical illnesses	Chronic primary insomnia
Toxic conditions	**Parasomnias**
Psychiatric disorders with hypersomnia	Disorders of arousal
Depression	Somnambulism
Other psychiatric disturbances	Somniloquy
Periodic hypersomnias	Night terrors
Kleine-Levin syndrome	Enuresis
Menstruation-associated syndrome	Nightmares and other dream alterations
Miscellaneous hypersomnias	Miscellaneous conditions
Sleep drunkenness	Nocturnal seizures
With nocturnal myoclonus	Cluster headache
With restless legs	Asthma
With CNS lesions	Cardiovascular symptoms
Idiopathic hypersomnias	Gastrointestinal disturbances
Insomnias	Painful erections
Psychiatric disorders with insomnia	Head banging
Affective disturbances	Bruxism

(Bonduelle and Degos, 1976; Fournier and Helguera, 1934; Kleitman, 1963; Miller, 1927; Roth, 1980; Spiller, 1926; Symonds, 1926). Brainstem trauma, cerebrovascular disease, neoplasms, and multiple sclerosis have also been associated with symptomatic narcolepsy in rare cases (Bonduelle and Degos, 1976; Roth, 1980).

Narcolepsy usually requires treatment with amphetamines or methylphenidate, whereas cataplexy, sleep paralysis, and hypnagogic hallucinations respond best to imipramine hydrochloride (Roth, 1980).

Sleep Apnea

Sleep apnea is a potentially life-threatening illness characterized by multiple episodes of nocturnal apnea, excessive snoring, and daytime sleepiness. The apnea is a product of insufficient air exchange and may be of central origin, reflecting inadequate stimulation of the respiratory muscles, a product of peripheral or occlusive conditions with obstruction of the oropharynx, or the result of mixed central and peripheral components. The patients may have frequent nocturnal awakenings and complain of nocturnal insomnia with daytime fatigue and somnolence. Systemic hypertension, cardiac arrhythmias, and morning headaches are common consequences of sleep apnea. Although extreme obesity may produce occlusive sleep apnea (Pickwickian syndrome), few sleep apnea patients are obese, and the diagnosis should be considered in any individual complaining of excessive daytime sleepiness. The diagnosis of sleep apnea is based on observation of a minimum of 30 episodes of apnea lasting for at least 10 seconds during a 7-hour period of sleep.

Relief of sleep apnea utilizes a variety of treatment modalities. Aggravating agents such as hypnotics and propranolol should be discontinued, sleeping upright may reduce symptoms, and loss of excessive weight should be encouraged. Protriptyline enhances ventilatory drive and may help patients with moderately severe apnea syndromes. Advanced sleep apnea may require tracheostomy to ensure adequate nocturnal ventilation (Chokroverty and Sharp, 1981; Guilleminault et al., 1973b; Walker and Cavenar, 1983; Williams et al., 1982).

Like narcolepsy, the central form of sleep apnea

may be idiopathic or may result from a variety of CNS disorders, including syringomyelia, posterior fossa neoplasms, bulbar poliomyelitis, brainstem infarction, Shy-Drager syndrome (a parkinsonian syndrome with prominent autonomic dysfunction), and olivopontocerebellar degeneration (Adelman et al., 1984; Chokroverty et al., 1984; Williams et al., 1982).

Toxic–Metabolic Hypersomnias

Tolerance to CNS stimulants (amphetamines, methylphenidate, caffeine) or their withdrawal may result in a paradoxical increase in daytime somnolence. Likewise, sustained use of depressants such as opiates, barbiturates, alcohol, antihistamines, and anxiolytics may result in excessive daytime sleep (Walker and Cavenar, 1983).

A wide variety of medical illnesses, including systemic infections, hormonal disorders, and environmental toxins, can also produce hypersomnia either directly or by disturbing nocturnal sleep (Williams et al., 1982).

Psychiatric Disorders with Hypersomnia

Insomnia is more characteristic of depression than hypersomnia, but in some cases the patient experiences a pathological increase in sleepiness, particularly early in the course of the depression. Sleep studies reveal a decreased latency to REM onset as in depression with insomnia (Williams et al., 1982).

Patients with personality disorders, dissociative disorders, hypochondriasis, and schizophrenia may complain of excessive sleepiness, but sleep studies reveal that the total daily amount of sleep seldom is increased (Williams et al., 1982).

Periodic Hypersomnias

Periodic hypersomnias are disorders of excessive sleep that recur at prolonged intervals. Kleine-Levin syndrome is a periodic hypersomnia that involves primarily adolescent males. The patients have irregular episodes lasting for a few days or weeks and characterized by increased somnolence, increased hunger, exaggerated sexual activity, and a confusional state with hallucinations, delusions, and poor attention and memory. The episodes recur at approximately 5-month intervals and eventually spontaneously disappear (Critchley, 1962; Critchley and Hoffman, 1942; Gallinek, 1962; Garland et al., 1965; Gilbert, 1964).

A syndrome sharing many of the features of the Kleine-Levin syndrome has been described in women, where the periodic sleep disturbance is temporally linked to the menstrual cycle (Sachs et al., 1982; Walker and Cavenar, 1983).

Miscellaneous Hypersomnias

In addition to the hypersomnias previously discussed, a variety of other disorders with excessive somnolence have also been described. *Sleep drunkenness* refers to a syndrome characterized by extended sleep with otherwise normal sleep architecture. The patients have difficulty awakening completely and are confused, incoordinated, and slow for the first few hours after arising (Roth et al., 1972).

Nocturnal myoclonus and the restless legs syndrome usually cause insomnia but in some cases may present as a compensatory daytime somnolence (Walker and Cavenar, 1983).

Excessive sleep may also occur with CNS lesions, particularly those involving the brainstem and diencephalon. Increased daytime sleepiness may follow trauma or may occur with tumors or infarctions affecting the brainstem, hypothalamus, or thalamus (Akert, 1965; Beal et al., 1981; Guilleminault et al., 1983; Hall and Danoff, 1975).

A few patients demonstrate an idiopathic hypersomnia unlike any of the primary or symptomatic hypersomnias described. Also called *slow-wave narcolepsy* or *hypersomnia with normal sleep,* the syndrome is characterized solely by increased daytime sleepiness. The sleep is of the slow-wave type and, unlike the sleep of narcolepsy, does not refresh the patient (Guilleminault and Dement, 1974).

Insomnias

Psychiatric Disorders

Depression is the most prevalent cause of insomnia, accounting for approximately 20 percent of patients referred to sleep disorder clinics with a chief complaint of inability to sleep (Coleman et al., 1982). Sleep during a major depressive episode is characterized by a decreased latency period between sleep onset and the beginning of the first REM period and by an increased density of REMs during REM periods (Coble et al., 1976; McCarley, 1982). The patients also have less total REM sleep and less deep sleep and complain of difficulty in falling and staying asleep as well as early morning awakening (Mendels and Hawkins, 1967). Insomnia is also common in mania but rarely is the dominant clinical feature.

Insomnia is a frequent complaint of patients with personality disorders and may occur in individuals with somatoform disorders, obsessive–compulsive disorders, or schizophrenia. Situational disturbances with anxiety also produce insomnia, and their greatest effect is on the time interval between retiring and sleep onset (Coleman et al., 1982; Kales and Kales, 1974, 1984; Reynolds et al., 1984).

Toxic–Metabolic Disorders

The most common toxic conditions with insomnia involve the use of CNS stimulants and the withdrawal of CNS depressants. Amphetamines, methylphenidate, and caffeine all produce increased arousal and diminished sleep. Withdrawal of alcohol or of sedative–hypnotic agents produces a withdrawal insomnia that may persist for up to 6 weeks following cessation of drug use. Even mildly sedating agents such as benzodiazepines, anticonvulsants, steroids, antipsychotic agents, antidepressant drugs, opiates, marijuana, and propranolol can be associated with insomnia when they are withdrawn (Kramer, 1982; Walker and Cavener, 1983).

A wide variety of medical conditions can produce disturbances of nocturnal sleep. Pain syndromes can be particularly disruptive and produce insomnia in patients with arthritis, headache disorders, and other chronic pain problems. Hyperthyroidism, pregnancy, gastrointestinal diseases, eating disorders, and cardiovascular disorders may also cause repeated awakening (Kales and Kales, 1984; Kramer, 1982; Walker and Cavenar, 1983).

Sleep Apnea

Sleep apnea, as noted earlier, usually presents with excessive daytime sleepiness, but some patients, particularly those with central type apneas have multiple nocturnal arousals and may have insomnia as their chief complaint (Guilleminault et al., 1976; Kramer, 1982; Walker and Cavenar, 1983).

Miscellaneous Disorders

Sleep-related periodic myoclonus is a syndrome characterized by difficulty in falling asleep and sustained nocturnal awakenings associated with repetitive myoclonic jerking of the legs. The jerking occurs every 20–40 seconds for periods of a few minutes to as long as 2 hours. The disorder occurs between age 30 and 60 and is a chronic, persistent problem (Guilleminault et al., 1975). Periodic nocturnal myoclonus must be distinguished from the common myoclonic jerks that occur just as one is falling asleep, myoclonic jerks occurring in the toxic–metabolic disturbances, epileptic myoclonic jerks, and flexor spasms associated with cervical spondylosis and other spinal cord diseases (Oswald, 1959).

The restless legs syndrome is an idiopathic disturbance characterized by creeping–crawling sensations in the distal lower extremeties that are most disagreeable when the patient is at rest and are relieved by walking. The sensations are most marked in the evening and night and may prevent the patient from sleeping (Ekbom, 1960). The restless legs syndrome and periodic nocturnal myoclonus may present with excessive daytime sleepiness if nocturnal insomnia is severe.

Brainstem lesions such as neoplasms and basilar artery strokes can produce almost complete loss of REM sleep, slow-wave sleep, or all phases of sleep (Cummings and Greenberg, 1977; Freemon et al., 1974; Guilleminault et al., 1973a, Hobson, 1975; Lavie et al., 1984). Similarly, degenerative brainstem disorders such as Parkinson's disease and progressive supranuclear palsy produce diminished REM sleep and decreased total sleep time (Bergonzi et al., 1975; Gross et al., 1978). Epileptic patients may have decreased sleep even in the absence of overt nocturnal seizures (Greenberg and Pearlman, 1968).

Chronic primary insomnia is an idiopathic sleep disturbance characterized by prolonged sleep latencies, diminished total sleep time, and decreased slow-wave sleep. The syndrome occurs in patients without identifiable psychiatric, neurological, or toxic–metabolic disturbances (Frankel et al., 1976).

Treatment of Insomnia

The treatment of insomnia is fraught with difficulty. Many sedative–hypnotics, although effective in the first few weeks of administration, soon lose efficacy and may even exaggerate sleep problems through tolerance and withdrawal effects. Benzodiazepine sedative agents have fewer side effects than do barbiturate or antihistaminic drugs but are not without adverse consequences and may lead to dependency and intellectual impairment and may exaggerate the effects of alcohol or other CNS depressants (Solomon et al., 1979). To the fullest extent possible, the clinician should direct efforts at eliminating the underlying cause of the insomnia (depression, sleep apnea, medical illness, stimulant use), encouraging the patient to regularize sleeping habits and avoiding the chronic use of soporifics.

Parasomnias

Parasomnias are a diverse group of disorders that occur during sleep or are exacerbated by sleep but do not necessarily result in either hypersomnia or insomnia (Table 17-1).

Disorders of Arousal

Sleep walking (somnambulism), sleep talking (somniloquy), enuresis (bedwetting), and night terrors (pavor nocturnus, incubus) are all disorders of nocturnal arousal (Broughton, 1966). Each of these nighttime events is initiated during Stage IV slow-wave sleep and represents automatic behavior with incomplete arousal. The patient is in a confusional state while the behavioral automatons are executed. Although sleep walking and sleep talking were originally suspected to be dream-related, they do not occur during REM sleep when dreams are most prevalent, and patients rarely report dream memories when awakened from a somnambulistic episode. Night terrors differ from nightmares in that the patient suddenly cries out and exhibits signs of acute anxiety such as tachypnea, tachycardia, diaphoresis, and dilated pupils. Frequently, the patient does not awaken and has no memory for the episode the following morning. If awakened at the time of the attack, the patient may give a vague description of an apprehensive feeling but lacks the detailed dream recall of patients awakened from REM sleep (Broughton, 1966; Fisher et al., 1973; Tassinari et al., 1972). Stage IV sleep and the associated disorders of arousal can be suppressed by administration of benzodiazepines (Fisher et al., 1973).

Nightmares and Other Dream Alterations

Nightmares are unpleasant dreams that, like most other dreams, occur in periods of REM sleep. The unpleasant quality usually correlates with the presence of anxiety or some situational disturbance (Walker and Cavenar, 1983). Occasionally, complex partial seizures may give rise to terrifying dreams as part of a complex psychosensory seizure (Boller et al., 1975; Epstein, 1979; Fuster et al., 1954). Epileptic sleep terrors respond to anticonvulsant therapy.

Dreaming and dream recall are affected by focal lesions of the nervous system. Amnestic patients with the Wernicke-Korsakoff syndrome have normal to low amounts of REM time and have little dream recall when awakened (Greenberg et al., 1968). Parietooccipital lesions produce diminished REMs, loss of EEG sleep spindles ipsilateral to the lesion, and impaired dreaming or dream recall (Epstein, 1979; Greenberg, 1966; Humphrey and Zangwill, 1951; Murri et al., 1984; Nielsen, 1955). Dreams and dream recall may be exaggerated by some brainstem lesions and, as noted earlier, abolished by others (Hobson, 1975).

Miscellaneous Conditions

Finally, there are a group of disorders whose occurrence is exaggerated during periods of nocturnal sleep. These include nocturnal seizures, cluster headache, asthma attacks, some cardiovascular and gastrointestinal symptoms, head banging (jactatio capitis nocturnus), and bruxism (tooth grinding). Penile erections occur during nocturnal REM periods and may occasionally be sustained and painful (Walker and Cavenar, 1983; Williams et al., 1982).

APPETITE DISTURBANCES

Profound loss of appetite (anorexia) or increased appetite (hyperphagia) may be produced by a number of neurological, medical, and psychiatric disorders (Table 17-2). Although hyperphagia frequently leads to obesity, the latter also has complex genetic, dietary, psychosocial, and activity-level determinants and is not considered separately here.

Anorexia

Loss of appetite is more commonly a product of idiopathic psychiatric conditions than of neurological or medical illness, but a few neuromedical diseases can produce anorexia and must be considered in the differential diagnosis. Hypothalamic lesions are more likely to cause hyperphagia than anorexia, but when the lateral hypothalamic region is involved, there may be a marked loss of appetite (Baur, 1954; Kraus, 1945; Martin et al., 1977; White and Hain, 1959). Tumors are the usual cause of hypothalamic injury, but appropriately placed vascular infarctions and infectious lesions may also produce anorexia. When such conditions occur in adolescents, they may be misdiagnosed as anorexia nervosa (Lewin et al., 1971). A related disorder is the diencephalic inanition syndrome that occurs in infants as a consequence of anterior hypothalamic neoplasms (Diamond and Averick, 1966; White and Ross, 1963). The patients typically have a clinical triad consisting of marasmus (severe weight loss), euphoria and nystagmus. The illness ends in death by the age of 2 years.

Anorexia is also seen in many degenerative brain diseases and may be particularly severe in the advanced stages of Alzheimer's disease and Huntington's disease.

Medical illnesses, including cardiopulmonary diseases, liver and kidney failure, endocrine disturbances, and infections may produce anorexia leading to severe loss of weight. Systemic cancer may have particularly profound effects on appetite, and neoplasms of prostrate, pancreas, lung, or gastrointestinal tract may present with weight loss as the first indication of their presence (Dally et al., 1979).

Depression is the most common cause of anorexia. The loss of appetite may accompany acute grief reactions and is a principal feature of major depressive episodes. The anorexia is accompanied by sleep disturbances, loss of libido, and neuroendocrinologic alterations consistent with limbic–hypothalamic–pituitary dysfunction (Chapter 14).

Anorexia nervosa is the most dramatic of the disorders of eating and weight control. Although actual loss of appetite is uncommon until the late phases of the dis-

TABLE 17-2. Disorders Producing Alterations in Appetite

Diminished appetite (anorexia)

Neurological disorders
Hypothalamic lesions
Advanced degenerative brain diseases

Systemic medical illnesses

Psychiatric disorders
Depression
Anorexia nervosa

Increased appetite (hyperphagia)

Neurological disorders
Hypothalamic lesions
Kleine-Levin syndrome
Bilateral temporal lobe injury (Klüver-Bucy syndrome)

Psychiatric disorders
Mania
Depression
Bulimia

orders, the patients take extreme measures to lose weight, including avoidance of high-calorie foods, self-induced vomiting, use of diuretics and laxatives, and excessive exercising. Despite these efforts, the patients manifest an intense fear of obesity and continue to feel as though overweight even when emaciated. The disorder commonly begins in adolescence, although onset may occur in the third decade and rarely even later. It involves males only very infrequently. In most cases there is a single episode that resolves with full recovery; a few patients have a relapsing and remitting course with recurrent episodes; and a few have an unremitting course ending in death by starvation. There is a familial predisposition to the disorder, and patients with urogenital abnormalities and Turner's syndrome appear to be particularly vulnerable to the development of anorexia nervosa. There is also a relationship between anorexia nervosa and affective disorder, and follow-up studies show an increased incidence of mood disturbances among patients with previous episodes of anorexia nervosa (Cantwell et al., 1977; Dally et al., 1979; *Diagnostic and statistical manual of mental disorders*, 1980; Kron et al., 1977).

A wide variety of clinical and metabolic alterations accompany anorexia nervosa (Table 17-3). Most of the changes appear to be secondary to the severe weight loss and occur with starvation of any etiology. The clinically evident abnormalities include hypothermia, dependent edema, bradycardia, hypotension, constipation, and the development of lanugo (Dally et al., 1979; *Diagnostic and statistical manual of mental disorders*, 1980). Many endocrinologic alterations have also been described in patients with anorexia nervosa. There are

diminished levels of thyroid-stimulating hormone (thyrotropin) (TSH), thyroxin (T4), luteinizing hormone (luteotropin) (LH), follicle-stimulating hormone (FSH), and gonadal steroids. There is a prepubertal LH secretory pattern, diminished responses to luteinizing hormone relasing hormone (LHRH), impaired dexamethasone-induced suppression of cortisol secretion, and decreased response to insulin-induced hypoglycemia. Plasma cortisol and growth hormone levels are elevated (Boyar et al., 1974, 1977; Dally et al., 1979; Garfinkel et al., 1975; Halmi and Sherman, 1975; Warren and Vande Wiele, 1973). Amenorrhea occurs in all females and is the feature least likely to normalize after weight has been restored. Cerebrospinal fluid abnormalities include decreased homovanillic acid and 5-hydroxyindoleacetic acid levels during the anorectic episode (Kaye et al., 1984). Studies of sleep architecture reveal decreased REM latency similar to but less marked than the shortened REM latency found in depression (Katz et al., 1984).

Treatment of anorexia nervosa depends on a combination of behavioral therapy, psychotherapy, and psychopharmacological treatment. In some cases crisis-oriented intervention and forced feedings may be required to prevent death from starvation.

Hyperphagia

Hyperphagia, the pathological increase in appetite, is a relatively rare symptom that may complicate neurological or psychiatric disorders. Lesions of the ventromedial hypothalamus commonly produce hyperphagia that may be associated with diabetes insipidus, rage, somnolence, hypogonadism, and/or memory loss (Baur, 1954; Beal et al., 1981; Bray, 1984; Bray and Gallagher, 1975; Haugh and Markesberry, 1983; Kirschbaum, 1951; Martin et al., 1977; Reeves and Plum, 1969). The Kleine-Levin syndrome (discussed earlier) is a product of presumed hypothalamic dysfunction characterized by periodic episodes of hyperphagia, somnolence, and altered sexual behavior in adolescent males (Critchley, 1962; Critchley and Hoffman, 1942; Gallinek, 1962; Garland et al., 1965; Gilbert, 1964). Hyperphagia is also seen in association with noncommunicating hydrocephalus and may be relieved by ventriculoperitoneal shunting (Krahn and Mitchell, 1984).

The Klüver-Bucy syndrome is a unique behavioral syndrome that was first described in monkeys subjected to bilateral anterior temporal lobectomy. The syndrome complex includes changes in dietary habits with bulimia, emotional placidity, psychic blindness, hypermetamorphosis (compulsive exploration of objects in the environment), hypersexuality, and hyperorality (Table 17-4) (Klüver-Bucy, 1939; Lilly et al., 1983).

TABLE 17-3.   Characteristics of Anorexia Nervosa

Clinical features

    Onset between adolescence and age 30 years
    Female predominance (95 percent)
    Mortality rate of 15–20 percent
    Familial predisposition
    Sleep alterations (decreased REM latency)
    Increased occurrence of urogenital abnormalities and Turner syndrome

Eating behavior

    Anorexia uncommon until late in clinical course
    Decreased high-calorie food, self-induced vomiting, use of laxatives
      and diuretics, excessive exercising,
      use of stimulants and appetite suppressants
    Intense fear of becoming overweight
    Disturbed body images, "feel fat" even when emaciated

Physical signs

    Hypothermia
    Dependent edema
    Cardiovascular changes

      Bradycardia
      Hypotension

    Lanugo (neonatal-like hair)
    Constipation

Endocrinologic alterations

    Amenorrhea
    Decreased TSH and T4
    Diminished levels of LH, FSH, gonadal steroids
    Prepubertal LH secretory pattern
    Diminished response to LHRH
    Increased plasma cortisol levels
    Impaired responsiveness to insulin-induced hypoglycemia
    Impaired dexamethasone-induced suppression of cortisol secretion
    Elevated growth hormone levels

Cerebrospinal fluid abnormalities

    Decreased homovanillic acid
    Decreased 5-hydroxyindoleacetic acid

In humans, the core symptoms are frequently complicated by the cooccurrence of amnesia, aphasia, dementia, or seizures (Lilly et al., 1983). The Klüver-Bucy syndrome may occur with any etiologic process producing bilateral temporal dysfunction and has been reported in herpes encephalitis, trauma, bitemporal surgery, paraneoplastic disorders, adrenoleukodystrophy, bilateral temporal infarction, Pick's disease, Alzheimer's disease, hypoglycemia, temporal lobe seizures, and toxoplasmosis (Table 17-5) (Cummings and Duchen, 1981; Liddell and Northfield, 1954; Lilly et al., 1983; Marlowe et al., 1975; Nakada et al., 1984; Narabayashi et al., 1963; Pilleri, 1966; Powers et al., 1980; Shoji et al., 1979; Shraberg and Weisberg, 1978; Terzian and Dalle Ore, 1955).

Hyperphagia may also occur in the course of affective disorders. Anorexia is the most common appetite alteration in depression, but a few patients have a paradoxical increase in appetite. Exaggerated hunger is routine in mania.

Bulimia is an idiopathic disorder manifest by episodic binge eating. The patients are aware that the eating pattern is abnormal and attempt to eat inconspicuously. They are fearful of not being able to stop eating voluntarily, and depressed mood and self-deprecatory thoughts are common following the binges. The binging is interspersed with programs for weight loss, including restrictive diets; self-induced vomiting; and use of cathartics, stimulants, and diuretics. The bulimia may coexist with anorexia nervosa (bulimorexia) or may occur as an independent disease entity. The disorder begins in adolescence or early adult life, occurs primarily in females, and has a chronic intermittent course. Most bulimics are of normal weight, but a few are obese and a few are slightly underweight (*Diagnostic and statistical manual of mental disorders,* 1980; Pyle et al., 1981; Russell, 1979). A few patients have improved with treatment with anticonvulsants, and monoamineoxidase (MAO) inhibitors have been successful in those with prominent depression and anxiety (Green and Rau, 1974; Stewart et al., 1984).

ALTERED SEXUAL BEHAVIOR

Three categories of altered sexual behavior are discussed: decreased sexual activity, increased sexual activity, and sexual deviations.

Decreased Sexual Activity

Decreased sexual drive may accompany both neurological and psychiatric disorders (Table 17-6). It is common among epileptics where it appears to be a product of several converging influences (Table 17-7). Hyposexuality—defined by a frequency of less than one episode of sexual behavior (masturbation or intercourse) per month—is present in 40–65 percent of patients with partial complex seizures (temporal lobe epilepsy) and 10 percent of patients with primary generalized seizures (Blumer, 1970a; Blumer and Walker, 1967; Johnson, 1965; Shukla et al., 1979; Walker and Blumer, 1977). In some cases a patient with occult seizure disorder may present with diminished libido and impotence as a chief complaint (Hierons and Saunders, 1966; Johnson, 1965). Such patients are likely to be misidentified as suffering from a psychogenic disorder if the neurological causes of reduced sexual drive are not considered.

Hyposexual epileptic patients have no interest in sexual activity, lack sexual fantasies, and—if the onset is prior to puberty—fail to develop any interest in sexual functions. At least four influences may contribute to this profound lack of sexual interest: the limbic lesion itself, the influence of drug therapy, endocrinologic alterations, and depression. Patients with temporal lobe epilepsy have a focal lesion of the limbic system, the anatomic substrate of emotional experience, including sexually oriented emotions, and the limbic dysfunction may interfere with sexual interest (Hierons and Saunders, 1966; Johnson, 1965). Blumer (1970a,b, 1977) has proposed that irritative temporal lobe foci produce hyposexuality analogous to the hypersexuality produced by destructive limbic lesions in the Klüver-Bucy syndrome. Anticonvulsant therapy may also contribute to

the diminished sexual drive. As shown in Table 17-8, barbiturate anticonvulsants may impair libido and diminish sexual arousal (Kaplan, 1979, 1983). A correlation has also been found between anticonvulsant therapy and reduced free serum testosterone activity, suggesting that anticonvulsants exert subtle homonal effects that may alter sexual drive (Toone et al., 1980). The onset of hyposexuality in some patients prior to initiation of anticonvulsant therapy and the significant reduction in sexual drive of patients with temporal lobe epilepsy compared with patients with primary generalized seizures requiring comparable drug therapy, however, suggest that other functions must also contribute to the hyposexuality of patients with temporal lobe foci (Hierons and Saunders, 1966; Johnson, 1965; Shukla et al., 1979). An endocrinologic influence that may contribute to the reduced sexual drive is the periodic elevation of serum prolactin that follows epileptic discharge (Collins et al., 1983; Dana-Haeri et al., 1983; Pritch-

TABLE 17-4.   Human Klüver-Bucy Syndrome

Core features
Emotional placidity
Hyperorality
Hypermetamorphosis
Dietary changes
Altered sexual activity
Psychic blindness (sensory agnosia)

Additional features common in humans
Aphasia
Amnesia
Dementia
Seizures

TABLE 17-5.   Differential Diagnosis of the Human Klüver-Bucy Syndrome

Herpes encephalitis
Amygdalotomy (bilateral)
Temporal lobectomy (bilateral)
Posttraumatic encephalopathy
Paraneoplastic limbic encephalitis
Adrenoleukodystropy
Bilateral temporal lobe infarction
Pick's disease
Alzheimer's disease
Hypoglycemia
Toxoplasmosis
Bilateral epileptic foci

TABLE 17-6.   Differential Diagnosis of Alterations in
                        Intensity of Sexual Drive

Decreased sexual drive

  Epilepsy
  Hypothalamic lesions
  Drug-induced changes
  Medical illnesses
  Depression
  Schizophrenia (chronic)

Increased sexual drive

  Neurological disorders
    Epilepsy
    Diencephalic lesions
    Kleine-Levin syndrome
    Bilateral temporal lobe injury (Klüver-Bucy syndrome)
    Frontal lobe syndromes

  Medical conditions and pharmacological agents
    Hyperthyroidism
    Cushing's disease and steroid administration
    Androgen administration
    Levodopa administration

  Psychiatric disorders
    Mania
    Schizophrenia (early stages)

ard et al., 1983; Trimble, 1978). Sustained hyperpro-
lactinemia leads to decreased libido and impotence, and
intermittent prolactin levels may have a similar effect.
Finally, depression is common in epileptics, and diminished libido may be a product of the affective disturbance (Betts, 1981).

Hypothalamic lesions also produce hyposexuality.
Naturally occurring lesions impair sexual interest, and
stereotactic lesions in the region of the ventromedial nuclei of the hypothalamus have been successfully utilized
to reduce sexual drive in patients with a variety of types
of sexually motivated criminal behavior (Dieckmann and
Hassler, 1977; Schneider, 1977).

Among other causes of hyposexuality, a large number of drugs impair sexual function. The impact may
be on libido, erection, or ejaculation as shown in Table
17-8. Psychotropic agents such as stimulants, antidepressants, neuroleptics, lithium, sedative–hypnotics, anxiolytics, and narcotics may all impair sexual function
in some patients (Hollister, 1975; Horowitz and Goble,
1979; Kaplan, 1979, 1983; Mitchell and Popkin, 1983;
Rees, 1983; Story, 1974). Likewise, many classes of
antihypertensive agents, estrogens, adrenal steroids, and
disulfiram may compromise sexual interest or performance (Kaplan, 1979). Trazodone and neuroleptic agents
have been associated with priapism (Gottlieb and Luskberg, 1977; Lanskey and Selzer, 1984; Scher et al.,
1983). Amoxapine and thioridazine have produced ejac-

ulatory disturbances (Kotin et al., 1976; Schwartz,
1982), and tricyclic agents may produce spontaneous
seminal emission (Breier et al., 1984).

A number of medical conditions can also impair
sexual behavior or diminish sexual drive. Testosterone
or thyroid deficiency, prolactin or estrogen excess,
chronic hepatic or renal disease, Addison's disease, debilitating cardiopulmonary failure, and systemic cancer
will also reduce libido and decrease sexual arousal (Horowitz and Goble, 1979; Kaplan, 1979; Renshaw, 1983).
Neuropathies causing autonomic dysfunction (e.g., diabetes) and local pelvic surgery frequently impair erection and ejaculation.

Among idiopathic psychiatric disorders, hyposexuality is a major feature of depressive episodes and is
common in chronic schizophrenia (Akhtar and Thomson, 1980).

Increased Sexual Activity

Increased sexual activity is normal in the face of
increased leisure time or when a novel partner is available. Abnormal hypersexuality, however, occurs with
a variety of neurological, drug-induced, and psychiatric disorders (Table 17-6) (Goodman, 1981). Although
epilepsy typically causes hyposexuality, there are a few
specific circumstances when sexual behavior may be increased in epileptic patients (Table 17-7). Hypersexuality has been noted to occur in the immediate postictal
period, following temporal lobectomy with successful
abolition of seizures, and occasionally in patients with
improved seizure control achieved with anticonvulsants
(Blumer, 1970b; Cogen et al., 1979; Walker and Blumer,
1977). Lobectomy frequently reverses the preoperative
hyposexuality of epileptic patients (Blumer, 1970b;
Cogen et al., 1979). Hypersexual behavior has also been
reported in the course of prolonged fugue states that occasionally occur as part of the interictal behavioral
changes of patients with limbic epilepsy (Mohan et al.,
1975). Genital sensations or coital-type movements may
occur in the course of seizures and simulate hypersexual
behavior. Ictal genital sensations include feelings of pleasurable stimulation or of frank orgasm (Erickson, 1945;
Hoening and Hamilton, 1960; Jacome et al., 1980; Remillard et al., 1983; Ruff, 1980; Warneke, 1976). Ictal
motor manifestations of a sexual nature that occur in
the course of psychomotor or petit mal seizures include
masturbation, coital movements and related verbalizations, and automatic disrobing (Currier et al., 1971;
Freeman and Nevis, 1969; Hooshmand and Brawley,
1969; Jacome and Risko, 1983; Spencer et al., 1983).
Hooshmand and Brawley (1969) suggested that ictal
disrobing can usually be distinguished from paraphilic

exhibitionism by the following criteria: exhibitionism occurs in males between ages 15 and 45 years and involves specific female victims, whereas ictal disrobing occurs in individuals of either sex at any age and occurs in diverse interpersonal circumstances.

Diencephalic injuries have also produced hypersexual behavior. The lesions have usually been inflammatory or neoplastic in origin and involve the medial thalamic, infrastriatal, and mesencephalic–diencephalic junction regions (Carpenter et al., 1982; Poeck and Pilleri, 1965). The Kleine-Levin syndrome is assumed to be a product of hypothalamic dysfunction and is manifest by periodic somnolence, hypersexuality, and hyperphagia (Critchley, 1962; Critchley and Hoffman, 1942; Gallinek, 1962; Garland et al., 1965; Gilbert, 1964).

The Klüver-Bucy syndrome was discussed previously with regard to the asociated bulimia (Tables 17-4 and 17-5). Animals with the Klüver-Bucy syndrome exhibit hypersexuality and altered sexual behavior, including interspecies copulation (Aronson and Cooper, 1979; Klüver and Bucy, 1939; Schreiner and Kling, 1953). Humans exhibit alterations in sexual interest but may have no increase in the quantity of sexual activity. Patients may be sexually disinhibited and publicly demonstrative, and a number have changed from heterosexual to homosexual preferences (Lilly et al., 1983; Marlow et al., 1975; Shraberg and Weisberg, 1978; Terzian and Dalle Ore, 1955). Some patients with other elements of the Klüver-Bucy syndrome, particularly those with dementing disorders, may have no change in sexuality or may be hyposexual (Lilly et al., 1983).

Frontal lobe syndromes resulting from damage to the orbitofrontal portion of the brain produce disinhibition, jocularity, poor judgment, and impulsivity (Chapter 6). Patients with orbitofrontal lesions (neoplasms, trauma, infarctions, infection) may make sexual jokes or openly solicit sexual activity. Despite the verbal hypersexuality, there is rarely an increase in actual copulation, although patients may masturbate openly, go about in the nude, or attempt to fondle members of the opposite sex.

Medical conditions and pharmacological agents can also produce increased sexual behavior (Table 17-8). Hyperthyroidism, Cushing's disease or exogenous steroid administration, and androgen excess may all cause heightened libido and increased sexual activity (Goodman, 1981; Kaplan, 1979). Levodopa has induced hypersexual behavior in parkinsonian patients either as one component of secondary mania or as an independent behavioral alteration (Bowers et al., 1971; Brown et al., 1978; Hyyppa et al., 1970; Goodwin, 1971; O'Brien et al., 1971; Shapiro, 1973).

Hypersexuality occurs in most, but not all, manic patients and consists of increased sexual thoughts and

TABLE 17-7. Altered Sexual Behavior in Epilepsy

Ictal

  Sensory seizures
    Genital sensations
    Orgasmic sensations

  Motor seizures
    Coital movements
    Exhibitionism (automatic disrobing)
    Masturbation

Interictal

  Hyposexuality
    Limbic dysfunction
    Depression
    Intermittent prolactin elevation
    Drug-related

  Hypersexuality
    Postictal
    Postlobectomy
    Improved seizure control

  Altered sexuality (occasional association)
    Fetishism
    Transvestism
    Voyeurism
    Exhibitionism
    Sadism
    Masochism
    Pedophilia
    Frotteurism
    Genital mutilation

statements, flirtation, and increased sexual contacts (Allison and Wilson, 1960; Tsuang, 1975). Schizophrenic patients may rarely have hypersexual behavior, particularly in the prodromal phase of their illness (Akhtar and Thomson, 1980).

Sexual Deviations

Sexual deviations (paraphilias) are a group of disorders in which unusual or bizarre imagery or acts are necessary for sexual excitement. Table 17-9 lists the paraphilias that have been identified. Sexual deviations include fetishism, transvestism, zoophilia, pedophilia, exhibitionism, voyeurism, masochism, and sadism, as well as a variety of atypical paraphilias (*Diagnostic and statistical manual of mental disorders,* 1980; Taska and Sullivan, 1983). Homosexuality is considered as a psychosexual disorder only if the behavior is ego-dystonic for the individual or represents a change in orientation of a formerly heterosexual person. Endocrinologic assessments of homosexuals reveal markers of sexual orientation that may reflect altered CNS function (Gladne et al., 1984).

TABLE 17-8.   Effects of Commonly Prescribed Drugs on Sexual Function

Drug	Effect on Sexual Function		
	Libido	Arousal or Erection	Orgasm or Ejaculation
Psychotropic Agents			
Amphetamines and cocaine	Enhanced with low doses; decreased with high doses	Decreased with chronic use	Increased with low doses; diminished with high doses
MAO-inhibiting antidepressants	—	—	Impaired
Tricyclic antidepressants	May be impaired	May be impaired	May be impaired; may cause spontaneous seminal emission
Trazodone	—	May cause priapism	—
Lithium carbonate	Impaired	Impaired	—
Neuroleptic agents	May be decreased	Impaired (rare priapism)	Retrograde ejaculation rarely
Sedative–hypnotics (alcohol, barbiturates, etc.)	Reduced	Reduced	—
Antianxiety agents (benzodiazepines, etc.)	—	Impaired with chronic usage	—
Narcotics	Impaired in high doses	Impaired in high doses	Impaired in high doses
Antihypertensive Agents			
Reserpine, α-methyldopa	Decreased	Decreased (common)	May be impaired
Diuretics	—	May be impaired	—
Clonidine	—	—	May block emission in males
Propranolol	May be decreased	May be decreased	—
Anticholinergic Agents	—	May be impaired	—
Hormonal Agents			
Androgens	Increased	Increased (men)	Increased (men)
Estrogens	Decreased—men; Variable—women	May cause impotence in men	Delay
Thyroxin	Increased	—	—
Adrenal steroids	Decreased in high doses	—	—
Miscellaneous			
Levodopa	May be increased	—	—
Disulfiram	—	Occasional impotence	Delayed

Data from Kaplan (1979, 1983) and Rees (1983).
1979 - Table 1   Page 205–211
1983 - Table 8   Page 191–192

Psychosexual disorders have been reported with a number of neurological illnesses (Table 17-10). Patients with temporal lobe epilepsy are particularly vulnerable to such deviations, although the percentage of affected individuals is small. Fetishism and transvestism are the two disorders most commonly reported (Davies and Morgenstern, 1960; Epstein, 1961; Hunter et al., 1963; Mitchell et al., 1954; Walinder, 1965). Rare instances of voyeurism, exhibitionism, sadism, masochism, pe-

dophilia, frotteurism, genital self-mutilation, and homosexuality have also been described (Kolarsky et al., 1967; Taylor, 1969).

The Gilles de la Tourette syndrome is a disorder manifest by involuntary tics and vocalizations beginning before the age of 15 years (Chapter 12). The motor behaviors frequently include copropraxia (lewd) gestures), and 50 percent have coprolalia. Obsessions and compulsions are a common part of the syndrome

TABLE 17-9.   Sexual Deviations

Disorder	Preferred Sexual Object or Activity
Fetishism	Nonliving objects
Transvestism	Cross-dressing (by heterosexual male)
Zoophilia (bestiality)	Animals
Pedophilia	Prepubertal children
Exhibitionism	Exposing genitals to an unsuspecting stranger
Voyeurism	Observes unsuspecting people who are naked, disrobing, or engaging in sexual activity
Masochism	Excited by being humiliated, bound, or beaten
Sadism	Excited by inducing humiliation or physical or psychological suffering
Atypical paraphilias	
Vampirism	Blood
Coprophilia	Feces
Urophagia	Urine
Klismaphilia	Enema
Frotteurism	Rubbing against others
Necrophilia	Corpse
Telephone scatologia	Obscene (lewd) telephone calls

TABLE 17-10.   Neurological Disorders Associated with Sexual Deviations (References in Text)

Sexual Deviation	Associated Neurological Disorder
Exhibitionism	Gilles de la Tourette syndrome
	Postencephalitic parkinsonism
	Frontal lobe syndromes
	Huntington's disease
	Multiple sclerosis
	Epilepsy
	Post-traumatic encephalopathy
Sadism	Epilepsy
	Postencephalitic parkinsonism
Frotteurism	Epilepsy
	Frontal lobe syndromes
Fetishism	Epilepsy
Pedophilia	Epilepsy
	Postencephalitic parkinsonism
	Frontal lobe syndromes
	Post-traumatic encephalopathy
	Dyslexia
	Klinefelter's syndrome
Masochism	Epilepsy
Voyeurism	Epilepsy
Zoophilia	Postencephalitic parkinsonism

and may include compulsive sexual touching of themselves or others or compulsive exhibitionism with repeated genital exposures (Comings and Comings, 1982; Shapiro et al., 1978).

Postencephalitic parkinsonism followed the epidemic of von Economo's encephalitis that persisted from 1919 to 1926. Pathologically, there were inflammatory changes in the rostral brainstem and diencephalon (Chapter 12). The parkinsonian state was accompanied by a variety of behavioral changes, including psychosexual disorders. The latter occurred in a majority of patients requiring psychiatric hospitalization and included homosexuality, pedophilia, exhibitionism, sadism, and zoophilia (Fairweather, 1947).

Frontal lobe syndromes can lead to public masturbation, exhibitionism, pedophilia, and frotteurism as part of the impulsive, disinhibited change in behavior. Frontal system alterations may also underlie the open masturbation and exhibitionism described in some patients with Huntington's disease and with multiple sclerosis (Langworthy et al., 1941; Lion and Kahn, 1938; Regestein and Reich, 1978; Rosenbaum, 1941).

Investigations of individuals arrested for sexually related crimes, particularly pedophilia, have revealed an increased prevalence of EEG abnormalities, neuropsychological deficits, dyslexia, cerebral blood flow abnormalities, and computerized tomographic (CT) scan changes (Berlin and Coyle, 1981; Graber et al., 1984; Small, 1966; Stafford-Clark and Taylor, 1949). A small number of pedophilics have been found to have elevated serum levels of testosterone (Berlin, 1983). These findings suggest that subtle neurological and endocrinologic abnormalities may contribute to some cases of idiopathic paraphilic behavior.

Sexual deviations may occur in schizophrenia, where they are frequently motivated by delusional ideas or precepts (Akhtar and Thomson, 1980). Paraphilias also occur in patients with pesonality disorders or may occur in absence of any other identifiable psychopathology (*Diagnostic and statistical manual of mental disorders* 1980).

REFERENCES

Adelman S, Dinner DS, Goren H, Little J, and Nickerson P. Obstructive sleep apnea in association with posterior fossa neurologic disease. *Arch Neurol*, 1984, *41*, 509–510.

Akert K. The anatomical substrate of sleep. *Progr Brain Res*, 1965, *18*, 9–19.

Akhtar S and Thomson JA Jr. Schizophrenia and sexuality: a review and a report of twelve unusual cases. *J Clin Psychiat*, 1980, *41*, 134–142, 166–174.

Allison JB and Wilson WP. Sexual behavior of manic patients. *South Med J*, 1960, *53*, 870–874.

Aronson LR and Cooper ML. Amygdaloid hypersexuality in male cats re-examined. *Physiol Behav*, 1979, *22*, 257–265.

Baur HG. Endocrine and other clinical manifestations of hypothalamic disease. *J Clin Endocrinol*, 1954, *14*, 13–31.

Beal MF, Kleinman GM, Ojemann RG, and Hochberg FH. Gangliocytoma of third ventricle: hyperphagia, somnolence and dementia. *Neurology*, 1981, *31*, 1224–1228.

Bergonzi P, Chinrulla C, Gambi D, Mennuni G, and Pinto F. L-Dopa plus decarboxylase inhibitor. Sleep organization in Parkinson's syndrome before and after treatment. *Acta Neurol Belg*, 1975, *75*, 5–10.

Berlin FS. Sex offenders: a biomedical perspective and a status report on biomedical treatment. In Greer JG and Stuart IR (Eds.): *The sexual aggressor*. New York, von Nostrand Reinhold Company, 1983, pp. 83–123.

Berlin FS and Coyle GS. Sexual deviation syndromes. *Johns Hopkins Med J*, 1981, *149*, 119–125.

Betts TA. Depression, anxiety and epilepsy. In Reynolds EH

and Trimble MR (Eds.): *Epilepsy and psychiatry*. New York, Churchill Livingston, 1981, pp. 60–71.

Blumer D. Changes of sexual behavior related to temporal lobe disorders in man. *J Sex Res*, 1970a, *6*, 173–180.

Blumer D. Hypersexual episodes in temporal lobe epilepsy. *Am J Psychiat*, 1970b, *126*, 83–90.

Blumer D. Treatment of patients with seizure disorder referred because of psychiatric complications. *McLean Hosp J*, 1977 (Special Issue), 53–73.

Blumer D and Walker AE. Sexual behavior in temporal lobe epilepsy. *Arch Neurol*, 1967, *16*, 37–43.

Boller F, Wright DG, Cavalieri R, and Mitsumoto H. Paroxysmal "nightmares." *Neurology*, 1975, *25*, 1026–1028.

Bonduelle M and Degos C. Symptomatic narcolepsies: a critical study. *Adv Sleep Res*, 1976, *3*, 313–332.

Bowers MR Jr, Van Woert M, and Davis L. Sexual behavior during L-dopa treatment of parkinsonism. *Am J Psychiat*, 1971, *127*, 1691–1693.

Boyar RM, Finkelstein JW, Kapen S, Weiner H, Weitzman ED, and Hellman L. Anorexia nervosa. Immaturity of the 24-hour lutenizing hormone secretory pattern. *New Engl J Med*, 1974, *291*, 801–865.

Boyar RM, Hellman LD, Roffwarg H, Katz J, Zumoff B, O'Connor J, Bradlow L, and Fukushima DK. Cortosol secretion and metabolism in anorexia nervosa. *New Engl J Med*, 1977, *296*, 190–193.

Bray GA. Syndromes of hypothalamic obesity in man. *Ped Ann*, 1984, *13*, 525–536.

Bray GA and Gallagher TF Jr. Manifestations of hypothalamic

obesity in man: a comprehensive investigation of eight patients and a review of the literature. *Medicine,* 1974, *54,* 301–330.

Breier A, Ginsberg EM, and Charney DS. Seminal emission induced by tricyclic antidepressant. *Am J Psychiat,* 1984, *141,* 610–611.

Broughton RJ. Sleep disorders: disorders of arousal? *Science,* 1966, *159,* 1070–1078.

Brown E, Brown GM, Kofman O, and Quarrington B. Sexual function and affect in parkinsonian men treated with L-dopa. *Am J Psychiat,* 1978, *135,* 1552–1555.

Cantwell DP, Sturzenberger S, Burroughs J, Salkin B, and Green JK. Anorexia nervosa. An affective disorder? *Arch Gen Psychiat,* 1977, *34,* 1087–1093.

Carpenter S, Yassa R, and Ochs R. A pathologic basis for Kleine-Levin syndrome. *Arch Neurol,* 1982, *39,* 25–28.

Chokroverty S, Sachdeo R, and Masden J. Autonomic dysfunction and sleep apnea in olivopontocerebellar degeneration. *Arch Neurol,* 1984, *41,* 926–931.

Chokroverty S and Sharp JT. Primary sleep apnea syndrome. *J Neurol Neurosurg Psychiat,* 1981, *44,* 970–982.

Coble P, Foster FG, and Kupfer DJ. Electroencephalographic sleep diagnosis of primary depression. *Arch Gen Psychiat,* 1976, *33,* 1124–1127.

Cogen PH, Antunes JL, and Correll JW. Reproductive function in temporal lobe epilepsy: the effect of temporal lobectomy. *Surg Neurol,* 1979, *12,* 243–246.

Coleman RM, Roffwarg HP, Kennedy SJ, Guilleminault C, Cinque J, Cohn MA, Karacan I, Kupfer DJ, Lemmi H, Miles LE, Orr WC, Phillips ER, Roth T, Sassin JF, Schmidt HS, Weitzman ED, and Dement WC. Sleep–wake disorders based on a polysomnographic diagnosis. *JAMA,* 1982, *247,* 997–1003.

Collins WCJ, Lanigan O, and Callaghan N. Plasma prolactin concentrations following epileptic and pseudoseizures. *J Neurol Neurosurg Psychiat,* 1983, *46,* 505–508.

Comings DE and Comings BG. A case of familial exhibitionism in Tourette's syndrome successfully treated with haloperidol. *Am J Psychiat,* 1982, *139,* 913–915.

Critchley M. Periodic hypersomnia and megaphagia in adolescent males. *Brain,* 1962, *85,* 627–656.

Critchley M and Hoffman L. The syndrome of periodic somnolence and morbid hunger (Kleine-Levin syndrome). *Br Med J,* 1942, *1,* 137–139.

Cummings JL and Duchen LW. Klüver-Bucy syndrome in Pick disease: clinical and pathologic correlations. *Neurology,* 1981, *31,* 1415–1422.

Cummings JL and Greenberg R. Sleep patterns in the "locked-in" syndrome. *Electroenceph Clin Neurophysiol,* 1977, *43,* 270–271.

Currier RD, Little SC, Suess JF, and Andy OJ. Sexual seizures. *Arch Neurol,* 1971, *25,* 260–264.

Dally P, Gomez J, and Isaacs AJ. *Anorexia nervosa.* London, William Heinemann Medical Books, 1979.

Dana-Haeri J, Trimble MR, and Oxley J. Prolactin and gonadotrophin changes following generalized and partial seizures. *J Neurol Neurosurg Psychiat,* 1983, *46,* 331–335.

Davies BM and Morgenstern FS. A case of cysticercosis, temporal lobe epilepsy, and transvestism. *J Neurol Neurosurg Psychiat,* 1960, *23,* 247–249.

Dement W, Rechtschaffen A, and Gulevich G. The nature of the narcoleptic sleep attack. *Neurology,* 1966, *16,* 18–33.

Diagnostic and statistical manual of mental disorders, 3rd ed. Washington, D.C., American Psychiatric Association, 1980.

Diamond EF and Averick N. Marasmus and the diencephalic syndrome. *Arch Neurol,* 1966, *14,* 270–272.

Dieckmann G and Hassler R. Treatment of sexual violence by stereotactic hypothalamotomy. In Sweet WH, Obrador S, and Martin-Rodriquez JG (Eds.): *Neurosurgical treatment in psychiatry, pain, and epilepsy.* Baltimore, University Park Press, 1977, pp. 451–462.

Eilenberg D and Wood LW. Narcolepsy with psychosis: report of two cases. *May Clin Proc,* 1962, *37,* 561–566.

Ekbom KA. Restless legs syndrome. *Neurology,* 1960, *10,* 868–873.

Epstein AW. Relationship of fetishism and transvestism to brain and particularly temporal lobe dysfunction. *J Nerv Ment Dis,* 1961, *133,* 247–253.

Epstein AW. Effect of certain cerebral hemispheric diseases on dreaming. *Biol Psychiat,* 1979, *14,* 77–93.

Erickson TC. Erotomania (nymphomania) as an expression of cortical epileptiform discharge. *Arch Neurol Psychiat,* 1945, *53,* 226–231.

Fairweather DS. Psychiatric aspects of the post-encephalitic syndrome. *J Ment Sci,* 1947, *93,* 201–254.

Fisher C, Kahn E, Edwards A, and Davis DM. A psychophysiological study of nightmares and night terrors. *Arch Gen Psychiat,* 1973, *28,* 252–259.

Fournier JCM and Helguera RAL. Postencephalitic narcolepsy and cataplexy. Muscles and motor nerves electrical excitability during the attack of cataplexy. *J Nerv Ment Dis,* 1934, *80,* 159–162.

Frankel BL, Coursey RD, Buchbinder R, and Synder F. Recorded and reported sleep in chronic primary insomnia. *Arch Gen Psychiat,* 1976, *36,* 615–623.

Freemon FR and Nevis AH. Temporal lobe sexual seizures. *Neurology,* 1969, *19,* 87–90.

Freemon FR, Salinas-Garcia RF, and Ward JW. Sleep patterns in a patient with a brain stem infarction involving the raphe nucleus. *Electroenceph Clin Neurophysiol,* 1974, *36,* 657–660.

Fuster B, Castells C, and Elcheverry M. Epileptic sleep terrors. *Neurology,* 1954, *4,* 531–540.

Gallinek A. The Kleine-Levin syndrome: hypersomnia, bulimia, and abnormal mental states. *World Neurol,* 1962, *3,* 235–243.

Garfinkel PE, Brown GM, Stancer HC, and Maldofsky H. Hypothalamic–pituitary function in anorexia nervosa. *Arch Gen Psychiat,* 1975, *32,* 739–744.

Garland H, Sumner D, and Fourman P. The Kleine-Levin syndrome. *Neurology,* 1965, *15,* 1161–1167.

Gilbert GJ. Periodic hypersomnia and bulimia. *Neurology,* 1964, *14,* 844–850.

Gladne BP, Green R, and Hellman R. Neuroendocrine response

to estrogen and sexual orientation. *Science*, 1984, *225*, 1496–1499.

Goodman JD. Nymphomania and satyriasis. In Mulé SJ (Ed.): *Behavior in excess*. New York, Free Press, 1981, pp. 246–263.

Goodwin FK. Psychiatric side effects of levodopa in man. *JAMA*, 1971, *218*, 1915–1920.

Gottlieb JL and Luskberg T. Phenothiazine induced priapism: a case report. *Am J Psychiat*, 1977, *134*, 1445–1446.

Graber B, Hartmann K, Coffman KA, Huey CJ, and Golden CJ. Brain damage among mentally disordered sex offenders. In Lief HI and Hoch Z (Eds.): *International Research in Sexology*. New York, Praeger Publishers, 1984, pp. 193–202.

Green RS and Rau JH. Treatment of compulsive eating disturbances with anticonvulsants. *Am J Psychiat*, 1974, *131*, 428–432.

Greenberg R. Cerebral cortex lesions: the dream process and sleep spindles. *Cortex*, 1966, *2*, 357–366.

Greenberg R and Pearlman C. Sleep patterns in temporal lobe epilepsy. *Comp Psychiat*, 1968, *9*, 194–199.

Greenberg R, Pearlman C, Brooks R, Mayer R, and Hartmann E. Dreaming and Korsakoff's psychosis. *Arch Gen Psychiat*, 1968, *18*, 203–209.

Gross RA, Spehlmann R, and Daniels JC. Sleep disturbances in progressive supranuclear palsy. *Electroenceph Clin Neurophysiol*, 1978, *45*, 16–25.

Guilleminault C, Cathala JP, aand Castaigne P. Effects of 5-hydroxytryptophan on sleep of a patient with brain-stem lesion. *Electroenceph Clin Neurophysiol*, 1973a, *34*, 177–184.

Guilleminault C and Dement W. Pathologies of excessive sleep. *Adv Sleep Res*, 1974, *1*, 345–390.

Guilleminault C, Eldridge FL, and Dement WC. Insomnia with sleep apnea: a new syndrome. *Science*, 193b, *181*, 856–858.

Guilleminault C, Eldridge FL, Phillips JR, and Dement WC. Two occult causes of insomnia and their therapeutic problems. *Arch Gen Psychiat*, 1976, *33*, 1241–1245.

Guilleminault C, Faull KF, Miles L, and van den Hoad J. Post-traumatic excessive daytime sleepiness: a review of 20 patients. *Neurology*, 1983, *33*, 1584–1589.

Guilleminault C, Raynal D, Weitzman ED, and Dement WC. Sleep-related periodic myoclonus in patients complaining of insomnia. *Trans Am Neurol Assoc*, 1975, *100*, 19–21.

Hall CW and Danoff D. Sleep attacks—apparent relationship to atlantoaxial dislocation. *Arch Neurol*, 1975, *32*, 57–58.

Halmi KA and Sherman BM. Gonadotropin response to LH-RH in anorexia nervosa. *Arch Gen Psychiat*, 1975, *32*, 875–878.

Haugh RM and Markesberry WR. Hypothalamic astrocytoma. *Arch Neurol*, 1983, *40*, 560–563.

Hierons R and Saunders M. Impotence in patients with temporal-lobe lesions. *Lancet*, 1966, *2*, 761–763.

Hisikawa Y and Kaneko Z. Electroencephalographic study of narcolepsy. *Electroenceph Clin Neurophysiol*, 1965 *18*, 249–259.

Hobson JA. Dreaming sleep attacks and desynchronized sleep enhancement. *Arch Gen Psychiat*, 1975, *32*, 1421–1424.

Hoening J and Hamilton CM. Epilepsy and sexual orgasm. *Acta Psychiat Neurol Scand*, 1960, *35*, 448–456.

Hollister LE. Drugs and sexual behavior in man. *Life Sci*, 1975, *17*, 661–668.

Hooshmand H and Brawley BW. Temporal lobe seizures and exhibitionism. *Neurology*, 1969, *19*, 1119–1124.

Horowitz JD and Goble AJ. Drugs and impaired male sexual function. *Drugs*, 1979, *18*, 206–217.

Humphrey ME and Zangwill OL. Cessation of dreaming after brain injury. *J Neurol Neurosurg Psychiat*, 1951, *14*, 322–325.

Hunter R, Logue V, and McMenemy WH. Temporal lobe epilepsy supervening on longstanding transvestism and fetishism. *Epilepsia*, 1963, *4*, 160–65.

Hyyppa M, Rinne UK, and Sonninen V. The activating effect of L-dopa treatment on sexual functions and its experimental background. *Acta Neurol Scand*, 1970, *46* (Suppl. 43), 223–224.

Jacome DE, McLain W Jr, and Fitzgerald R. Postural reflex gelastic seizures. *Arch Neurol*, 1980, *37*, 249–251.

Jacome DE and Risko MS. Absence status manifested by compulsive masturbation. *Arch Neurol*, 1983, *40*, 523–524.

Johnson J. Sexual impotence and the limbic system. *Br J Psychiat*, 1965, *111*, 300–303.

Kales A, Cadieux RJ, Soldatos CR, Bixler EO, Schweitzer PK, Prey WT, and Vela-Bueno A. Narcolepsy–cataplexy. I. Clinical and electrophysiologic characteristics. *Arch Neurol*, 1982, *39*, 164–168.

Kales A and Kales JD. Sleep disorders. *New Engl J Med*, 1974, *290*, 487–499.

Kales A and Kales JD. *Insomnia*. New York, Oxford University Press, 1984.

Kaplan HS. *Disorders of sexual desire*. New York, Simon and Schuster, 1979.

Kaplan HS. *The evaluation of sexual disorders*. New York, Brunner-Mazel, 1983.

Katz JL, Kuperberg A, Pollack CP, Walsh BT, Zumoff B, and Weiner H. Is there a relationship between eating disorder and affective disorder? New evidence from sleep recordings. *Am J Psychiat*, 1984, *141*, 753–759.

Kaye WH, Ebert MH, Raleigh M, and Lake R. Abnormalities in CNS monoamine metabolism in anorexia nervosa. *Arch Gen Psychiat*, 1984, *41*, 350–355.

Kirschbaum WR. Excessive hunger as a symptom of cerebral origin. *J Nerv Ment Dis*, 1951, *113*, 95–114.

Kleitman N. *Sleep and wakefulness*. Chicago, University of Chicago Press, 1963.

Klüver H and Bucy PC. Preliminary analysis of functions of the temporal lobes in monkeys. *Arch Neurol Psychiat*, 1939, *42*, 979–1000.

Kolarsky A, Freund K, Machek J, and Polak O. Male sexual deviation. *Arch Gen Psychiat*, 1967, *17*, 735–743.

Kotin J, Wilbert DE, Verburg D, and Soldinger SM. Thioridazine and sexual dysfunction. *Am J Psychiat*, 1976, *139*, 82–84.

Krahn DD and Mitchell JE. Case report: bulimia associated

with increased intracranial pressure. *Am J Psychiat*, 1984, *141*, 1099–1100.

Kramer PD. Insomnia: importance of the differential diagnosis. *Psychosomatics*, 1982, *23*, 129–137.

Kraus JE. Morphologic aspects and genesis of disorders of the adenohypophysis. *Arch Pathol*, 1945, *40*, 191–207.

Krishnan RR, Volow MR, Miller PP, and Carwile ST. Narcolepsy: preliminary retrospective study of psychiatric and psychosocial aspects. *Am J Psychiat*, 1984, *141*, 428–431.

Kron L, Katz JL, Gorzynski G, and Weiner H. Anorexia nervosa and gonadal dysgenesis. *Arch Gen Psychiat*, 1977, *34*, 332–335.

Langworthy OR, Kolb LC, and Androp S. Disturbances of behavior in patients with disseminated sclerosis. *Am J Psychiat*, 1941, *98*, 243–249.

Lansky MR and Selzer J. Priapism associated with trazodone therapy: case report. *J Clin Psychiat*, 1984, *45*, 232–233.

Lavie P, Pratt H, Scharf B, Peled R, and Brown J. Localized pontine lesion: nearly total absence of REM sleep. *Neurology*, 1984, *34*, 118–120.

Lewin K, Mattingly D, and Mills RR. Anorexia nervosa associated with hypothalamic tumour. *Br Med J*, 1972, *2*, 629–630.

Liddell DW and Northfield DWC. The effect of temporal lobectomy upon two cases of an unusual form of mental deficiency. *J Neurol Neurosurg Psychiat*, 1954, *17*, 267–275.

Lilly R, Cummings JL, Benson DF, and Frankel M. The human Klüver-Bucy syndrome. *Neurology*, 1983, *33*, 1141–1145.

Lion EG and Kahn E. Experiential aspects of Huntington's chorea. *Am J Psychiat*, 1938, *95*, 717–727.

Marlowe WB, Mancall EL, and Thomas JJ. Complete Klüver-Bucy syndrome in man. *Cortex*, 1975, *11*, 53–59.

Martin JB, Reichlin S, and Brown GM. *Clinical neuroendocrinology*. Philadelphia, FA Davis Company, 1977.

McCarley RW. REM sleep and depression: common neurobiological control mechanisms. *Am J Psychiat*, 1982, *139*, 565–570.

Mendels J and Hawkins DB. Sleep and depression. *Arch Gen Psychiat*, 1967, *16*, 344–354.

Miller E. Mental dissociation: its relation to catatonia and the mechanism of narcolepsy. *Brain*, 1927, *50*, 624–630.

Mitchell JE and Popkin MK. Antidepressant drug therapy and sexual dysfunction in men: a review. *J Clin Psychopharmacol*, 1983, *3*, 76–79.

Mitchell W, Falconer MA, and Hill D. Epilepsy with fetishism relieved by temporal lobectomy. *Lancet*, 1954, *2*, 626–630.

Mohan KJ, Salo MW, and Nagaswami S. A case of limbic system dysfunction with hypersexuality and fugue state. *Dis Nerv Syst*, 1975, *36*, 621–624.

Murri L, Arena R, Siciliano G, Mazzotta R, and Muratorio A. Dream recall in patients with focal cerebral lesions. *Arch Neurol*, 1984, *41*, 183–185.

Nakada T, Lee H, Kwee IL, and Lerner AM. Epileptic Klüver-Bucy syndrome: case report. *J Clin Psychiat*, 1984, *45*, 87–88.

Narabayashi H, Nagao T, Saito Y, Yoshida M, and Nagahata M. Stereotaxic amygdalotomy for behavior disorders. *Arch Neurol*, 1963, *9*, 1–16.

Nielsen JM. Occipital lobes, dreams and psychosis. *J Nerv Ment Dis*, 1955, *121*, 50–52.

O'Brien CP, DiGiaconno JN, Fahn S, and Schwartz GA. Mental effects of high-dosage levodopa. *Arch Gen Psychiat*, 1971, *24*, 61–64.

Oswald I. Sudden bodily jerks on falling asleep. *Brain*, 1959, *82*, 92–103.

Pilleri G. The Klüver-Bucy syndrome in man. *Psychiat Neurol Basel*, 1966, *152*, 65–103.

Poeck K and Pilleri G. Release of hypersexual behaviour due to lesion in the limbic system. *Acta Neurol Scand*, 1965, *41*, 233–244.

Powers JM, Schaumburg HH, and Gaffney CL. Klüver-Bucy syndrome caused by adreno-leukodystrophy. *Neurology*, 1980, *30*, 1131–1132.

Pritchard PB III, Wannamaker BB, Sagel J, Nair R, and DeVillier C. Endocrine function following complex partial seizures. *Ann Neurol*, 1983, *14*, 27–32.

Pyle RL, Mitchell JE, and Eckert ED. Bulimia: a report of 34 cases. *J Clin Psychiat*, 1981, *42*, 60–64.

Rees JMH. Sexual dysfunction and prescribed psychotropic drugs. In Wheatley D (Ed.): *Psychopharmacology and sexual disorders*. New York, Oxford University Press, 1983, pp. 138–147.

Reeves AG and Plum F. Hyperphagia, rage and dementia accompanying a ventromedial hypothalamic neoplasm. *Arch Neurol*, 1969, *20*, 616–624.

Regestein QR and Reich P. Pedophilia occurring after onset of cognitive impairment. *J Nerv Ment Dis*, 1978, *166*, 794–798.

Remillard GM, Andermann F, Testa GF, Gloor P, Aube M, Martin JB, Feindel W, Guberman A, and Simpson C. Sexual ictal manifestations predominate in women with temporal lobe epilepsy: a finding suggesting sexual dimorphism in the human brain. *Neurology*, 1983, *33*, 323–330.

Renshaw DC. Sexuality in old age, illness, and disability. In Wheatley D (Ed.): *Psychopharmacology and sexual disorders*. New York, Oxford University Press, 1983, pp. 88–100.

Reynolds CF, Taska LS, Sewitch DE, Restifo K, Coble PA, and Kupfer DJ. Persistent psychophysiologic insomnia: preliminary research diagnostic criteria and EEG sleep data. *Am J Psychiat*, 1984, *141*, 804–805.

Rosenbaum D. Psychosis with Huntington's chorea. *Psychiat Quart*, 1941, *15*, 93–99.

Roth B. *Narcolepsy and hypersomnia*. New York, S Karger, 1980.

Roth B, Nevisimalova S, and Rechtschaffen A. Hypersomnia with "sleep drunkenness." *Arch Gen Psychiat*, 1972, *26*, 456–462.

Roy A. Psychiatric aspects of narcolepsy. *Br J Psychiat*, 1976, *128*, 562–565.

Ruff RL. Orgasmic epilepsy. *Neurology*, 1980, *30*, 1252–1253.

Russell G. Bulimia nervosa: an ominous variant of anorexia nervosa. *Psychol Med,* 1979, *9,* 429–448.

Sachs C, Persson HE, and Hagenfeldt K. Menstruation-related periodic hypersomnia: a case study with successful treatment. *Neurology,* 1982, *32,* 1376–1379.

Scher M, Krieger TN, and Juergens S. Trazodone and priapism. *Am J Psychiat,* 1983, *140,* 1362–1363.

Schneider H. Psychic changes in sexual delinquency after hypothalamotomy. In Sweet WH, Obrador S, and Martin-Rodriquez JG (Eds.): *Neurosurgical treatment in psychiatry, pain, and epilepsy.* Baltimore, University Park Press, 1977, pp. 463–468.

Schreiner L and Kling A. Behavioral changes following rhinencephalic injury in the cat. *J Neurophysiol,* 1953, *16,* 643–659.

Schwartz G. Case report of inhibition of ejaculation and retrograde ejaculation as side effects of amoxapine. *Am J Psychiat,* 1983, *139,* 233–234.

Shapiro AK, Shapiro ES, Bruun RH, and Sweet RD. *Gilles de la Tourette syndrome.* New York, Raven Press, 1978.

Shapiro SK. Hypersexual behavior complicating levodopa (L-dopa) therapy. *Minn Med,* 1973, *56,* 58–59.

Shoji H, Teramoto H, Satowa S, Satowa H, and Narita Y. Partial Klüver-Bucy syndrome following probable herpes simplex encephalitis. *J Neurol,* 1979, *221,* 163–167.

Shraberg D and Weisberg L. The Klüver-Bucy syndrome in man. *J Nerv Ment Dis,* 1978, *166,* 130–134.

Shukla GD, Srivastava ON, and Katiyar BC. Sexual disturbances in temporal lobe epilepsy: a controlled study. *Br J Psychiat,* 1979, *134,* 288–292.

Small JG. The organic dimension of crime. *Arch Gen Psychiat,* 1966, *15,* 82–89.

Solomon F, White CC, Parron DL, and Mendelson WB. Sleeping pills, insomnia and medical practice. *New Engl J Med,* 1979, *300,* 803–808.

Sours JA. Narcolepsy and other disturbances in the sleep-waking rhythm: a study of 115 cases with review of the literature. *J Nerv Ment Dis,* 1963, *137,* 525–542.

Spencer SS, Spencer DD, Williamson PD, and Mattson RH. Sexual automatisms in complex partial seizures. *Neurology,* 1983, *33,* 527–533.

Spiller WG. Narcolepsy occasionally a post-encephalitic syndrome. *JAMA,* 1926, *86,* 673–674.

Stafford-Clark D and Taylor FH. Clinical and electroencephalographic studies of prisoners charged with murder. *J Neurol Neurosurg Psychiat,* 1949, *12,* 325–330.

Stewart JW, Walsh T, Wright L, Roose SP and Glassman AH. An open trial of MAO inhibitors in bulimia. *J Clin Psychiat,* 1984, *45,* 217–219.

Story NL. Sexual dysfunction resulting from drug side effects. *J Sex Res,* 1974, *10,* 132–149.

Symonds CP. Narcolepsy as a symptom of encephalitis lethargica. *Lancet,* 1926, *2,* 1214–1215.

Taska RJ and Sullivan JL. Sexual dysfunctions and deviations. In Cavenar JO Jr and Brodie HKH (Eds.): *Signs and symptoms in psychiatry.* Philadelphia, JB Lippincott, 1983, pp. 553–573.

Tassinari CA, Mancia D, Bernadina BD, and Gastaut H. Pavor nocturnus of nonepileptic nature in epileptic children. *Electroenceph Clin Neurophysiol,* 1972, *33,* 603–607.

Taylor D. Sexual behavior and temporal lobe epilepsy. *Arch Neurol,* 1969, *21,* 510–516.

Terzian H and Dalle Ore G. Syndrome of Klüver-Bucy. *Neurology,* 1955, *5,* 373–380.

Toone BK, Wheeler M, and Fenwick PBC. Sex hormone changes in male epileptics. *Clin Endocrin,* 1980, *12,* 391–395.

Trimble MR. Serum prolactin in epilepsy and hysteria. *Br Med J,* 1978, *2,* 1682.

Tsuang MT. Hypersexuality in manic patients. *Med Aspects Hum Sex,* 1975, *9,* 83–89.

Walinder J. Transvestism, definition and evidence in favor of occasional deviation from cerebral dysfunction. *Internat J Neuropsychiat,* 1965, *1,* 567–573.

Walker AE and Blumer D. Long term behavioral effects of temporal lobectomy for temporal lobe epilepsy. *McLean Hosp J,* 1977, Special Issue, 85–103.

Walker JI and Cavenar JO Jr. Sleep disorders. In Cavenar JO Jr and Brodie HKH (Eds.): *Signs and symptoms in psychiatry.* Philadelphia, JB Lippincott, 1983, pp. 267–294.

Warneke LB. A case of temporal lobe epilepsy with an orgasmic component. *Can Psychiat Assoc J,* 1976, *21,* 319–324.

Warren MP and Vande Wiele RL. Clinical and metabolic features of anorexia nervosa. *Am J Obstet Gynecol,* 1973, *117,* 435–449.

White LE and Hain RF. Anorexia in association with a destructive lesion of the hypothalamus. *Arch Pathol,* 1959, *68,* 275–281.

White PT and Ross AT. Inanition syndrome in infants with anterior hypothalamic neoplasms. *Neurology,* 1963, *13,* 974–981.

Williams RL, Derman S, and Karacan I. Disorders of excessive sleep and the parasomnias. In Zales MR (Ed.): *Eating, sleeping, and sexuality.* New York, Brunner-Mazel, 1982, pp. 150–185.

Zarcone V. Narcolepsy. *New Engl J Med,* 1973, *288,* 1156–1166.

Index

Page numbers in *italics* indicate illustrations.
Page numbers followed by *t* indicate tables.